UNITED STATES RECOMMENDED DAILY ALLOWANCES (U.S. RDAs) For Labeling Purposes Recommendations for Adults and Children Over 4 Years

MANDATORY NUTRIENTS

D1473298

Protein	
Quality equal to or greater than casein	45 g
Quality less than casein	65 g
Vitamin A	5,000 IU
Vitamin C	60 mg
Thiamine	1.5 mg
Riboflavin	1.7 mg
Niacin	20 mg
Calcium	1.0 g
Iron	18 mg

OPTIONAL NUTRIENTS

Vitamin D	400 IU
Vitamin E	30 IU
Vitamin B_6	2.0 mg
Folacin (folic acid)	0.4 mg
Vitamin B_{12}	6 μg
Phosphorus	1.0 g
Iodine	150 μg
Magnesium	400 mg
Zinc	15 mg
Copper	2 mg
Biotin	0.3 mg
Pantothenic acid	10 mg

TABLE OF EQUIVALENTS

COMMON UNITS OF WEIGHT

METRIC SYSTEM	ENGLISH SYSTEM	CONVERSIONS BETWEEN SYSTEMS
1 kilogram (kg) = 1000 grams (g)	1 pound (lb) = 16 ounces (oz)	1 pound = 454 grams
1 gram = 1000 milligrams (mg)		1 ounce = 28.35 g (usually rounded to 28 or 30)
1 milligram = 1000 micrograms (μg)		2.2 pounds = 1 kilogram

COMMON UNITS OF VOLUME

METRIC SYSTEM	ENGLISH SYSTEM	CONVERSIONS BETWEEN SYSTEMS
1 liter (L) = 1000 milliliters (mL)	1 gallon (gal) = 4 quarts (qt)	1.06 qt = 1 liter (L)
	1 qt = 2 pints (pt)	1 qt = 946 mL
	1 pt = 2 cups (c)	1 c = 237 mL
	1 c = 8 fluid oz	1 tbsp = 15 mL
	1 c = 16 tablespoons (tbsp)	1 tsp = 5 mL
	1 T = 3 teaspoons (tsp)	

COMMON UNITS OF LENGTH

METRIC SYSTEM	ENGLISH SYSTEM	CONVERSIONS BETWEEN SYSTEMS
1 meter (m) = 100 centimeters (cm)	1 foot (ft) = 12 inches (in)	1 inch = 2.54 cm
1000 meters = 1 kilometer (km)	1 yard (yd) = 3 feet	39.37 in = 1 m

NUTRITION

PRINCIPLES, ISSUES,
AND APPLICATIONS

NUTRITION

PRINCIPLES, ISSUES, AND APPLICATIONS

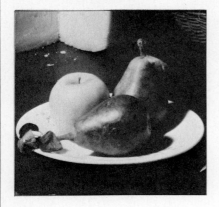

Eleanor R. Williams
University of Maryland

Mary Alice Caliendo
University of Maryland

McGRAW-HILL BOOK COMPANY
New York St. Louis San Francisco Auckland Bogotá Hamburg
Johannesburg London Madrid Mexico Montreal New Delhi
Panama Paris São Paulo Singapore Sydney Tokyo Toronto

This book was set in Optima by Black Dot, Inc.
The editors were Rhona Robbin, James S. Amar, and David Dunham;
the designer was Joan E. O'Connor;
the production supervisor was Charles Hess.
The photo editor was Inge King.
The cover photograph was taken by DeMarco/Tomaccio Studio.
The drawings were done by Fine Line Illustrations, Inc.
Von Hoffmann Press, Inc., was printer and binder.

PART-OPENING PHOTO CREDITS

PART I   Left, Jean Baptiste-Simeon Chardin, "La Brioche," *Art Resource.*
  Right, Frans Hals, Nicolas Van Heussen "A Woman Selling Fruit," *The Bettmann Archive.*
PART II   Left, Adrian Van Ostade, "The Fish Seller," *The Bettmann Archive.*
  Right, Annibale Carracci, "The Bean Eater," *Art Resource.*
PART III   Left, The Milkmaid after a Painting by Jan Vermur, *The Bettmann Archive.*
  Right, Henri Fantin-LaTour "Still Life with Flowers and Fruit," *The Metropolitan Museum of Art.*
PART IV   Left, Jean Baptiste-Simeon Chardin, "Nutura Morta," *Art Resource.*
  Right, Willem Kalf, "Still Life," *The Metropolitan Museum of Art.*
PART V   Left and right, Juan Sanchez Cotan, "Quince, Cabbage, Melon, and Cucumber,"
  San Diego Museum of Art.

NUTRITION: PRINCIPLES, ISSUES, AND APPLICATIONS

1 2 3 4 5 6 7 8 9 0 V N H V N H 8 9 8 7 6 5 4

ISBN 0-07-070510-0

LIBRARY OF CONGRESS CATALOGING IN PUBLICATION DATA

Williams, Eleanor R.
  Nutrition: principles, issues, and applications.

  Bibliography: p.
  Includes index.
  1. Nutrition. I. Caliendo, Mary Alice. II. Title.
TX354.W485   1984   613.2   83-17510
ISBN 0-07-070510-0

Contents

v

PART II   THE ENERGY NUTRIENTS

PREFACE

Americans are bombarded with information about nutrition—some of it scientifically sound, but much of it half-true, misleading, or downright false. Given this situation the first college nutrition course should enable students to find answers to their pressing questions, while also challenging them to use scientific facts and principles to critically analyze nutrition information abounding in the popular media. This book is designed for use in such a course—a beginning course, requiring no prerequisites, which is offered to majors and/or nonmajors.

In our experience, an integrated approach to nutrition science, relevant practical applications, and current issues motivates students to become thinkers rather than passive regurgitators of facts. For this reason, each chapter provides those concepts and scientific principles students need in order to analyze current issues in nutrition. Those questions and concerns that capture the interests of today's students are integrated into the scientific discussions. Many chapters open with brief case studies designed to excite student curiosity.

OVERVIEW

Serving as an orientation to the text, the Introduction provides students with an overview of the relationships between nutrition and health, discusses the kinds of issues the book addresses, and reviews some basic biological and chemical concepts pertinent to the study of nutrition. Chapter 1 briefly describes the United States food system, a topic not commonly found in other texts, and invites students to examine factors that govern their own access to food, as well as factors determining which foods they find acceptable. Chapter 2 focuses on one of the questions beginning nutrition students most frequently ask: "How do I know whether my diet is nutritionally adequate?" Students need not wait until the end of the course to find answers to this question. They all are familiar with foods and the question can initially be answered in terms of foods, rather than in terms of nutrients. Chapter 2 therefore explains the proper uses of the RDAs and of the Basic Four, the Exchange System, and the U.S. Dietary Guidelines in planning diets. Reasons for conflicts among scientists regarding the U.S. Dietary Guidelines are presented, thereby introducing students to the first of many controversies in nutrition that they will enounter in the text.

Part Two (Chapters 3 to 8) covers carbohydrates, lipids, proteins, and energy balance and imbalance. Chapters on carbohydrates, lipids, and proteins describe their basic chemical structures; their digestion, absorption, and metabolism; food sources; human requirements; and interrelationships. The relationships of carbohydrates and lipids to disease are discussed in a separate chapter, pointing out controversial aspects. A separate chapter also addresses energy imbalances: overweight and underweight. Because we assume that most students using this textbook will not have previously studied chemistry or physiology, terms are defined and concepts explained when they are introduced. Illustrations lead students step by step through complex processes at the point of discussion in order to enhance understanding of basic principles.

Vitamins, minerals, and water are discussed in Part Three (Chapters 9 to 13). Each vitamin or mineral is discussed separately, including functions, food sources, effects of deficiency or excessive intake, human requirements, and interrelationships. Issues of current concern are addressed regarding each nutrient. Review charts are included at the end of each chapter as study aids for students.

Part Four, Nutrition throughout the Life Cycle, describes the special nutritional needs and concerns of pregnancy and lactation (Chapter 14), infancy and childhood (Chapter 15), and the later years (Chapter 16). Among the topics of current interest discussed in this section are diet and hyperactivity and drug-nutrient interactions. Part Five, Food Safety and Adequacy at Home and Abroad, is devoted to discussion of consumer concerns of food labeling, additives, and toxicants (Chapter 17) and world food problems (Chapter 18). Controversies about nitrites and saccharin in the United States and the bottle-feeding problem in developing countries are highlighted in these chapters.

SPECIAL FEATURES

Several pedagogical aids are designed to help students sharpen their skills in evaluating nutrition information. Chapter 5 is devoted to discussion of evidence for the relationships of dietary lipids and carbohydrates to various diseases. This chapter features a discussion in Box 5–1 of research in nutrition. Students learn the rudiments of experimental design and gain basic insights into the uses and limitations of animal studies, human metabolic studies, and intervention trials in nutrition reserach. This chapter also discusses the conflict among nutritional scientists concerning advice the public should be given about dietary fat and cholesterol. As is the case whenever conflicts are discussed in this text, arguments on both sides are presented along with rationales behind each view. In our experience, students feel less frustrated in reaching decisions regarding personal dietary guidelines when they understand the reasons for disagreement among scientists.

Another pedagogical tool, "Nutrition in the News," features excerpted newspaper and magazine articles on topics related to each chapter. Questions following the news items in "Ask Yourself" sections are designed to stimulate student evaluation of the information in the excerpts and ultimately to encourage students to think more critically about nutrition information they encounter in popular sources.

Other aids to student learning include brief sections entitled "A Closer Look" in which interrelationships among nutrients are treated (as in Chapters 8 and 9, for example) or in which attention is focused on practical applications (as in Chapters 1, 3, 11, and 12). Boxed materials are integrated into the ongoing discussion in the text and emphasize current issues or practical aspects of a topic. Examples include Box 3–2: Misconceptions about the Digestive Tract, Box 6–2: Vegetarian Diets, Box 7–2: Misconceptions about Food and Energy, Box 8–1: Recognizing Unsound Claims about Weight Reducing Diets, Box 9–1: False Vitamins, Box 10–2: Saving Vitamins and Minerals in Foods, Box 11–1: Is Vitamin A the Answer to Acne?, and Box 13–1: Hair Analysis as an Assessment Tool.

Ongoing attention is paid to nutrition for athletes. Carbohydrate loading and the athlete's requirements for protein, energy, water, and sodium are discussed in chapters devoted to each of these nutrients. The problems of alcohol consumption and nutrition also appear at appropriate places in the text. The initial discussion of alcohol appears in the carbohydrate chapter, continues in Chapter 13, centering around alcohol's effects on vitamin and mineral nutrition, and culminates in Chapter 14 with the discussion of fetal alcohol syndrome.

A numbered summary ending each chapter is designed to aid student review. Sections at ends of chapters entitled "For Discussion and Application" encourage students to study their own diets and include activity suggestions to promote further exploration and discussion. Suggested readings invite students to investigate further.

A comprehensive Glossary appears at the end of the book, including all terms that have been defined in the text.

The Appendixes provide extensive tables on nutrients in foods as well as directions for recording and calculating one's dietary intake. Other tables include the Recommended Dietary Allowances, the Exchange Lists, Height–Weight Tables, U.S. RDA tables, and a table of Energy Expenditure for Physical Activity. In addition, sections are included on chemical structures, laboratory tests used in nutritional assessment, methods of measuring protein quality, and calculation aids.

SUPPLEMENTS

Both an instructor's manual and a test bank *prepared by the authors* are available. The instructor's manual includes, for each chapter, a brief overview and a key points section reviewing important principles and concepts. A teaching suggestions section provides (a) assistance in identifying common student problems and concerns, (b) discussion topics, and (c) answers to "Ask Yourself" questions in the "Nutrition in the News" boxes. At the back of the manual is (a) an annotated list of available films, filmstrips, videotapes, and audiotapes, (b) transparency masters for use in the course, and (c) a ministudy guide, consisting of a set of learning objectives and short answer questions which constitute a student self-test, organized by chapter. Instructors may duplicate the study guide for their students.

The test bank provides multiple-choice, true-false, essay, and matching-format questions with their answers. In addition, two separate final exams of 50 questions each are included.

ACKNOWLEDGMENTS

The authors wish to acknowledge those who helped prepare the manuscript: Johanna Aydelotte, Maxine Barish, Patricia Byrdsong, Susan Coles, Carlie Dozier, Claudia Jiminez, Margaret Reese, and Susan Yarus. We owe a large debt of gratitude to the following reviewers who gave us invaluable suggestions, criticisms, and perspectives: Judith V. Anderson, The University of Michigan; Carol W. Bishop, Solano Community College; Marjorie Caldwell, University of Rhode Island; Kate Clancy, Syracuse University; Marie Z. Cross, University of Kansas; Mary C. Donne, West Valley College; Christine DuPraw, San Diego Mesa College; Dean C. Fletcher, Washington State University; Bella Freeman, University of Dayton; Joan Gussow, Teachers College, Columbia University; Frances M. LaFont, University of Illinois; Phylis B. Moser, University of Maryland; Nell B. Robinson, Texas Christian University; Judith B. Roepke, Ball State University; Jeanne M. Singer, Teachers College, Columbia University; Joanne Spaide, University of Northern Iowa; Paul Stake, University of Connecticut; and William Yamanaka, University of Washington.

Finally, we realize that, despite our best efforts, some errors of fact, emphasis, or interpretations may have occurred. We therefore invite students and teachers to send us any criticisms or suggestions for improvement that can be included in later printings or editions.

Eleanor R. Williams
Mary Alice Caliendo

NUTRITION

PRINCIPLES, ISSUES, AND APPLICATIONS

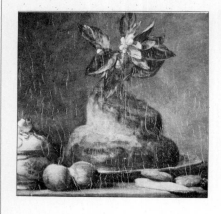

PART I

ASSUMING RESPONSIBILITY FOR FOOD CHOICES

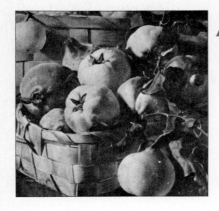

American supermarkets carry huge numbers of food items—from 10,000 to 12,000 items in an average store; more in "fancy" supermarkets. Put yourself into Zoltan's shoes. Zoltan is a college junior greatly interested in technology who reads science fiction for relaxation. He has perfected a robot that can choose items completely at random from a supermarket that carries 13,473 different food items. Each day the robot delivers to Zoltan's door 12 food items—his diet for that day. Each day the 12 items chosen by the robot are entirely different. How would you feel if you had to eat only foods obtained in this way? How would you plan meals using this system? Do you think you would enjoy such a diet? Would it be a nutritionally adequate diet?

The absurdity of this situation is readily apparent. Whether or not such a diet might be nutritionally adequate is beside the point, for no one eats this way. Each of us likes to have some say about what we eat—in fact, many of us would probably become belligerent if we were in Zoltan's shoes. Many foods chosen by our robot would be those we were completely unfamiliar with or disliked.

How can you plan a diet that is attractive, that you enjoy eating, but which is, at the same time, a healthful diet? That is the focus of the first section of this book. The Introduction lays the groundwork, showing how nutrition relates to health, and explaining basic terms pertaining to the science of nutrition. Chapter 1 will give you greater insight into those factors governing your ability to obtain foods as well as those that determine which foods you are inclined to accept from those available. As you become more aware of influences on your food choices, you may wish to assume greater responsibility for consciously choosing those that provide you with a nutritionally sound diet. Chapter 2 offers practical guidelines that can assist you in making such choices.

NUTRITION TODAY: AN INTRODUCTION

NUTRITION AND HEALTH
THE SCIENCE OF NUTRITION: A REVIEW OF BASIC CONCEPTS
A WORD TO STUDENTS

A recent issue of a national news magazine sported the following headline: "America's Great New Food Craze." The feature article described how the American "meat and potatoes" mentality had changed, and how we now paid more attention to food, devoting more time and energy to its preparation, demanding and enjoying more fresh foods, more locally grown foods, and a greater variety of foods. Many supermarkets today stock foods unheard-of a few years ago—such as tofu (soybean curd), bean sprouts, alfalfa sprouts, kiwi fruit, a variety of hot peppers, and fresh seafood [1].

NUTRITION AND HEALTH

Paralleling the rising interest in enjoyment of food as both a pastime and a creative outlet has been an unprecedented increase in concern about the relationship of food and nutrition to health. Many supermarkets have responded, giving information about calories, fat, and sodium in specific foods. Food companies have begun to promote many foods as "nutritious," while only a decade earlier they protested that nutrition wouldn't "sell." Many restaurants now respond to greater demands for lower calorie foods by serving more fish, salads, and vegetables [1].

On the other hand, not all Americans can afford to experiment with gourmet foods and new taste sensations. Rising food costs coupled with declining employment force many people to restrict food expenditures. In fact, the number

3

of people obtaining a portion of their daily food from charitable organizations has escalated in recent years. Fixed costs such as rent or mortgage payments and utilities take precedence over food when income is restricted. A great many Americans, consequently, are constantly alert to ways of saving money on food. At the same time, they need to know how to obtain a nutritious diet while spending limited amounts. This textbook will increase your awareness of how foods can supply your body's nutrient needs and points out how economic, psychological, social, and cultural factors influence an individual's choices of foods. It also suggests ways of obtaining a nutritionally adequate diet at relatively low cost. Practical questions are discussed regarding nutrition for infants, children, adolescents, young, middle-aged, and older adults, and athletes. Problems given special attention include weight control, the world food situation, and how to determine whether or not one is well-nourished.

Almost everyone would like to be healthy. Indeed, the public's recent surge of interest in nutrition developed along with a heightened concern about general health. The chances are good that young adults today are more concerned about having healthy bodies than were their parents when they were the same age. You may, for example, feel a little guilty when you fail to exercise regularly because the importance of exercise is so frequently emphasized, both in the popular media and by health professionals. You may have been one of many children who pressured their parents to stop smoking upon learning in school of its dangers to health. You also may be aware that today many health professionals promote greater *personal responsibility* for health than in the past. As costs of medical care escalate, *preventing* diseases becomes more attractive than trying to cure them. Nutrition is an essential component of attempts to prevent disease. But what exactly do we mean by nutrition?

Nutrition means different things to different people. To many among the general public, the word *nutrition* triggers an image of foods that are "good for you." To the nutrition scientist, however, nutrition is the *process* by which foods consumed are converted into, and are used to maintain, living tissue. To the educator, nutrition encompasses, in addition, all those processes that make foods available and acceptable to people. The term *foods* refers to those substances which, when consumed, furnish nutrients needed to synthesize and maintain body tissues. *Nutrients* are those substances in foods the body needs to build and sustain body tissues. In this book, we shall use the definitions of both the nutrition scientist and the educator, taking into account not only the chemical and physiological processes by which "food becomes you," but also those factors that influence *what* you eat, *how much* you eat, and the circumstances under which you eat—your food habits. What is the relationship of your food habits to health?

Evidence is building that the way people live—their lifestyle—is largely responsible for their state of health. One study illustrated that length of life was associated with routine habits of living. *Daily* habits studied were:

1. Eating breakfast
2. Eating regular meals and not eating between meals
3. Eating moderate amounts of food so as to maintain desirable weight
4. Consuming alcohol in moderation or not at all

5. Engaging in some kind of exercise
6. Sleeping 7 to 8 hours
7. Avoiding cigarette smoking

Men who followed six to seven of these habits could expect, at age 45, to live 33 more years, while those who followed three or less could expect to live only 22 more years [2]. The significance of the 11 years' difference between the two groups is pointed up by the fact that *all* the medical progress made in the United States between 1900 and 1970 increased the number of years a man aged 45 could expect to live by only 4—not 11—years [3]. Moreover, those men who followed all or nearly all the seven health practices were found to be healthier at an older age than those who followed few of them [4]. Obviously, "taking care of yourself," with an emphasis on establishing regular, moderate food habits, pays off in health benefits.

For some time nutrition scientists have studied the role of diet in preventing such diseases as heart disease, stroke, cancer, diabetes, tooth decay, and weight problems—overweight and underweight. This book gives you the opportunity to examine your own food habits in relationship to what is *currently known* about preventing these diseases.

Not only will you study your food habits as they may relate to chronic disease, but you will also become more aware of factors that influence your food choices. What influence do psychological, cultural, and social factors have on your food habits? To what extent does your economic condition affect your choices? What is the influence of your ethnic background on your food preferences? Where do foods that you eat originate? How much is locally grown, and how much shipped great distances? How "energy-intensive" is your diet from the view of the amount of resources required to produce it? How might a change in our ability to obtain fossil fuels (oil, gas, and coal) affect your diet? Should you be concerned about loss of topsoil from our nation's farms? About loss of farmlands to shopping centers and parking lots? Answers to these questions should broaden your view of your own diet in relation to family, national, and global issues concerning food.

Once you have examined your food habits, will you be asked to throw them all out and start afresh? No, not at all. There are many ways to select a healthful diet. People vary widely in their food preferences, and need not deny themselves favorite foods to have an adequate diet. Furthermore, food is one of the pleasures of life and should continue to be so even when nutritious choices are made. In addition, abrupt changes in food habits usually do not last. If you decide to make changes in your food habits, this book will assist you in deciding what changes are sensible for you to achieve the goals you set for yourself.

While the unprecedented increase in public concern about nutrition during the last decade is welcome and gratifying to professional nutritionists, there is, unfortunately, a drawback. Self-styled "nutritionists" have jumped at the opportunity to promote sales of books and magazine articles promoting fad diets—those wildly popular for a few weeks or months, fading away when a new one captures the public's interest. Other "nutritionists" promote the sale of expensive supplements such as protein supplements or vitamin and mineral pills, promising extravagant health benefits. The chief motivation for all this activity is financial profit. As a result, myths and half-truths about nutrition abound.

Most "nutritionists" appearing on television are self-taught; they have not studied the science of nutrition in recognized universities. These "nutritionists" frequently make claims having no scientific validity. Well-trained nutrition scientists find that these claims range from those that are unsubstantiated, but harmless, to those that are flagrantly false and dangerous. Yet nutrition scientists are apt to project a dull, ponderous image on television because they cannot in good conscience make the kinds of sensational, dramatic statements that television audiences are accustomed to hearing from self-styled "nutritionists."

How can you learn to tell the difference between those who are responsible and scientifically sound and those who are untrained, misleading, and irresponsible? The primary way is to develop and exercise critical judgment. To reach this objective, you need to know how the body functions, and the roles that nutrients play in those functions. The more you understand about nutrition and your body, the more you can logically question claims made about the effects of diet on the body. Additionally, you need to learn how scientists find out how nutrients affect the body. If you know whether or not a scientific study is well designed and properly executed, you will be better equipped to judge whether or not a claim is based on scientific facts or on conjecture and wishful thinking. This book guides you through the complex functions of nutrients in the body and their interrelationships. In addition, it describes the rudiments of scientific methods used in nutrition to help you judge when to be skeptical of claims made about diet and health.

You may be somewhat confused at first to find that sometimes investigators in the field of nutrition publicly disagree about a particular question involving diet and health. Usually in such cases different investigators disagree as to *how much* scientific evidence should be amasssed before a policy or guideline is set for the public to follow. When research evidence fails to provide absolute certainty as to the consequences of having the public follow a specific course or guidelines, scientists are bound to disagree on what the public should be advised to do. In these controversial areas, this book lays out the arguments on various sides of the issues to help you choose a reasonable course to follow. Among the issues examined are what guidelines should be given the public about diet.

THE SCIENCE OF NUTRITION:
A REVIEW OF BASIC CONCEPTS

To understand what we know today about the relationship between nutrition and health requires some basic knowledge of chemistry, anatomy, and physiology. The authors realize that many of their readers have little or no background in these areas. Therefore, we present some important basic concepts in biology and chemistry in the pages which follow to enhance your understanding of nutritional concepts. Terms are defined and concepts explained when they are introduced and appear again in the glossary at the end of the book. Examples are used to

TABLE 1. PERCENT OF NUTRIENTS IN A VARIETY OF FOODS

	COOKED SPINACH	COOKED GROUND BEEF	BAKED POTATO	CHEDDAR CHEESE	RAW ORANGE
	PERCENT				
Water	92.0	54.2	75.1	37.0	86.0
Proteins	3.0	24.2	2.6	25.0	1.0
Fats	0.2	20.2	0.1	32.1	0.1
Carbohydrates	3.6	0	21.0	2.1	12.2
Minerals	1.1	1.3	1.1	3.7	0.6
Vitamins	0.1	0.1	0.1	0.1	0.1

SOURCE: Watt, B.K., and A. L. Merrill, *Composition of Foods*, Agriculture Handbook No. 8, USDA, Washington, D.C.: 1963.

illustrate new concepts whenever possible, and numerous practical applications of interest to the reader are included.

Nurturing Components of Food

''You are what you eat'' means, not that your body is made up of hamburgers and potato chips, but that the foods you eat supply nutrients. Classes of nutrients in foods include carbohydrates, fats, proteins, water, vitamins, and minerals. The body can manufacture (synthesize) certain nutrients in the amounts needed, but can make only limited amounts of others. Still other nutrients cannot be made at all by body tissues. Those the body is unable to manufacture, or cannot synthesize in sufficient quantities, are called *essential nutrients*, meaning that it is *essential that these be in the diet*. Those the body can synthesize in amounts needed are called *nonessential nutrients*, even though they are just as important metabolically to normal body functions as the essential nutrients. In other words, both kinds of nutrients are needed for normal functioning of the body.

Foods differ in the proportion of nutrients they supply. Table 1 indicates amounts of carbohydrates, proteins, fats, vitamins, minerals, and water in several common foods. Notice that many foods are high in water content, and that the amount of minerals and vitamins in foods tends to be small compared with the amount of carboyhydrate, protein, or fat. We will see later, however, that vitamins and minerals are vital to normal body functions even though they are needed in small amounts.

Basic Chemical Facts about Nutrients

All nutrients are chemical substances, and all except minerals are compounds. A *compound* is a substance that can be broken down into simpler components. Water, for example, is a compound that can be decomposed to its basic elements, hydrogen and oxygen. An *element* is one of the 103 or so pure chemical substances which combine to make up chemical compounds. Elements are not easily broken down chemically. All minerals, such as calcium, iron, phosphorus, and magnesium, are elements.

An *atom* is the smallest unit of an element having the chemical properties of that element. An atom is made up of a *nucleus* containing positively charged *protons* and uncharged *neutrons*, with negatively charged *electrons* orbiting around the nucleus. The number of electrons equals the number of protons, with the result that the atom itself is an uncharged particle. The atoms of a given element are alike in that they have the same number of protons, neutrons, and electrons. The number of electrons in an atom determines its chemical properties. Atoms of carbon, hydrogen, and oxygen are illustrated in Figure 3-2.

A *molecule* is the smallest part of a substance as it normally exists, regardless of whether it is a compound or an element. The element oxygen, for example, normally exists as two atoms of oxygen joined together to form a molecule commonly designated as O_2. The compound water exists as two atoms of hydrogen joined to one atom of oxygen to form the molecule designated as H_2O.

All nutrients except minerals and water are *organic compounds*, meaning that they contain the element *carbon*. Organic compounds are important in the study of nutrition because by far the largest number of compounds in our bodies and in food are organic compounds.

Importance of Nutrients to Cells

The body is made up of skin, bones, muscles, brain, nerves, organs (liver, heart, lungs, kidneys, pancreas), blood vessels, digestive tract, urinary tract, and reproductive tract. The basic unit of each of these body parts is the cell.

The Cell   All cells have common constituent parts even though a nerve cell, for example, bears no resemblance to a muscle cell in size, shape, or function. A typical cell is diagrammed in Figure 1. Note in this figure the cell membrane, the nucleus, cytoplasm, endoplasmic reticulum, ribosomes, mitochondria, and lysosomes. The *nucleus* contains the genes or the hereditary material which directs the activities of the cell. For example, the genes direct the synthesis of proteins in the cell's *ribosomes*, which are attached to the *endoplasmic reticulum* (ER). The ER is a system of membranes, categorized as either rough or smooth, through which cellular materials are transported. Only the rough ER has ribosomes attached. The *mitochondria* have been called the powerhouse of the cell because they are centers of energy production obtained from the oxidation of carbohydrates, fats, and proteins. The *lysosomes* contain powerful enzymes that digest foreign matter; if the lysosome membrane is broken the released enzymes can destroy the cell.

Cells are organized into specific tissues such as liver or muscle tissues. They grow by reproducing themselves (increasing cell number) or by enlarging (increasing cell size). Growth occurs in infancy, childhood, adolescence, during pregnancy, and upon recovery from an accident or illness during which there has been loss of body tissues (bone fractures, serious burns, feverish illnesses).

Cells require nutrients to be able to fulfill many divergent needs. Among these are the need for energy, growth, repair, and regulation of body processes.

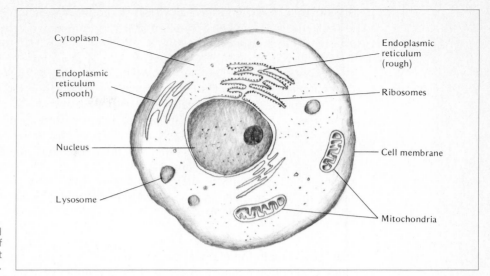

Cytoplasm

Endoplasmic
reticulum
(smooth)

Nucleus

Lysosome

Endoplasmic
reticulum
(rough)

Ribosomes

Cell membrane

Mitochondria

FIGURE 1. A typical cell, showing some of its important components.

Energy Needs *The cell's fundamental and primary need is for energy.* Consequently, the body will use its own tissues for energy if too little is in the food consumed each day. Energy is needed to build new tissues and support normal activities of organs, muscles, and nerves. In nutrition the energy unit is the *kilocalorie*, abbreviated *kcal*, and called the calorie in popular writing. The kilocalorie is defined as the amount of heat required to raise the temperature of one kilogram (1000 g) of water 1°C. The kilocalorie is therefore 1000 times larger than the smaller gram calorie used in chemistry and physics. Older nutrition textbooks frequently capitalize the word, Calorie, to designate the kilocalorie, but we shall simply call it kilocalorie.

Cells obtain energy, or kilocalories, from carbohydrates, fats, proteins, and alcohol. Each gram of carbohydrate in a slice of bread, for example, provides 4 kcal when body cells use it for energy. Each gram of protein provides 4 kcal, each gram of fat 9 kcal, and each gram of pure alcohol, 7 kcal when the body obtains energy from them.

Growth Nearly all nutrients are involved in supporting growth of new tissues. Carbohydrates and fats are important especially as sources of energy to support growth. Proteins provide amino acids without which growth cannot occur. Most vitamins and minerals also are needed for normal growth to occur.

Repair of Tissue Many cells in the body of the child or adult are torn down daily and must be replaced. A cell in the lining of the intestinal tract, for example, exists only about 3 days. At end of that time, it is sloughed off and must be replaced by a new cell. This need for replacement of tissues is called the *maintenance requirement*, meaning that nutrients are constantly required to maintain body tissues in their normal state by synthesizing new cells to replace old ones. Most tissues in the body are subject to this "wear and tear" phenomenon, but some tissues are torn down faster than others. In adults, for example, the basic protein forming the structure of bones, collagen, is torn down very slowly, while in infants it is torn down more rapidly.

Regulation of Body Processes Many nutrients play roles in regulating certain vital functions in the body. For example, cells shrink and die if suddenly a large proportion of the water normally held within the cell is withdrawn. Sodium and potassium are minerals which are part of a complex mechanism which *regulates* the vital distribution of fluid in and around body cells. Some nutrients play a role in enhancing the absorption of other nutrients. Vitamin D, for example, increases the absorption of calcium. Many vitamins are necessary to regulate aspects of the complex process by which energy is obtained by the body from the breakdown of carbohydrates, fats, and proteins. The roles of regulating body processes involve vitamins, minerals, and proteins more frequently than carbohydrates or fats.

Conversion of Food to Body Tissues

How, then, does food become a part of your body? We have seen that food furnishes the body with nutrients it cannot itself synthesize (as well as with many that it *can*), and that cells use these nutrients to obtain energy and support growth and repair of tissues. Nutrients also help the cell regulate certain vital processes. For food to supply nutrients to the cells, it must first be *digested*, meaning that it must be broken down to simpler units. These simple substances must then be *absorbed* into the blood. The blood carries nutrients and oxygen to the cells and removes waste products (carbon dioxide and other chemical wastes). *Metabolism* is the process by which nutrients are used by cells to replace worn-out tissues, to build new cells and tissues, or to perform normal cell functions. Metabolism also includes all processes in which components of cells are torn down, and those by which cells rid themselves of wastes.

Homeostasis

During health, the body maintains an internal environment in which the concentration of many different substances in body fluids (blood, lymph, and tissue fluid) is maintained within narrow limits. This remarkable state, called *homeostasis*, is achieved by the interactions of the nervous system, enzymes, and hormones.

The Nervous System The nervous system consists of the brain, the spinal cord, and nerves that reach all parts of the body. Nerves control the functions of organs or particular tissues by use of electrical impulses. The brain integrates messages from the nerves and decides upon the appropriate response, but these complex maneuvers occur unconsciously.

Enzymes Enzymes are proteins produced by cells that catalyze (increase the speed of) chemical reactions. Without enzymes, body cells, tissues, and organs could not survive because chemical reactions vital to life would occur too slowly

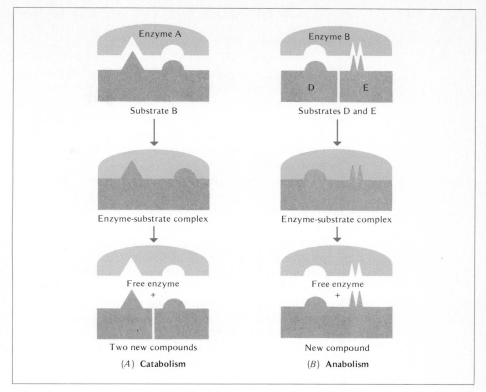

FIGURE 2. Enzyme action. Enzymes join the substrate, temporarily forming an enzyme-substrate complex. This close association allows the enzyme to catalyze the *breakdown* of a compound, in the case of some enzymes *(A),* or the *synthesis* of a new compound, in the case of others *(B).*

or not at all. Enzymes are necessary for digestion of food and for the metabolism of nutrients within the body.

Some enzymes require minerals or vitamins to function properly. If the needed mineral or vitamin is missing, the enzyme cannot do its job. Although enzymes are not used up in the reactions they catalyze, they are nevertheless eventually destroyed in the body and require replacement. Dietary lack of needed amino acids, vitamins, or minerals can result in failure to synthesize the active form of some enzymes required for normal body functions. The mode of action of enzymes is illustrated in Figure 2.

Most enzymes are named for the substance they act upon, called the *substrate,* and nearly all enzyme names end in *-ase.* For example, *sucrase* is the enzyme that speeds up the breakdown of *sucrose* (table sugar) during digestion. Sucrose is the substrate upon which sucrase acts.

Hormones   Hormones are substances secreted into the blood by specialized cells in response to a stimulus and are circulated to a specific target organ. For example, the hormone insulin is secreted by the pancreas whenever blood glucose levels increase above normal. Insulin travels in the blood and causes muscle and adipose tissue (fat storage) cells to remove glucose from the blood, thus lowering blood glucose and restoring homeostasis.

A WORD TO STUDENTS

As we've noted, today's student of nutrition is faced with the task of sorting out much information from many sources, including the news media. Special features of this book are designed to help you sharpen your critical thinking skills and to develop an appreciation of the various sides of many current issues.

Boxed material is set off from the text throughout the book. These inserts explore important issues, questions, fallacies, or applications.

Brief discussions labeled *A Closer Look* appear in most chapters. These focus on important nutrient interrelationships or provide additional information on practical applications.

Nutrition in the News features excerpts from newspapers and magazines that focus primarily on unresolved issues in nutrition. These are followed by author-developed questions designed to help you critically evaluate the nutrition information you encounter in the media.

Sections at the end of each chapter entitled *For Discussion and Application* contain questions and activities designed to encourage examination of your own food and exercise habits, to foster insights and investigation into issues in nutrition, and to further your knowledge and experience in the field of nutrition.

The authors hope that reading this text will give you a solid foundation in nutrition and make you more fully aware of important food and nutrition-related issues. We hope also that you will learn how to critically evaluate claims made about food and nutrition. Lastly, we hope you will be motivated to examine your lifestyle and make informed decisions about whether to modify or change particular aspects of it in relation to food and exercise. If you decide to make changes, this book should guide you in how to plan and maintain a reasonable, moderate diet. We would be gratified also if this book increases your interest in the field of nutrition.

1 INFLUENCES ON FOOD CHOICES

How did you decide what to have for your evening meal yesterday? Were you completely free to choose anything you wanted for that meal? Can you pinpoint any constraints on your choices? Did you eat only enough to satisfy your physiological hunger, or were there other factors—psychological or social—that influenced the amounts or kinds of food you ate?

Increasing your understanding of factors that influence your food habits will make you more aware of the extent to which you control what and how much you eat and the extent to which your eating behavior is influenced by other factors. Such an awareness may motivate you to think about how you might gain more control. In this chapter, we will examine the myriad influences on food choices in our complex society.

You probably realized when you thought about yesterday's evening meal that you were *not* free to choose whatever foods you wanted. If you ate in a cafeteria or restaurant, your choices were limited to the foods offered. If someone cooked the meal for you at home, you may or may not have had something to say about which foods were served. If you prepared the meal yourself, you were limited to the foods available in your house or apartment. Food choices are influenced by all those factors that govern the availability and acceptability of foods. Let's examine those factors, beginning with the more global ones.

INFLUENCES ON AVAILABILITY OF FOOD

Ecological Influences

Climate and local growing conditions influence the kinds of food grown in specific regions of the world. Wheat is the staple crop of North America and central Europe, where the climate is ideal for its production, while rice is favored by the wet climates of southeastern Asia. Corn requires specific growing conditions found in the midwestern United States, Mexico, Central America, Indonesia, Thailand, Argentina, and the Balkan States of Europe [1]. Populations living near oceans or rivers generally harvest and consume more fish than those living far inland. Many tropical regions grow fruits that are locally available all year round.

While normal conditions of the soil, rainfall, and weather foster production of specific foods, climatic conditions also bring about disasters in the food supply. Droughts, storms, and floods all take their toll, sometimes producing famine, but nearly always producing increases in food prices so that some people lose access to some foods. When weather deviations are widely different from normal, yields of grains—the foundation of the diet in most of the world—are lowest [2]. Although one may believe that humans are at the mercy of weather, geographers have pointed out that people themselves can causes droughts and famines by making seemingly small modifications of the environment which "set the stage for . . . natural occurrences (hurricanes, tornadoes, blizzards, or flooding) that not only destroy crops but the environmental matrix for food production" [3]. The study of how we can avoid contributing to the development of droughts and floods is vital to our understanding of how we can increase a population's access to food.

Food availability also varies with seasonal changes. For example, even though the food system in the United States makes many fresh fruits available throughout the year, berries, cherries, plums, melons, and peaches are available in most markets only during the summer. Today in many parts of the world changes in seasons greatly affect the variety of foods accessible to specific populations.

The Food System

How an individual obtains food depends upon the system by which food is produced and conveyed from the farm or factory to the consumer. This system strongly influences the kinds and amounts of foods available. Today's food system in the United States is highly complex compared with that prior to the beginning of this century. In earlier times farmers lived on their own land, produced most of the foods their families consumed, and marketed their crops within the local region. Each farmer decided which specific crops and how much of each should be planted, taking into account local conditions of soil and weather and the prevailing market situation. Land was plentiful and little capital was required since farmers did not have to buy machinery or fertilizer. The power required to work the land came from human labor and that of animals raised on the farms. Most food processing occurred in the farm home. Industrial processing generally

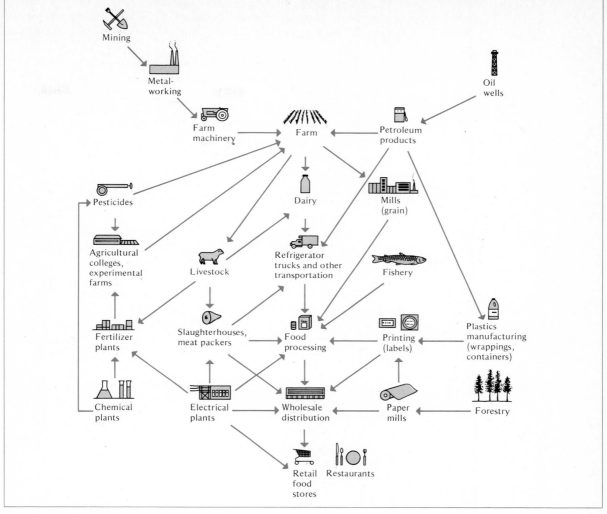

FIGURE 1-1. A flow chart depicting the U.S. food system. On the input side of the farm are industries that supply such items as fuel, fertilizer, and machinery. On the output side of the farm are the food processing industries. (Source: Heady, E. O., "The Agriculture of the U.S.," *Scientific American,* 235(3):107, 1976.)

was limited to flour milling, vegetable canning, and cheese making and was confined to the immediate region. Under this system people consumed almost exclusively those foods grown within a limited region.

Today, although still the basic source of our foods, farmers are only one part of an intricate food system. This system is sometimes referred to as "agribusiness," and consists of three components [4] (Figure 1-1). First, so-called "input" industries supply farmers with machinery, tools, seeds, fertilizers, pesticides, and fuel for machines. Second, farmers use these inputs to produce crops. Frequently, they choose to specialize in producing only one or two kinds of grain or legume, and/or one kind of livestock [5]. Third, food processing industries buy and transport farm products to various plants where they process them (milling grains, slaughtering animals, preparing various specialty meat and processed food items, canning, freezing, dehydrating, packaging, and labeling). Finally the finished products are transported, often over great distances, to wholesale distributors who transport them to retail stores, restaurants, and other food-serving institutions[4].

This system has developed fairly recently—largely since World War II—and has been highly productive. For example, the productivity of each farm worker has increased enormously, with each on-farm worker now feeding 50 people[6]. (This does not count the number of workers required in the input industries, however.) The U.S. food system makes more than 10,000 different food items available to consumers in modern supermarkets. In addition, U.S. agriculture has the capacity to export large amounts of grains and other commodities. In 1979 the United States exported 87 percent of world soybean exports and 67 percent of world grain exports [7].

The U.S. food system is not without its problems. Among concerns are that the system (1) is highly energy-intensive; (2) results not only in pollution of lakes and streams, but also in soil erosion; (3) diminishes the number of small farms; and (4) results in increased prices for consumers. Box 1-1 examines each of these problems briefly.

Human beings have always gained their sustenance from the products of the soil, lakes, streams, and oceans. Our myopic view of how we get our food—"from the supermarket"—blinds us to our utter dependence on the earth and on farmers. In our preoccupation with producing as high yields as possible, we have behaved as if we could afford to ignore the damage to our basic means of sustenance—the land, and resources needed to renew it and keep it productive.

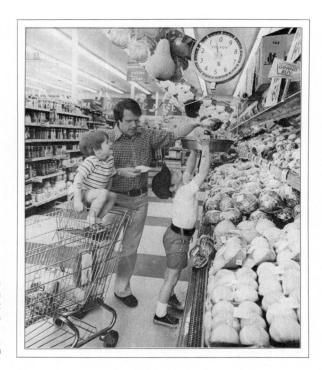

The modern supermarket is an important component of the United States food system. *(James H. Karales/Peter Arnold, Inc.)*

Concerns about the U.S. Food System

No food system is perfect. From the viewpoint of the possible long-term consequences of continuing our present food system, critics have voiced several concerns.

Energy Use The great productivity of U.S. agriculture depends upon fossil fuels (petroleum, coal, and natural gas) which in the past were inexpensive and seemingly plentiful. Fossil fuels are used not only to manufacture and run farm machinery, irrigation systems, and to transport farm products, but also to produce pesticides (made chiefly from petroleum) and fertilizer (made chiefly from natural gas). Energy from fossil fuels is required at every point of the food system represented in Figure 1-1. Energy use is particularly high for processing and packaging foods. Frozen foods are highly energy-intensive [6], while metal cans, glass jars, and other forms of packaging are often more expensive than the monetary value of the food itself [8].

The U.S. food system, overall, is estimated to consume 9 kcal of energy to produce 1 kcal from food. One study pointed out that if the entire world were fed using a system like ours, 80 percent of the world's entire energy expenditure would have to be used just to produce food [9]. Obviously our system can survive only as long as inexpensive energy sources are obtainable, but fossil fuel sources are becoming depleted [6]. If the present U.S. system is to survive, other cheap energy sources must be made available before fossil fuel supplies become exhausted, and methods of reducing the energy loss in the food systsem must be vigorously pursued [9,10].

Pollution and Soil Erosion Food production requires other resources than fuel. Productive soils, adequate water resources, and unpolluted streams, rivers, lakes, and oceans are needed to supply human populations with a varied diet, including fish and shellfish. Although the very high yields of crops in U.S. agriculture have been most closely associated with increasing fertilizer applications, pollution problems are related to heavy fertilizer use. The runoff, as rains wash over soils, can pollute well waters, streams, and lakes, producing in the latter overgrowth of algae. These processes in turn deplete the water of oxygen and destroy fish life [11].

Loss of topsoil is estimated to range between 9 and 12 tons per acre annually, while new topsoil forms under good farming conditions at a rate of only 1.5 tons per acre per year. Generally farmers have ignored soil conservation practices because of incentives to produce ever greater crop yields. Farmers' heavy indebtedness in the face of rising costs for machinery, fertilizers, and fuel tend also to discourage soil conservation practices [12]. While no good farmer wants to despoil the land, many farmers find they are unable to fulfill their roles as protectors of the ecological health of their land.

Decline in Number of Small Farmers A striking effect of the development of our present food system is the decline in the number of farms, and the increase in their size [13]. The largest farms, although they are relatively few, account for a very high percentage of agricultural-product sales. This rapid change from smaller to larger farms occurred largely because the kind of farming we have described requires large outlays of capital for purchase of equipment and machinery as well as fertilizers, pesticides, herbicides, and fuel. The farmer with large land holdings can establish credit and obtain needed funds, while the smaller farmer has greater difficulty doing so.

Another reason for the predominance of large farms lies in the increasing concentration of buying power among a small number of large corporations that purchase farm products. Because the buyer can cut costs to a minimum by reducing the number of farmers he or she buys from, a buyer prefers to deal with larger, not smaller, farmers. For some products, notably broiler chickens and vegetables for canning or freezing, small producers have little or no access to markets as a result of this system [14].

What are the consequences of this trend for big farms to get bigger, and for small ones to disappear? One consequence is that the production of many foods will be highly concentrated among a small number of large farms, increasing the power of large producers to affect prices. Another effect of more large farms is that fewer young people will be able to acquire farms, since large amounts of capital will be required to buy land and machinery. Those who wish to live on their own small farms because they believe this provides them with a better quality of life are apt to be forced by economic reality to farm only part-time, supporting themselves with nonfarm jobs [13].

Increased Consumer Prices An important criticism of the U.S. food system is that it increases prices consumers must pay for food. Higher profits by the food processing and retailing industries—the middlemen between farmers and consumers—resulted in increased consumer food prices of 35 percent between 1948 and 1972, and 21 percent between 1974 and 1978 [15].

Increases in profits in the processing and retailing sector of the food system are made possible in large part by increasing concentration within these industries—that is, only a small number of companies dominate processing and marketing for specific foods. The member companies are then said to form an *oligopoly*. The advantage of such consolidation is that the large corporation increases its power to set prices without having to worry so much about what its competitors will do [16].

Those food companies making greatest profits tend to be oligopoly members manufacturing *differentiated products*—that is, similar products that retain some distinctive differences [15], such as breakfast cereals or snack foods. According to agricultural economist John M. Connor, successful product differentiation often allows a food company to sell a new product at a higher price than a competitor who sells a close substitute [15]. This position has been challenged by food manufacturers, however. It is clear, though, that gaining acceptability for a new differentiated product today involves concentrated advertising, an additional cost the consumer bears.

Consumers influence the food system by where they choose to shop for food and the choices they make there. The great variety of high kilocalorie–low nutrient foods on supermarket shelves would not be there if no one bought them. Consumers should take their responsibilities seriously because their choices are extremely influential on the U.S. food system.

There are signs that Americans are thinking seriously about alternatives to some parts of our current food system. The annual meeting of the Society of Nutrition Education in the summer of 1981 was devoted to the theme "Access to Food." The society approved resolutions to promote: (1) increased production and use of local fruits and vegetables; (2) increased education of professionals and the public on the benefits of and methods of achieving a more regional, seasonal diet; and (3) methods of stemming the current loss of prime farmland to non-food-producing purposes (shopping centers, etc.) [17].

One suggested way farmers might reduce their costs is by adopting some of the practices used in organic farming. These practices include avoiding or severely restricting the use of synthetic fertilizers, pesticides, growth regulators, and livestock feed additives. Crop rotations and use of animal manures, mechanical cultivation, and biological pest control maintain soil productivity. A study of organic farming by the USDA (U.S. Department of Agriculture) found that this method is less costly because of its reduction in use of petrochemical-based fertilizers and pesticides, as well as its reduction in total fossil fuel use. The report also found that organic farming results in less soil erosion, less nutrient runoff from soil into lakes and streams, and less pesticide pollution. The report suggests that conventional farmers could profitably adopt *some* practices used by organic farmers, but does not advocate large-scale conversion to organic farming. Substituting organic sources of fertilizers for chemical fertilizer on a wide scale would be limited by both availability and cost. The study suggests that small farms or those larger ones producing mixed crops and large numbers of animals might be best suited to this method [18].

A CLOSER LOOK

Are "organic foods"—many of which are marketed in small food cooperatives, health food stores, or farmer's markets—better for you than those you find in the supermarket? To avoid confusion in terminology, it is preferable to refer to these foods as *organically grown foods*—that is, they are grown by the methods described in the discussion of organic farming. Since a large percentage of organically grown foods in the United States is marketed through conventional channels, most of us have been consuming them whether or not we are aware of it [18].

In chemistry, the term "organic" encompasses all compounds that contain carbon (except for carbon dioxide and salts, such as carbonates). Nutritionists, when discussing organic foods, frequently maintain that "all foods are 'organic' because they are composed of organic compounds containing carbon" [19]. This statement is correct when one uses the chemical definition, but producers of organically grown foods use a broader, philosophical definition of the word. Organic farming is concerned with organizing use of land and resources for food production in such a way as to produce healthy plants and animals while maintaining soil quality and balance, and avoiding environmental damage. The definition of organic used by organic farmers, therefore, is closer to: "constituting a whole whose parts are mutually dependent or intrinsically related" [20]. [By permission. From *Webster's Third New International Dictionary*, copyright 1981 by Mirriam-Webster, Inc., publisher of the Mirriam-Webster Dictionaries, p. 1590, definition **5b**(1).]

Consumers who believe in the philosophical tenets of organic farming can and do indicate their support by purchasing organically grown foods. Some individuals may buy them in the belief that they are nutritionally superior to conventionally grown foods, but so far, research studies fail to support this belief [18]. More rigorous studies are needed on this question, however. Meanwhile, consumers should not be led to believe that organically grown foods are nutritionally superior. Nevertheless, they should have the option of choosing these foods if they prefer them.

Farmer's markets are common in many parts of the country, offering consumers the opportunity to purchase fresh produce directly from the producer, avoiding costs for middlemen. Increasing farmer access to local markets, especially in the northeast where agricultural land is under development pressure, can help retain food-growing capacity in various parts of the country [21].

Another way to increase consumer access to affordable food is through food co-ops. Many of these consumer-run co-ops started in the 1960s and are still in business throughout the country. They offer lower prices because many are nonprofit, have low overhead, and little in the way of packaging costs. The foods they sell are generally traditional, minimally processed foods.

As inflation and food prices continue to be high, more people are gardening, and canning or freezing their excess production. More consumers are patronizing discount food stores that offer fewer services but lower prices than supermarkets. Food systems are dynamic and change as economic, social, and political conditions change.

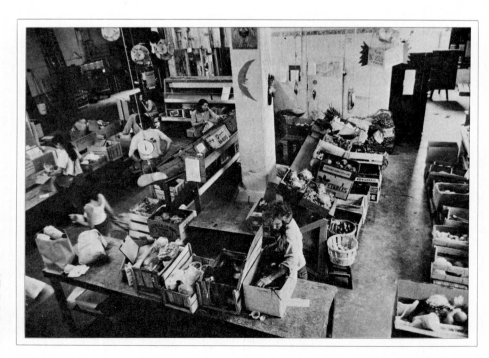

Consumer-run food cooperatives (co-ops) offer traditional, minimally processed foods, many of which are unavailable in supermarkets. *(Jim Harris/Stock, Boston, Inc.)*

We have dwelt at some length on the U.S. food system because it is probably the most pervasive influence on American food habits. For example, are you in the habit of going to the refrigerator or vending machine for a soft drink when you feel thirsty? The U.S. food system has made soft drinks widely available and has advertised them so effectively that many consumers equate thirst with soft drinks. This brings us to a discussion of advertising, an integral part of the U.S. food system.

Advertising

Foods are the most highly advertised among all consumer products in the United States [22]. Advertising consists of any strategy that influences consumers to choose among brands or to consume a specific product. Some growers' associations, for example, advertise to increase total consumption of such products as citrus fruit or milk, but do not promote a specific brand. Companies in an oligopoly often advertise to take sales for similar products away from one another, not primarily to promote higher total consumption of a product.

Food advertising has been divided into "pull" and "push" promotional techniques [22]. *Pull advertising* is directed to the consumer, and includes messages projected by radio, television, newspapers, magazines, discount coupons, free sample distribution, recipes and promotions on packaging, and incentives such as contests, premiums, and trading stamps. *Push techniques* are aimed at the retailer to obtain favorable amounts of space and locations on shelves, and end-of-aisle displays for specific products. Consumers are usually unaware of these techniques, which include promotions at retailer trade fairs and conventions, advertising in trade publications, and discounts, rebates, and reimbursement to the retailer for local advertising [22].

Highly processed foods account for most food advertising. In 1978 six food-product groups accounted for only 20 percent of the consumer food dollar, but 50 percent of all media advertising. These groups were soft drinks, breakfast cereals, candy and other desserts, oils and salad dressings, coffee, and prepared foods [22]. Soft drinks alone used up $260 million in advertising in 1978, about 13.5 percent of media advertising for food that year [23]. By way of comparison, food-product groups accounting for more than 50 percent of the consumer food dollar received less than 8 percent of national media advertising in 1978 [22]. These groups were made up of highly perishable foods, and included fresh poultry, fish, meats, eggs, fruits, vegetables, and dairy products. However, these foods were and are highly advertised by retail stores in local newspapers, making up about 40 percent of such advertising [22].

Generally the largest food companies spend the most on advertising. Large companies that produce differentiated products rely upon advertising when establishing a new product. Think, for example, of all the snack items on a supermarket shelf. A new snack item could hardly find a place on the shelf today without a sizeable advertising expenditure to alert the consumer to its existence. A small company, to accomplish its goal of getting its snack item on the shelf, would have to match the advertising expenditure of the big companies.

Retail outlets promote food sales using techniques of which many consumers

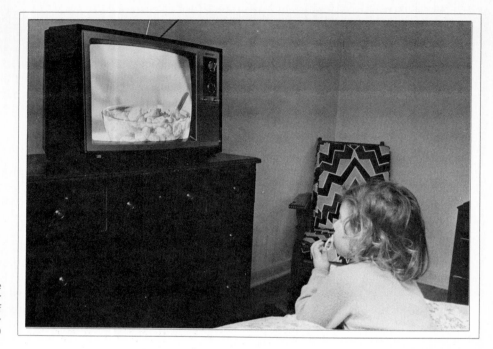

Children frequently are the targeted audience for television advertising of breakfast cereals. *(Randy Matusow)*

may be unaware. Usually supermarkets place items in locations likely to catch the eye of consumers. Items intended to attract children are placed on lower shelves. Next time you are in a supermarket, notice the number of children who ask for items they see on the low shelves. End-of-aisle displays draw attention to certain products. Notice the amount of space provided to different items in a supermarket —this fact alone has an impact on purchasers. Items placed at checkout counters are there to encourage impulse buying, as are displays in which items are placed together that might be used together—such as salad dressings and salad greens.

How much does food advertising cost consumers? One estimate for 1981, looking only at expenditures on food for home use, found that advertising accounted for between 3 and 4 cents per consumer dollar spent on food [22]. For a family spending $3000 per year on food for home use, this would amount to $90 to $111 per year. What benefits does the consumer receive from advertising to weigh against the costs? For one thing, advertising revenues finance commercial television and radio, and reduce prices of magazines and newspapers to consumers. Advertising may also reduce time required for shopping since it can inform consumers where to find bargains. It also helps new manufacturers to compete by expanding their sales sufficiently to reach a high-volume, low-cost level [16].

Critics of advertising claim that much advertising is wasteful, however. Since consumers have a limited capacity for quantity of food they can consume, and since the population of the United States is not growing rapidly, there is always a limited market for a specific food product. As noted earlier, companies forming

KELLOGG TESTS AREA'S TASTE FOR PRICEY FERMENTED MILK

R. E. Bucklin, *The Washington Post,* August 5, 1982

There are 77 different kinds of yogurt crowding the coolers at Safeway, but Kellogg Co. figures that's not enough. . . .

In the next few weeks Kellogg will use Washington and Baltimore supermarkets to begin the national roll-out of "Whitney's," a new brand that Kellogg officials claim will be "the Häagen-Dazs of yogurt."

Kellogg's marketing strategy is to make Whitney's the highest-priced fermented milk money can buy, selling it for 62 to 65 cents for six ounces while house brands go for 40 cents for eight ounces.

The up-market introduction began with a black-tie dinner at the Four Seasons Hotel earlier this summer for 125 grocery trade representatives.

"It's not unusual to hold a trade dinner," explained Dave Brenner, director of market development for Kellogg's yogurt division. "It is unusual perhaps for it to be black tie. We wanted to establish the evening as something different. We're trying to establish this product as a step above."

Although Kellogg won't say how much it has budgeted to promote its new high-class yogurt, supermarket industry representatives who attended the formal bash agreed that the company is "going to spend one heck of a lot of money. . . ."

The new product has been "engineered" for a smoother, richer, more textured taste than its competitors, said Brenner. "It will come in a cup which looks as though it was designed by Tiffany's. . . ."

By aiming for the very top of the yogurt strata with a product costing twice as much per ounce as its lowest-priced competitors, Kellogg hopes to grab a new segment of a market now dominated by Dannon. . . .

The potential for profit in the fast-growing yogurt market first attracted Kellogg several years ago. In 1980, Kellogg acquired Le Shake, whose claim to distinction is that its yogurt is so runny you can drink it.

Four years of research and 2,200 taste tests later, Kellogg is now ready to introduce Whitney's.

Safeway and other supermarket chains expect to make room for the new product on their overflowing yogurt shelves if they are satisfied with Kellogg's advertising and promotion plans.

Women and children are the major buyers of yogurt, according to Brenner's market research, and Kellogg will be targeting its promotional efforts toward them.

ASK YOURSELF:

Are consumers demanding a new, richer yogurt? If not, how does the manufacturer of Whitney's plan to create a demand for it? The article says supermarkets will make room for the new products "if they are satisfied with advertising and promotion plans." What would satisfy them? The new product is "smoother and richer." What ingredients might you expect to find in this new product if you had the opportunity to check the label?

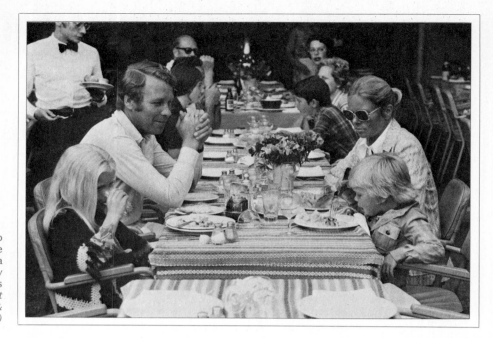

Family outings to restaurants are more frequent today than a decade ago, particularly when both parents work. (© *John Garrett 1980/Woodfin Camp & Assoc.*)

an oligopoly therefore advertise chiefly to take customers away from each other. The result is that the consumer pays more for a product simply because it is advertised. Other criticisms of advertising are that it creates desires for frivolous products, distorts tastes, is often offensive, and may misinform consumers [16]. Clearly, advertising is neither "all bad" nor "all good." Consumers must decide for themselves whether to buy highly advertised foods and beverages. Furthermore, one is apt to be influenced less by advertising as one becomes more aware of the techniques used.

Economic Influences

Economic factors exercise a pervasive influence on one's access to foods. In 1981, the U.S. population as a whole spent about 16.7 percent of its income on food; about 12.3 percent was spent on food for home use, while the rest was spent on food away from home [24]. When income is low, however, the percentage that must be spent for food is usually greater than the average. For example, data from the 1965 Household Food Consumption Survey showed that households making less than $4000 per year spent about 42 percent for food [25]. Recent increases in food prices due to inflation and other factors, coupled with the rise in unemployment, have caused many families and individuals to sharply curtail their food expenditures. Many find that they can no longer afford some of their favorite foods, such as meats, certain cheeses, and fresh fruits and vegetables.

An important economic trend is the rapid growth in number of families with two incomes; an estimated 50 percent of all married women now work outside the home. This fact results in some changes in food choices. For example, the extra income allows more individuals or families to eat out more frequently. The amount they are willing to pay when eating out affects their food choices. Foods available in fast-food restaurants, for instance, tend to be more limited than those offered in expensive restaurants. Moreover, working mothers, because they have less time to devote to planning and preparing meals, may rely more heavily on frozen, canned, or otherwise prepackaged convenience foods than on foods ''made from scratch.''

Among families or individuals living below the poverty level, high food prices are particularly damaging. Frequently, after the rent and utilities are paid, money left over may be inadequate to provide an adequate diet. Although the federal Food Stamp Program may adequately supply the food needs for some families, others fall between the cracks and receive little, if any, aid.

The very poor are limited in their food purchases by more than just lack of money for food. They often lack transportation as well, which may force them to shop at the corner grocery store [26]. Prices at these small local stores frequently are higher, and choices of foods are more restricted than in many supermarkets [26]. Low-income consumers often have a low educational level; consequently, they are apt to be less assertive than the affluent about their rights as consumers. If taken advantage of, legal counsel or professional help is often out of reach for them. Economic factors obviously exert a tremendous influence on the amounts and varieties of foods accessible to individuals and families.

INFLUENCES ON THE ACCEPTABILITY OF FOOD

Nowhere in the world do human beings eat all the foods available to them. Among those foods available, what influences an individual to choose or accept certain foods, and reject others? Cultural factors play important roles in determining behavior toward food—what foods people eat, and how, when, where, and how much they consume. These cultural factors, therefore, have nutritional consequences; few people choose foods solely or even chiefly for their nutritive value.

Cultural Influences

Culture refers to the ''learned way of life shared by the members of a society, consisting of the totality of tools, techniques, social institutions, attitudes, beliefs, motivations, and systems of values known to the group'' [27]. A *cultural group* refers to a group of people who share the same learned bahaviors. Each human group develops its own system of deciding what animals and plants are to be eaten, how they are to be prepared, and how they are to be distributed among men, women, and children.

Psychological Meanings of Food Within a cultural group, food becomes overlaid with complex psychological meanings from the moment of birth. One does not give food alone to someone else, but communicates attitudes and feelings with it as well. Early feeding experiences allow the baby to learn about

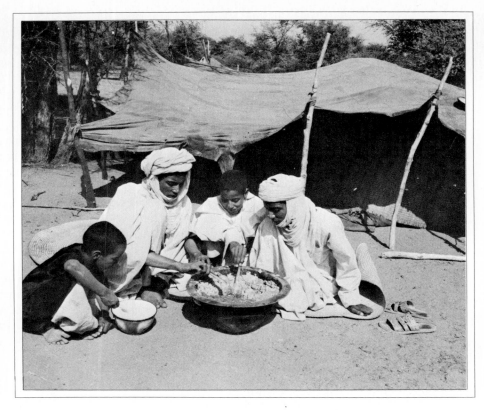

A nomadic Tuareg
family enjoys a staple
food, millet stew, by
their tent in the Niger
Republic.
*(© Marc & Evelyne
Bernheim/Woodfin
Camp & Assoc.)*

others, and about the world around him or her. Margaret Mead, the anthropologist, stated it this way:

> An individual's basic attitudes toward food stem from early feeding experiences. . . . Food may be regarded by the baby as something delightful, plentiful and always there, something very hard to get for which it is necessary to fight, something which is uncertain and undependable, and about which one must always be anxious, something to which one can respond for itself, or only as a part of the mother-child relationship; all this is conveyed to babies by the ways they are fed. . . . It is possible to associate a background of generous, ungrudging child feeding with an adult's emotional security regarding food whereby he can go for a long time without. Conversely, a child who experiences a rigidly austere or very meager diet throughout infancy may have a conditioning which produces the same adult strength. Or it may be developed by austerity in diet imposed after a generously indulged infancy. It is therefore not possible to say that any single-patterned way of feeding infants results inevitably in certain specified food behavior in adults, but it is possible to say that the particular way children of any society are fed and weaned has significance for the food behavior of that society [28]. (Reproduced by permission of UNESCO.)

Foods become associated with pleasant or unpleasant experiences, and therefore take on symbolic meanings. Under stress, people often revert to foods associated in their childhood with security. For example, a nurse who was undergoing severe psychological difficulty began to go early to the hospital where she worked so that she could have for breakfast old-fashioned hot oatmeal that the cook had prepared by long, slow cooking. Later, she realized that she had associated this food with her mother and the warmth and security surrounding early childhood breakfasts. In the same way, a food dislike is often associated with the perception that the food once made the individual ill. The experience often results in lifelong rejection of this food. Feeding problems with children quickly develop because of psychological links to foods. Children who are rewarded for eating a food that "is good for you" (e.g., broccoli) with a promise of dessert ("a food you really like") develop a lifelong conflict. They must choose between doing what is right versus doing what they enjoy [29]. Obviously, this situation is likely to result in a child perceiving that desserts are uncommonly good and desirable, while broccoli and other vegetables are not. Techniques for preventing such feeding problems are discussed in Chapter 15.

As noted above, people become strongly attached to foods that were customarily served in their homes from early childhood. Staple foods, sometimes called "cultural superfoods" [30], frequently take on great psychological and emotional significance. Rice, for example, is an important dietary component in parts of the southern United States, particularly in South Carolina and Louisiana, where it is easily grown. Cornbread, cornmeal mush, and hominy—either whole

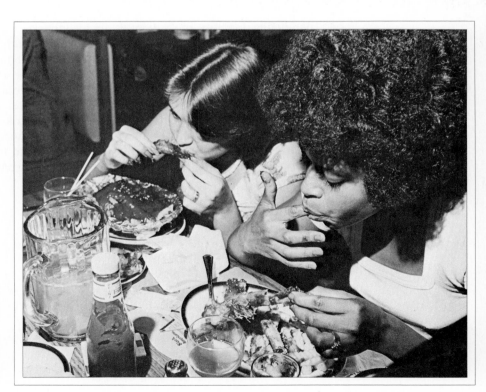

Ethnic restaurants cater to the desire for foods that specific groups of people "grew up on." These women enjoy the offerings of a soul food restaurant. *(© David Sheffield 1978/Woodfin Camp & Assoc.)*

or as grits—have long been preferred foods in the South. Wheat bread was a component of practically every meal in the Midwest and parts of the southwestern United States until after World War II. Foods common to the region in which one grew up often are among one's favorite foods.

In the same way, familiar foods that one particularly enjoys are often the ethnic foods of one's family. Families whose ancestors came from eastern Europe may enjoy cold borscht (soup made from beets) in the summertime, while those from Lebanon might favor tabouli (a salad made from cracked wheat, parsley, mint, green onions, lemon juice, and oil). What are some of the ethnic foods of your own family?

Favorite foods are often associated with celebrations, such as birthdays or homecomings. Today, when you return home after an absence, are some of your favorite foods served in celebration of your homecoming? What circumstances do you associate with those foods that you want most after an extended absence from home? Were some of them regional or ethnic favorites in your family? Associations with experiences of security and pleasure in family situations probably account for some of your preferences, but your own perceptions of flavor, odor, and texture of food undoubtedly are also important factors.

Human beings are born with a preference for sweetness—in other words, individuals do not have to *learn* to like sweet foods [31]. In adults, taste buds exist on the tongue, but during infancy and childhood they are also present in the cheeks and throat [32]. Children between the ages of 3 and 12 years frequently show strong dislikes for some foods, but these tend to decline as they become older, paralleling the loss of taste buds in the cheeks and throat. Although individuals vary in their responses to flavors, odors, and textures of foods, preferences for sour, bitter, or salty flavors can be learned. Small children quickly learn to like the bitter taste of beer, for example, if those adults around them obviously enjoy it. In fact, children quickly learn which foods are desirable by observing which foods their parents and siblings relish most.

Psychological associations with foods may play a role in obesity. Some individuals are driven to eat when they are under stress or when they experience anxiety, depression, or rejection. One of the challenges in feeding infants and young children is to avoid allowing foods to be used to assuage these and other feelings.

Food and Social Status   Nearly all cultures regard some foods as symbols of status. In some parts of Africa, for example, meat is viewed as a luxury item that "sweetens the mouth." In those areas, meat is the fare of men of high status, but is never served to women or children [33].

An example of the social and prestige value of food in the United States is described by Vance Packard in *The Status Seekers*. He tells of a man who, during his lifetime, made various changes in his eating habits as he climbed the social ladder.

As a lad, this man had grown up in a poor family of Italian origin. He was raised on blood sausages, pizza, spaghetti, and red wine. After completing high school, he went to Minnesota and began working in logging camps, where anxious to be accepted he soon learned to prefer beef, beer, and beans, and he shunned "Italian" food. Later, he went to a Detroit industrial plant, and eventually became a promising young executive. This was in the days when it was still fairly easy for a non-college man to rise in industry. In his executive role he found himself cultivating the favorite foods and beverages of other executives: steak, whiskey, and seafood. Ultimately, he gained acceptance in the city's upper class. Now he began winning admiration from people in his elite social set by going back to his knowledge of Italian cooking, and serving them, with the aid of his manservant, authentic Italian treats such as blood sausage, pizza, spaghetti, and red wine [34]. (Reproduced by permission of Vance Packard.)

White bread became a high-status food in Europe at the time when only wealthy people could afford it. As lower-class people began to acquire more wealth, they too consumed white bread until it became a common food. Unfortunately, this food is less nutritious than the whole wheat from which it is obtained (see Chapter 3).

The manner in which food is served also carries connotations of status. For example, a governess in Edwardian England would have been humiliated had she been served with the other servants, but neither did she expect to eat with the family on all occasions. Another example comes from the Near East. An American fuel corporation, in an effort to improve the health, nutrition, and working efficiency of its employees, built a modern canteen and included a cafeteria where delicious food was available at a very reasonable cost. But it was soon evident that the workers were very resentful of this. Why? In the Near East only beggars stood in line for food. Having to pass through the cafeteria line suggested to them that they were like beggars, dependent on their employer's goodwill for their food [35].

To many in the United States steak is a status symbol, while hamburger carries little prestige value. To other Americans who are highly health conscious, and who regard the most desirable diet to be one which includes whole grains, homemade breads, cheeses, and fresh fruits and vegetables, steak is not a status symbol. This emphasizes that attitudes toward foods frequently arise out of a belief system.

Food Beliefs People within a cultural group develop specific beliefs about the value of certain foods, and the particular circumstances under which foods should or should not be consumed. In many parts of the world, children are never fed eggs or meat because it is believed this practice will make thieves of them. The logic is that since these foods are scarce and very expensive in these cultures, if children become accustomed to them, they must in the future steal to obtain them [36]. You may think that similar beliefs about food do not exist in the United States since we are a "more scientific" nation. A great many food beliefs common in the United States are not substantiated by scientific evidence, however. These include beliefs that fish is brain food, meat is necessary for muscular work, oysters increase sexual potency, and fish and ice cream eaten together cause illness. Can you think of some others?

The fact that so many people in the United States take up fad diets indicates a willingness to believe claims about foods or combinations of foods, even though most of these do not produce the desired results. Sellers of vitamin and mineral supplements have convinced many Americans that foods alone cannot supply all the nutrients needed because "soils have become depleted" and "processing devitalizes foods" [37]. Many buyers of pills may not believe all the sales pitch, but take vitamin or mineral pills as "insurance"—just to be sure they obtain these nutrients. These notions are misguided because a variety of basic foods can and do supply all needed nutrients, as will be demonstrated in the following chapters. (See Box 10–1).

Other groups of Americans form subcultures in which beliefs about food and health deviate to a greater or lesser degree from that of the "average" American. This is not a new phenomenon, but one which has existed since the beginning of the nation. During the 1960s, however, the number of such groups expanded tremendously. For many of these groups, diet is determined by a basic philosophy. For example, among Zen macrobiotic adherents, one is to balance the *yin* components of the diet with *yang* components, embracing Chinese philosophy. In this philosophy, Nature and human beings are viewed to include opposite forces such as calmness (*yin*) versus activity (*yang*). In Nature, spring is *yin*, while autumn is *yang*, for example. Among foods sugar, oil, and fruits are *yin*, while fowl, meats, and eggs are *yang*. Grains represent the perfect balance between *yin* and *yang*. The Zen macrobiotic follower attempts to balance the diet according to *yin* and *yang*, therefore, and not according to nutritional principles [38]. This example makes clear how, in some subcultures, diet is determined by a complex philosophy. The Zen macrobiotic diet may or may not be nutritionally adequate, depending upon how restrictive food choices are [38].

In other instances, however, the philosophy determining a diet is simpler and easier to grasp. One writer has pointed out that many people who believe strongly that the foods they choose affect their health shop at health food stores or small food co-ops rather than supermarkets [39]. They are willing to pay more for so-called health and organic foods because they consider them more beneficial in several respects. For example, they avoid highly processed foods because they wish to avoid additives and the nutrient depletion that sometimes accompanies processing. They share an interest in protecting the environment against pollution with pesticides. They believe that their simpler diet of minimally processed foods is healthier than the general American diet. These beliefs are reinforced by their subculture—those who are drawn together because of their similar views concerning foods and health [39]. Generally, diets in this subculture are apt to be nutritionally adequate if a wide variety of foods are included.

The professional nutritionist who counsels people about diet must understand thoroughly the belief system of the individuals or groups involved to know what suggestions about diet are apt to be acceptable. Such a professional needs to be nonjudgmental about the client's belief system.

Lifestyle Influences

Although nearly all the factors we have discussed influence your preferences for and actual choices of foods at some time in your life, your actual style of living (or lifestyle) greatly affects your daily food choices. In the United States, lifestyles may change fairly frequently. For example, if you move from your home to a college campus, your food choices may change as you adjust to foods served in dormitory dining rooms, those you prepare for yourself in the small dormitory kitchen, and those popular among students in inexpensive restaurants. If you take an apartment with other students, your food patterns may change as you prepare most of your own food—perhaps for the first time. Convenience foods may then form a larger part of your diet. As you graduate and become part of the work force, you may eat away from your home or apartment more frequently. When you marry, your food habits may change as you and your spouse work out how foods are to be provided. Foods served at home are apt to be different if both of you work than if one of you remains at home all day.

Despite the fact that lifestyle changes often result in food habit changes, you usually continue to make individual choices among foods. These choices are influenced by the factors we have discussed. Cultural factors, among others, determine what foods you find acceptable, while the food system and economic factors largely determine what foods are available to you. You can decide whether or not health is a primary concern and whether or not you want to make those food choices that are most likely to contribute to good health. This is the topic of the next chapter.

SUMMARY

1 Food choices are influenced by a great many factors. Foods available to a population are governed by climate and local growing conditions as well as by the kind of food system existing in a locality.

2 The U.S. food system today consists of (a) input industries that supply machinery and other farming needs to the farmer; (b) modern farms requiring little human labor, but much use of machinery and fuel resources; and (c) industries that buy, process, package, and distribute farm products.

3 Concerns expressed about the U.S. food system are that it is highly energy-intensive, results in soil erosion and water pollution, diminishes the number of small farms, and results in increased consumer prices.

4 Foods are more highly advertised than any other consumer product. Highly processed foods account for most food advertising, and the largest food companies do most food advertising.

5 Economic circumstances play a major role in determining an individual's or a group's access to foods.

6 Among those foods available, individual choices are governed by learned psychological associations with foods, familiarity with foods due to one's ethnic or regional background, personal taste preferences, one's concern with social status, one's belief system

concerning foods, and one's lifestyle. An individual's food choices are apt to change as some of these influences on food choices change.

FOR DISCUSSION AND APPLICATION

1 To observe how food patterns have changed over generations, talk to your parents and grandparents or aunts and uncles about foods they usually ate as children, when the big meal of the day was, what foods were served for breakfast and for the noon and evening meals, and for celebrations. What foods did they produce or gather themselves? Ethnic food differences should become apparent in this exercise.

2 Watch children's TV shows on Saturday morning for 1 hour. Document how many commercials are shown during the hour, and how many are for food. Of those that are for food, how many are high in sugar, fat, or salt?

3 Find out what foods are produced in the part of the country where you live. What problems do farmers face in your part of the country? Are local farmer's markets available where the farmer sells directly to

consumers? What efforts are made to encourage gardening in the cities or towns in your region of the country? Do some farmers in your region use some organic farming techniques? If you are attending a land-grant university, find out if the county extension agents frequently are asked for information about organic farming techniques, soil conservation techniques, etc.

SUGGESTED READINGS

Empty Breadbasket? The Coming Challenge to America's Food Supply and What We Can Do About It. The Cornucopia Project, 33 East Minor Street, Emmaus, Pa., 18049, 1981.

Wilson, C. S. (ed.), *"Food—Custom and Nurture,"* Journal of Nutrition Education, 11(suppl. 1), 1979. An annotated bibliography of sociocultural and biocultural aspects of nutrition.

Sanjur, D., *Social and Cultural Perspectives in Nutrition,* Englewood Cliffs, N.J.: Prentice-Hall, Inc., 1982. This text emphasizes topics including the influence of sociotechnological forces, food preferences, and food ideology in determining food habits. It includes sections on the dietary patterns of selected ethnic groups in the United States.

The Problem of Changing Foods Habits. Report of the Committee on Food Habits, 1941–1943. National Academy of Sciences Bulletin No. 108, Washington, D.C., 1945. This is a classic publication. It is perhaps as relevant today as it was when it was first published.

Fitzgerald, T. K., *Nutrition and Anthropology in Action,* Assen, Netherlands: Van Gorcum, 1976. This collection of papers provides interesting reading on an anthropological approach to the study of nutrition.

2 CHOOSING AN ADEQUATE DIET

One of the first questions that comes to mind when one begins to study nutrition is "How do I know whether or not I'm eating a nutritionally adequate diet?" It's possible that you feel confused about whether or not you need to reduce the amount of fat, cholesterol, sugar, or salt in your diet since conflicting statements by scientists in this regard have been in the news. Perhaps you are thinking that you *can't* plan an adequate diet until you know all about the nutrients. But you have been eating *food* for a long time, so this chapter focuses on patterns of food choices most likely to provide an adequate diet. You are introduced to the Recommended Dietary Allowances (RDAs) and to such guides as the Four Food Groups and the Exchange System. Advantages, limitations, and proper use of these guides are discussed. In addition, guidelines promulgated in recent years to help people choose healthful diets are presented. Controversial aspects of these guidelines are discussed, indicating reasons for disagreements about them. Even though you have yet to advance very far into the study of nutrition, you still can plan a diet that is nutritionally adequate.

The first question that needs to be addressed concerns the amounts of nutrients needed by the body.

HOW MUCH OF EACH NUTRIENT DOES THE BODY NEED?

Recommended Dietary Allowances (RDAs)   Amounts of proteins and many of the vitamins and minerals recommended in the diet of normal people have been set by the Food and Nutrition Board of the National Academy of Sciences (Appendix A). The RDAs were originally set in the early 1940s and have been revised every 5 years since that time, taking into account with each revision our increasing knowledge of human needs for nutrients. The recommendations are set for males and females of different age groups, and are intended for healthy people, not for those who are ill. Illnesses often increase one's needs for nutrients.

The amounts of nutrients set are termed *recommended allowances* and not *requirements* because they are *not* the *minimal* amounts needed, below which people could not maintain normal body functions and might develop deficiency symptoms. Because of genetic differences, individuals vary in their minimal requirements, some having higher requirements than others. The RDAs are set at amounts that are high enough to cover the needs of practically all those (97 to 98 percent) in the population of healthy individuals. The notion found in some writings for popular consumption that *many* people require higher amounts of nutrients than the RDAs is incorrect.

The RDAs do not answer our question completely as to how much of each nutrient the body needs because no recommendations are set for carbohydrates, fats, cholesterol, or dietary fiber (the indigestible portion of plants). There is insufficient evidence on which to base a recommendation for dietary fiber, and conflict among authorities about the amount of fats, cholesterol, and carbohydrate that should be recommended to the general public. This conflict is discussed below.

No RDAs have been set for certain vitamins and minerals for which there is too little information yet to set RDAs. Instead, a *range* of values is given for these (Appendix A), thought to represent adequate but safe intakes.

For those nutrients for which there are RDAs, then, we can say that for normal, healthy people if the diet furnishes at least the amounts recommended by the RDAs, the chances are very good that the diet is nutritionally adequate in those nutrients. Only about 2 to 3 percent of the population will need more than the RDA for a specific nutrient.

A CLOSER LOOK

Because the RDAs cover the needs of practically *all* healthy people, it is inappropriate to conclude that an *individual* has an inadequate diet if it is found that he or she routinely consumes less than the RDA for a nutrient. Let us take iron as an example. Suppose we found that Lisa, who is 23 and healthy, routinely consumes only 10 mg/day of iron, while the RDA for women her age is 18 mg/day. We cannot legitimately conclude that Lisa needs more than 10 mg/day of iron in her diet for good health without doing some blood studies to determine whether or not her iron status is normal (Chapter 13). Lisa may be among those women who require less iron than the RDA, in which case her blood studies would indicate normal values. We *can* say, however, that if Lisa routinely consumes the RDA of 18 mg of iron per day, the chances are very good that she is consuming sufficient iron to meet her needs. We can also say that any individual's *chances* of having an *inadequate* intake of a nutrient are increasingly greater as the intake falls progressively below the RDA for the nutrient.

The Conflict about Dietary Guidelines

In recent years more and more people have become interested in nutrition, and frequently express the desire for guidance about how they should choose foods for good health. The United States, however, has no official agency responsible for setting national food and nutrition policy.

The U.S. Dietary Goals   It was into this vacuum that the Senate Select Committee on Nutrition and Human Needs published *Dietary Goals for the United States* in February 1977 [1]. The Senate Select Committee was formed in 1968 with authority to conduct investigations and hearings concerning current problems in nutrition. At the outset, the Select Committee worked chiefly on programs designed to alleviate hunger in the United States, but by 1975 it shifted its concerns to overnutrition as the major nutrition problem in the United States. *Dietary Goals for the United States*, therefore, was formulated by staff members of the Senate Select Committee, based on their evaluation of current scientific knowledge, using nutrition scientists as consultants.

The goals, unlike the RDAs, made specific recommendations for intakes of carbohydrate, fat, cholesterol, sugar, and salt in the hope·that such dietary changes would decrease the incidence of heart disease and other degenerative diseases. Some aspects of their recommendations were criticized by scientists and industry; on the basis of these criticisms revised dietary goals were published in December 1977 [2]. The revised goals recommended:

1. Avoiding overweight
2. Reducing cholesterol consumption to about 300 mg/day
3. Limiting sodium consumption by reducing salt intake to about 5 g/day
4. Changing consumption of fats and carbohydrates as shown in Figure 2-1. The significant change suggested was that the amount of fat be decreased and the amount of carbohydrate increased.

The revised goals were criticized by industry groups apt to be detrimentally affected by adherence to the goals (dairy, meat, egg, sugar, and salt industries) and also by some nutrition scientists. Some scientists pointed out that the goals failed to warn against dangers of overconsumption of alcohol, and overlooked the importance of dietary iron in preventing anemia, and of fluoridation in preventing tooth decay [3]. Some authorities also expressed the opinion that the recommendations for modifying fat and cholesterol consumption were premature, since evidence is lacking that such a change would, in fact, result in lowering the

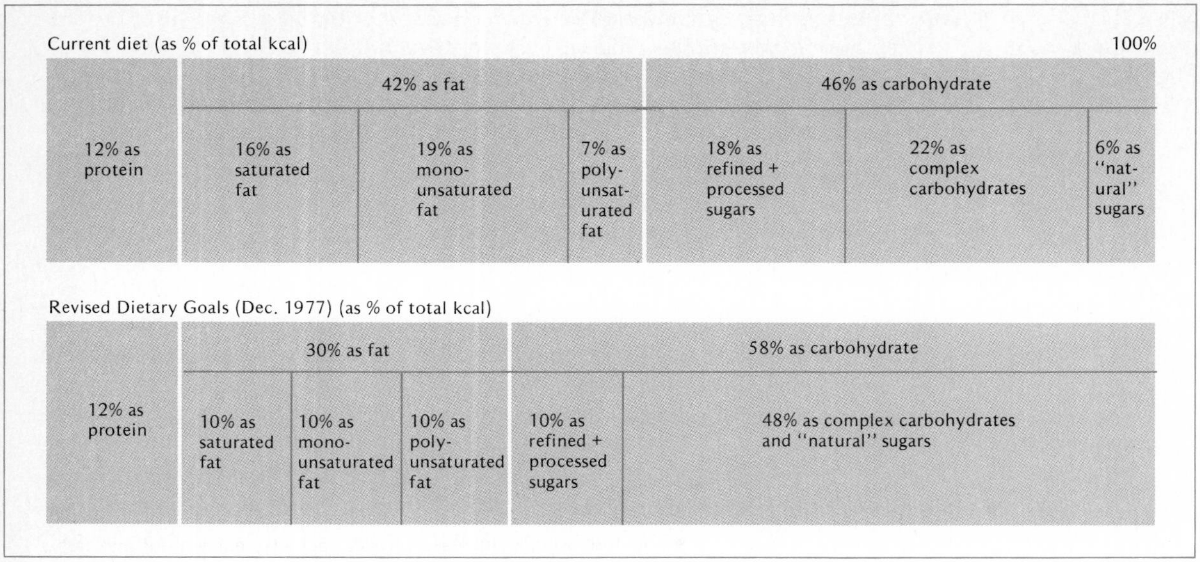

Current diet (as % of total kcal)   100%

12% as protein	42% as fat				46% as carbohydrate		
	16% as saturated fat	19% as mono-unsaturated fat	7% as poly-unsaturated fat	18% as refined + processed sugars	22% as complex carbohydrates	6% as "natural" sugars

Revised Dietary Goals (Dec. 1977) (as % of total kcal)

12% as protein	30% as fat				58% as carbohydrate
	10% as saturated fat	10% as mono-unsaturated fat	10% as poly-unsaturated fat	10% as refined + processed sugars	48% as complex carbohydrates and "natural" sugars

FIGURE 2-1. Comparison of current American diet with recommendations in the revised *Dietary Goals for the United States*, 1977.

incidence of heart disease [3,4]. This argument was made despite the fact that many official groups[1] around the world had made similar recommendations regarding fat intake for the general public [5].

The Dietary Guidelines Soon after publication of the *Dietary Goals*, the U.S. Department of Health, Education and Welfare published a report entitled *Healthy People: Health Promotion and Disease Prevention* [6]. This report was followed in early 1980 by *Nutrition and Your Health, Dietary Guidelines for Americans* [7], a joint publication of the U.S. Department of Agriculture and the then Department of Health, Education and Welfare. Both these publications supported in essence the same guidelines (Table 2-1). The *amount* by which reductions should be made in fat, cholesterol, sugar, or salt intake do not appear in these guidelines, as was done in the *Dietary Goals*, but the reader is told what food choices to make to follow the guidelines.

Food and Nutrition Board Report By the Spring of 1980, then, dietary guidelines for the general public had been developed and were widely publicized by the two governmental agencies that promulgated them. Against this background, a furor developed when the Food and Nutrition Board of the National

[1]Among such groups were The American Heart Association, 1973; The American Health Foundation, 1972; U.S. Inter-Society Commission for Heart Disease Resources, 1970; New Zealand Heart Foundtion, 1973; government of The Netherlands, 1973; U.S. White House Conference, 1973; Australian National Heart Foundation, 1974; Federal Republic of Germany, 1975; Australian Academy of Sciences, 1975; Royal College of Physicians & British Cardiac Society, 1976; Norwegian Ministry of Agriculture, 1975; and Canadian Health & Welfare Department, 1975.

Academy of Sciences published *Toward Healthful Diets* in June 1980 [8]. This report agreed with *Dietary Guidelines for Americans* that the general public should consume a wide variety of foods, maintain ideal weight, avoid too much sodium (salt), and consume alcohol only in moderation. The report disagreed with the *Dietary Guidelines for Americans* regarding recommendations for fat and cholesterol intake, however. The public consequently was faced with conflicting advice: Government agencies advised decreased intakes of fat and cholesterol, while the Food and Nutrition Board advised that such changes were not needed.

TABLE 2-1. DIETARY GUIDELINES FOR AMERICANS

GUIDELINES	HOW TO IMPLEMENT GUIDELINES
Eat a variety of foods	• Include foods daily from fruits; vegetables; whole grain and enriched breads, and cereals; milk, cheese, and yogurt; meats, poultry, fish, eggs, and legumes (dry peas and beans)
Maintain ideal weight	• To improve eating habits: Eat slowly, prepare smaller portions, avoid "seconds"
	• To lose weight: Increase physical activity, eat less fat and fatty foods, eat less sugar and sweets, avoid too much alcohol
Avoid too much fat, saturated fat, and cholesterol	• Choose lean meat, fish, poultry, dry peas, and beans as protein sources
	• Moderate use of eggs and organ meats (such as liver)
	• Limit intake of butter, cream, hydrogenated margarines, shortenings, and coconut oil, and foods made from these.
	• Trim excess fat off meat
	• Broil, bake, or boil rather than fry
	• Read labels carefully to determine both amount and types of fats in foods
Eat food with adequate starch and fiber	• Substitute starches for fats and sugars
	• Select foods that are good sources of fiber and starch such as whole-grain breads and cereals, fruits and vegetables, beans, peas, and nuts
Avoid too much sugar	• Use less of all sugars, including white and brown or raw sugars, honey, and syrups
	• Eat less of foods containing sugars such as candy, soft drinks, ice cream, cakes, cookies, pies
	• Read food labels. If sucrose, glucose, fructose, maltose, dextrose, or lactose appear *first* on label, there is a large amount of sugar in product
	• Remember, *how often* you eat sugar is as important as *amount* you eat.
Avoid too much sodium	• Learn to enjoy unsalted flavors of foods
	• Cook with only small amounts of added salt
	• Add little or no salt at table
	• Limit intake of salty foods such as potato chips, pretzels, salted nuts and popcorn, condiments (soy sauce, steak sauce, garlic salt), cheese, pickled foods, cured meats
If you drink alcohol, do so in moderation	• Moderate consumption of alcohol is one or two drinks a day

SOURCE: USDA and USDHEW, *Nutrition and Your Health, Dietary Guidelines for Americans*, Washington, D.C.: U.S. Government Printing Office, February 1980.

It is important to understand the basis for the disagreement. To understand thoroughly requires knowledge of the metabolism of fats and other lipids in the body, and the evidence we have concerning diet and diseases of the heart and blood vessels. These are discussed in Chapters 4 and 5. However, at this stage, it is possible for the reader to understand the *models* used by the two groups in deciding what advice to give.

Advice about fat and cholesterol in the diet is related in large part to the possible involvement of these substances in a disease of the arteries, atherosclerosis, and heart disease. Atherosclerosis is a disease in which cholesterol and other substances accumulate inside artery walls, eventually obstructing the flow of blood in the vessels, resulting in heart attacks or strokes. (See Chapter 5 for a more thorough discussion.) An important hypothesis in the study of heart disease is that high intakes of fat and cholesterol in the diet contribute to high levels of blood cholesterol, which contribute to atherosclerosis and therefore to heart disease. Many scientists assume that lowering the present high intake of fat and cholesterol in the diet is apt to decrease the occurrence of heart disease, although it has been impossible, so far, to *prove* that this would occur.

Public Health vs. Medical Model   The basis for the conflicting advice about dietary fat and cholesterol is that the government agencies, in setting *Dietary Guidelines for Americans*, used the *public health model* as a basis for their advice on fat and cholesterol, while the Food and Nutrition Board used the *medical model*. The Board, however, used the public health model as a basis for their advice to the public on intakes of kilocalories, salt, and alcohol. The Board's report does not make clear why the medical model is used only in regard to fat and cholesterol and not to the other food components.

In using the public health model, an agency or other group studies all the evidence available on the relationship, in this case, of dietary fat and cholesterol to disease. The group then decides on a recommendation that they believe would benefit the entire population without doing harm. Such a recommendation might have little effect on some *individuals* in the population (for example, some individuals maintain normal blood cholesterol levels regardless of their dietary intake), but could have very important effects on the population as a whole. The reasoning is that the chances are good, based on present knowledge, that if the population as a whole decreased its present high intake of fat and cholesterol, the *average* serum cholesterol levels in the population would decrease sufficiently to result in a significant reduction in the occurrence of heart disease and deaths from it [9]. An additional aspect of the public health model is that the chances are viewed as good that the proposed dietary change might *prevent* the development of atherosclerosis and heart disease in young people in the population. Scientists who support the *Dietary Guidelines for Americans* recognize that *proof* is lacking that a decreased intake of fat and cholesterol will either decrease the occurrence of heart disease or prevent atherosclerosis and heart disease, but they believe that the chances are good that this might happen [10].

The Food and Nutrition Board, on the other hand, takes the view that because, at this stage, we cannot *prove* that the proposed dietary changes will either decrease or prevent heart disease, we should not recommend a decrease in fat and cholesterol in the diet of the general population [8]. The Board recommends that people who have increased chances of having heart disease (those who are obese, have high blood pressure or diabetes, or who have a family history of heart disease) should have their blood cholesterol and other blood lipid levels determined, and should be treated by a physician if the levels are high. Presumably, diet would be an important aspect of treatment. Other people would not need to alter their intakes of fat and cholesterol unless they are so sedentary that they need a relatively low kilocalorie diet to maintain ideal weight, in which case lowering the fat intake is recommended as an important way to diminish the kilocalorie intake. This approach of advocating that only these people with symptoms or who have attributes that increase their chances of illness need change their food intake, and then only as advised by a physician, is the *medical model.*

Scientists who subscribe to the public health model regarding dietary fat and cholesterol point out that the medical model might be "too little and too late." Their argument is that atherosclerosis and heart disease develop slowly and silently over a 20-to-40-year period. By the time symptoms develop, extensive atherosclerosis has occurred, which can be reversed only slightly, if at all, by treatment. Attempting to prevent atherosclerosis by lowering fat and cholesterol in the diet is viewed as a preferable approach by this group [8].

The Food and Nutrition Board report makes no recommendation about decreasing sugar in the diet except for those who need to consume relatively low kilocalorie intakes. The Board does not explain why, in their dietary recommendations, they failed to consider the role of diet in the development of dental decay. Sugar is widely implicated as a cause of dental decay (Chapter 5).

Given the opposing views of scientists, what should Americans do, then, about fat and cholesterol in the diet? One answer is given by G. Timothy Johnson, M.D., in his syndicated newspaper column:

> Most heart specialists take a "safe" approach: Since fats and cholesterol are not needed by the body in large amounts (none of us needs those calories) and since some of us will benefit by cutting down on fats and cholesterol, the best general advice is to do so. In other words, until final evidence on the role of diet is in, we play it safe and hedge our bets.
>
> If you want to follow the course of periodic blood testing for fat and cholesterol levels and tailor your diet accordingly, well and good. But most of us won't, and so the best general advice is for all of us to cut down on fat and cholesterol [11].

Having gained some insights into the basis of the disagreement, you can decide for yourself whether you prefer to follow the medical model or the public health model.

Politics explains some of the continuing controversy surrounding dietary guidelines. The U.S. Department of Agriculture (USDA) and the Department of Health and Human Services that originally published the dietary guidelines are both in the executive branch of the federal government. As administrations change, top positions in these agencies are usually filled by those in sympathy with the views of the new administration. *Dietary Guidelines for Americans* was published during the Carter administration. The Reagan administration stopped distributing these guidelines free of charge, and decided not to publish *Food/2* which advised readers on how to decrease fat and cholesterol in the diet. (A professional organization has published *Food/2* and *Food/3*. See Suggested Readings.) In recent years the extent to which the USDA has directed its efforts to farmers and the food processing industries, on the one hand, and to general consumers, on the other, has varied from administration to administration.

In evaluating positions taken by different groups on controversial issues, ask yourself: "Who takes each position?" "What is the background, training, or expertise of members of the group?" "What do they stand to gain or lose if the policy they advocate is adopted?" Regardless of official positions taken by different groups on dietary guidance, you are free to decide for yourself what guidelines you will follow.

Report on Diet, Nutrition and Cancer In addition to *Dietary Goals for the United States* and *Dietary Guidelines for Americans*, other guidelines recently came from the Committee on Diet, Nutrition and Cancer of the National Academy of Sciences [12]. This committee reviewed current scientific research regarding the relationship of diet to cancer at the request of the National Cancer Institute. It recommended that Americans reduce their fat intake to 30 percent of total kilocalories because studies completed so far point to high fat consumption as more closely related to cancer of the colon and breast than any other dietary component. In addition, they recommended that Americans (1) frequently consume whole-grain products, citrus fruits, and carotene-rich and cruciferous vegetables (cabbage, cauliflower, broccoli, brussel sprouts); (2) minimize intake of salt-cured, salt-pickled, and smoked foods; and (3) avoid excessive alcohol consumption, especially in conjunction with cigarette smoking.

The committee emphasized that vitamin A and vitamin C supplements cannot be assumed to take the place of carotene-rich foods, citrus fruits, or cruciferous vegetables since the evidence analyzed focused on *food*, and not on nutrients. Factors in these foods other than vitamins, such as dietary fiber or interactions of nutrients, may account for their effects. Salt-cured and smoked foods should be minimized because a greater incidence of cancer of the stomach and esophagus is associated with consumption of these foods. Excessive alcohol consumption is associated with cancer of the mouth, esophagus, stomach, and respiratory tract. The committee concluded:

> It should be made clear that the weight of evidence suggests that what we eat during our lifetime strongly influences the probability of developing certain kinds of cancer but that it is not possible, and may never be possible, to specify a diet that protects all people against all forms of cancer [12].

The committee indicated that these guidelines will likely be revised as new evidence accumulates.

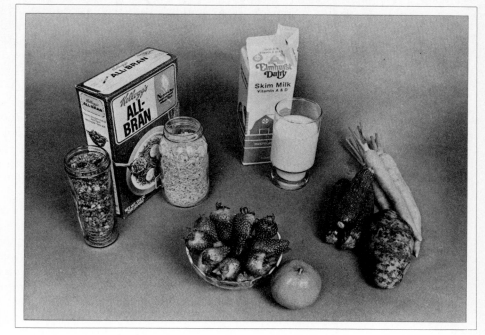

Foods low in kilocalories but high in nutrients are said to be of high nutrient density. Emphasizing choices of these foods increases the likelihood of a nutritionally adequate diet when the total kilocalorie need is low. *(Randy Matusow)*

HOW DOES ONE PLAN AN ADEQUATE DIET?

In planning an adequate diet, one needs to accomplish the following: (1) avoid excessive intake of kilocalories; (2) consume a wide variety of foods daily; and (3) practice *moderation* in food consumption to avoid too high an intake of any one food, nutrient, or contaminant. This means, among other things, that you would moderate your intake of sugar, total fat, saturated fat, cholesterol, alcohol, and salt.

A rough way to estimate your need for kilocalories is the one many dietitians use: Calculate 30 to 35 kilocalories per kilogram of body weight. Additional ways of estimating your kilocalorie needs are discussed in Chapter 7.

Exactly what is meant by moderation in food consumption has not been defined to the satisfaction of all nutritionists. *Dietary Guidelines for Americans* [7] suggests that one or two alcoholic beverages per day appear not to be harmful to adults, but makes no suggestions about amounts of other foods or nutrients (Table 2-1). *Dietary Goals for the United States* [2] suggests specific amounts and types of fats and carbohydrates (Figure 2-1). An activity at the end of Chapter 3 shows you how to calculate the percentage of your kilocalorie intake that comes from protein, fat, carbohydrate, and alcohol.

Dietary Goals also recommends that salt (sodium chloride) intake should be about 5 g per day (about 1 tsp), while the Food and Nutrition Board in *Toward Healthful Diets* suggests a range of 3 to 8 g of salt per day.

Daily Food Guide (Four Food Groups)   To encourage consumption of a wide variety of foods and to increase the possibilities of choosing foods that will provide needed protein, vitamins, and minerals, the USDA publishes a Daily Food Guide, often called the Basic Four or Four Food Groups. The most recently published version of this guide includes five groups (Table 2-2), but the first four groups are the same as in previous editions.

Although the Daily Food Guide when first established in 1956 appeared to provide the RDA for all nutrients set at that time except iron and thiamine, the most recent RDAs include many more nutrients than were included in 1956. One group of investigators calculated the nutritive value of menus published as examples of well-planned diets based on the Daily Food Guide, and compared the values with the 1974 RDAs [13]. The menus were found to meet or exceed the RDAs for the adult male in protein, vitamin A, vitamin C, riboflavin, vitamin B_{12}, calcium, phosphorus, and iodine. They failed to meet the RDA, however, for vitamin E, thiamine, vitamin B_6, folacin, magnesium, zinc, and iron. To improve the Daily Food Guide, these investigators suggested that all the bread and cereal in the diet should be whole grain (increasing the intake of vitamin E, vitamin B_6, folacin, magnesium, and zinc), that two servings per day of dried beans and/or nuts should be consumed (to supply vitamin B_6, magnesium, zinc, and iron), and that 1 tbsp of fat or oil should be added to furnish vitamin E. An additional suggestion was that one dark-green vegetable should be consumed daily. In using the Daily Food Guide, then, one would improve the chances of planning an adequate diet by using these suggestions whenever possible.

The newest Daily Food Guide was published in an attractive bulletin called *Food/1* [14]. Although the guide itself does not mention kilocalories, sugar, fat, or salt, the bulletin *Food/1* includes suggestions similar to those in Table 2-1 for lowering the intake of these food components and increasing the fiber intake.

In attempting to use the Daily Food Guide to evaluate the adequacy of a diet, one encounters some problems. One is that food chosen could be high in kilocalories, fat, sugar, and/or salt. For example, a person could choose apple pie, counting the apples as fruit, and the crust as fulfilling the bread or cereal group. Another problem is that people could consistently over- or underestimate serving sizes, or could choose foods of low nutritive value in a group (for example, a cup of cooked mushrooms is much lower in nutritive value than a cup of cooked spinach). Also, foods such as casserole dishes, pizza, and tacos require that one divide them up into food groups, guessing at what fraction of a serving belongs in each group.

It is possible, however, to use food groups effectively in planning adequate diets, as in the Exchange System described below. Obviously, the diet will be better planned if you know the nutrient composition of foods and choose those that supply protein, vitamins, and minerals without causing the diet to be too high in kilocalories, fat, sugar, or salt. Your ability to do this should improve as you progress in the study of nutrition.

An important practical way to use food groups in dietary planning was developed by the American Dietetic Association and is called the Exchange System.

TABLE 2-2. USDA DAILY FOOD GUIDE

FOOD GROUP	NO. OF SERVINGS A DAY	SIZE OF SERVING	NOTES
Vegetable and fruit group	4	½ c or a typical portion, such as 1 orange, 1 potato, etc.	Include one good source of vitamin C a day. Include deep-yellow or dark-green vegetables frequently for vitamin A. Include unpeeled fruits and vegetables for dietary fiber.
Bread and cereal group	4	1 slice bread; ½ to ¾ c cooked cereal, rice, macaroni, noodles; 1 oz ready-to-eat cereal	Include *some* whole-grain bread or cereals. Others should be enriched or fortified products.
Milk and cheese group	Children under 9: 2–3 servings Children 9–12: 3 servings Teens: 4 servings Adults: 2 servings Pregnant women: 3 servings Nursing mothers: 4 servings	8 oz milk or yogurt 1 oz cheddar or Swiss cheese = ¾ c milk ½ c ice cream = ⅓ c milk ½ c cottage cheese = ¼ c milk	Portions noted give about the same amount of calcium, but varying amounts of kilocalories.
Meat, poultry, fish, and bean group	2	2–3 oz lean cooked meat, poultry, fish 1 egg = 1 oz meat ½ to ¾ c cooked dry beans = 1 oz meat 2 tbsp peanut butter = 1 oz meat ¼ to ½ c nuts, sesame, or sunflower seeds = 1 oz meat	Try to vary choices among these foods as each has distinct nutritional advantages. Cholesterol and vitamin B_{12} occur only in foods of animal origin, and not in plant foods.
Fats, sweets, and alcohol group	No specific recommendation. Choose foods in first four groups, then add additional foods from those groups or choose some foods from this group to reach kilocalorie level needed	—	This group includes butter, margarine, mayonnaise, and other salad dressings; candy, sugar, jams, jellies, sweets of all kinds; soft drinks, alcoholic beverages, and unenriched, refined bakery products. These foods tend to be low in nutrients relative to their kilocalorie contribution.

SOURCE: *Food*, Home and Garden Bulletin No. 228, Washington, D.C.: USDA, 1979.

Exchange System   The Exchange System provides a way of controlling certain aspects of the diet such as kilocalories, fat, and sugar while choosing a wide variety of foods. The system was originally designed as an aid in planning diabetic diets, but is equally useful in planning ordinary diets. The Exchange Lists are in Appendix B, and advantages of the use of the Exchange System in planning diets are given in Box 2-1.

The Concept of Nutrient Density   A concept underlying successful planning of adequate diets is that generally the foods chosen should contribute large amounts of needed nutrients relative to the number of kilocalories in the food. Most Americans need to be on their guard to prevent gaining excessive amounts of body fat, while a great many Americans have already gained too much and need to lose fat. Using the Exchange Lists in Appendix B allows one to choose foods that are high in nutrients but relatively low in kilocalories because foods low in fat appear in boldface type (except in the fat group itself), and no foods high in added sugar appear in the Exchange Lists, requiring a person to become highly conscious of choices of those foods. Foods that are high in nutrients but relatively low in kilocalories are said to have *high nutrient density*, while those high in kilocalories but with few nutrients are said to have *low nutrient density*. A sensible rule to follow is to minimize the number of *low nutrient density* foods in the diet. One system devised to calculate the nutrient density of foods appears in Appendix O.

Frequently, methods of preparing or serving foods decrease the nutrient density by adding large amounts of fat or sugar. For example, Table 2-3 illustrates the lower nutrient density of apple pie compared with plain apple, of fried

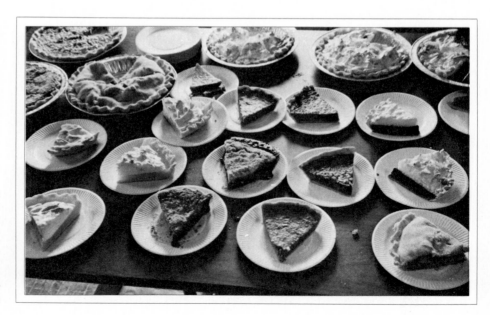

Foods high in kilocalories but low in nutrients are said to be of low nutrient density. These foods should be consumed infrequently when the total kilocalorie need is low.
(David Strickler Monkmeyer)

The Exchange System is centered on six groups of foods, called Exchange Lists (Appendix B). Foods in a given list are similar in carbohydrate, protein, fat, and kilocalorie content. One food can be substituted or *exchanged* for another *in the same list*, but it is essential to take note of serving sizes for each food. To begin to plan a diet, you need to decide how many exchanges from each group to include. *Dietary Guidelines for Americans*, the *Daily Food Guide*, and the • U.S. Senate's *Dietary Goals for the United States* may be used to help you make this decision.

To begin, notice that the groups of foods making up the Exchange Lists are milk, vegetables, fruit, bread (cereals and starchy vegetables), meat (cheese and dried beans), and fat. No sugars, syrups, jams, jellies, cakes, pies, cookies, or alcohol are included. The salt content of foods is ignored.

Advantages of using the Exchange System in planning diets include the following:

1 Use of sugar, foods high in sugar, and alcohol must be consciously chosen. Since planning is done without sugary foods or alcohol, the basic diet is apt not to have its nutritive value diluted by large amounts of sugar or alcohol.

2 The Exchange System encourages choosing a wide variety of foods, while at the same time allowing control of the kilocalorie intake.

3 One learns the carbohydrate, protein, fat, and kilocalorie value of foods while using the Exchange Lists.

4 Attention is drawn to foods that are either low in fat or high in polyunsaturated fat because these foods are printed in boldface type.

The Exchange System is an excellent system to use in planning weight reduction diets. Additions to the basic foods listed in Appendix B make it possible also to use the Exchange System for vegetarian diets [15] and to include Chinese [16] and other ethnic foods.

potatoes compared with plain baked potato, and of peanut brittle compared with plain peanuts.

The food of lowest nutrient density is probably sucrose (white sugar) because it is so highly purified. It supplies only kilocalories with only tiny amounts of iron and zinc (Table 2-3). On the other hand, the molasses left behind when sucrose is crystallized contains some vitamins and minerals (Table 2-3), blackstrap molasses having more nutrients than light molasses. Brown sugar, which consists of sucrose to which some molasses adheres, and honey both contain more nutrients than sucrose. Although blackstrap molasses is the only one of these sweeteners containing a significant amount of nutrients, its strong flavor prevents its wide usage in foods. Furthermore, very high intakes of any of these sweeteners are apt to contribute relatively more kilocalories than nutrients, and all can contribute to dental decay. It is obvious, however, that if one is going to consume some cookies, cakes, sweet breads, or other baked products, making them from brown sugar, honey, or molasses furnishes more nutrients than white sugar.

TABLE 2-3. COMPARISON OF SOME NUTRIENTS IN 100-kcal PORTIONS OF FOODS*

FOOD (100-kcal PORTIONS)	PROTEIN, g	CALCIUM, mg	MAGNESIUM, mg	ZINC, mg	IRON, mg	THIAMINE, mg	RIBOFLAVIN, mg	VITAMIN B₆, mg	PANTOTHENIC ACID, mg	FOLACIN, mg	VITAMIN C, mg
Apple (1 med.)	0.4	12.5	12.5	0.10	0.50	0.05	0.04	0.05	0.25	6.3	8.0
Apple pie	0.9	3.8	1.3	0.03	0.13	0.008	0.008	0.02	0.05	0.8	0.5
Baked potato (plain)	2.9	10.7	32.1	0.29	0.79	0.14	0.05	0.36	0.57	14.3	21.4
French fried potatoes (frozen, reheated)	1.6	4.5	13.6	0.14	0.36	0.005	0.009	0.09	0.22	4.5	9.1
Peanuts	11.5	30.8	76.9	1.38	0.92	0.14	0.06	0.15	0.92	12.3	0
Peanut brittle	1.3	8.3	u	u	0.58	0.04	0.008	u	u	u	0
White sugar (2 tbsp) (granulated)	0	0	0	0.01	0.03	0	0	0	0	0	0
Brown sugar (2 tbsp)	0	22.6	u	u	0.91	0.002	0.009	u	u	u	0
Honey (1½ tbsp)	0.15	1.5	1.5	0.03	0.15	tr	0.015	tr	0.06	0	tr
Light molasses (2 tbsp)	0	70.0	18.0	u	1.8	0.02	0.02	u	u	u	0
Blackstrap molasses (2.2 tbsp)	54	300.0	115.6	u	7.1	0.04	0.09	u	u	u	0
White bread, not enriched	3.1	28.6	7.1	0.29	0.29	0.03	0.03	0.01	0.14	4.3	0
White bread, enriched†	3.1	28.6	7.1	0.29	0.86	0.09	0.07	0.01	0.14	4.3	0
Whole wheat bread	3.9	38.5	15.4	0.62	1.23	0.09	0.05	0.06	0.31	13.9	0

*Symbols used: tr = trace; u = unknown but thought to be present; 0 = absent or below detection level.

†"Enriched" bread has added iron, thiamine, riboflavin, and niacin.

SOURCE: Table 2 of the appendix, from *Bogert's Nutrition and Physical Fitness* by George M. Briggs and Doris Calloway. Copyright 1979 by W. B. Saunders. Reprinted by permission of W. B. Saunders, CBS College Publishing, Philadelphia.

NUTRITION IN THE NEWS

FOOD NOTES. SELECTIVE EATING HABITS

The New York Times, September 8, 1982

Americans appear to listen selectively to advice about healthful eating habits, if the latest figures from the Department of Agriculture are an accurate gauge. . . .

Health concerns probably played some role in the decline of beef consumption, down from 97.8 pounds to 78.8 pounds per person per year, but cost was probably the most important factor, as beef prices rose significantly in the five-year period. So shoppers replaced some of the beef with much less expensive pork, which has as much fat as beef. Pork consumption rose over 10 pounds per person during that period, from 54.6 pounds to 65.

Americans were also eating almost 10 pounds [more] of chicken a year each; consumption jumped from 42.7 pounds per person to 51.7 pounds. Not only is chicken a less expensive alternative to beef, but it is also considered more healthful because it has much less fat than beef or pork.

Americans are making such changes as drinking more low-fat milk and less whole milk and using more margarine and less butter, but the overall consumption of fat is 34 percent higher than in 1910 and consumption of complex carbohydrates from starches, such as flour and cereal, has decreased 43 percent. Calorie and protein consumption have remained fairly constant. It is the increase in fat consumption and the decrease in carbohydrate consumption that "Dietary Guidelines for the United States," a Government publication, and the recent report of the National Academy of Sciences on the relationship between diet and cancer are trying to reverse. . . .

ASK YOURSELF:

How does the American public learn about issues regarding nutrition and health? What information did you have about recommendations for dietary fat and carbohydrate before you began this course? How did you obtain that information? By newspapers? Magazines? TV?

SUMMARY

1 In planning an adequate diet, one should avoid excessive kilocalorie intake, consume a wide variety of foods, and practice moderation in foods consumed. The Basic Four Food Groups, *Dietary Guidelines for Americans*, and the Exchange System may be used as aids in reaching these goals. Food of high nutrient density should be stressed in dietary planning.

2 The Recommended Dietary Allowances indicate the intake of protein, vitamins, and minerals that appear to cover the needs of almost all healthy Americans.

3 The *Dietary Guidelines for Americans* and the *Dietary Goals for the United States* advocate consuming less sugar, fat, cholesterol, salt, and alcohol than the average American has been consuming. The recommendation to decrease fat and cholesterol intake has been challenged by some scientists who believe that evidence is insufficient to recommend this change for all Americans.

4 A report from the Committee on Diet, Nutrition and Cancer of the National Academy of Sciences recommended decreasing fatty foods, salt-cured and salt-pickled foods, and alcohol, while increasing the intake of whole grains, carotene-rich foods, and cruciferous vegetables (cabbage, cauliflower, broccoli, brussels sprouts) in an effort to decrease the incidence of cancer.

FOR DISCUSSION AND APPLICATION

1 Recall all the food you ate within the past 24 hours. Write these down, including an estimate of amounts consumed.

a. What problems did you find in recalling all you ate? Do you believe the list to be an accurate account of what you ate?

b. How well did your intake for 1 day meet the Daily Food Guide (Table 2-2)?

c. What problems do you encounter in using this guide? Was any one of these food groups omitted entirely in your food selections? Does it appear that you now consume a wide variety of foods?

2 Using the above list of foods, how well did your intake for 1 day meet the *Dietary Guidelines for Americans* (Table 2-1)? What further information do you need to enable you to follow these guidelines?

3 To begin your acquaintance with the Exchange System, use Appendix B to list the number of exchanges you consumed in 24 hours from each exchange list. For this purpose, use a table set up as follows:

NUMBER OF EXCHANGES IN LISTS

Food	1	2	3	4	5			6
					lean	med.	fat	

Using the Exchange System, calculate the number of kilocalories and the number of grams of protein, carbohydrate, and fat you consumed in 24 hours.

Compare the number of grams of protein with that in the RDAs (Appendix A) for your age and sex.

SUGGESTED READINGS

Dietary Goals for the United States (2d ed.), U.S. Senate Select Committee on Nutrition and Human Needs. Washington, D.C., 1977. This publication contains the rationale for development of the dietary goals.

Food/1, U.S. Department of Agriculture, 1979. Superintendent of Documents, U.S. Government Printing Office, Washington, D.C., 20402. Stock No. 001-000-03881-8. This is a colorful booklet offering food, nutrition advice, and recipes.

Food/2, A Dieter's Guide, The American Dietetic Association, P.O. Box 91403, Chicago, Ill., 60693. The guide originally meant to be published by USDA. This section treats weight loss and includes low calorie recipes.

Food/3, Eating the Moderate Fat & Cholesterol Way, The American Dietetic Association, P.O. Box 91403, Chicago, Ill., 60693. A 16-page booklet includes guidance and recipes on lowering dietary fat and cholesterol.

Ideas for Better Eating—Menus and Recipes to Make Use of the Dietary Guidelines, U.S. Department of Agriculture, 1981. This pamphlet offers menus and recipes to help the lay person apply the dietary guidelines to personal eating habits.

Cummings, C., and V. Newman, *Eater's Guide: Nutrition Basics for Busy People*, San Diego, Calif.: Wellspring Applications, 1980. This book offers practical nutrition advice based on the dietary guidelines. Recipes are included.

PART II

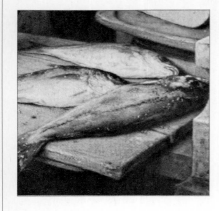

PART II

THE ENERGY
NUTRIENTS

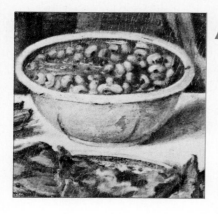

Americans are obsessed with body weight; for many, the obsession begins in early childhood. Most weight-conscious individuals soon learn that kilocalories (Calories) are the culprits. This obsession with body weight and kilocalories easily obscures recognition of the body cells' absolute dependence for life and function on sources of kilocalories or energy. Too often, the disorder called anorexia nervosa, in which an individual deliberately starves, is the tragic result.

This section discusses those nutrients—carbohydrates, alcohol, fats, and proteins—from which the body obtains energy or kilocalories. Separate chapters treat carbohydrates and alcohol (Chapter 3), fats and other lipids (Chapter 4), and proteins (Chapter 6). Each chapter offers practical guidance for including appropriate amounts and sources of these energy nutrients in the diets of normal young to middle-aged adults.

The energy nutrients interest us for reasons other than as sources of kilocalories. Chapter 5 considers carbohydrates, fats, and other lipids as they relate to heart disease, cancer, diabetes, and tooth decay, while Chapter 6 discusses vegetarian diets and protein-calorie malnutrition. The place of carbohydrates and protein in the diets of athletes is taken up in Chapters 3 and 6, respectively.

Once you understand how the body obtains energy from foods, you are ready to consider how much energy the body needs and how to estimate those needs (Chapter 7). Finally, Chapter 8 is devoted to the causes and treatment of overweight and obesity, at one extreme, and of underweight, including anorexia nervosa, at the other.

Upon completing the chapters in Part II, you should be better able to critically assess information appearing in the popular press and electronic media concerning energy nutrients and weight control diets.

CARBOHYDRATES

Greg has always had a "weight problem." He has tried the Scarsdale Diet, the Beverly Hills Diet, and the Liquid-Protein Diet but was unable to stay on any one of these very long. Greg firmly believes that bread, cereals, spaghetti, and potatoes are "fattening" and almost never eats them. He would not, as a consequence, be able to follow *Dietary Guidelines for Americans*, the Daily Food Guide, or the Exchange System, discussed in the previous chapter, in planning his diet. Is he justified in his belief? Might his practice of excluding these foods from his diet have any nutritional consequences?

Carmen is serious about running, and plans to enter a marathon race soon. She has heard about carbohydrate loading, and wonders if she should try it as a means of increasing her chances of winning. Is carbohydrate loading clearly beneficial to athletes? Might there be any adverse side effects?

In this chapter we will address these questions and others in our discussion of the importance of carbohydrates as an energy source, its food sources, the changing patterns of carbohydrate consumption, how the body uses carbohydrates, and amounts of carbohydrates recommended in the diet. We will focus additional attention on the effects of refining and processing on the nutritive value of high-carbohydrate foods, and the relationship of dietary carbohydrate to the problems of lactose intolerance and hypoglycemia. Finally, because alcohol is a significant kilocalorie source for many and is obtained by fermenting carbohydrates, a discussion of the absorption, metabolism, and possible benefits and hazards of alcohol is also included in this chapter.

IMPORTANCE OF CARBOHYDRATES IN THE DIET

Carbohydrates are substances many of which contain carbon, hydrogen, and oxygen in the general ratio of one water molecule for each carbon atom, indicated by the formula $(CH_2O)_n$. Originally these substances were thought of as hydrates (referring to water) of carbon, hence the name *carbo-hydrates*. The carbohydrates include sugars, starches, and most of the components of dietary fiber. *Dietary fiber* includes those parts of plant foods that are indigestible in the upper part of the small intestine.

Starches and sugars are important in the diets of all nations as relatively inexpensive sources of energy. In most national diets cereal grains are chief sources of starch because they are easily grown, produce high yields per unit of land, are easy to store and transport, and will grow in most parts of the world. Specific grains have become the staple crop in varying regions of the world because climatic and soil conditions favor production of one grain over another. Wheat is the staple grain in the United States, not because Americans prefer it, but because conditions favor its growth over other grains—rice, for example.

The production of carbohydrate by plants ranks as one of the wonders of the world, illustrating the interdependence of animals, including the human animal, and plants. *Chlorophyll*, the pigment in green plant leaves, is essential for this process, called *photosynthesis*, which is illustrated in Figure 3-1. Chlorophyll converts energy from the sun into sugars and starch, using carbon dioxide from the air and water from the soil and air. In the process, oxygen is released. Animals consume oxygen to support activities vital to life, and give off carbon dioxide which is essential for plant life, completing the cycle. Animal wastes also provide nitrogen and minerals which are essential for plant growth.

COMPOSITION OF CARBOHYDRATES

Carbohydrates are divided into monosaccharides, disaccharides and polysaccharides. The suffix *-saccharide* means sugar, while the prefix *mono-* means one, *di-* means two, and *poly-* means many. The monosaccharide molecule therefore consists of a single sugar, the disaccharide molecule of two sugar molecules, linked together, and the polysaccharide molecule of many sugar molecules linked together.

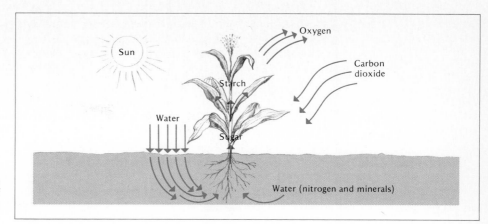

FIGURE 3-1. The synthesis of carbohydrates by green plants.

Simple Sugars (Monosaccharides)

Monosaccharides are the basic carbohydrate units. The term *simple sugars* implies that these are the fundamental or simplest form of carbohydrates. For our purposes, the most important monosaccharides are glucose, fructose, and galactose.

Structure of Monosaccharides Glucose, fructose, and galactose are alike chemically in that they contain 6 carbon atoms, 12 hydrogen atoms, and 6 oxygen atoms per molecule, and therefore have the general formula $C_6H_{12}O_6$. These sugars are called *hexoses* because they have six carbons. (The suffix *-ose* refers to sugars.) To understand how these sugars differ, it is necessary to examine their chemical structures. But first, let's look at how atoms form compounds, and how the structure of compounds is represented in chemical shorthand.

In the Introduction to this book, we pointed out that the number of electrons in an atom determines its chemical properties. The outermost electrons circling around the nucleus of each atom are called *valence electrons*; they are the ones that determine how the atom will combine with others to form compounds. Figure 3-2 shows the valence electrons for carbon, hydrogen, and oxygen, and an arbitrary electronic abbreviation for each.

Carbohydrates, like all nutrients except for water and minerals, are organic compounds—that is, they contain carbon. Carbon atoms have the ability to form *covalent bonds* with one another and with hydrogen and oxygen. When a covalent bond forms, electrons are shared between two atoms. Using electronic symbols, Figure 3-3 indicates how valence electrons are shared in the organic compound ethyl alcohol, and how this is designated in the structural formula.

Glucose, fructose, and galactose differ from one another in degree of sweetness and in their roles in metabolism. These different properties are due to structural differences, shown in Figure 3-4. The ring structure is shown for each sugar because chemically this structure accounts for all the chemical properties of these sugars.

Glucose Glucose is present in fruits, honey, and corn syrup. It is one of the sugar molecules in each of the important disaccharides in nutrition: sucrose (table

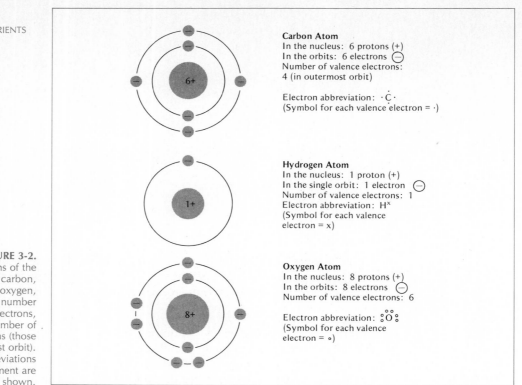

FIGURE 3-2. Representations of the atoms of carbon, hydrogen, and oxygen, showing only the number of protons and electrons, including the number of valence electrons (those in the outermost orbit). Electronic abbreviations for each element are shown.

Carbon Atom
In the nucleus: 6 protons (+)
In the orbits: 6 electrons ⊖
Number of valence electrons:
4 (in outermost orbit)

Electron abbreviation: ·Ċ·
(Symbol for each valence electron = ·)

Hydrogen Atom
In the nucleus: 1 proton (+)
In the single orbit: 1 electron ⊖
Number of valence electrons: 1
Electron abbreviation: Hˣ
(Symbol for each valence electron = x)

Oxygen Atom
In the nucleus: 8 protons (+)
In the orbits: 8 electrons ⊖
Number of valence electrons: 6

Electron abbreviation: ₒ̈Ȯₒ
(Symbol for each valence electron = o)

sugar), lactose, and maltose (discussed below). Glucose is also the sugar found in blood. The importance of maintaining blood glucose levels and mechanisms the body has for doing so are discussed in the section on metabolism.

Fructose Fructose is in fruits, honey, and high-fructose corn syrups used commercially to sweeten soft drinks and other foods. Recently promoters claimed

FIGURE 3-3. Electronic and structural formulas for ethyl alcohol. The two carbons share one pair of electrons, each carbon furnishing one of the pair. Each hydrogen furnishes one electron of each pair it shares with carbon. Oxygen shares one pair of electrons with carbon and one pair with hydrogen. Each pair of shared electrons represents one covalent bond, indicated in the structural formula by a line.

Electron Formula

Electrons from C: •;
from H: x; and from
O: ∘.
H: hydrogen
C: carbon
O: oxygen

Structural Formula

Each covalent bond is designated by a line.

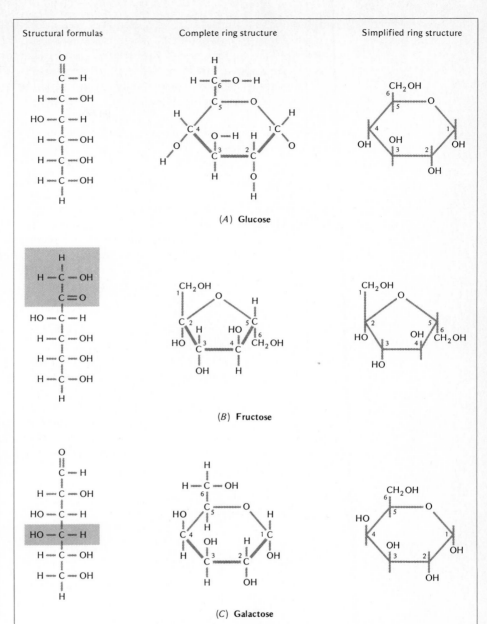

| Structural formulas | Complete ring structure | Simplified ring structure |

(*A*) **Glucose**

(*B*) **Fructose**

(*C*) **Galactose**

FIGURE 3-4. Structural differences among glucose, fructose, and galactose. Fructose and galactose differ from glucose only in the configurations around carbons 1 and 2 for fructose, and carbon 4 for galactose. The simplified ring structure omits the Cs and Hs, but a carbon is understood to be at each angle of the ring, and one H is understood to be at the end of each vertical line opposite —OH.

that fructose is useful in weight-reducing diets because it is sweeter than sucrose. Theoretically less of it could be used to attain the same sweetness as attained with sucrose, thereby cutting down on total kilocalorie consumption. But fructose is markedly sweeter than sucrose only in dilute solution. Temperature, acidity, and presence of other sugars or other substances all influence the relative sweetness of fructose [1]. Using fructose in cake, pudding, and cookies resulted in products that were even less sweet than when made with sucrose [2]. The relative sweetness of varying substances from several studies was compiled by Paul and Palmer [1], and appears in Table 3-1. Although fructose is sweeter than sucrose, there is no evidence of its practical benefit for individuals who need to watch their weight, since so many factors influence its sweetness.

Galactose   Galactose does not occur as such in foods, but it is one of the sugars in milk sugar or *lactose*.

Double Sugars (Disaccharides)

A disaccharide is made up of two monosaccharide units. In forming disaccharides, a molecule of water is removed as the two sugars join, as indicated in Figure 3-5. This process is called *condensation*. The reversal of this process, *hydrolysis*, is the addition of one molecule of water per molecule of disaccharide, which produces the monosaccharides that make up the disaccharide.

Three disaccharides are important in nutrition and foods: sucrose, lactose, and maltose.

Sucrose   A molecule of sucrose, or common white table sugar, is made up of one molecule of glucose and one of fructose (Figure 3-5). Sucrose is obtained commercially from sugar beets and sugar cane, and is the sugar present in brown sugar, molasses, maple syrup, and, to a small extent, in fruits. Sucrose furnishes energy (kilocalories), but no nutrients. Molasses, the substance left behind during the processing of sucrose, contains vitamins and minerals that were present in the original sugar cane or beets (see Table 2-3, and the discussion in Chapter 2 on nutritive value). Because readers frequently want information on the different kinds of sugars and other sweeteners on the market, Table 3-2 explains how various sweeteners are obtained.

TABLE 3-1.   RELATIVE SWEETNESS OF VARIOUS SUBSTANCES IN SOLUTIONS OF MODERATE INTENSITY*

SUBSTANCE	RANGE OF SWEETNESS RATINGS
Saccharin	306–675
Dulcin	90.7–265
Fructose	1.15–1.16
Sucrose	1.00
Glucose	0.61–0.79
Galactose	0.59–0.67
Maltose	0.46–0.47
Lactose	0.30–0.38

*Sucrose is used as the standard, and assigned a rating of 1.00; higher numbers therefore indicate greater sweetness while lower numbers indicate less sweetness than sucrose. Dulcin and saccharin are noncaloric sweeteners, and are shown here for comparison. In more dilute solutions than used here, fructose has ranked 1.7.

SOURCE: Selected from Paul, P.C., and H.H. Palmer, *Food Theory and Applications*, New York: John Wiley & Sons, Inc., 1972, p. 43.

TABLE 3-2. PRODUCTION OF VARIOUS SUGARS AND SWEETENERS

Sucrose, or common white table sugar, is obtained from sugar cane or sugar beet juice. Workers evaporate the juice until it becomes so highly concentrated that crystals of sucrose come out of the solution [6]. Sucrose is refined and purified until it is about 99.9% pure sucrose; it is therefore of low nutrient density.

Raw sugar is unwashed and unrefined sucrose left when the molasses is spun off the sugar. Raw sugar contains extraneous matter, and is not allowed on the market in the United States for reasons of sanitation and safety [6].

Turbinado sugar is raw sugar from which extraneous matter and most of the molasses has been removed [6]. It is marketed in the United States chiefly in health food stores and other specialty shops.

Brown sugars are more highly refined than raw or turbinado sugar, and are of varying colors, from yellow to dark brown, depending upon how much molasses or syrup they contain. Brown sugars are usually made by adding highly refined molasses-flavored syrup to white sugar [6] (see Chapter 2 for discussion of its nutritive value).

Invert sugar is a mixture of equal weights of glucose and fructose obtained commercially by treating a solution of sucrose with heat and acid, or with the enzyme invertase. It is useful commercially in candies because it will not crystallize, and it also keeps baked goods and confections moist [6]. It is not widely available for home use.

Honey is formed by the honey bee from plant nectars. It is chiefly a mixture of glucose and fructose formed by the bee's enzyme, honey invertase, acting upon sucrose in the nectars.

Corn syrup is obtained by breakdown of cornstarch using acid, alkali, or enzymatic catalysts, and is a mixture of dextrins, maltose, and glucose. Corn syrup is used in soft drinks, and in canned and brewed products.

High-fructose corn syrup is obtained by treating the glucose in corn syrup with an enzyme, an isomerase, which converts some of the glucose to fructose. The syrup contains both *glucose and fructose* and is used by manufacturers to sweeten foods, especially soft drinks. Currently, three types are available. One is 42% fructose, one is 55% fructose, and the last is 90% fructose. Only the first two are widely sold to food manufacturers [3].

Molasses is the liquid from which sucrose has crystallized. The sugar in molasses is, therefore, sucrose. Molasses can be obtained in a light-colored form or as the dark, blackstrap molasses. The darker form is richer in minerals than the lighter (see Table 2-3 and the discussion about nutritive value in Chapter 2).

Maple syrup is obtained from the sap of the hard maple tree by boiling the sap to concentrate it. The sugar then crystallizes out of the syrup. The sugar in maple syrup is sucrose.

The food industry uses more sucrose, corn syrup, and high-fructose corn syrup in foods than other sweeteners.

FIGURE 3-5. Formation of sucrose, a disaccharide, from condensation of one molecule of glucose with one molecule of fructose. In forming sucrose, the linkage between glucose and fructose occurs between carbon 1 of glucose and carbon 2 of fructose.

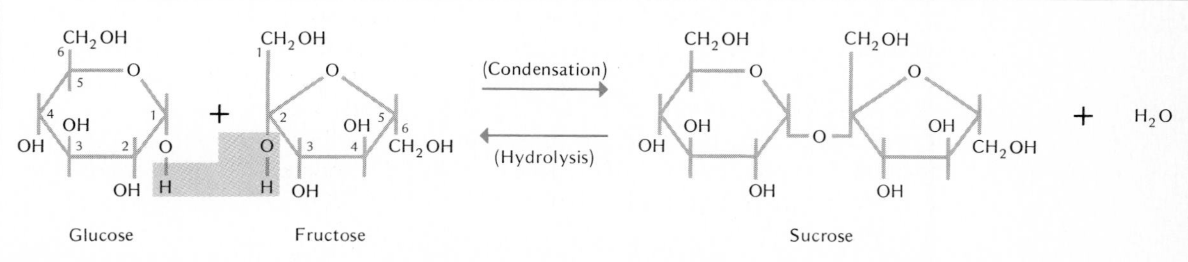

Lactose Lactose is milk sugar and has the distinction of being the least sweet of all the sugars. Table 3-1 indicates that sucrose is approximately three times sweeter than lactose. Interestingly, milk, the food on which infant mammals depend for survival, contains lactose rather than a sweeter sugar as its sole carbohydrate. A molecule of lactose is formed by the condensation of one molecule of glucose with one of galactose.

Maltose Very little maltose occurs naturally in foods, but maltose is a breakdown product of starch digestion, discussed later in this chapter. Mixtures of maltose and glucose may be used in baby formulas or baby foods, and in bread making. A molecule of maltose is made up of two glucose units.

To recapitulate: Each molecule of a disaccharide is made up of two monosaccharides linked together after removal of a molecule of water. Hydrolysis produces the two sugars that make up the disaccharide. The monosaccharides making up specific disaccharides are:

$$\text{Glucose + fructose} \underset{\text{hydrolysis}}{\overset{\text{condensation}}{\rightleftharpoons}} \text{sucrose} + H_2O$$

$$\text{Glucose + galactose} \underset{\text{hydrolysis}}{\overset{\text{condensation}}{\rightleftharpoons}} \text{lactose} + H_2O$$

$$\text{Glucose + glucose} \underset{\text{hydrolysis}}{\overset{\text{condensation}}{\rightleftharpoons}} \text{maltose} + H_2O$$

Complex Carbohydrates (Polysaccharides)

Starches Starches occur in plants such as potatoes and other tubers or roots (tapioca, arrowroot), and cereal grains (wheat, rice, oats, corn). In these plants starch exists as granules which take up water and expand when heated. Starches isolated from these plants have different physical characteristics. For example, when cooked in water and cooled, cornstarch forms a rigid gel that leaves sharp edges when cut with a knife, while tapioca flows together again after a knife passes through.

In spite of different physical characteristics, the starch in potatoes, tapioca, cereal grains, and other plants is similar chemically. All starches are composed of glucose molecules linked together to form very large starch molecules. The number of glucose molecules vary from 400 to several hundred thousand.

Two forms of starch molecules exist. In one, called *amylose*, glucose molecules form a straight chain, while in the other, called *amylopectin*, branches form (Figure 3-6). While these two forms are significant in food preparation because they contribute to differences in physical characteristics, they are of little significance in normal nutrition because the body easily digests both forms to glucose.

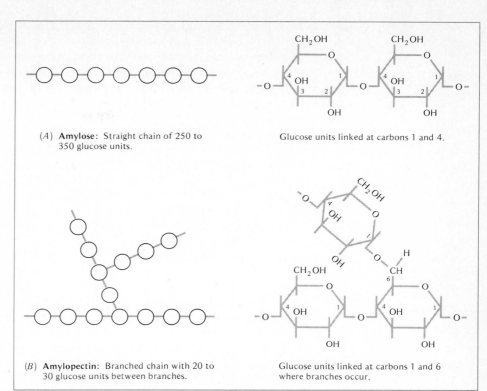

(A) **Amylose:** Straight chain of 250 to 350 glucose units.

Glucose units linked at carbons 1 and 4.

FIGURE 3-6. Diagram of the two forms of starch: amylose, the straight-chain form, and amylopectin, the branched form. In the simple diagrams on the left, —O— represents a glucose molecule. Glucose units are linked at carbons 1 and 4 in amylose and in the straight-chain portion of amylopectin. Where branches occur in amylopectin, the linkage is between carbons 1 and 6.

(B) **Amylopectin:** Branched chain with 20 to 30 glucose units between branches.

Glucose units linked at carbons 1 and 6 where branches occur.

Dextrins Dextrins are breakdown products of starch. They are only about one-fifth the size of the starch molecules from which they come, but are still made up only of glucose units. They are formed during digestion or during commercial manufacturing of corn syrup, of which they are a part.

Glycogen Foods contain very little glycogen, although shellfish and animal livers may furnish small amounts. Glycogen has been called animal starch, and is manufactured in the liver and muscles from glucose. The glycogen molecule is similar to amylopectin, but its molecule is even more highly branched. Liver glycogen serves as a source of stored energy which the liver can easily break down when needed to maintain the blood glucose level or to use for energy. Muscle glycogen serves as stored energy for muscle activity. The importance of glycogen to the body is explained in the section below on metabolism.

  Glycogen occurs in greatest *concentration* in the liver, but the largest *amount* in the body is in muscles because their mass is greater than that of liver.

Dietary Fiber Much current interest centers around dietary fiber because of speculations that low intakes of this substance in industrialized countries may be related to the occurrence of heart disease and certain intestinal diseases, including cancer of the colon. The possible relationship between fiber intake and these diseases is discussed in Chapter 5. At this point we will define dietary fiber and discuss its components and food sources.

Dietary fiber may be defined as those components of plant cell walls and other plant polysaccharides that resist digestion by enzymes *of the upper intestinal tract*. This does *not* mean that components of dietary fiber are not digested *anywhere* in the human intestinal tract. In fact, enzymes produced by bacteria in the colon *do* digest, absorb, and metabolize some components of dietary fiber, and the human body appears to absorb some of the products of bacterial metabolism (chiefly some fatty acids). The extent of this absorption appears to be relatively small, and varies among individuals. This is an area of continuing research activity. In the past, writers and physicians often used imprecise terms such as roughage or bulk when referring to indigestible materials in foods.

Components of dietary fiber include cellulose, hemicelluloses, pectins, gums and mucilages, and lignin. Of these, only lignin is not a carbohydrate. Let's examine each of these briefly.

Cellulose is widely distributed among plants, and is the only component of dietary fiber having a fibrous structure—that is, forming threadlike filaments. Like starch, the basic unit of cellulose is glucose, forming a straight-chain, unbranched structure like that of amylose. The crucial difference between amylose and cellulose, accounting for the easy digestibility of amylose but not of cellulose by the human intestinal tract, lies in the different kind of linkages between the glucose molecules (Figure 3-7). A cellulose molecule contains 3000 or more glucose units [4].

Hemicelluloses are frequently called *pentosans* because they are made up chiefly of a variety of 5-carbon sugars (pentoses), but they also contain hexose sugars. The molecule is small, compared with cellulose, for it contains only 150 to 200 sugar units. However, hemicellulose molecules differ widely in the specific sugars they contain [4].

Pectins and hemicelluloses form the matrix of the plant cell wall into which cellulose fibers are embedded. Pectins generally occur in smaller amounts in most cell walls than other components of dietary fiber. However, citrus fruit rinds contain 30 percent pectin, apple skins 15 percent, and onion skins 11 to 12 percent. Pectin is well known for its ability to form gels in preparing fruit jams or jellies [4].

FIGURE 3-7. Differences in the linkage between glucose units in (a) starch and (b) cellulose. Enzymes produced in the human upper small intestines are unable to break the β-linkage, but easily break the α-linkage. Cellulose, therefore, is indigestible in the upper intestinal tract, while starch is easily digested.

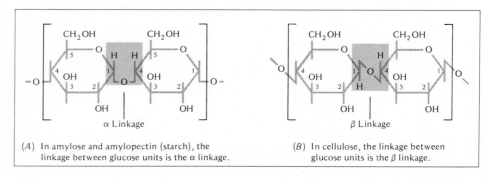

(A) In amylose and amylopectin (starch), the linkage between glucose units is the α linkage.

(B) In cellulose, the linkage between glucose units is the β linkage.

Plant *gums* and *mucilages* are not components of cell walls, but are included in dietary fiber because they share properties with some cell-wall components. Plant gums are exudates of plants that form protective coverings at sites where injuries occur. They include gum arabic, karaya gum, and gum tragacanth. Mucilages exist in plant seeds to protect them from drying out. They include guar and carob gums. Many of the gums and mucilages are used in small concentrations in certain foods as thickeners and stabilizers. Some are also used as laxatives. Carrageenan is a gel-forming substance obtained from seaweed, and is often used in chocolate milk [4].

Derivatives of Carbohydrates

Sugar Alcohols A constant search goes on commercially for sweeteners that may furnish fewer kilocalories than sugars, or may have other advantages, such as a lessened tendency to produce dental decay. Sugar alcohols, such as *sorbitol*, *mannitol*, and *xylitol* have been used in recent years as sweeteners in some dietetic products and in "sugarless" gums.

Sorbitol occurs naturally in small amounts in many vegetables and fruits, but is obtained commercially from sucrose. At one time, sorbitol was used in dietetic foods because it was thought the body did not utilize it. We know now, however, that sorbitol furnishes the same number of kilocalories as sucrose, although it is absorbed more slowly than sucrose. Its slow absorptive rate is apt to keep blood glucose levels sufficiently elevated after eating to result in postponing hunger sensations a longer time than if sucrose is consumed. This explains its use in dietetic foods designed for weight control, but diabetics are advised not to use such products [5]. Sorbitol is only about 60 percent as sweet as sucrose. An undesirable side effect is that diarrhea and flatulence (gas) may result from its use, especially if consumed in amounts of 1 to 2 oz per day (25 to 50 g) [6].

Mannitol is less well metabolized than glucose or sucrose, and has about one-half the kilocalorie value of those sugars. It is about half as sweet as sucrose.

Xylitol is obtained commercially from wood pulp, corncobs, or straw, but it occurs naturally in many fruits and vegetables. It is of special interest to manufacturers of "sugarless" gum because it does not support the bacterial growth that results in dental decay. However, the Food and Drug Administration is currently reviewing its safety as a food ingredient since there have been reports that it may cause cancer. Many manufacturers have voluntarily withdrawn its use in gums and other foods while the review is in progress. Xylitol is about as sweet as sucrose.

Nonnutritive Sweeteners

Many people are convinced that using sweeteners that furnish few or no kilocalories helps them to control body weight. In addition, individuals with diabetes can enjoy the sweet flavor of these products free of the worry that doing so will elevate their blood sugar levels. At present only saccharin and aspartame are approved synthetic sweeteners in the United States. (See Chapter 17 for a discussion of saccharin.) *Aspartame* was approved for use in foods such as breakfast cereals and powdered beverages in 1981. In 1983, it was approved for use in soft drinks. It cannot be used in baked products because it decomposes at high temperatures. It is not, strictly speaking, a nonnutritive sweetener because it furnishes 4 kcal/g, just as sugars do. But because aspartame is about 180 times sweeter than sucrose, it provides only about 0.1 kcal for the same degree of sweetness found in 1 tsp of sucrose. Aspartame is a synthetic compound made up of the amino acid aspartic acid and a derivative of a second amino acid, phenylalanine.

CARBOHYDRATES IN FOOD

Our discussion so far has pointed out some food sources of starch, sugars, and some components of dietary fiber. But which foods are high and which low in

FIGURE 3-8. Percentage of carbohydrate in selected foods. (Source: Watt, B.K., and A.L. Merrill, *Composition of Foods, Raw, Processed, Prepared,* Agriculture Handbook 8, Washington, D.C.: USDA, 1963.)

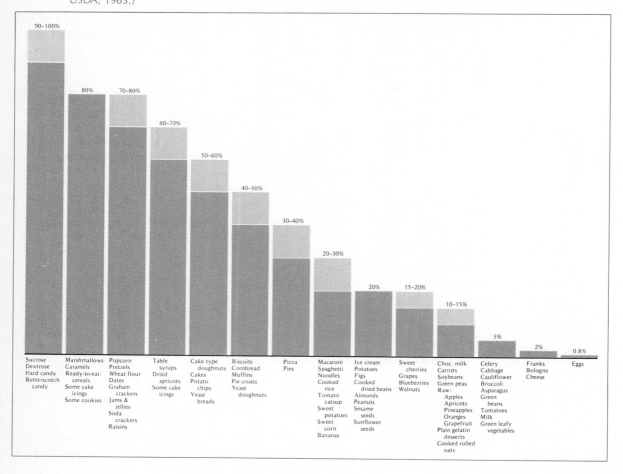

carbohydrates? To answer this question, nutritionists frequently report the percentage of the weight of a food that is due to carbohydrate. The total weight of a food is due largely to water, carbohydrates, fats, and proteins, with relatively small proportions of total weight coming from minerals and vitamins. Values for percentage of carbohydrate in a food are therefore obtained from those food composition tables reporting weights of these components in 100-g portions of the food. Figure 3-8 shows the percentage of carbohydrates (the concentration) in many commonly used foods. Knowing only the *concentration* of carbohydrate in a food may be misleading, however, since it is more practical to know how much you get from one or several servings of food. Appendix C lists carbohydrate in foods according to serving sizes, but it also gives the weight in grams for one serving. Using the weight of a serving, you can calculate the grams of carbohydrate if you know the concentration (from Figure 3-8). For example, 1 c of milk weighs 245 g and is 5 percent carbohydrate. One cup therefore furnishes 245 g × .05 = 12 g of carbohydrate.

Sugar in foods is of interest particularly because it is "hidden" in many processed foods. Appendix E lists the sugar concentration in many foods, including breakfast cereals. Food companies often do not list on the label the amount of sugar in a product because they are not required to do so. They must list the ingredients in order of predominance, however, listing that ingredient present in largest amount first. See Chapter 17 for more information on reading labels, particularly regarding sugars in foods.

The amount of dietary fiber in foods is technically difficult to determine, and only recently have some values been made available. Most tables of food composition in current use provide values only for "crude fiber," which are inaccurate values because the measuring method used destroys much of the dietary fiber. Table 3-3 indicates that foods highest in dietary fiber include bran and bran cereals, whole wheat flour and bread, legumes (beans), corn, nuts, vegetables, and fruits. Values for "crude fiber" tend to be much lower than the total dietary fiber in a food. A careful study of Table 3-3 reveals that puffed wheat and shredded wheat are higher in dietary fiber than other cereals (not counting All-Bran), and that potato chips are much higher in dietary fiber than other forms of potatoes. This occurs because the puffing, toasting, and browning processes used in producing these foods result in formation of substances that are indigestible, and which therefore actually increase the dietary fiber in these foods [7].

It is instructive to examine changes in intakes of various carbohydrates that have occurred among Americans over many years.

CHANGING PATTERNS OF CARBOHYDRATE CONSUMPTION

At the outset, it's important to point out that the information we have on changes in U.S. food consumption since early in this century come from data gathered by the U.S. Department of Agriculture. These data are actually for foods that

TABLE 3-3. TOTAL DIETARY FIBER AND CRUDE FIBER IN SOME FOODS (IN g/100 g)

FOOD	TOTAL DIETARY FIBER	CRUDE FIBER
FLOUR, BREAD, AND CEREALS		
White flour	3.2	.3
Whole wheat flour	7.9	2.3
Bran	44.0	9.1
White bread	2.7	.2
Whole wheat bread	8.5	1.5
All-Bran	26.7	7.8
Grapenuts	7.0	—
Rice Krispies	4.5	.6
Puffed Wheat	15.4	2.0
Shredded Wheat	12.3	2.3
Sugar Puffs	6.1	—
Special K	5.5	—
VEGETABLES		
Broccoli (cooked)	4.1	1.5
Brussels sprouts (cooked)	2.9	1.6
Cabbage (cooked)	2.9	.8
Lettuce (raw)	1.5	.5
Onions (raw)	2.1	.6
Baked beans	7.3	1.4
Frozen peas (raw)	7.8	1.9
Carrots (cooked)	3.7	1.0
Turnips	2.2	.9
Potatoes (raw)	3.5	.5
French fries	3.2	.6
Potato chips	11.9	1.6
Tomatoes (raw)	1.4	.5
Sweet corn (cooked)	4.7	.7
FRUITS		
Apples (flesh)	1.4	.6
Apple peels	3.7	—
Bananas	1.8	.5
Cherries	1.2	.4
Grapefruit (canned)	0.4	.2
Peaches	2.3	.6
Pears (flesh)	2.4	
Pears (peels)	8.6	—
Strawberries (raw)	2.1	1.3
NUTS		
Brazils	7.7	3.1
Peanuts	9.3	2.4
Peanut butter	7.6	1.8

Figures for crude fiber, markedly lower than those for total fiber, are poor indicators of the total fiber in foods.

SOURCES: 1. For total dietary fiber: Southgate, D.A.T., B. Bailey, and A.F. Walker, "A Guide to Calculating Intakes of Dietary Fiber," *Journal of Human Nutrition*, 30:303, 1976.
2. For crude fiber: Watt, B.K., and A.L. Merrill, *Composition of Foods: Raw, Processed and Prepared*, Handbook No. 8, Washington, D.C.: USDA, 1963.

"disappeared" from consumer markets, and do not reflect any losses in processing, or any wastage. This means that, although the figures are called "consumption" figures, they do not represent amounts actually consumed, but instead are amounts that were *available* for consumption.

Consumption of carbohydrates available to the American public decreased markedly from 1909, when the USDA first recorded consumption, to about 1974. The decline was due chiefly to decreased consumption of flour and cereal products which fell from about 300 lb per person per year in 1909 to 142 lb per person per year in 1970. Since about 1960, a slight increase in total carbohydrate consumption occurred due to an increased use of sugars and other sweeteners [8].

Sources of American carbohydrate consumption have changed significantly since 1909. Figure 3-9 indicates that in 1909 only about 32 percent of our carbohydrate intake came from sugars, while in 1980 about 53 percent came from sugars.

A CLOSER LOOK

A noteworthy change is that early in this century, most of the sucrose and other sweeteners used were added to foods at home, but today about 70 percent of sugars consumed are added by the manufacturer. Soft drinks now provide about 20 to 25 percent of the sucrose consumed by Americans, about seven times as much as was in beverages at the turn of the century [8].

The practical significance of these changes is that grains, breads, and potatoes, the consumption of which has decreased, contribute many nutrients to the diet, as well as dietary fiber, while sucrose and other caloric sweeteners, which have increased in consumption, tend to be low in nutrients relative to the kilocalories they provide. Furthermore, diets high in refined carbohydrates tend, at the same time, to be low in dietary fiber. The potential for decreasing the nutrient density of the diet by replacing grains, bread, and potatoes with high-sugar foods should be recognized by anyone interested in good nutrition.

FIGURE 3-9. Changes in percentage of carbohydrate available from starch or sugars in the U.S. food supply from 1909 to 1980. (Source: Drawn from data in Welch, S.O., and R.M. Marston, "Review of Trends in Food Use in the United States, 1909 to 1980," Reprinted by permission from *Journal of the American Dietetic Association,* 81:120, 1982.)

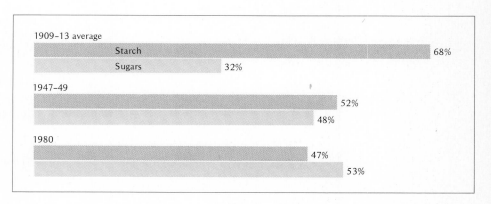

The sucrose (table sugar) consumption in the United States today is double that of 100 years ago, but has not increased markedly since 1925. In fact, sucrose consumption has declined slowly since the late 1960s when use of corn syrups, including high-fructose corn syrup, began to increase (Table 3-4). The total use of sucrose plus other nutritive sweeteners was about 130 lb per person per year in 1979. It has been projected that by 1985 sucrose consumption will have dropped to about 69 lb and total corn sweeteners increased to about 62 lb per person per year [3].

The intake of dietary fiber has diminished markedly in the United States since early in this century (Figure 3-10). Routine use of highly refined breads and cereals has contributed to the lower intake of dietary fiber in this and other affluent countries. Box 3-1 makes clear how the milling process results in losses of dietary fiber and vitamins and minerals. Chapter 5 discusses the possible effects of low fiber intakes on the occurrence of diseases of the colon and other diseases.

How does the body utilize food carbohydrates? How important are carbohydrates in the normal functions of the body? To answer these questions, we need to

TABLE 3-4. PER CAPITA U.S. CONSUMPTION OF CALORIC SWEETENERS, 1963–1979, IN POUNDS

	1963	1979
Sucrose	97.3	91.1
Corn sweeteners	14.2	37.2
Honey and syrups	1.8	1.5
Total	113.3	129.8

Corn sweeteners include glucose and regular corn syrup (containing dextrins, maltose, and glucose). In 1968, high-fructose corn syrups were introduced, and by 1979 15.4 lb of the 37.2 lb of corn sweeteners were high-fructose syrups. Notice that sucrose consumption declined as corn sweeteners increased.

SOURCE: Sugar and Sweetener Report, National Economics Division, Economics, Statistics, and Cooperatives Service, SSR-vol. 5, No. 7, Washington, D.C.: USDA, September 1980.

FIGURE 3-10. Trends in dietary fiber available for consumption in 1909–1913 compared with 1957–1959 to the present day. Dietary fiber from cereal consumption declined by 55 percent, from potatoes by 45 percent, while total dietary fiber declined by 33 percent. (Source: Drawn from data in Bingham, S., and J.H. Cummings, "Sources and Intakes of Dietary Fiber in Man," in Spiller, G.A., and R.M. Kay (eds.), *Medical Aspects of Dietary Fiber*, New York: Plenum Medical Book Co., 1980, p. 273.)

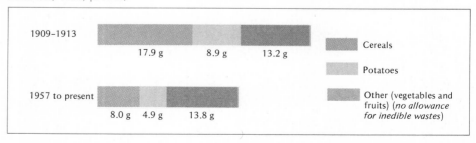

Nutritive Losses in Refining Grains

Grains in their natural, unmilled state consist of three distinct parts: the endosperm, the germ, and the outer coating or bran. The outer bran layers contain dietary fiber, many minerals, and many of the B vitamins (Figure 3-11). The largest part of the grain is called the endosperm and consists chiefly of starch embedded in a protein matrix. The amount of starch in the endosperm is much greater than the amount of protein. The germ, a small part of the grain, is necessary for the germination or reproduction of the plant, because it is the plant embryo. It is highly nutritious, as indicated in Figure 3-11.

When white flour is made from whole wheat, the bran and germ are removed. The manufacturer is able to make a finer flour when the bran is removed. In addition, removing the germ produces a flour that stores longer, since the germ contains fat that can become rancid. However, as the diagram indicates, removing the bran removes B vitamins, dietary fiber, and many minerals, while removing the germ removes not only B vitamins, but also vitamin E, essential fatty acid, and many minerals.

The primary ingredient in both white and whole wheat flour is starch, but obviously

FIGURE 3-11. Diagram of a grain of wheat, including the nutrients in its components: the bran, endosperm, and germ.

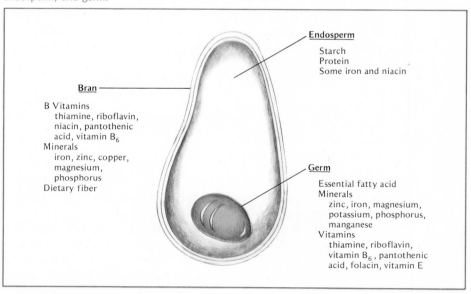

Endosperm
Starch
Protein
Some iron and niacin

Bran
B Vitamins
    thiamine, riboflavin,
    niacin, pantothenic
    acid, vitamin B$_6$
Minerals
    iron, zinc, copper,
    magnesium,
    phosphorus
Dietary fiber

Germ
Essential fatty acid
Minerals
    zinc, iron, magnesium,
    potassium, phosphorus,
    manganese
Vitamins
    thiamine, riboflavin,
    vitamin B$_6$, pantothenic
    acid, folacin, vitamin E

whole wheat flour, which contains not only the endosperm but the germ and most of the bran, contains many more nutrients than white flour.

White *enriched* flour consists of white flour to which three B vitamins, thiamine, riboflavin, and niacin, and one mineral, iron, are added at approximately the levels they occur in whole wheat. However, none of the other vitamins and minerals noted in the diagram that occur in whole wheat are added during enrichment of flour. (*Fortified* foods, such as ready-to-eat breakfast cereals, may have additional nutrients added, as discussed in Chapter 17.)

There is no question that whole wheat flour is more nutritious than white flour, even enriched white flour (see Table 2-3). But whether or not substituting whole wheat for white enriched bread would markedly improve the nutritive value of a diet depends upon how much bread is consumed. Some people in the United States consume so little bread that little improvement would result. If, however, one routinely consumes two or more slices per day,

plus a serving of cereal or rice, using whole-grain rather than white, enriched products would definitely increase the nutritive value of the diet.

In general, whole wheat bread is more expensive than white bread. At first, this might seem strange, since it must cost more to remove so much of the grain when making white flour than *not* to remove it. But high competition among white bread manufacturers forces them to keep prices as low as possible, while manufacturers charge whatever consumers will pay for more specialized breads, such as whole wheat. Another factor is that whole wheat bread is made in smaller batches, so the economy of mass production is lost. Furthermore, if whole wheat bread is made without additives that extend the shelf life, the manufacturer must bear the cost of stale loaves returned by retailers. The nation's bakers would, no doubt, quickly produce relatively inexpensive whole-grain bread if the majority of consumers refused to buy white and insisted on whole-grain bread.

discuss how the body digests, absorbs, and metabolizes carbohydrates. Before we turn our attention specifically to how the body uses carbohydrates, let's first examine generally what happens during digestion, absorption, and metabolism in the body.

DIGESTION, ABSORPTION, AND METABOLISM: SOME BASIC CONCEPTS

Digestion

Digestion occurs in the digestive tract, shown in Figure 3-12. *Digestion* is the process by which complex substances in foods are converted to simpler ones that can cross from the intestinal lumen to the blood.

The digestive tract is, in effect, a tube extending from the mouth to the anus. Digestion occurs in the mouth and stomach and in the *lumen* of the small intestines, that is, in the hole that runs through the tube (Figure 3-12). During digestion, as food passes along the digestive tract, two processes serve to reduce it from complex to simpler substances—one is mechanical and the other chemical. *Mechanical* processes include grinding by the teeth and mixing and

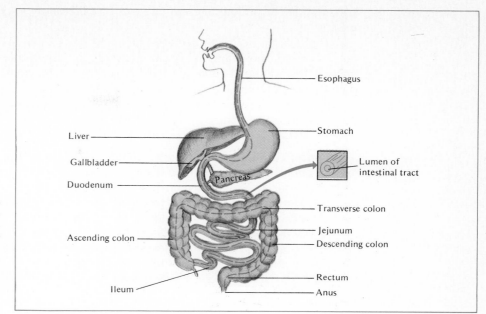

Esophagus

Stomach

Liver

Gallbladder

Lumen of
intestinal tract

Duodenum

Pancreas

Transverse colon

Jejunum

Ascending colon

Descending colon

Rectum

Ileum

Anus

FIGURE 3-12. The digestive tract. The dotted line indicates the path taken by food after it is consumed. Secretions from the liver, gallbladder, and pancreas empty into the duodenum where they aid in digestion.

churning brought about by alternate contraction and relaxation of muscles in the stomach and intestinal wall. *Chemical* processes involve the action of enzymes secreted in *saliva* (in the mouth) and in gastric (stomach), pancreatic, and intestinal juices. Other secretions, such as the stomach's *hydrochloric acid* and the liver's *bile* help enzymes accomplish their task of chemically converting foods to simple substances that can pass into the blood.

The complex digestive process begins as one masticates food. As the teeth mechanically grind the food, salivary secretions, including *mucus*, moisten the food, making it easier to swallow. Rhythmic contractions of muscles in the esophagus propel the moistened food toward the stomach. At the juncture of the esophagus and stomach, a *sphincter* muscle opens, allowing the food to pass into the stomach. There, powerful contractions of stomach muscles reduce the food further to smaller particles. At the same time, gastric juices mix in thoroughly with the food, converting it to a souplike mixture called *acid chyme*. Digestive enzymes secreted by the stomach operate best in an acidic environment.

Acid chyme leaves the stomach in little spurts, governed by the sphincter muscle located between the stomach and duodenum. Introduction of acid chyme into the duodenum in small, spaced amounts is one means of ensuring efficient digestion in the small intestines. The entry of acid chyme into the duodenum triggers release of pancreatic and intestinal juices, both of which contain many digestive enzymes. Bile also enters the duodenum from its storage place in the gallbladder. Bile is strongly alkaline, as are the pancreatic secretions. Muscle contractions of the intestinal wall rapidly mix chyme with bile and pancreatic secretions until the chyme becomes alkaline in reaction. Enzymes secreted by the pancreas and small intestines all operate most efficiently in an alkaline environment.

The digestion of carbohydrates, fats, and proteins all takes place chiefly in the duodenum and jejunum. Specific enzymes are responsible for the digestion of each of these nutrients. Bile, although it contains no enzymes, is required for the digestion of fats.

Box 3-2 discusses some common misconceptions about digestion.

Absorption

Absorption consists of the passage or transport of digestive products into the blood circulation. The human intestinal tract is designed so that its total absorptive surface is larger than half a basketball court [11]. This design is as follows: The lining or mucosa of the intestinal lumen exists in hundreds of folds. Each fold is covered with thousands of *villi*; furthermore, the surface of each cell on each villus contains *microvilli*, called the *brush border* (Figure 3-13). This system causes the surface area of a section of intestine on the inside, or mucosal side, to be about 600 times that of its smooth exterior [11].

Figure 3-13 also shows that each villus is equipped with a capillary (small

FIGURE 3-13. The mucosa of the intestine illustrating progressively smaller sections. Large folds *(a)* greatly increase the surface area which is further increased by small projections called villi *(b)*. The cells of each villus have on their surface microvilli or the brush border *(c)*, which further increase the surface area.

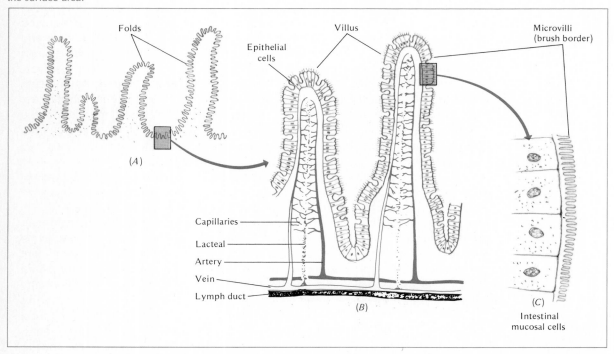

3-2 BOX — Misconceptions about the Digestive Tract

Indigestion Sometimes a normal person says: "Something I ate last night gave me indigestion. I was miserable all night." Is it likely that the food itself was the chief cause of the misery? Most often it is not. It is more likely that the person's emotional state was the underlying cause. More than any other body system, the gastrointestinal tract is affected by worry, fear, anxiety, hostility, depression, and conflicts. Individual responses to emotional factors may range all the way from occasional gastric discomfort, quickly forgotten, to chronic ulcers of the stomach or duodenum. A person may say he or she has "indigestion" when suffering from one of the following symptoms after eating: frequent belching, bad taste or bad breath, heartburn (burning sensation in the chest), bloating, nausea, or pain. Most often these symptoms result from slowing down or speeding up of the normal mechanical movements of the stomach or intestines, or to spasms of the sphincter muscles. Normally a person is unaware of the activity of the sphincters, or of the movements of the stomach or intestines. Strong emotions, however, can either stop or greatly speed up normal stomach or intestinal movements, resulting in various symptoms that make the person conscious that something is not quite as it should be. Physicians working in college health services hear frequent complaints of digestive problems from students faced with difficult exams, the possibility of failing a course, or serious personal problems. The basic remedy in these cases is to help students learn to deal in a positive way with the underlying emotional reactions to their problems, but this is not always easy to do. While the physician is attempting to help with the emotional response, he or she may advocate avoidance of highly spiced or seasoned foods, smoking, alcohol, and caffeine, all of which can exacerbate the problem.

Ulcers The cause or causes of stomach or duodenal ulcers are not completely understood. One authority states: "It seems likely that inheritance, personality, and society are the three largest factors having to do with the development of duodenal ulcers today" [9]. Generally, ulcer patients tend to cover up strongly held feelings by appearing to others to be calm and cool. People who have a genetic predisposition to ulcers are most apt to develop them if they have very strong feelings which they learned early in life not to express. In effect, then, they take out their feelings on themselves. For normal health, one needs not only a good inheritance, a good diet supporting normal growth, development, and maintenance of body tissue, but also healthful ways of expressing oneself emotionally.

Mucus Some popular writing advocates avoiding foods that "produce mucus." Mucus is a slippery secretion produced all along the digestive tract from the mouth through the colon. Mucus acts as a lubricant, and is known to protect the walls of the stomach and intestines from attack by powerful digestive enzymes. The idea that certain foods produce more mucus than others and therefore should be avoided has no scientific validity. Any admonition to severely restrict the variety of foods included in the diet is apt to increase the chances of having a nutritionally inadequate diet.

Restriction of Simultaneous Consumption of Certain Foods Another notion found in some popular writing is that carbohydrates should be eaten alone in one meal while proteins should be eaten alone in another, or that certain combinations, such as fruit and cereals, should never be eaten in the same meal. Advocates of such eating patterns often claim that the human gastrointestinal tract is unable to properly digest certain combinations of foods. Nothing could be further from the truth. The human digestive system is marvelously well equipped to digest combinations of all sorts of foods. While moderation in total amount of food consumed in a day, and in amount eaten at one meal is a good rule to follow, fortunately one does not need to be concerned that particular combinations of foods cannot be digested.

Constipation Constipation is a disorder in which defecation is not frequent enough for comfort, and in which the stools may be abnormally hard and dry. Symptoms include a dull headache, foul breath, coated tongue, abdominal discomfort, and mental depression. These symptoms are known to result from the presence of unevacuated feces in the descending colon and rectum, and not from any toxic substances absorbed into the blood. Packing the rectum with cotton produces symptoms of constipation which disappear immediately when the cotton (or feces) are removed from the rectum.

Constipation results most frequently from failure to consume sufficient dietary fiber and fluid, along with failure to establish regular bowel habits. The human digestive tract is designed to accommodate a certain amount of dietary fiber. The desire to defecate is brought about by the passage into the rectum of feces of

sufficient bulk to stimulate the nerve endings in the wall of the rectum. It is possible, however, to voluntarily restrain evacuation of the bowel, especially if little dietary fiber is present to cause a bulky stool. Repeated refusal to evacuate the bowel eventually results in reduced muscle tone in the wall of the rectum, and the rectum is then able to hold a larger fecal mass without the desire to defecate. Regular use of laxatives prevents occurrence of the normal stimulus to the nerve endings because there are never any formed stools. Laxatives, therefore, never really solve the problem.

Inclusion in the diet of sufficient dietary fiber and fluid, and establishment of a regular schedule for evacuation, based on one's own physiological inclination, will prevent and cure constipation in most normal people.

The idea of autointoxication, often seen in the popular press, is another myth. It is true that very small amounts of poisonous substances are produced in the colon as bacteria attack some amino acids that have escaped digestion. Very little, if any, of these are absorbed—thus there is no harmful effect [10]. Admonitions to eat only certain foods and avoid others to prevent autointoxication are without merit, and should be ignored.

It is useful to realize the extent to which emotions can effect the normal functions of the gastrointestinal tract, and the extent to which myths about digestion abound, even today. Many untruths are published in the field of nutrition, and the beginning student soon becomes aware that publication does not guarantee credibility.

blood vessel) and a lacteal (small lymph vessel). (*Lymph* is a clear fluid contained in lymph vessels, and is like blood in composition except that it contains no red blood cells and has a lower amount of protein than blood.) Nutrients picked up by the *capillaries* flow into the *portal vein* to the liver. Those picked up by *lacteals* flow into the *thoracic duct*, a large lymph vessel, which passes upward through the diaphragm into the chest area. The thoracic duct continues upward alongside the esophagus to the neck where it enters the left subclavian vein. Nutrients absorbed via lymph, therefore, enter the *general* blood circulation (at the subclavian vein), while those absorbed via capillaries are carried directly to the liver, and, from there, are put into the general circulation. Cells needing specific nutrients pick them out of the blood as it flows through tissues.

Forms of Transport   The task of absorption is to get nutrients from the lumen side of the intestinal mucosal cells to the capillaries or lacteals on the opposite side of the cell (Figure 3-14). The membrane of the microvilli is made up of a layer of lipid (fatty material) held between two layers of protein. Small pores in the membrane allow water and a few small substances such as chloride ions to pass through. Most molecules are too large to pass through the pores, however. Fatty substances can pass easily through this membrane, but water-soluble substances cannot, except for those small enough to pass through the pores.

A special mechanism helps larger water-soluble nutrients, such as sugars and amino acids, to cross the membrane. This mechanism consists of protein carriers existing in the membrane which pick up the nutrient on the lumen side of the cell and carry it across the cell membrane to the cell interior. When the concentration of nutrients in the lumen is higher than that inside the mucosal cells, this process is called *facilitated diffusion* and does not require energy. This situation exists only a very short time after a meal, however, for water rapidly moves in the direction needed to equalize the concentration on either side of the mucosal cell membranes. Continued absorption at this stage means that these water-soluble nutrients must be able to cross the membrane against a concentration gradient—that is, from a lower concentration in the lumen to a higher concentration in the mucosal cells. This process requires not only special protein carriers, but also uses *energy,* and is called *active transport.* Active transport is the chief mode of absorption for glucose and amino acids [11,12].

Most absorption occurs in the duodenum and jejunum, but some nutrients are absorbed from the ileum, as you will see later.

Foods are not completely digested. Substances left undigested may be attacked by the bacteria (called *microflora*) that live in the colon. By-products of bacterial attacks on undigested portions of food are gases and fatty acids, some of

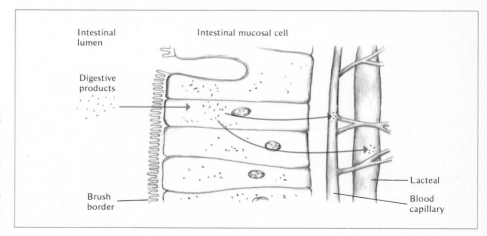

FIGURE 3-14. Absorption consists of transporting products of digestion from the intestinal lumen across the intestinal mucosal cells to the capillaries or the lacteals. Abosrption is completed when products of digestion reach the circulating blood.

which are absorbed. The body also absorbs from the colon large amounts of water and the minerals sodium and potassium. As food residues pass through the colon, they become progressively less fluid until formed stools accumulate in the descending colon and rectum. Feces consist of undigested portions of food, residues from sloughed-off intestinal cells and secretions, bacteria (dead and alive), and water.

Metabolism

Metabolism involves all those processes by which nutrients become part of body tissues, are used for energy, or otherwise perform their functions. Additionally, metabolism refers to those processes in which body compounds or structures are torn down and their products excreted. Metabolism therefore covers two phases: *anabolism*—the synthesis or building up of body components, and *catabolism*—the breakdown of body components to substances that usually are excreted. Most catabolic waste products are lost via the kidneys (in the urine), or via the lungs (as carbon dioxide and water). Small amounts of metabolic wastes are lost through the skin in sweat. Although feces represent waste, they are not primarily *metabolic* wastes, but are chiefly undigested food residues.

Metabolism occurs in every body cell. Complex processes of metabolism involve synchronized activities of enzymes and hormones (synthesized in the cells) with required nutrients supplied in the diet. The study of metabolism of specific nutrients should further your insights into and appreciation of the complexities of the body's use of nutrients.

THE BODY'S USE OF CARBOHYDRATES

Carbohydrate Digestion

The goal of the digestion of carbohydrates is to convert them to simple forms the body can absorb, namely to the monosaccharides glucose, fructose, and galactose. We can paint a clearer picture of how carbohydrate digestion occurs by tracing the digestion of the carbohydrates in a whole wheat raisin muffin. Figure 3-15 indicates the specific carbohydrates in the muffin.

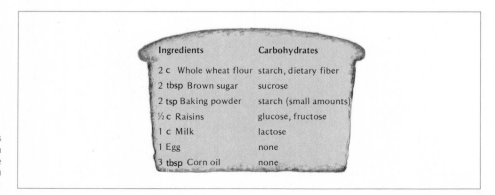

Ingredients	Carbohydrates
2 c Whole wheat flour	starch, dietary fiber
2 tbsp Brown sugar	sucrose
2 tsp Baking powder	starch (small amounts)
½ c Raisins	glucose, fructose
1 c Milk	lactose
1 Egg	none
3 tbsp Corn oil	none

FIGURE 3-15. Ingredients in a whole wheat raisin muffin, indicating the specific carbohydrate(s) furnished by each.

Digestion in the Mouth   The taste and odor of the muffin trigger saliva secretions. As one chews the muffin, it mixes with the saliva forming a moist mass that can be swallowed. Digestion of the starch in the muffin begins in the mouth, but is not completed there. The only digestive enzyme in the mouth is *salivary amylase*, secreted by the salivary glands. This enzyme attacks starch and converts it to dextrins and a little maltose, but only if the food is kept in the mouth long enough for sufficient digestion to occur. On swallowing the bite of muffin, the acidity of the stomach secretions stops the action of salivary amylase. (Stomach secretions are triggered also by taste and smell of food.) Since the stomach secretes no enzymes that digest carbohydrates, no further digestion of starch occurs there. Stomach hydrochloric acid catalyzes hydrolysis of a small amount of sucrose in the muffin, however, producing some glucose and fructose.

Digestion in the Small Intestines   The remaining digestion of starch and sugars in the muffin occurs in the duodenum and jejunum. Starch digestion is completed by the action of two enzymes: *pancreatic amylase*, which converts starch and dextrins to maltose; and *maltase*, which converts maltose to glucose (Table 3-5). Sucrose is digested by *sucrase* and lactose by *lactase*, producing the sugars of which these disaccharides are composed (Table 3-5). Fructose and glucose from the raisins require no digestion. The final products of digestion of the mixture of carbohydrates in the muffin are therefore three monosaccharides: glucose, fructose, and galactose.

Dietary fiber remains undigested and moves on down to the colon. There, bacteria attack it, converting some of it to fatty acids, which may be absorbed. The remainder of the dietary fiber is excreted in the feces.

Physicians rarely encounter individuals who have low levels of intestinal sucrase or maltase. A great many people have low lactase levels, however.

Lactose Intolerance [13,14]

The enzyme lactase occurs abundantly in all newborn infants, and remains abundant until the child is 3 or 4 years of age. After that age 60 to 90 percent of

TABLE 3-5.   DIGESTION OF CARBOHYDRATES

ORIGIN OF ENZYME	ENZYME	SUBSTRATE*	PRODUCTS FORMED
Salivary glands in mouth	Salivary amylase	Starch	Mostly dextrins, and a little maltose
Pancreas	Pancreatic amylase	Starch and dextrins	Maltose
Small intestines	Maltase	Maltose	Glucose
Small intestines	Sucrase	Sucrose	Glucose and fructose
Small intestines	Lactase	Lactose	Glucose and galactose

*Substrate is the substance an enzyme acts upon.
Nearly all the digestion of carbohydrates occurs in the duodenum and jejunum. The bulk of starch digestion results from the action of pancreatic, not salivary, amylase. The end products of digestion of a mixture of the most commonly occurring carbohydrates in foods are glucose, fructose, and galactose.

non-Caucasians have low lactase activity, while this is the case in only 5 to 15 percent of Caucasians. Individuals having low lactase activity are said to have *lactose intolerance*. The problem is thought to be inherited, and apparently has appeared over the ages among people who traditionally have not consumed milk after infancy. Northern European countries traditionally have continued milk consumption beyond infancy.

In cases of low lactase activity, undigested lactose moves down the small intestines, drawing fluids into the intestinal lumen due to its osmotic effect. The osmotic effect is due to the tendency to equalize the concentration of dissolved substances between the blood and the intestinal contents. If an unusually high concentration of sugar occurs in the lower small intestines, water is drawn in from the blood to dilute the sugar concentration. When this happens, the intestines become distended and the individual feels bloated. As the undigested lactose reaches the colon, bacteria attack it, producing gases and acids. The individual is apt to experience diarrhea, flatulence (gas), and abdominal cramps.

When physicians test an individual for lactose intolerance, they generally give a dose of pure lactose (equivalent to the amount in 1 or 2 qt of milk), and check the blood glucose levels at intervals afterwards. A lack of elevation of blood glucose after the dose indicates inability to absorb lactose. However, large numbers of people report no symptoms of discomfort despite showing no rise in blood glucose after the lactose dose.

In a practical sense, then, most lactose-intolerant people can consume some milk and should be encouraged to do so since milk is highly nutritious. The most effective milk source for lactose-intolerant individuals is probably that containing predigested lactose, which is available in many supermarkets. Yogurt is somewhat lower in lactose than regular milk, and cheddar cheese contains many of the same nutrients as milk, but contains no lactose. Cheddar cheese tends to be high in fat and kilocalories, however. Some lactose-intolerant individuals tolerate milk better with meals than by itself.

Now let's return to a consideration of how sugars are absorbed.

Absorption of Sugars

The largest amount of monosaccharide from the digestion of carbohydrates in the muffin we were discussing earlier is glucose—from starch, sucrose, lactose, and glucose in raisins. Smaller amounts of galactose result from the digestion of lactose. Glucose and galactose are transported across the intestinal mucosal cell membrane by *active transport*, a system, you recall, that requires energy. These two sugars utilize the same carrier protein to aid them in crossing the membrane. Fructose, on the other hand, does not utilize active transport, but instead uses *facilitated diffusion*—that is, it requires a carrier, but is not transported against a concentration gradient. Although the mechanisms by which monosaccharides are absorbed are incompletely understood, the normal individual very efficiently absorbs practically all the glucose, galactose, and fructose after a meal.

Once the monosaccharides are inside intestinal mucosal cells, they move across the cell and enter the capillaries located just beyond the cell's basement

HOW DIET CAN AFFECT MOOD AND BEHAVIOR

Jane E. Brody, *The New York Times*, November 16, 1982

The timing and contents of meals, as well as the consumption of certain individual nutrients, can have subtle and occasionally dramatic effects on mood and behavior, according to a series of new studies described at the Massachusetts Institute of Technology. . . .

. . . Several studies demonstrated that eating carbohydrates can raise the level of a brain chemical, serotonin, that is associated with feeling relaxed, calm, sleepy, less depressed and less sensitive to pain.

This may be why so many people report that they binge on carbohydrates when they feel anxious or depressed, noted Dr. Judith J. Wurtman, a cell biologist and nutritionist at M.I.T. . . .

"It may also explain why high-protein, low-carbohydrate weight-reduction diets usually fail," she went on. "These diets induce a serotonin deficiency in the brain which is turn could trigger carbohydrate cravings to correct the imbalance." . . .

The research reported here is largely an outgrowth of neurochemical studies by Dr. Richard Wurtman, Dr. John D. Fernstrom, also of M.I.T., and others that found that the consumption of certain nutrients can change the levels of brain chemicals that transit messages between nerve cells. These neurotransmitters, as they are called, regulate a wide variety of brain activities and can affect both mood and performance. The nutrients are actually the chemical precursors, or parents, of neurotransmitters, which cannot be given directly because they do not cross into the brain from the blood.

For example, tryptophan, an amino acid found in protein foods like meat, chicken and fish, is the precursor of serotonin, a neurotransmitter that induces sleep and acts as an antidepressant. When tryptophan is given or when foods are eaten that raise the blood levels of tryptophan, serotonin levels in the brain increase.

Although tryptophan is a constituent of protein, it is the consumption of carbohydrate foods that actually raises tryptophan levels in the blood and brain. This occurs because other amino acids in protein successfully compete with tryptophan for passage into the brain, and brain levels of tryptophan and, in turn, serotonin, fall when protein is eaten.

Carbohydrate foods like sweets, bread, pasta, and rice, on the other hand, result in removal from the blood of the competing amino acids and a consequent increase in tryptophan and serotonin levels in the brain. . . .

Dr. [Judith] Rapoport [of the National Institute of Health] also reported that, contrary to the popular impression, sugar had a calming effect on the children she studied, a finding that fits in with the known effects of carbohydrates on serotonin levels in the brain.

This raises serious questions about the use of low-sugar diets to treat hyperactive children and to calm prison inmates. Although one such plan, sometimes called the Oklahoma prison diet, has been instituted in a number of prisons, Dr. Richard Wurtman said it was not based on scientifically derived facts and made no biological sense in light of the sedating effect of carbohydrates. . . .

ASK YOURSELF:

Based on this report, does it seem logical that including a certain amount of high-carbohydrate foods in a low kilocalorie diet for weight loss might prevent binge eating? What questions does this very brief report raise in your mind about this area of research? What further information would you like to have on this topic? (See Suggested Readings.)

membrane (Figure 3-14). The capillaries carry them to the portal vein, through which they reach the liver.

Now that we have seen how the products of carbohydrate digestion enter the blood, we are ready to consider metabolism of carbohydrates.

Carbohydrate Metabolism

In the following discussion of carbohydrate metabolism, you will see how the body maintains normal blood glucose levels and why that is crucial. You will also learn how energy is obtained from glucose, how glycogen stores are maintained, and how glucose is converted to fat. The central importance of the liver in carbohydrate metabolism will become obvious.

The Fate of Sugars   We noted earlier that glucose, fructose, and galactose from carbohydrate digestion all reach the liver by way of the portal vein. Upon reaching the liver, fructose and galactose are converted by liver cells to glucose. The liver then uses this glucose in the same way it uses glucose from fruits, or from starch digestion. Glucose may be used (1) to maintain the blood glucose level, (2) to produce energy needed by cells, (3) to maintain glycogen stores, or (4) to form fat stores.

Maintenance of Blood Glucose Levels   Normal blood glucose levels are important for a feeling of well-being because the brain and other nervous tissue are dependent on glucose for energy, since glycogen is not stored in nervous tissue. In an emergency, nervous tissue can use other substances for energy (such as ketones, which result from incomplete oxidation of fatty acids in the liver), but ordinarily these tissues use only glucose. If the blood glucose level falls to a low enough level, central nervous tissue becomes very excitable and the person feels nervous, dizzy, or faint. Unusually low blood glucose, usually defined as below 30 to 50 milligrams of glucose per 100 milliliters of blood (30 to 50 mg/100 mL), is called *hypoglycemia* (*hypo* = low; *glyc* = sugar; *-emia* = in the blood). On the other hand, unusually high blood glucose levels—hyperglycemia (*hyper* = high) are also undesirable because this condition causes fluid to be withdrawn from body cells, dehydrating them. Hyperglycemia is a sign of diabetes.

Normally, the blood glucose levels on arising in the morning, called the fasting level, is between 80 to 100 mg/100 mL of blood. After eating a meal containing carbohydrates, one's glucose level normally rises to 130 to 140 mg/100 mL at 1 hour, but returns to the fasting level 2 hours after the meal.

Some popular nutrition books claim that huge numbers of American suffer from hypoglycemia. Let's look at expert medical opinion regarding this claim.

Hypoglycemia   If blood glucose levels fall to low levels (30 to 50 mg/100 mL) the brain becomes deprived of its energy source and the person experiences some of the following symptoms: lightheadedness, jitteriness, fatigue, inability to concentrate, dizziness, irritability, stomach pains, sweating, crying jags, headaches, and feeling cold. Some people experience these symptoms after drinking alcoholic beverages, or after heavy exercise. If the blood levels become exceedingly low, fainting, coma, and death may ensue.

Those who claim that vast numbers of people suffer from hypoglycemia advocate a diet low in sugars and starches and high in protein for those who have one or more of the above symptoms. Medical experts in hypoglycemia point out, however, that many people who have these symptoms *do not have unusually low blood glucose levels at the time they experience the symptoms*. It is important to realize that the symptoms described may originate from psychological causes, or from physiological disorders having no relationship to hypoglycemia.

If one *does* have such symptoms, one should obtain competent medical evaluation to determine their cause. Trying to counteract the symptoms by dietary manipulation alone without medical diagnosis can, in many cases, mean that an underlying disorder goes undiagnosed and uncorrected. For example, hypoglycemia in many cases is a forerunner of diabetes, and should be properly treated at an early stage. Furthermore, some types of hypoglycemia are made worse by the high-protein diet advocated in popular books because amino acids can trigger the release of insulin, which in some people brings about hypoglycemia. Anyone who routinely or frequently experiences symptoms of hypoglycemia should receive a thorough examination from a competent physician, preferably one who specializes in diabetes and hypoglycemia. One should never rely upon a popular book for treatment of medical disorders.

A person in good health easily maintains normal blood glucose levels, but the complexity of the mechanism for doing so becomes apparent as one examines it.

Mechanisms of Control   The liver is the chief organ in the body for control of the blood glucose level. Directly after a meal containing carbohydrates, the liver stores any excess glucose as glycogen. As time elapses after a meal, body cells remove glucose from the blood to use for energy, and blood levels gradually decline. The liver then obtains glucose from (1) breakdown (catabolism) of liver glycogen to form glucose, (2) certain amino acids obtained either from food or from catabolism of some body protein, (3) glycerol from the catabolism of body fat, or (4) lactic acid from muscle exercise. Muscles produce lactic acid from the catabolism of muscle glycogen to form glucose, and further catabolism of glucose to lactic acid. The lactic acid is then sent to the liver by way of the blood. The sources used by the liver to form blood glucose are summarized in Figure 3-16.

The body maintains normal blood glucose levels even when there is no carbohydrate in the diet, by converting noncarbohydrate substances (amino acids and glycerol) to glucose. This process is called *gluconeogenesis* and occurs in the liver and kidneys. During total starvation, for example, gluconeogenesis is the chief mechanism used to maintain blood glucose levels, using amino acids and glycerol from the catabolism of body tissues. This mechanism accounts in part for the survival of animals, including humans, through periods of famine.

Hormones also play critically important roles in controlling blood glucose. Of particular importance are *insulin* and *glucagon*. Insulin, secreted by the pancreas whenever the blood glucose level rises, causes muscles and adipose

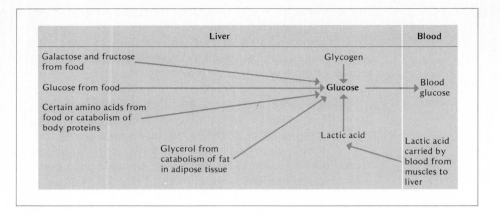

tissue (fat stores) to take up glucose from the blood. In addition, this hormone promotes storage of glycogen in the liver, and stimulates conversion of glucose to fat in adipose tissue. The effect of insulin is therefore to *lower* the blood glucose level.

Glucagon is secreted also by the pancreas, but its effect is opposite to that of insulin. When blood glucose levels fall toward the low side, glucagon raises these levels by stimulating glycogen breakdown and gluconeogenesis. Other hormones that play a role in increasing the blood glucose levels include *epinephrine*, synthesized by the adrenal glands. Epinephrine release occurs in response to fright or anger, and triggers glycogen breakdown in the liver, apparently to provide a burst of energy for an emergency.

The kidneys play a role in regulating blood glucose levels when the level is unusually high. Normally, as glucose filters into the fluid in the kidneys that eventually forms urine, it is reabsorbed into the blood so that none is excreted in the urine. But if blood glucose levels are higher than about 170 to 180 mg/100

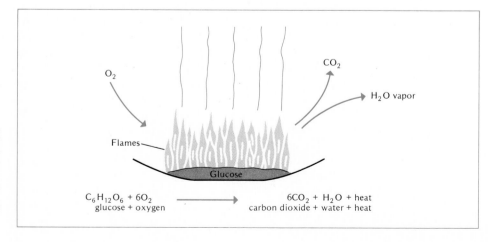

FIGURE 3-17. Complete burning (oxidation) of glucose in the laboratory uses up oxygen and produces CO_2 (carbon dioxide) and H_2O (water). Energy is released in the form of heat.

mL, excessive amounts will be excreted in the urine. The routine appearance of glucose in the urine is detrimental because it causes losses of body fluids which result in dehydration, and is a sign of diabetes.

Maintaining normal blood glucose levels ensures that tissues have access to glucose as an energy source, if and when it is needed. Body cells generally are not *dependent* on glucose for energy, however. It is important to realize that *the body's paramount need is for energy*. Body cells therefore are able to obtain energy from several sources. Most cells, except nervous tissue, can and do use fatty acids for energy, and all cells except those in the liver can obtain energy from ketones, the incomplete oxidation products of fats. Nevertheless, the major use the body makes of dietary carbohydrates is as a fuel. Body cells may use glucose directly for energy, or may convert it to body fat, which it later uses for fuel. Let's first examine how the body uses glucose directly for energy.

Splitting Glucose for Energy   The overall process by which glucose is converted to energy is called *oxidation*. Oxidation occurs whenever oxygen is used up in a reaction. If you burn pure glucose in the laboratory, oxygen is consumed, and carbon dioxide (CO_2) and water (H_2O) are produced. The energy locked within the glucose molecules is released as *heat* (Figure 3-17). Body cells also oxidize glucose to CO_2 and H_2O, but the glucose does not burn with a flame. Instead, body cells use enzymes to catalyze stepwise breakdown of glucose to simpler chemical compounds until, finally, CO_2 and H_2O are produced.

A critical difference between the oxidation of glucose outside and inside the body is that the body captures the energy released from the glucose molecules in the form of high-energy chemical bonds in specific compounds, the most important of which is *ATP* (adenosine *triphosphate*). When cells need energy, their enzymes catalyze the breaking of the high-energy bonds of ATP; the released energy is used to drive chemical reactions, muscular activity, or nerve transmissions.

Anabolic reactions, such as building up glycogen from glucose, or building up muscle proteins from amino acids, require energy and therefore use up ATP. Catabolic reactions, such as the breakdown of carbohydrates, proteins, or fat, may use up some ATP, but produce far more than they use.

The oxidation of glucose by body cells for energy produces some heat (the body is not 100 percent efficient in capturing the energy released in the form of ATP). Some of the heat is used to maintain the body temperature, but most of it is dissipated through the skin. You have probably noticed how a lecture room may be cold when you arrive early for a lecture, but that after 100 students sit in the room for awhile, the room may become uncomfortably warm. Dissipation of body heat is necessary for maintenance of normal body temperature.

Figure 3-18 indicates how all body cells obtain energy from glucose. Glucose, a 6-carbon compound, is broken down in several steps to two molecules of pyruvate, a 3-carbon compound. Pyruvate, in turn, is converted to acetyl coenzyme A (abbreviated acetyl CoA), a 2-carbon compound. In this process, a small amount of ATP is produced, and some hydrogen atoms (indicated by $\cdot \overset{\cdot\cdot}{H} \cdot$ and CO_2 are released.

Next, acetyl CoA enters the Krebs cycle. This cycle consists of carbohydrate

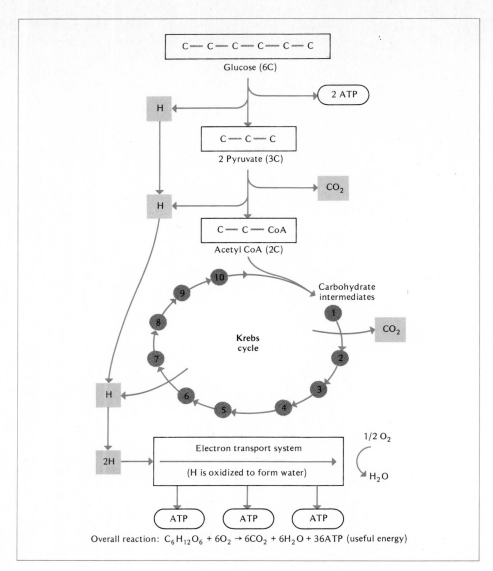

FIGURE 3-18. The oxidation of glucose to obtain energy.

Overall reaction: $C_6H_{12}O_6 + 6O_2 \rightarrow 6CO_2 + 6H_2O + 36ATP$ (useful energy)

derivatives or intermediates, designated here by numbers ①through ⑩. Compound ⑩ combines with acetyl CoA to form compound ①, which is converted to ②, etc., until compound ⑩ is regenerated. In this process, CO_2 is released and so are hydrogen atoms. All the hydrogen released in the entire process of glucose oxidation is oxidized through the electron transport system to form H_2O. In this process, ATP is produced. Complete oxidation of one glucose molecule produces 36 ATPs, 6 molecules of CO_2, and 6 molecules of H_2O. The CO_2 enters the blood and is carried to the lungs where it is exhaled.

Acetyl CoA, the Krebs cycle, and the electron transport system are also involved in the metabolism of fats and protein for energy, as will be made clear in

Chapters 4 and 6. For those who wish more detail regarding the oxidation of glucose than is given in Figure 3-18, Appendix K gives such information.

Maintaining Glycogen Stores   We have observed that whenever more carbohydrate is supplied in the diet than is needed immediately for energy, both the liver and muscles synthesize glycogen from the extra glucose. Normally the body stores only a limited amount of glycogen. A man weighing 70 kg (154 lb) stores about 350 g, or about ¾ lb. This is enough to supply his body with energy for about 13 hours only, if it were the only source of energy used. Glycogen stores therefore require constant replenishing from dietary carbohydrates, and quickly disappear as one fasts (starves) or consumes a very low carbohydrate diet.

Liver glycogen stores are quickly converted to glucose to be used for energy or to supply blood glucose. Muscle glycogen, however, is used only to supply the muscle with energy via glucose, and does not directly increase the blood glucose level. We have already noted that the lactic acid from muscular exercise can be converted by the liver to glucose, so muscles contribute to blood glucose only indirectly.

Liver glycogen stores are important to protect the entire body against bacterial toxins or such toxic agents as alcohol and other chemicals. An important function of the liver is to remove or destroy toxic agents before they reach other vital organs, and the liver is best able to do this when it has a good supply of glycogen [15].

A CLOSER LOOK

The fact that a good supply of liver glycogen diminishes the amount of fat the liver catabolizes demonstrates an important relationship between carbohydrate and fat. If the liver lacks glycogen, and little carbohydrate is in the diet, the body breaks down fat for energy. The liver is therefore forced to catabolize fats, but without carbohydrate it cannot oxidize fats completely. Instead, it forms ketones, the products of incomplete fat oxidation. Ketones enter the blood from the liver, and most body cells use them for energy. When blood levels become so high in ketones that they are excreted in the urine, however, the individual is said to have ketosis. Symptoms of ketosis include excessive urination, dizziness upon rising from a recumbent position, bad breath, fatigue, and sometimes nausea and lack of appetite. Adequate carbohydrate in the diet and consequent adequate glycogen in the liver prevent ketosis. Ketosis is discussed further in Chapter 4, since the condition is related to fatty acid metabolism.

A good supply of liver glycogen also "spares protein." Protein is the sole source of amino acids needed to build body protein, but if the body needs *energy*, and can't get it elsewhere, it will use amino acids to form glucose (gluconeogenesis). As mentioned earlier, the body's energy need takes precedence over all other needs. Sufficient carbohydrate in the diet maintains liver glycogen stores as a ready source of glucose to supply energy and to maintain blood glucose levels. Under these conditions the protein in the diet will not be used for energy, but will be spared to be used for its unique function—to build body protein.

At the beginning of this chapter, Carmen was raising questions about whether she, as an athlete, should investigate "carbohydrate loading" as a method of increasing her endurance. These questions are addressed in Box 3-3.

Converting Glucose to Fat Carbohydrates consumed in amounts greater than needed to supply energy are converted to body fat, but this is also the case when excessive amounts of fat or protein are consumed. Contrary to Greg's beliefs, described at the beginning of the chapter, carbohydrates are not more "fattening" than fats or protein. Starchy foods such as potatoes, spaghetti, and bread are lower in kilocalories than many people think, but adding butter, sour cream, and sauces rapidly increases the kilocalorie level, as noted in Table 3-6. Actually, fats are more apt to run up the number of kilocalories than carbohydrates because, on a weight basis, they contribute more than twice the kilocalories of carbohydrates (9 kcal/g vs. 4 kcal/g). By avoiding starchy foods in his diet, Greg is also excluding excellent sources of the B vitamins, many minerals, and dietary fiber. He may also, by excluding these foods, be consuming a diet that is very high in fat, a dietary pattern that may well promote his tendency toward being overweight and may be related to coronary heart disease (see Chapter 5).

How does the body convert carbohydrate to fat? The process actually involves some of the metabolic steps you are already familiar with from our discussion of glucose metabolism. Figure 3-19 points out how the body breaks glucose down to acetyl CoA, as if it were oxidizing it for energy, and then builds fatty acids from the acetyl CoA units. Glycerol, needed to join with the fatty acids to form fats (triglycerides), also comes from catabolism of glucose. The cells can break down stored fat to fatty acids and glycerol, but only the glycerol—and not the fatty acids—can be reconverted to glucose (indicated by the dotted line in Figure 3-19).

Conditions under which glucose is apt to be converted to triglyceride in the body include times when the body cells have all the kilocalories they need. Any

TABLE 3-6. COMPARISONS OF ENERGY (kcal) VALUE OF CARBOHYDRATE FOODS ALONE AND WITH USUAL ACCOMPANIMENTS

FOOD	kcal	ADDITION OR SUBSTITUTION	TOTAL kcal
1 med. boiled potato	90	2 tsp butter	155
1 large baked potato	140	2 tbsp sour cream	205
1 slice bread	65	1 tbsp jelly	120
1 c plain spaghetti	155	Tomato sauce and cheese	260
4 saltine crackers	50	1 oz cheddar cheese	165
1/12 of an angel food cake	135	2 tbsp uncooked icing	285
1 c cornflakes (no sugar)	95	1 c sugar-frosted cornflakes*	155
1 corn tortilla	65	1 beef taco*	160

*For these two foods, the food in the right-hand column is substituted for the one in the left-hand column.

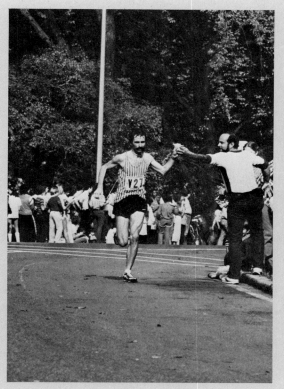

BOX
3-3

Carbohydrate Loading

The practice of carbohydrate loading for athletes engaged in endurance contests has become popular recently. What is the basis for this dietary regimen? First, it is necessary to understand that during light to moderate exercise, when large amounts of oxygen are available, muscles use primarily fatty acids for energy. However, during vigorous, prolonged exercise, such as marathon running, oxygen becomes less available to muscles, whereupon they switch to using more carbohydrate for energy.

The basic assumption behind carbohydrate loading is that an increase in the amount of glycogen stored in muscles will increase the athlete's endurance. Studies in which samples of muscle have been analyzed for glycogen show that athletes consuming the usual mixed diet will have about 1.5 grams of glycogen per 100 grams of muscle (1.5 g/100 g). If an athlete switches to a diet high in carbohydrates for several days, the amount increases to about 2.5 g/100 g of muscle. However, if the athlete undergoes the carbohydrate loading procedure, the amount of glycogen in the muscles increases to 5.0 g/100 g of muscle [16]. When following the loading procedure, athletes first exercise their muscles so as to exhaust all their glycogen stores from day 6 through day 4 before a competition, while consuming a diet low in carbohydrate, but high in fat and protein. This is followed by light exercise and a diet high in carbohydrates on days 3 through 1 before a competition. On the day of competition, athletes eat as desired.

There are reasons to be concerned about the carbohydrate loading routine. One is that for each gram of glycogen stored, 2.7 g of water are stored with it. Glycogen loading is therefore apt to result in weight gain, decreasing the athlete's efficiency because it increases the

Some long distance runners find that carbohydrate loading improves endurance, but this technique should be used *only* under the supervision of an experienced sports physician or other athletic expert. *(Peter Arnold)*

work load of the heart. The muscles may also feel heavy and stiff as a result [16].

Glycogen is deposited in the heart as well as the skeletal muscles by the loading routine. Persons having any indication of heart problems are well advised to avoid the procedure, but unfortunately we know too little at present to say whether or not possible heart damage can occur in seemingly normal people.

Another reason for concern is that the low-carbohydrate diet used early in this routine is very high in fat, and may therefore increase the possibility of developing atherosclerosis, a disease of the arteries associated with coronary heart disease [16] (see Chapters 4 and 5). In addition, the possibility that carbohydrate depletion may result in heart arrythmias (abnormal heartbeat) is currently under study.

Furthermore, it has been shown that the endurance of a well-trained athlete is much less apt to be improved by glycogen loading than that of a less well-trained athlete. This is because a slower rate of utilization of glycogen, which occurs in the better trained athlete, is more effective in increasing endurance than a faster rate, typical of the less well-trained. Therefore, the total amount of glycogen present in muscles is by no means the only important factor increasing endurance [16].

What should Carmen, who was mentioned at the beginning of the chapter, do about carbohydrate loading? First, she should seek out a sports physician or other athletic expert who has had experience with carbohydrate loading. Many such experts have found that modifications of the routine described here are effective, such as elimination of the phase in which exhaustion of glycogen stores occur.

If Carmen decides to try carbohydrate loading, it is recommended that she consume at least 100 g of carbohydrate while on the low-carbohydrate diet to prevent ketosis and the fatigue and loss of body fluids that accompany it [17]. While she is on the high-carbohydrate diet, she should choose bread, cereals, fruits, and vegetables, and not high-sugar foods because the former foods are higher in nutrient density.

Generally, it is recommended that carbohydrate loading be used only two or three times a year at most, and probably not at all by very young teenagers and preteens [18].

excess carbohydrate will then be converted to fat. Another circumstance is when insulin secretion is sufficient to favor triglyceride synthesis. This occurs after almost every meal. Body tissues, including body fats, are in a *dynamic state*—that is, they are constantly being built up and torn down. Some carbohydrate is converted to body fat nearly every day in the life of a normal individual. It is not

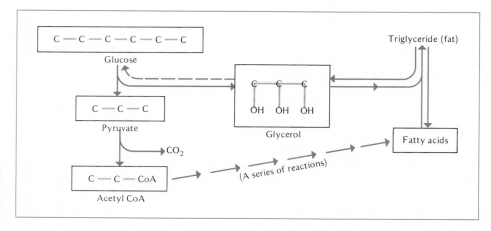

FIGURE 3-19. Conversion of carbohydrate to fat in the liver and adipose (fat storage) tissue.

necessary for there to be an excessively high carbohydrate intake to trigger formation of body fat. For *excessive* body fat to *accumulate*, however, there must be excessive kilocalorie consumption—a higher intake than one expends. So, while some conversion of food carbohydrate to body fat probably takes place every day in a normal adult, an equal amount of fat is quickly torn down if the person maintains a normal amount of body fat.

HOW MUCH CARBOHYDRATE IS SUGGESTED?

No RDA has been set for carbohydrates, but the Food and Nutrition Board notes that a *minimal* intake of 50 to 100 g/day prevents ketosis, and that intakes "considerably above this minimal level are desirable" [19].

Dietary Goals for the United States recommended that total carbohydrate intake be increased from 46 to 58 percent of total kilocalories, and that only 10 percent of total kilocalories should come from refined carbohydrates. Following these goals would mean that most Americans would cut their refined and processed sugar intakes by one-half, while doubling their complex carbohydrate and "natural sugar"—mostly fruit—intake. The guidelines in *Dietary Guidelines for Americans*, set by the U.S. Department of Agriculture and the Department of Health and Human Services, also recommended decreasing sugar intake and increasing complex carbohydrates. Doing so would increase dietary fiber and the intake of many vitamins and minerals. The Committee on Diet, Nutrition and Cancer of the National Academy of Sciences emphasized the importance of including fruits, vegetables, and whole-grain cereal products in the diet (Chapter 2).

Although human beings seem to be born with an appreciation of sweet foods, many people have become accustomed to unusually high sugar intakes. It is possible to "unlearn" the preference for very sweet foods. Some practical suggestions for increasing complex carbohydrates and decreasing refined sugar in the diet appear in Table 3-7.

ALCOHOL

About 90 percent of college students are believed to be alcohol users, while 30 percent or more reach a state of intoxication as often as once a month or more [20]. Low intakes of alcohol may be beneficial. People who drink one or (at most) two drinks of wine or other alcoholic beverage a day tend to have higher levels of high density lipoproteins (HDL) in their blood, substances that may be protective against heart disease [21] (see Chapter 3). But although a little may be good, a lot more is not better, for alcohol is a toxic drug.

In this section we discuss how the body absorbs and metabolizes alcohol, its toxic effects, and suggestions for moderating its use. Chapter 12 discusses how alcohol consumption influences the absorption, metabolism, and excretion of vitamins and minerals, while Chapter 13 discusses alcohol use in pregnancy.

The alcohol in beverages is ethyl alcohol, or ethanol (Figure 2-3). It is a

TABLE 3-7. SUGGESTIONS FOR INCREASING COMPLEX CARBOHYDRATES AND DECREASING REFINED SUGAR IN DIET

TO INCREASE COMPLEX CARBOHYDRATES

1. Increase number of main dishes containing starchy foods, such as rice and beans, macaroni and cheese, spaghetti and meat sauce, and tortillas and beans.
2. Choose more whole-grain breads, pasta, and cereals to increase dietary fiber.
3. Increase number of servings of bread and cereals, while cutting down on fat and sugar intake. Learn to enjoy the flavor of whole-grain breads without added butter or margarine. Home-baked breads are so good, it is easy to eat more of them.
4. Eat potatoes frequently, but with little fat. Potatoes are good sources of vitamin C, iron, and many other nutrients.

TO DECREASE REFINED SUGAR

1. Read food labels carefully, and avoid foods having one or several sugars or caloric sweeteners (such as corn syrup) listed among the first few ingredients.
2. Use fruit as the only sweetener on breakfast cereal.
3. Use juice-packed canned fruit in place of that packed in heavy (sugar) syrup.
4. Drink water or unsweetened fruit juice in place of a soft drink when you are thirsty.
5. When baking, cut down on amount of sugar in sweet breads, cookies, and cakes. Some cakes will fail if a large amount of sugar is not used. Find a recipe using lower amounts!
6. Consume fruit (without added sugar) in place of high-sugar desserts.
7. Substitute crackers, bread, popcorn, raw vegetables, or fruit for high-sugar snacks.

by-product of the oxidation of sugars for energy by yeast enzymes. Types of alcoholic beverages include wines, beers, and hard liquors (distilled spirits). Wines are made from the juice of grapes, berries, or other fruits, dandelions, honey, or rice. The alcohol content of wines varies from 9 to 20 percent, the higher percentages occurring in sherry, port, and sake. Beers are made from malt (barley grains) and vary in alcohol content from 3.2 to 4.5 percent for light beers to 6 to 7 percent for darker beers. Since high accumulations of alcohol stop yeast growth, the high concentrations of alcohol in hard liquors are achieved by distilling the fermented products of grains, sugar cane, molasses, or fruit juices. Examples of hard liquors are gin, rum, whisky, vodka, and brandy. "Proof" is a measure of the alcohol content of hard liquors. By dividing the proof in half, one finds the alcohol content in percentage—that is, 80 proof whisky is 40 percent alcohol.

Absorption

Although alcohol can be absorbed from the stomach, it is most efficiently absorbed from the duodenum and jejunum, probably because of the vast absorptive area there. Consuming food before drinking alcohol decreases the rate and extent of alcohol absorption. Studies suggest that delaying gastric emptying by consuming foods high in carbohydrates, fats, and dietary fiber reduces alcohol absorption [22]. This dilutes the concentration of alcohol in the stomach, delaying its absorption there and further delaying its entry into the duodenum where absorption is more rapid.

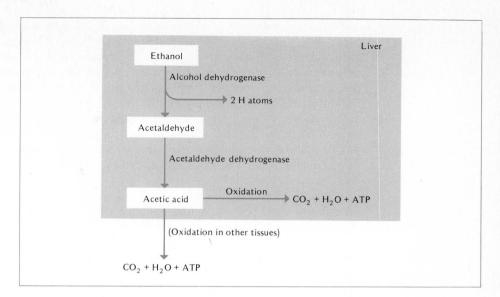

FIGURE 3-20. Oxidation of ethanol in the liver.

Metabolism

Ethanol is foreign to body tissues in the sense that they are unable to synthesize or store it, as they can synthesize and store carbohydrates and fats. The only way the body disposes of alcohol is to oxidize it, for only small amounts are lost through the lungs, sweat, and the kidneys. Practically all the ethanol oxidation in the body takes place in the liver [23].

The liver begins its oxidation of ethanol using the enzyme alcohol dehydrogenase, forming acetaldehyde while releasing two hydrogen atoms. A second liver enzyme, acetaldehyde dehydrogenase, oxidizes acetaldehyde to acetic acid, which is eventually oxidized to carbon dioxide and water by the liver and other body tissues (Figure 3-20). Much of the tissue damage in alcoholics comes from the hydrogen atoms and unoxidized acetaldehyde from the first reaction [23].

Although oxidation of ethanol outside the body yields 7 kcal per gram, the yield appears to be somewhat less when large quantities of alcohol are consumed and metabolized. This is because a second system of ethanol oxidation comes into play under these circumstances. This system is less efficient than the alcohol dehydrogenase system, and wastes some energy as heat, producing fewer than 7 kcal/g [23]. Nevertheless, alcohol oxidation *does* provide the body with kilocalories, even though not always as many as 7 kcal/g.

The liver metabolizes alcohol slowly, at an average rate of about 0.1 g/kg body weight/hour. An average 70-kg man will require about 2 hours to metabolize the alcohol in a 12-oz bottle of beer and 3 hours to metabolize that in a manhattan or martini. Individuals who are accustomed to drinking routinely adapt so as to metabolize alcohol somewhat more rapidly.

Excessive alcohol that the liver cannot metabolize enters the bloodstream and quickly reaches the brain. At first this results in a state of euphoria, often accompanied by release of inhibitions. The blood alcohol level increases rapidly as increasing amounts of alcohol are consumed over a short time period. As blood levels reach 0.10 to 0.15 pecent—the legal intoxication level in most states—poor eye and muscle coordination develop and speech and walking may be affected. Continued rapid increase in the blood alcohol level results in complete loss of control and eventually in coma. Death can result from respiratory failure as blood alcohol levels reach 0.5 percent or higher.

Dangers of heavy alcohol consumption include the risks of automobile or industrial accidents, serious liver disease, stroke, cancer of the mouth, throat, or esophagus and perhaps the liver, and injury to the absorptive surfaces of the stomach and small intestines. In addition, there is the danger of becoming addicted to alcohol.

Since alcohol is a toxic drug, it is important to control its use. Remember that the smaller your body and the less alcohol you are accustomed to, the less alcohol you can tolerate. Eat some food and wait awhile before you accept a drink; then drink it very slowly. Don't let people talk you into drinking more than you can tolerate and never take alcohol with drugs. At parties alternate drinks with plain soda or other mixers without alcohol.

SUMMARY

1 Carbohydrates include sugars, starches, and most of the components of dietary fiber, the portions of plants that are not digested by enzymes in the upper small intestines.

2 Carbohydrates are classified as monosaccharides, disaccharides, and polysaccharides. The most important monosaccharides are glucose, fructose, and galactose. The most important disaccharides are sucrose, maltose, and lactose, while the most important polysaccharides are starch, glycogen, and most of the dietary fiber components.

3 Americans today consume significantly more sugar and less starch than they did in 1909, and the largest amount of sugar consumed today is added by the manufacturer and not by the consumer at home.

4 The liver may use glucose for energy to support its own activities, to maintain the blood glucose level, to synthesize glycogen, or to synthesize fat. All body cells can use glucose for energy. Muscle cells also use it to synthesize glycogen, while adipose cells use it to synthesize fat.

5 The liver plays a central role in maintenance of the blood glucose level by obtaining glucose from glycogen breakdown, or by converting certain amino acids, glycerol, or lactic acid to glucose.

6 Insulin and glucagon are hormones that act to help regulate the level of blood glucose. Insulin tends to lower blood glucose levels, while glucagon tends to raise it.

7 When glucose is used for energy, it is oxidized in a stepwise manner to form carbon dioxide, water, and energy in the form of ATP (adenosine triphosphate).

8 Ethanol, the alcohol in beverages, is obtained by yeast fermentation of carbohydrates. In small amounts, it may be beneficial, but large does are toxic to tissues.

FOR DISCUSSION AND APPLICATION

1 Food Intake Record. As an ongoing activity in your study of nutrition, follow the directions in Appendix L for recording your 3-day food intake. You can then conveniently study various aspects of your diet as you progress through this textbook.
After totaling your 3-day intake of kilocalories and carbohydrates, evaluate it as follows:
(1) Calculate the percentage of your total kilocalorie intake that came from protein, fat, carbohydrate (abbreviated CHO), and alcohol. Multiply total grams of protein intake by 4, total grams of fat by 9, total grams of CHO by 4, and total grams of *pure* alcohol by 7 to obtain kilocalories from each. Add these together to get total kilocalories. (Upon completing your calculations, the percentages should add up to 100 percent.)

Then calculate the percentage of your total kilocalorie intake that came from each as follows:

$$\frac{\text{kcal from CHO}}{\text{total kcal intake}} \times 100 = \text{\% of total kcal furnished by CHO}$$

Follow the same procedure in estimating the percentage of total kilocalories that came from protein and fat.

(2) Compare the percentages you obtained with recommendations in *Dietary Goals for the United States* (Chapter 2).

(3) List the sources of sugar in your 3-day food intake. What problems do you encounter in doing this? Explain.

(4) From your knowledge of the specific sugars that occur in foods, list the sugars you consumed and their sources.

(5) You did not estimate your intake of dietary fiber. From your knowledge of food sources of dietary fiber, which foods in your 3-day record contributed dietary fiber? Would you estimate that your usual intake of dietary fiber is low? High? Defend your estimate.

2 Bring to class labels from soups, condiments (catsup, seasoning sauces, etc.), convenience foods (frozen, dried, or canned), and note all forms of sugar listed on the labels.

3 Study the sugar content of foods in Appendix E. Calculate the *amount* of sugar you would obtain from one serving (1 oz or 28 g) of several of the ready-to-eat breakfast cereals (follow directions in the introduction to Appendix E to do this calculation).

SUGGESTED READINGS

Smith, J. J., *Food for Sport*, Palo Alto, Calif.: Bull Publishing Co., 1976. This book provides information on the relationship between diet and athletic performance, including sections on the pregame meal and basic or nontraditional diets for the athlete.

Cavaiani, Mabel, *The High Fiber Cookbook*, Chicago: Contemporary Books, Inc., 1980. This book guides the reader to increase dietary fiber in usual recipes by using more fruit, vegetables, nuts, and whole-grain flours. Also included is general cooking information.

Wurtman, Richard J., "Nutrients that Modify Brain Function," *Scientific American*, 246(4):50–59, 1982. This article summarizes in a clear, concise way the research done in diet related to neurotransmitters, the subject of Nutrition in the News in this chapter.

4

FATS AND OTHER LIPIDS

Barry, although only in his early twenties, was concerned because many of his close relatives had died of heart disease. He decided to try a very low fat diet, said to be of possible benefit in preventing such disorders. He found that he had to eat many times during the day, and noticed that he consumed much more food than usual. Yet he lost weight on this diet. What properties of fat account for these changes when dietary fat intake is drastically reduced?

In an African country, an investigator found vitamin A deficiency among children, despite the fact that they ate large amounts of vegetables high in vitamin A value. Observing that their fat intake was unusually low, he cured their vitamin A deficiency simply by increasing fat in the diet. What explains this phenomenon?

In the early 1940s, infants fed skim milk formulas (devoid of fat) grew poorly, developed scaliness of the skin (eczema), and showed increased susceptibility to infection. Adding certain sources of fat to the diet caused all these symptoms to

94

disappear. What component of fat is necessary in the diet to prevent these symptoms?

A physician recommended that a patient decrease his intake of saturated fat and cholesterol. What *are* these substances, and what foods will the patient have to cut down on?

This chapter will address these questions as it examines the substances in foods classified as lipids and their properties, and discusses how they are modified in food processing and how they behave in the body. It will also consider changing patterns of fat consumption in the United States, and present recommendations for fat and cholesterol intake.

LIPIDS IN FOODS

Lipids are defined as substances that do not dissolve in water but dissolve in ether, chloroform, or other similar solvents. Among the lipids that will be discussed in this chapter are fats (technically called triglycerides), cholesterol, and phospholipids, such as lecithin. Since there is much current interest and discussion of fat (triglyceride) and cholesterol in foods, Figures 4-1 and 4-2 provide a picture of the amounts of these two lipids in many foods.

Fat (Triglyceride) in Foods

Cooking oils, butter, and margarines are high in fat. These, along with the fat on the outer part of meat, are the so-called visible fats, since you can easily see how much of these you eat. But much of the fat in foods is hidden. Figure 4-1 gives the percentage of fat in foods, beginning with oils and shortenings which are 100 percent fat (they contain no water). Butter, margarines, and mayonnaise are about 80 percent fat since they contain water and other substances. Hidden fats are present in the muscle part of meat as "marbleized fat"; even if you trim off the visible fat, the lean meat still contains from 4 to 15 percent fat. Other foods containing hidden fats are cakes, pies, cookies, doughnuts, Danish pastry, nuts, ice cream, olives, avocadoes, cheeses, and peanut butter. Whole milk, which is about 3.5 percent fats, contains 8.5 grams of fat per cup. Other milks are lower in fats; for example, "2 percent milk" contains 4.9 grams and "1 percent milk" contains 2.4 grams of fat per cup, respectively. Skim milk contains a mere 0.2 grams of fat per cup. Foods very low in fat include most vegetables and fruits, grains, beans, plain bread, and pasta (spaghetti, macaroni, etc.), and a few desserts such as angel food cake and gelatin desserts.

Cholesterol in Foods

Cholesterol occurs only in foods of animal origin. Brains, kidneys, and liver contain the largest amounts of cholesterol among foods, but egg yolk is probably more frequently eaten than these foods, and is the largest single source of cholesterol in most American diets (Figure 4-2). Other sources of cholesterol in the diet are meats, poultry, some kinds of fish and shellfish, and dairy products.

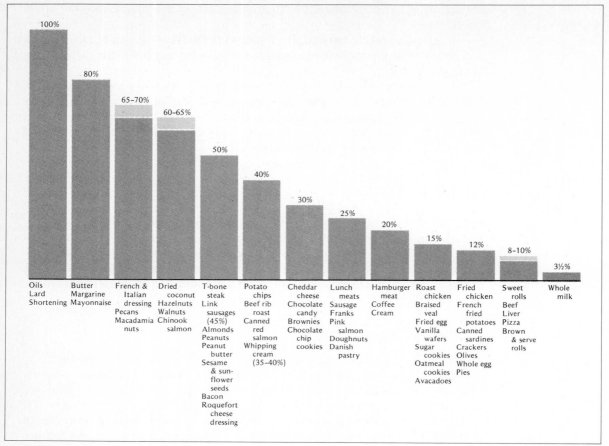

100%													
	80%												
		65–70%											
			60–65%										
				50%									
					40%								
						30%							
							25%						
								20%					
									15%				
										12%			
											8–10%		
												3½%	
Oils Lard Shortening	Butter Margarine Mayonnaise	French & Italian dressing Pecans Macadamia nuts	Dried coconut Hazelnuts Walnuts Chinook salmon	T-bone steak Link sausages (45%) Almonds Peanuts Peanut butter Sesame & sun- flower seeds Bacon Roquefort cheese dressing	Potato chips Beef rib roast Canned red salmon Whipping cream (35–40%)	Cheddar cheese Chocolate candy Brownies Chocolate chip cookies	Lunch meats Sausage Franks Pink salmon Doughnuts Danish pastry	Hamburger meat Coffee Cream	Roast chicken Braised veal Fried egg Vanilla wafers Sugar cookies Oatmeal cookies Avacadoes	Fried chicken French fried potatoes Canned sardines Crackers Whole egg Pies	Sweet rolls Beef Liver Pizza Brown & serve rolls	Whole milk	

FIGURE 4-1. Percentage (by weight) of fat (triglyceride) in foods. (Source: Watt, B.K., and A.L. Merrill, *Composition of Foods, Raw, Processed, Prepared*, Agriculture Handbook 8, Washington, D.C.: USDA, 1963.)

IMPORTANCE OF FAT (TRIGLYCERIDE) IN THE DIET

The mass media have focused increasing attention on research examining the possible relationships between an overabundance of dietary fat and health problems. This topic will be discussed in Chapter 5. Before the reader considers such relationships, however, it is necessary to understand first why fat is such an important nutrient.

Benefits of Fat

Concentrated Source of Energy   Fats are important as a concentrated source of energy or kilocalories. Fats furnish 9 kcal/g, while carbohydrates and proteins furnish only 4 kcal/g. A diet very low in fat becomes quite bulky because greater quantities of food must be consumed to achieve one's kilocalorie need. For example, 1 cup of cooked macaroni furnishes 190 kcal, while 1 cup of rich ice cream furnishes 350 kcal. Obviously then it is necessary to consume much more food per day if the diet is almost free of fat than if 42 percent of the total kilocalories comes from fat, as in the usual American diet. This is why Barry, when following the very low fat diet mentioned at the beginning of the chapter, found he had to eat so much food. Apparently he was not able to eat a large enough amount of food, however, to prevent weight loss, a common experience on such a diet.

Accumulating Body Fat   Is there any advantage to accumulating fat in the body? Normally, fat accumulates in adipose (fat) cells under the skin (subcutaneous fat) and around the kidneys, holding them in place and protecting them against jarring and jostling. A certain amount of subcutaneous fat helps to keep the body warm, since fat is a poor heat conductor and prevents loss of body heat. Emaciated (extremely thin) people, such as those with anorexia nervosa (see Chapter 8) must wear warm clothing even in summer because they lack subcutaneous fat. On the other hand, very fat people need to avoid strenuous exercise in hot weather because their fat layers prevent adequate dissipation of body heat. Body temperature may rise to dangerous levels as a result. From the standpoint of regulating body temperature, it is preferable to avoid either too little or too much accumulation of body fat.

Body fat accumulations represent nature's method of providing animals

FIGURE 4-2. Cholesterol content of foods. (Source: Feeley, R.M., P.E. Criner, and B.K. Watt, "Cholesterol Content of Food," Reprinted by permission from *Journal of the American Dietetic Association,* 61:134, 1972.)

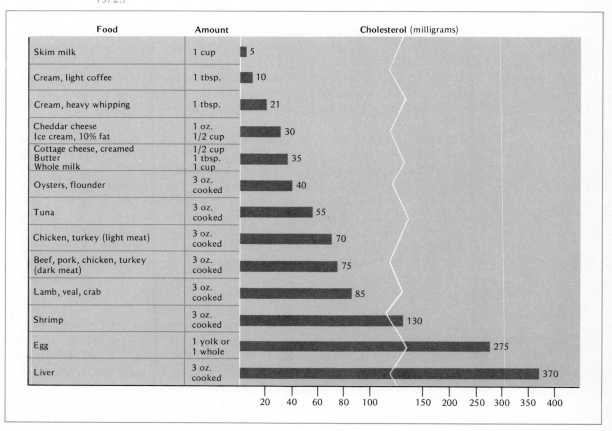

(including human beings) with stored energy, ready to be used whenever food is too scarce to meet the energy need. Fat is an ideal source of emergency energy because a great deal of energy is concentrated into a relatively small mass. Only ¼ lb of pure fat will furnish 1000 kcal, compared with a little more than ½ lb of pure carbohydrate. Obviously, using a more concentrated rather than a less concentrated form of energy as the storage form means that animals need to carry less weight around to ensure having a ready supply of energy. The body is able to accumulate a great deal of adipose tissue, while the amount of glycogen stored in the body is limited, as discussed in Chapter 3.

A person who has a good store of body fat therefore has an advantage over a thin person in case of an emergency in which food is unavailable for long periods. Historically, adequate fat stores were essential to survival, since the food supply was often erratic. Today, however, food is available in abundant amounts to most Americans, and large accumulations of adipose tissue are actually thought to be detrimental rather than advantageous (Chapter 8).

Satiety Value   The case of Barry demonstrates another benefit of fat in the diet. He found that, on his very low fat diet, he had to eat very frequently throughout the day. (This could be an advantage or a disadvantage, depending on how much time he had to devote to eating, and how much he enjoyed the food allowed on the diet). Foods very low in fat have poor *satiety value*. In other words, one doesn't feel satisfied very long after eating them. On the other hand, foods high in fat remain in the stomach longer, preventing the feeling of hunger that occurs when the stomach is empty. A fatty meal (50 g of fat) gradually leaves the stomach over 4 to 6 hours, for example [1]. Eating too large an amount of foods high in fat can result in discomfort in individuals who have adapted to a relatively low fat intake of 10 to 20 percent of total kilocalories. The discomfort is probably due to the slow motility of the stomach resulting from the high fat intake.

Palatability   Fats provide a characteristic tactile sensation or "mouth feel" that contributes to the enjoyment of certain foods. The creamy smoothness of ice cream, hollandaise sauce, and whipped cream is due to the fat. The rich, velvety feeling on the tongue of chocolate cake, and the crisp texture of butter cookies also come from the fat. To demonstrate how unaware you may be of the contribution of fat to the palatability of food, pop some popcorn without adding fat before, during, or after the popping. Can you manage to eat a cup of it? Do you *enjoy* eating it? One reason Barry may be losing weight on his low-fat diet is that he may find the food so unpalatable that he can't eat enough to maintain his weight. In general, at least 15 to 20 percent of the kilocalories need to be present as fat for a diet to be palatable.

Flavor   In addition to palatability, many fats are prized for their characteristic flavors. Certain fats have been traditionally preferred by specific ethnic or regional groups. For example, olive oil is the favorite fat of Mediterranean populations, while peanut oil is used by the Chinese, and butter by Scandinavians. Fats take up other flavors readily, creating endless possibilities for the adventurous chef to develop subtle flavorings in foods. For this reason, many chefs are reluctant to specialize in low-fat, low-kilocalorie creations because the opportunities to develop enticing blends of flavors are drastically diminished when fat is limited. Populations do learn to accept new and different fats, however, as demonstrated by the wide use of margarines and almost flavorless cooking oils in the United States since 1945.

Aid in Absorbing Fat-Soluble Vitamins   Fat must be present in the intestines at the proper time and place to aid in absorption of the fat-soluble vitamins (vitamins A, D, E, and K). Carotene in dark-green and yellow vegetables is converted, after absorption, to vitamin A, but is poorly absorbed if insufficient fat is present at the time of absorption. This explains why the children described at the beginning of the chapter were deficient in vitamin A, even though they consumed large amounts of carotene. The amount of fat in their diets, approximately 7 percent of the kilocalories, was insufficient to permit adequate absorption of carotene [2]. Persons like Barry who are consuming very low fat diets should consume at least 10 to 15 percent of their calories as fat to permit normal absorption of carotene and the fat-soluble vitamins.

Essential Fatty Acid   One of the most important reasons to include some fat in the diet is to supply linoleic acid, the *essential fatty acid*. As we noted in the Introduction, an essential nutrient is one that must be obtained from food because the body is unable to synthesize it, at least in the amounts needed. Absence of an essential nutrient will produce specific symptoms, and in the case of many nutrients, results eventually in serious disability or death.

Linoleic acid deficiency has never been observed to occur in population groups consuming their usual diets, but has occurred in specialized situations in which fat has been almost totally excluded from the diet. One example of such a situation was the unintentional exclusion of linoleic acid when formulas based on skim milk were fed to infants, described at the beginning of this chapter. At that time, physicians were unaware of the body's need for linoleic acid, but infant formulas today all contain an adequate amount.

Another example of an unusual situation resulting in linoleic acid deficiency involved infants and adults who had to be fed parenterally, that is by a catheter which empties into a large vein near the heart. For this purpose it was necessary to use a liquid formula devoid of fat. The patients developed severe scaly dermatitis (skin inflammation) that cleared up completely when linoleic acid was given by mouth. One of the tests for deciding that a nutrient is essential in the diet is to document that symptoms that develop in its absence completely disappear upon feeding the pure nutrient.

Several years ago linoleic, linolenic, and arachidonic acids all were thought to be essential in the diet. We know now, however, that arachidonic acid is synthesized in the body from linoleic, and that there is too little arachidonic acid in foods, anyway, to meet body needs. Therefore, linoleic acid is the one required in the diet. While at present linolenic acid is considered not to be essential, at least one case of linolenic acid deficiency was reported to result in nervous system damage in a child. The symptoms were relieved by giving pure linolenic acid [3]. Scientific work continues on whether or not linolenic acid is a dietary essential. It should be understood that normal diets adequate in linoleic acid are also adequate in linolenic acid.

Linoleic and arachidonic acids function in the body as important components of the normal structure of cell membranes. These fatty acids are therefore vital for the normal function of nearly all cells. Arachidonic acid appears to be more important than linoleic acid in cellular metabolic functions, but the body easily obtains arachidonic as needed from linoleic. Arachidonic acid, in addition to its structural functions, is used to form hormonelike substances called *prostaglandins*, which appear to have a wide range of uses in the body.

The amount of linoleic acid needed in the diet is relatively small. The amount recommended is 2 percent of total kilocalories for adults, 3 percent for full-term infants and 4.5 percent for premature infants. But how much is this in terms of food? Figure 4-3 shows you how to find out. Safflower, sunflower, and corn oils are high in linoleic acid, but certain margarines and walnuts also contain relatively large amounts (Appendix C).

To recap: Fats (triglycerides) are important in the diet for satiety value and for palatability and flavor. They are important in the body as an aid in absorption of fat-soluble vitamins and carotene, and as sources of kilocalories and of linoleic acid, the essential fatty acid. In addition, they provide protective padding for vital organs, and help regulate the body temperature by acting as insulators under the skin.

Sharon, a college student, wondered how much corn oil would provide her with the recommended amount of linoleic acid. She first marshalled the facts:

After considering these facts, she calculated the daily intake of corn oil needed to supply the recommended amount of linoleic acid:

FACTS

(a) 2 percent of total kcal intake should come from linoleic acid for the adult

(b) 1 g of any pure fat, including linoleic acid, supplies 9 kcal

(c) corn oil contains 7.8 g linoleic acid per tablespoon (3 teaspoons) (Appendix C)

(d) Sharon needs 2000 kcal/day to maintain her normal weight.

CALCULATIONS

(1) 2000 kcal × 2% = 2000 kcal × .02 = 40 kcal needed in the form of linoleic acid

(2) 40 kcal ÷ 9 kcal/g = 4.4 g of linoleic acid

(3) if 3 teaspoons of corn oil contain 7.8 g linoleic acid, x teaspoons contain 4.4 g. Solve for x.

(4) Answer: $1^2/3$ (1.6) teaspoons of corn oil contain 4.4 g of linoleic acid.

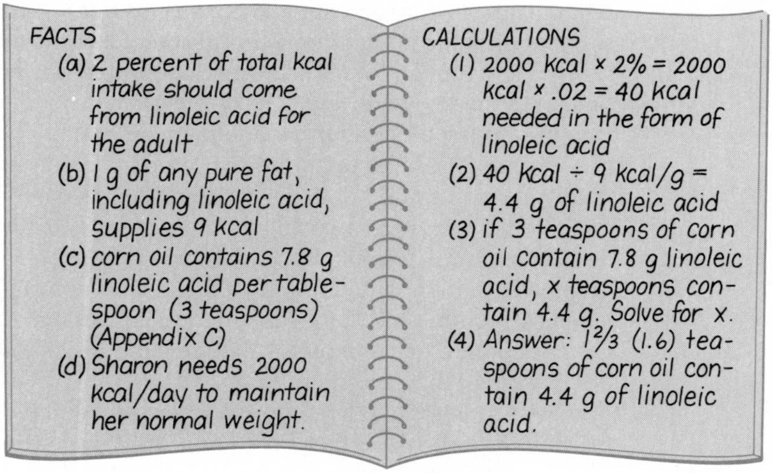

If Sharon considered other fatty foods as her sole source of linoleic acid, she would find the following amounts would meet her recommendation:

$1\frac{1}{3}$ tsp. safflower oil; $2\frac{1}{3}$ tsp. mayonnaise; $4\frac{1}{4}$ tsp. vegetable shortening; 44 tsp. butter (very low in linoleic acid).

FIGURE 4-3. Estimating amounts of foods that furnish the linoleic acid recommendation for an adult each day.

COMPOSITION OF FATS

In discussing linoleic acid, we did not mention that this fatty acid is one of the *polyunsaturated* fatty acids. To be an informed consumer today one needs to understand terms such as saturated, unsaturated and polyunsaturated fat, hydrogenated fat, and cholesterol. Furthermore, knowledge of fat composition is needed to appreciate the processes of fat digestion, absorption, and metabolism.

At the outset, it is essential to realize that the term *fat* is properly applied only to *triglycerides*. Triglycerides are one of several lipids of interest in nutrition. While fat is a lipid, all lipids are not fats (triglycerides).

Triglycerides are formed in food and in the body by the chemical reaction of three fatty acid molecules and one glycerol molecule, as indicated in Figure 4-4. *Glycerol* is a molecule in which three carbon atoms are joined. Each carbon atom has an —OH group, made up of one oxygen atom attached to one hydrogen atom. The —OH group is called a hydroxyl group. *Fatty acids* consist of chains of carbon atoms hooked together with an acid (—COOH) group at the end of their molecules. The remaining carbon atoms have hydrogen atoms (—H) attached. When a triglyceride forms, as illustrated in Figure 4-4, the —OH of the glycerol combines with the —H (hydrogen) of the fatty acid, the water formed splits out, and the carbon of glycerol joins a carbon of the fatty acid through oxygen (O). When a fatty acid has become joined in this way to each of the three glycerol carbons, a new compound called a triglyceride forms.

Mono- and *diglycerides* are derived from triglycerides. Monoglycerides have only one fatty acid molecule attached to either the middle carbon or one of the end carbons of glycerol (Figure 4-5). These compounds are produced from triglyceride during digestion, discussed later in this chapter. They are also added to some foods by the manufacturer because they are good emulsifying agents. Emulsifying agents help hold two liquids that do not usually mix, such as oil and water, in close association so they do not separate.

The fatty acids that occur most commonly in foods are listed in Table 4-1.

Saturated and Unsaturated Fatty Acids

The first group of fatty acids listed in Table 4-1 is *saturated* fatty acids. As explained in Chapter 3, carbon has four valence electrons and has a tendency to

FIGURE 4-4. Formation of triglyceride (fat) from glycerol and fatty acids. *Only the —COOH (acid group) of the fatty acid is shown, written HO—$\overset{\overset{\textstyle O}{\|}}{C}$. The —R indicates the rest of the molecule. —R_1, R_2, and R_3 signify that each fatty acid is different in structure from the others, as is the case in most food fats.

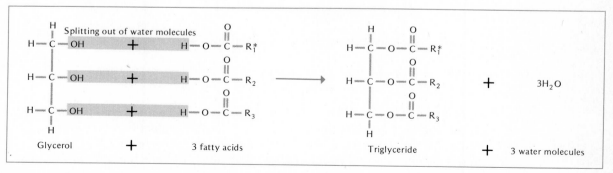

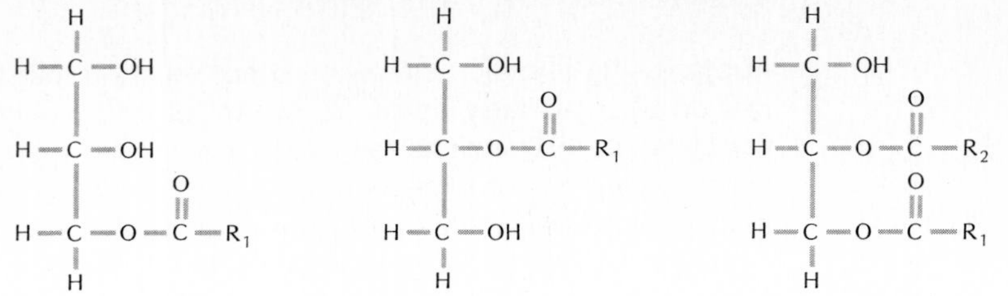

FIGURE 4-5. Mono- and diglycerides. The fatty acid attached to the glycerol in a monoglyceride may be attached either to one of the end carbons (a), or to the middle carbon (b). In a diglyceride, two fatty acids are attached to the glycerol molecule (c).

(A) Monoglyceride   (B) Monoglyceride   (C) Diglyceride

TABLE 4-1. CLASSIFICATION, CHEMICAL COMPOSITION, AND FOOD SOURCES OF FATTY ACIDS IN FOODS

CLASSIFI- CATION	COMMON NAME	NO. OF CARBONS AND DOUBLE BONDS*	FORMULA†	FOOD SOURCES
Saturated	Butyric	4:0	$CH_3CH_2CH_2COOH$	Butter
	Caproic	6:0	$CH_3(CH_2)_4COOH$	Butter
	Caprylic	8:0	$CH_3(CH_2)_6COOH$	Coconut oil, butter
	Capric	10:0	$CH_3(CH_2)_8COOH$	Palm oil, butter, coconut oil
	Lauric	12:0	$CH_3(CH_2)_{10}COOH$	Coconut oil, butter
	Myristic	14:0	$CH_3(CH_2)_{12}COOH$	Butter, coconut oil, nutmeg fat
	Palmitic	16:0	$CH_3(CH_2)_{14}COOH$	Beef, pork, and lamb; most vegetable fats
	Stearic	18:0	$CH_3(CH_2)_{16}COOH$	Beef, pork, and lamb; most vegetable fats
	Arachidic	20:0	$CH_3(CH_2)_{18}COOH$	Peanut oil and lard
Monoun- saturated	Palmitoleic	16:1	$CH_3(CH_2)_5CH=CH(CH_2)_7COOH$	Butter and seed oils
	Oleic	18:1	$CH_3(CH_2)_7CH=CH(CH_2)_7COOH$	Olive oil, meats, and most other fats and oils
Polyun- saturated	Linoleic	18:2	$CH_3(CH_2)_4CH=CHCH_2CH=$ $CH(CH_2)_7COOH$	Corn, cottonseed, soybean, sunflower, safflower oils; poultry, walnuts
	Linolenic	18:3	$CH_3CH_2(CH=CHCH_2)_2CH=$ $CH(CH_2)_7COOH$	Soybean oil, other vegetable oils, egg yolk
	Arachidonic	20:4	$CH_3(CH_2)_4(CH=CHCH_2)_4$ $(CH_2)_2COOH$	Very little in foods

*First figure indicates number of carbons; figure after colon indicates number of double bonds.

†To save space. $(CH_2)_4$, for example, means the group $—\overset{\displaystyle H}{\underset{\displaystyle H}{C}}—$ occurs four times in the formula.

form covalent bonds. Each carbon atom in a correctly written chemical formula must have four covalent bonds, since each single covalent bond represents the sharing of one pair of electrons, each atom contributing one to the pair. Many fatty acids have some double bonds. A double covalent bond represents the sharing of two pairs of electrons between the two atoms involved. *Saturated* fatty acids have only single covalent bonds between the carbon atoms in the chain, and each carbon atom holds all the hydrogen of which it is capable (Figure 4-6). *Unsaturated* fatty acids, on the other hand, have one or more double bonds between carbons. Less than the full load of hydrogen is held by the carbons having a double bond between them, and the double bond is said to be the point of *unsaturation*.

The unsaturated fatty acids having only one double bond are classified as *mono*unsaturated (*mono-* means "one"), while those having two or more double bonds are classified as *poly*unsaturated (*poly-* means "many" or "more than one"). Table 4-1 lists food sources of specific saturated, monounsaturated, and polyunsaturated fatty acids. Generally, foods high in saturated fats include beef, pork, lamb, coconut and palm oils, butter, whole milk, cream, and hydrogenated fats. Those high in polyunsaturated fats include most salad or cooking oils, special margarines, and walnuts.

FIGURE 4-6. Differences among saturated, monounsaturated, and polyunsaturated fatty acids. (a) In a saturated fatty acid, each carbon (C) holds all the hydrogen (H) of which it is capable, and there are single covalent bonds between carbon atoms. (b) In a monounsaturated fatty acid, one pair of carbon atoms holds only half as much hydrogen as is possible, forming a double covalent bond (══). (c) In a polyunsaturated fatty acid, more than one double bond occurs in the C chain.

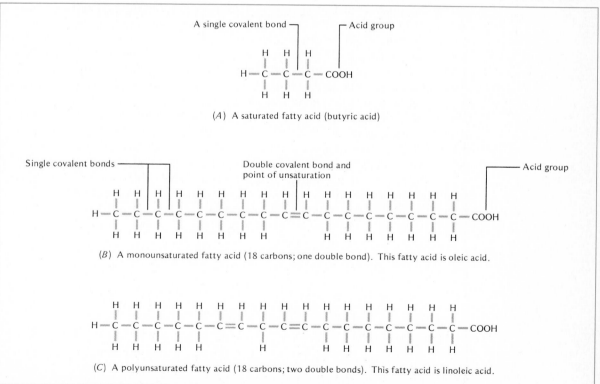

(A) A saturated fatty acid (butyric acid)

(B) A monounsaturated fatty acid (18 carbons; one double bond). This fatty acid is oleic acid.

(C) A polyunsaturated fatty acid (18 carbons; two double bonds). This fatty acid is linoleic acid.

The amount of saturated and polyunsaturated fats in the diet is of interest because of their possible relationship to the blood cholesterol level and coronary heart disease. Saturated fatty acids in the diet raise blood cholesterol levels, while polyunsaturated fatty acids lower it. Persons in a population having high blood cholesterol levels have a greater chance of developing coronary heart disease than those with low levels [4] (see Chapter 5).

The ratio of dietary polyunsaturated fat to saturated fat in the diet (the P/S ratio) is used by physicians and nutritionists in counseling people who are advised to lower their blood cholesterol values. To calculate the P/S ratio, divide grams of dietary polyunsaturated fat by the grams of dietary saturated fat. An optimal ratio is thought to be 1, while a ratio below 1 indicates relatively too much saturated fat in the diet. Values for saturated fatty acids and the polyunsaturated fatty acid, linoleic acid, in foods can be found in Appendix C.

Hydrogenation of Fats

Hydrogenation is a commercial process used to convert oils or softer fats into more nearly solid or plastic forms that can be spread or molded. Margarines and shortenings are made by this process. During hydrogenation, the manufacturer adds hydrogen to fats or oils having double bonds, causing some of the bonds to break, and allowing the carbons to take up additional hydrogen (Figure 4-7). In the process, the fat becomes more highly saturated.

Hydrogenation of fats also causes some of the unsaturated fatty acids to become *trans* fatty acids. *Trans* fatty acids still retain their double bonds, but differ in physical shape from the original fatty acid (Figure 4-8). An *isomer* is one of two or more substances having the same molecular formula but showing different properties because of different spatial arrangements of the atoms in the molecule. Most unsaturated fatty acids occurring naturally in foods are *cis* isomers, while hydrogenation of unsaturated fats produces many *trans* isomers. Because of their different shapes, investigators are trying to find out if high intakes of *trans* fatty acids contribute to coronary heart disease or other diseases [5]. Some investigators believe the *trans* fatty acids may function in the body in much the same way as do saturated fats, but work is just beginning on this question.

Manufacturers are required to state on the label which specific fats have been *added* to a food, allowing the consumer to decide whether or not a product meets his or her requirements. For example, if a person has been told by a

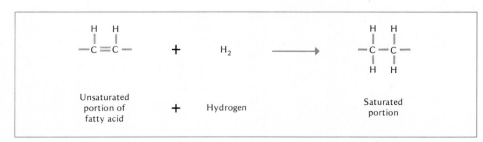

FIGURE 4-7.
Hydrogenation. Some of the unsaturated portions of the fatty acids become saturated, as hydrogen atoms add onto the carbons after the double bond is broken.

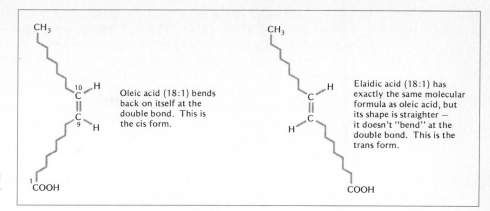

Oleic acid (18:1) bends back on itself at the double bond. This is the cis form.

Elaidic acid (18:1) has exactly the same molecular formula as oleic acid, but its shape is straighter — it doesn't "bend" at the double bond. This is the trans form.

FIGURE 4-8. Cis and trans isomers of fatty acids.

physician to reduce her intake of saturated fat, she would want to avoid a cracker for which the label ingredient list states "vegetable shortening (contains one or more of the following: partially hydrogenated soybean oil; palm oil; coconut oil)." Notice that if the label had merely stated "vegetable oil," that would not help the consumer because palm and coconut oils are vegetable oils, but highly saturated. The manufacturer is allowed to list two or three different fat sources that *may* be in the product because it is economically important for the manufacturer to be able to use the fat source that is least expensive at a given time. The kind of fat naturally present in a food, such as that in milk, does not appear on the label.

PROPERTIES OF FAT

When a chef chills a pot of oxtail soup, then removes the solidified fat from the surface she makes use of several properties of fat: (1) A specified volume of fat is lighter in weight than is the same volume of water, therefore the fat floats on the surface of water; (2) fats are insoluble in water; and (3) fats become liquid when heated to their specific melting points, but solidify at some temperature below the melting point that is characteristic of each fat. The chef could observe an additional physical property if she placed some of the removed fat on a plain sheet of paper. A translucent spot would form, typical of greasy substances.

Whether or not a fat is liquid or solid at room temperature depends partly upon its fatty acid composition. Fats that are liquid at room temperature are called oils, and are liquid for one of two reasons: either they are high in unsaturated fatty acids, as is the case for olive, corn, safflower, cottonseed, and soybean oils; or they are high in short- or medium-chain saturated fatty acids, as in coconut oil. (Short-chain fatty acids are those containing two to four carbons, while medium-chain ones contain six to 10 carbons.) On the other hand, fats having long-chain saturated fatty acids (more than 12 carbons per molecule) are more apt to be solid at room temperature. Hydrogenation, as it increases the degree of saturation of a fat and the number of *trans* fatty acids, also causes a fat to become more nearly solid.

Fats also have characteristic smoke points. The smoke point is the temperature at which visible fumes are given off, indicating that chemical decomposition of the fat has begun. Heating a fat to its smoke point breaks down some of the triglyceride to free fatty acids and glycerol. Further heating causes breakdown of the glycerol, forming a compound called *acrolein*. Acrolein has a pungent, unpleasant odor and is highly irritating to the eyes and mucous membranes. Fats chosen for deep-fat frying should be those with high smoke points, such as corn, cottonseed, and peanut oils. Butter and lard are unsuitable for deep-fat frying because they decompose at relatively low temperatures.

Sometimes consumers ask whether or not fats used in frying foods commercially might be harmful when consumed. Studies with laboratory rats indicate no toxic effects when fats actually used commercially for frying were fed at high levels. Only so-called "laboratory-heated fats," which have been heated alone at temperatures between 200 to 300°C for several days have been demonstrated to be toxic to experimental animals. Fats used in frying foods have not been subject to such extreme treatment, and toxicity does not seem to be a problem [6]. Nutritionists are concerned about fried foods because of their high kilocalorie and high fat content.

Unsaturated fatty acids, such as those in olive, corn, soybean, and safflower oils, are more subject to spoilage than saturated fatty acids due to the ease with which oxygen can cause their double bonds to split, resulting in short-chain compounds with disagreeable flavors and odors. The resulting fat is said to be rancid. Whether or not consumption of rancid fat is harmful is not known, but the flavors and odors prevent most people from consuming them. Manufacturers stand to lose money if their products containing fat become rancid quickly, and often add *antioxidants* to prevent this reaction with oxygen. Antioxidants tend to take up oxygen themselves, preventing the fat from doing so.

Most unsaturated oils contain vitamin E, which is a natural antioxidant present in the sources from which oils are obtained. Some manufacturers, therefore, do not add additional antioxidants to oils, but these oils should be protected against oxidation by refrigerating them in the store and at home. Commonly added antioxidants include propyl gallate, BHA (butylated hydroxyanisole), and BHT (butylated hydroxytoluene).

LIPIDS OTHER THAN FAT

So far we have dwelt on fats (triglycerides), but other lipids are equally necessary for normal body functions. The fat-soluble vitamins (vitamins A, D, E, and K) are classified as lipids, but are discussed in a separate chapter (Chapter 11). Most important among lipids are cholesterol and phospholipids.

Cholesterol

Cholesterol is a lipid so important that the body can manufacture all it needs and is therefore not dependent on dietary cholesterol. Cholesterol plays many important roles in the body: (1) It is an important structural component of all the membranes in body cells, and is absolutely necessary for normal development of brain and other nervous tissue. Cholesterol is the chief substance in skin that makes it impervious to water. (2) The breakdown of cholesterol by the liver produces bile salts without which digestion of fats could not occur. (3) Cholesterol is a *precursor* to several important compounds, meaning that it is a substance from which other compounds are synthesized. Many hormones, including the sex hormones, are synthesized in the body from cholesterol. In addition, *7-dehydrocholesterol* is synthesized from cholesterol. This compound is present in the skin and, when exposed to ultraviolet light (sunlight), produces vitamin D.

Interest in cholesterol in the diet centers around observations that high levels of cholesterol in the blood increase one's chances of developing coronary heart disease (see Chapter 5).

Cholesterol should not be confused with fat (triglyeride). The chemical structure of cholesterol is not even remotely like that of triglyceride (Figure 4-9).

As mentioned earlier, cholesterol occurs only in *animal* foods, and sources are shown in Figure 4-2 and in Appendix F.

Phospholipids

Like cholesterol, phospholipids are important structural components of all cell membranes. Without them, cells would be unable to survive. They are essential components of the structure of brain and other nervous tissue. Phospholipids are also important in the structure of liproproteins, the substances that carry triglyceride and cholesterol in the blood.

Lecithin is probably the phospholipid best known to general readers. A molecule of lecithin contains one molecule of glycerol and two fatty acid molecules, joined in the same way as in triglycerides. Lecithins differ from triglycerides, however, because phosphate and choline are attached to the third carbon of the glycerol molecule (Figure 4-10). Although extravagant claims are made for lecithin in popular magazines and books, research studies do not support the claim that lecithin granules or capsules will lower blood cholesterol levels or otherwise improve health. Few harmful effects of lecithin consumption have been reported, except that the fatty acids increase the kilocalorie intake. The human body is able to synthesize all the phospholipids it needs, including lecithin, and therefore is not dependent on dietary sources.

FIGURE 4-9. Cholesterol and cholesterol esters. Cholesterol belongs to the class of lipids called sterols. The body synthesizes this complex molecule from the 2-carbon compound, *acetate,* the active form of which is *acetyl CoA* (Chapter 3).

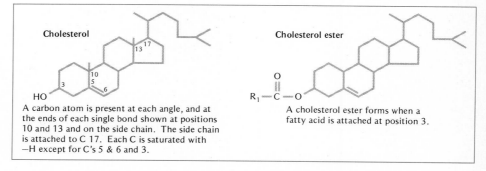

Cholesterol

A carbon atom is present at each angle, and at the ends of each single bond shown at positions 10 and 13 and on the side chain. The side chain is attached to C 17. Each C is saturated with —H except for C's 5 & 6 and 3.

Cholesterol ester

A cholesterol ester forms when a fatty acid is attached at position 3.

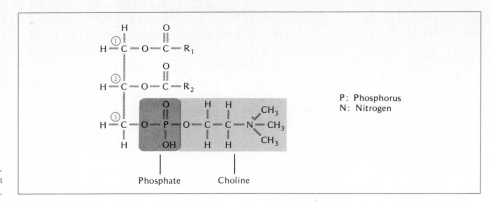

FIGURE 4-10.
Lecithin, a
phospholipid.

Lipids other than triglyceride generally furnish very little of the energy need of the body, although it is possible that some of the fatty acids in lecithin, for example, if consumed in large quantities, could be used for energy. Triglycerides are clearly the only important energy source among the lipids in foods.

DIGESTION

The goal of fat digestion is to convert fat to simpler forms that the body can absorb, chiefly to monoglycerides, fatty acids, and glycerol. Because triglycerides and most of the digestion products are insoluble in water, the body uses bile salts to make them more soluble in the watery medium of the intestines.

We shall follow the digestion of lipids in a muffin, as we followed the digestion of carbohydrates in Chapter 3. These lipids might include those shown in Figure 4-11. Fats in this recipe come from oil, milk, and egg. If the oil is corn, cottonseed, or safflower oil, the fatty acids are likely to be long-chained polyunsaturated ones, while the whole milk triglycerides contain small amounts of medium- and short-chain fatty acids. The egg furnishes chiefly monounsaturated fats, but also provides rather large amounts of cholesterol. Eggs also contain phospholipids, including lecithin.

FIGURE 4-11. Lipids present in the ingredients in a muffin recipe. (Source of values: *Composition of Foods. Dairy and Egg Products,* Agriculture Handbook No. 8-1, revised 1976; *Fats and Oils,* Agriculture Handbook No. 8-4, revised 1979. Agriculture Research Service, USDA, Washington, D.C.)

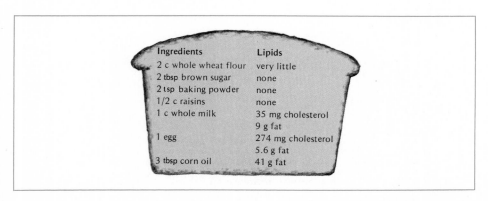

No fat digestion occurs in the mouth, and no significant amount occurs in the stomach. However, a lipase secreted by glands in the throat may emulsify some fats in the stomach. In addition, *gastric lipase* (secreted in the stomach) is active in the infant, but digests little fat in the adult [7]. Its digestive function is limited to triglycerides containing short- and medium-chain fatty acids. The presence of fat in the acid chyme stimulates release of the hormones *cholecystokinin-pancreozymin* (CCK-PZ) and *gastric inhibitory polypeptide* (GIP) when chyme begins to enter the duodenum from the stomach. These hormones decrease the motility of the stomach and decrease the rate of stomach emptying. After a meal very high in fat, several hours may lapse before the stomach empties.

If we now consider the fats and other lipids in the muffin, we realize that little change occurs until they enter the duodenum. There they encounter the very powerful enzyme from the pancreas, *pancreatic lipase*. This enzyme attacks the fats in the oil, milk, and eggs, producing chiefly monoglycerides, fatty acids, and glycerol [7] (Figure 4-12). This enzyme catalyzes the removal of fatty acids (FA) attached to either position 1 or 3 on the triglyceride molecule. It cannot remove FA from position 2. Therefore, in step 3 (Figure 4-12), a different enzyme—an

FIGURE 4-12. Digestion of fat by pancreatic lipase.

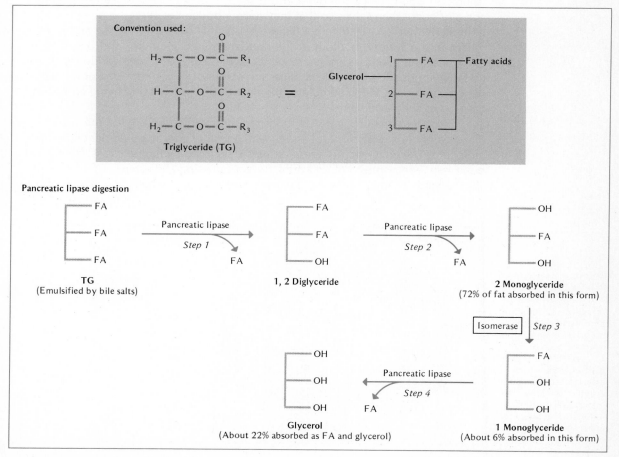

isomerase present in the small intestine—moves the FA of the 2-monoglyceride to position 1. Pancreatic lipase then is able to remove the FA (step 4). The chief products of pancreatic lipase digestion are therefore monoglycerides, glycerol, and fatty acids, although some diglycerides are also formed. Unsaturated fatty acids in triglycerides (such as in corn oil) are digested more rapidly than saturated ones. An *intestinal lipase*, situated just inside the intestinal mucosal cells, breaks the fatty acid off the 2-monoglyceride as it is absorbed, freeing glycerol and a fatty acid.

Bile, secreted by the liver, must be present in the small intestines for fat digestion to take place. Bile salts, formed from the breakdown of cholesterol in the liver, act as emulsifying agents. An emulsifying agent is capable of keeping two nonmixing liquids such as oil and water from separating. As you know from previous experience, when you pour oil into water, the oil particles join together and soon collect on top of the water. Adding an emulsifying agent, such as egg yolk or bile salts, and shaking the mixture causes the oil layer to break up into tiny oily particles dispersed throughout the water. The emulsifying agent (emulsifier) is able to accomplish this seeming miracle because one end of its molecule is soluble in water, while the other end is soluble in oil. The emulsifier molecules actually orient themselves so that they form a bridge between the oil and water, holding the two phases together (Figure 4-13). Bile salts emulsify the fat from the muffin in the watery medium of the duodenum and jejunum, and by doing so allow the water-soluble lipases to get close enough to the triglycerides to digest them. Without bile salts, little fat digestion occurs. The hormone cholecystokinin-pancreozymin (CCK-PZ) stimulates the flow of bile when acid chyme containing fat reaches the duodenum.

Cholesterol occurring free in foods requires no digestion, but some cholesterol exists in foods as cholesterol esters, with one fatty acid attached per cholesterol molecule. The enzyme *cholesterol esterase*, secreted by the pancreas, breaks the bond between cholesterol and the fatty acid, freeing cholesterol for absorption.

Lecithin is attacked by *pancreatic phospholipase*, which breaks one of the

FIGURE 4-13.
Emulsification of fat. An emulsifier disperses fat or other lipids into tiny droplets, surrounding each droplet with a shell of water. In effect, this allows the fat to move easily in a watery medium. This is accomplished because one end of the emulsifier molecule is soluble in water, while the other end is soluble in fat, or other lipids.

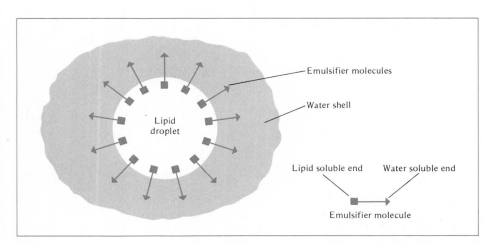

TABLE 4-2. LIPID DIGESTION*

WHERE IT OCCURS	SUBSTRATE	ENZYME AND ITS ORIGIN	PRODUCTS OF DIGESTION
Stomach	Triglycerides containing short- and medium-chain fatty acids	Gastric lipase	Some fatty acids and glycerol in infants. May start hydrolysis of emulsified fats in adults
Duodenum and jejunum	Triglycerides	Pancreatic lipase	Monoglycerides, fatty acids, and glycerol. Small amounts of diglycerides
Duodenum and jejunum	Cholesterol esters	Pancreatic cholesterol esterase	Cholesterol and free fatty acid
Duodenum and jejunum	Lecithin	Pancreatic phospholipase	Fatty acid and lysolecithin

*Bile salts are necessary for the digestion of triglycerides and cholesterol.

fatty acids off. The remaining part of the lecithin is called *lysolecithin*, and is absorbed as such. Lecithin, then, appears to be absorbed chiefly as lysolecithin and a fatty acid, although it is possible that lecithin and other phospholipids are completely broken down to glycerol, fatty acids, and other components during digestion.

Lipid digestion is summarized in Table 4-2.

ABSORPTION OF FATS AND OTHER LIPIDS

The absorption of fats and other lipids involves the passage of their digestion products across the membrane of the intestinal mucosal cell, their modification within the mucosal cell, and their transport finally into the circulating blood.

Role of Bile Salts

Bile salts are necessary not only for *digestion* of triglycerides and cholesterol, but also for their *absorption*. The products of fat digestion, monoglycerides and fatty acids, are insoluble in water, as is cholesterol. Bile salts emulsify these digestion products as they form, and help them travel through the watery medium of the intestinal lumen to reach the intestinal mucosal cells. Upon reaching the mucosal cells, the bile salts release the lipid substances which diffuse passively across the cell membrane. The bile salts remain in the lumen and move down to the ileum where most of them are absorbed by the portal vein and returned to the liver. There is therefore an *enterohepatic* circulation of bile salts (*entero* refers to the intestines, while *hepatic* means the liver). The enterohepatic circulation is a system whereby bile salts are conserved in the body; generally only about 3 percent of the bile salts are lost through the feces each day, while 97 percent are reabsorbed [8] (Figure 4-14).

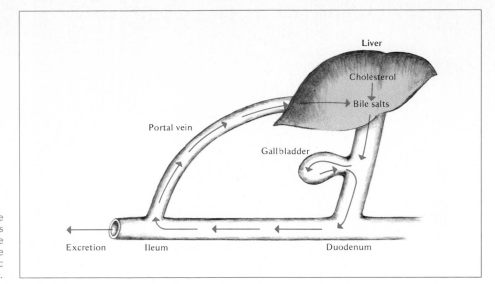

Inside the Mucosal Cells

What happens to the products of lipid digestion inside the mucosal cells? *Intestinal lipase*, located just inside the intestinal mucosal cells, breaks down monoglycerides as they enter the cell to fatty acids and glycerol. Glycerol and those fatty acids of less than 12 carbons immediately enter the portal blood and are carried to the liver. The absorption of fatty acids having 12 carbons or more in their chains is more complicated, however. These fatty acids are again formed into triglycerides within the mucosal cells. Since triglycerides are insoluble in water, the cell tucks them into little packages called *chylomicrons*. The outer coating of chylomicrons consists of protein which is soluble in water. These cellular processes are summarized in Figure 4-15.

Some artificially made medium-chain triglycerides (MCT) are absorbed without being digested and do not require bile. However, these do not exist naturally in foods. Food triglycerides that contain short- and medium-chain fatty acids also contain some long-chain fatty acids.

Cholesterol, as it is freed from bile acids, crosses the intestinal mucosal cell membrane mostly as free cholesterol. Inside the mucosal cell, it is linked again to fatty acid, forming cholesterol esters (see Figures 4-9 and 4-15). Cholesterol esters, because of their insolubility, also require help in getting out of the cell, and they are placed with triglycerides inside the chylomicrons.

Chylomicrons, carrying triglycerides and cholesterol esters, pass from the mucosal cells into the *lacteals* (small lymph vessels), which empty into the *thoracic duct* and enter the blood at the *subclavian vein* in the neck region. This is the route of absorption taken by all fat-soluble nutrients, and is called the *lymphatic route* of absorption (Figure 4-16).

Normally, 95 percent of the fat in the usual American diet is absorbed [7]. Persons in whom bile flow from the liver or gallbladder to the duodenum is

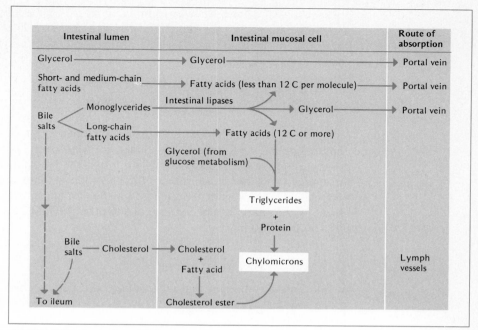

FIGURE 4-15. Absorption of lipids.

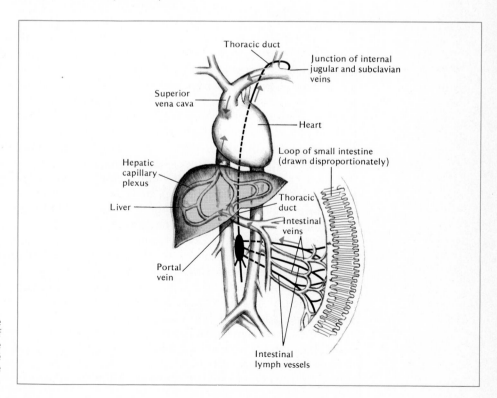

FIGURE 4-16. The lymphatic route of absorption—the route used by fat-soluble nutrients to reach the blood.

obstructed will absorb fat very poorly. Diseases of the pancreas that prevent secretion of lipase into the duodenum can also prevent fat absorption. Inadequate fat absorption ususaly results also in inadequate absorption of the fat-soluble vitamins, A, D, E, and K.

METABOLISM AND STORAGE

Metabolism, as mentioned previously, includes both *anabolism*, in which compounds are synthesized, and *catabolism*, in which compounds are broken down. In the section below we shall consider: (1) the catabolism of triglycerides for energy, and the circumstances under which ketones are produced; (2) the synthesis of nonessential fatty acids; (3) the storage of triglycerides in adipose tissue; (4) the anabolism of cholesterol and phospholipids; and (5) the transport of lipids in the blood.

Catabolism of Fats for Energy

At one time we thought that glucose was the body's chief energy source. We know now that fatty acids are equally important as energy sources and, in fact, are preferred sources for some organs in the body. In the discussion of carbohydrate loading in Chapter 3, we mentioned that the muscles use fatty acids as their primary energy source when the athlete engages in light to moderate exercise.

In order to produce energy from triglycerides, regardless of whether they come from food or body fat stores, the body first breaks them down to *fatty acids* and *glycerol*. Triglyceride originating in food is catabolized by an enzyme, lipoprotein lipase, which is present in cells lining the blood vessels. This enzyme removes triglyceride from the chylomicrons which, you recall, carry triglyceride from the intestinal cells to the blood. Liproprotein lipase then breaks the removed triglycerides down to fatty acids and glycerol, allowing tissues to take up fatty acids as needed for energy. Triglycerides stored in adipose cells (fat storage cells) are catabolized within those cells by a lipase to fatty acids and glycerol, both of which enter the blood. Again, the fatty acids are picked up by tissues as needed for energy. Most body cells except brain and nervous tissue are able to use fatty acids for energy. Glycerol resulting from catabolism of triglycerides circulates in the blood to the liver where it is converted to glucose, if needed, or is catabolized for energy.

When fats are used for energy, they produce more than twice the energy of carbohydrates or protein. The reason for this becomes clear when one examines the process by which catabolism of fat produces energy (Figure 4-17). The triglyceride is first broken down to glycerol and fatty acids. The fatty acid chain is then broken down in a stepwise fashion—two carbons at a time—to produce acetyl CoA. The process by which fatty acids are catabolized to acetyl CoA is called beta oxidation. Each acetyl CoA then enters the Krebs cycle and energy is obtained from it as described in Chapter 3.

A fatty acid containing 18 carbons will yield nine acetyl CoA molecules via

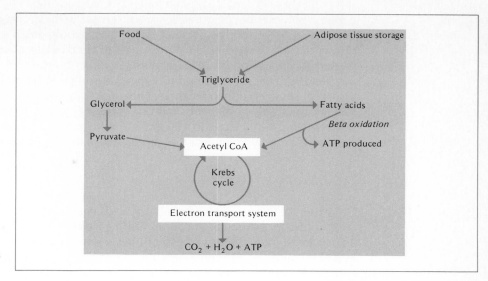

FIGURE 4-17. Use of fats
(triglycerides) for energy.

beta oxidation. A triglyceride made up of three 18-carbon fatty acids therefore would produce 27 acetyl CoA molecules, plus one from glycerol catabolism, giving a total of 28. One glucose molecule, in contrast, yields only two acetyl CoA molecules. Each acetyl CoA molecule metabolized via the Krebs cycle and the electron transport system (respiratory chain) produces 12 molecules of ATP. In addition, the process of producing each acetyl CoA molecule from a fatty acid, results in production of 5 more ATPs as the electrons released in the reactions go through the electron transport system.

Ketosis A special condition occurs in the body when excessive amounts of fatty acids are catabolized by the liver in the absence or near-absence of carbohydrate. These conditions prevail in: (1) starvation (when glycogen stores are depleted, and stored body fat becomes the chief energy source); (2) when a high-fat, very low carbohydrate diet is consumed; and (3) in an individual with untreated diabetes mellitus (whose body cells cannot use carbohydrate). Under these circumstances, the liver soon becomes flooded with fatty acids coming from either stored fat or from the diet. The liver cannot oxidize them efficiently to carbon dioxide, water, and ATP because it lacks the carbohydrate derivatives needed for this oxidation (review Figure 3-18). The result is that the liver produces compounds called *ketones* which it cannot oxidize, so it puts them in the blood. Other body tissues *can* oxidize ketones for energy but only to a certain extent. As the liver continues to put them in the blood, the blood level of ketones rises until they are excreted in the urine. This condition, in which blood ketone levels are high and ketones appear in the urine, is called *ketosis*.

A person who has ketosis will notice some of the following symptoms: (1) greater volume of urine than usual, (2) depressed appetite, (3) nausea, (4) excessive tiredness, (5) dizziness, and (6) bad breath. The symptoms may in some cases be mild, and appear not to be harmful for normal people over a short time period, but can become serious over longer periods. People who have an inherited tendency to the disorder called gout should avoid ketosis because the uric acid levels of the blood and urine tend to become elevated in ketosis. Gout is caused by deposition of uric acid crystals in the joints.

Ketosis is dangerous when prolonged elevation of blood ketones (which are acids) causes the blood to become acidic, resulting eventually in death. This may happen in untreated diabetics but not in normal people. Ketosis rapidly disappears when as little as 65 to 100 g of carbohydrate are utilized by the body per day. Low-carbohydrate diets that produce ketosis are discussed in Chapter 8.

Anabolism of Lipids

Nonessential Fatty acids   All the fatty acids needed except linoleic acid can be synthesized in the body. In addition to their use as energy sources, these fatty acids can be used in the synthesis of triglycerides and stored in adipose tissue or as components of phospholipids and other complex lipids important to cell membranes and to brain and nervous tissue.

Building Fat Stores   We know that body fat is stored whenever excessive kilocalories are consumed either as carbohydrates, fat, or protein. In Chapter 3 we saw that when carbohydrate supplies excessive kilocalories, the conversion of carbohydrate to fat involves the catabolism of glucose to acetyl CoA, which is then used to build up fatty acids. The fatty acids are then combined with glycerol to form triglyceride. This process takes place in both the liver and adipose tissue cells.

Figure 4-18 indicates that fatty acids from food triglycerides may enter adipose tissue or muscle cells soon after the food is eaten. Triglyceride reaching

FIGURE 4-18. Conversion of food triglyceride (fat) to body fat.

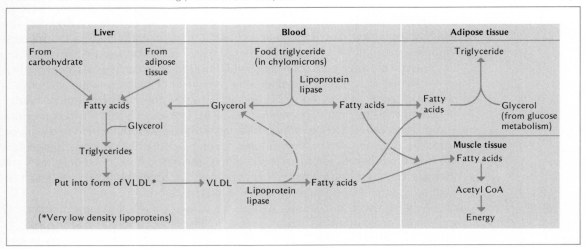

the adipose tissue in chylomicrons is catabolized to fatty acids and glycerol by lipoprotein lipase, present in the blood vessels nourishing the muscle and fat cells. Those fatty acids entering fat cells may be formed into triglyceride and stored. Those entering muscles are catabolized for energy. The liver also synthesizes triglyceride but does not store it. Instead, the liver puts fat into the blood in a carrier called VLDL (very low density lipoproteins), discussed below in the section on lipid transport in the blood. This carrier is attacked by lipoprotein lipase, releasing the triglycerides, and breaking them down to glycerol and fatty acids. The fatty acids enter the adipose cells and are used there for triglyceride synthesis.

The fatty acid composition of stored fat varies with the diet. Triglycerides synthesized by liver cells from carbohydrate contain mostly saturated fatty acids. Those triglycerides synthesized by adipose cells from dietary fat reflect the composition of the fat. For example, one study showed that a high polyunsaturated fat diet fed over a 5-year period resulted in an increase in linoleic acid in the men's adipose tissue from 11 to 32 percent of the total fatty acids [9]. Whether or not it is beneficial to have more or less polyunsaturated fat in adipose tissue is unknown.

Since fats are the most concentrated energy sources in foods, high intakes may contribute to obesity, the accumulation of excessive body fat stores (see Chapter 8).

Anabolism From Acetyl CoA   One way to sum up anabolism of lipids in the body is to observe the central role played by the 2-carbon compound, acetyl CoA. This molecule is used by the body in the synthesis of fatty acids, cholesterol, and ketones. Fatty acids, in turn, are used in the synthesis of triglycerides and phospholipids. Cholesterol also is involved in many anabolic reactions, discussed earlier in this chapter. Figure 4-19 indicates the important uses the body makes of acetyl CoA.

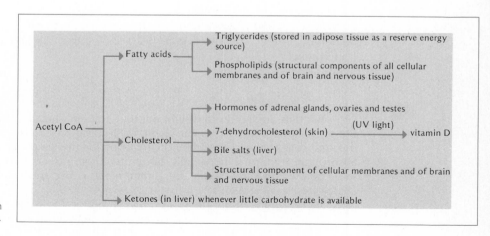

FIGURE 4-19. Anabolism of lipids from acetyl CoA.

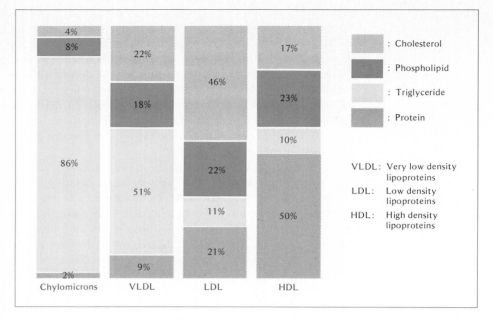

FIGURE 4-20.
Lipoproteins in the blood
and their relative
percentage of
components. (Source:
Drawn from values in
Mayes, P.A., "Lipids," in
Martin, D.W., Jr., P.A.
Mayes, and V.W.
Rodwell, *Harper's
Review of Biochemistry*,
18th ed., Lange Medical
Publications, Los Altos,
Calif., 94022, 1981,
p. 194, table 16-3.)

Transport of Lipids in the Blood

We have noted that triglycerides and cholesterol, because they are insoluble in water, must be put into the form of chylomicrons before they can be moved out of the intestinal mucosal cells into the lymph and finally into the blood. Chylomicrons are one of several such carriers used by the body to transport lipids. These carriers are called *lipoproteins* because they have an outer coating of protein and carry various lipids inside. A detailed discussion of lipoproteins is inappropriate here, but the reader needs some information about them because blood lipoprotein levels are frequently mentioned in the mass media in relation to coronary heart disease.

Lipoproteins are classified according to their density. The lower density ones contain a relatively low amount of protein, while the higher density ones are higher in protein content. Figure 4-20 shows the composition of the various lipoproteins.

A CLOSER LOOK

Chylomicrons are lighter in weight per unit volume (they are the least dense) than the other lipoproteins. They carry chiefly food triglyceride from the intestinal mucosal cells to the general blood circulation via the lymphatic route of absorption. In normal individuals, *lipoprotein lipase* clears chylomicrons out of the blood within 6 to 8 hours after a fatty meal; consequently, chylomicrons are absent from fasting blood.

The remaining lipoproteins are present in blood to some extent at all times. As Figure 4-20 indicates, VLDLs carry primarily triglyceride. Most of the VLDLs are synthesized by the liver, and are the vehicle for transporting triglyceride from the liver, since this organ normally accumulates no fat.

LDLs (low-density lipoproteins) carry cholesterol to peripheral tissues, including the artery walls. LDLs actually enter tissue cells and are broken down to their component parts within the cells. High blood levels of LDLs have been associated with increased chances of heart disease (see Chapter 5).

HDLs (high-density lipoproteins) carry both triglyceride and cholesterol, but are of special interest because high blood levels are associated with decreased chances for having heart disease [10]. The way in which HDLs protect against heart disease is not thoroughly understood, but two mechanisms have been proposed. One is that HDLs transport cholesterol away from the arteries and other peripheral tissues to the liver where it is catabolized to bile salts. The other is that HDLs block the uptake of LDLs by local tissues, including artery walls. [11]. Further research should clarify the functions of HDLs.

An additional lipid, not shown in Figure 4-20, that may appear in blood is free fatty acids. Free fatty acids are transported in the blood attached to albumin, a protein. Ordinarily, the blood level of free fatty acids is low, but becomes elevated whenever large amounts of stored fat are catabolized for energy. This is the case in starvation, or in a person who has untreated diabetes mellitus.

We have seen that fat is important in the diet to provide a source of energy and the essential fatty acid, and to aid in absorption of fat-soluble vitamins. It is also important for satiety. Cholesterol and phospholipids, although important in the body, do not need to be provided in food. Let us now look at how our uses of fat have changed over the years, and at recommendations that are made concerning fat intake.

CHANGING PATTERNS OF FAT CONSUMPTION

The data we have on fat consumption, like those for carbohydrate consumption, do not take into account any wastage. Instead, they reflect fats *available* to the American consumer. Figure 4-21 indicates that today a larger amount of fat is available to each American than was the case early in this century. In 1980, 169 g (about ⅓ lb per day) of fat was available per person per day compared with 125 g in 1909 (about ¼ lb per day). Another way of looking at fat availability is that in 1909 fat accounted for about 32 percent of the total kilocalories in the diet, while in 1980 it accounted for 43 percent [12].

A striking change since 1909 has been the increasing percentage of the total fat available from vegetable sources rather than from animal sources. At the end of World War II, vegetable fat made up about 26 percent of the total fat available, while in 1980 it made up 43 percent of the total fat. The great increase in use of hydrogenated shortenings and margarines made from vegetable oils, accompanied by decreased use of butter and lard, account for this change [12]. Beef, poultry, and fish availability all have increased since 1909, however the proportion of total fat from animal sources has gradually declined since 1909 (Figure 4-21).

Concern about our increasing fat intake relates to the prevalence of diseases or disorders such as obesity, heart disease, and cancer. The possible relationship of heart disease and cancer to fat consumption is discussed in Chapter 5.

PERSONAL HEALTH. THE EXACT ROLE OF TRIGLYCERIDES IS DEBATABLE, BUT IT PAYS TO KEEP AN EYE ON THEIR LEVELS

Jane E. Brody, *The New York Times*, October 20, 1982.

"The doctor said my cholesterol was O.K. but my triglycerides were too high. What does that mean?" The questioner was not sure whether to worry. . . . If all Americans were tested at least one in 20 would be found to have triglyceride, or fat, levels in their blood that are generally regarded as "too high." . . .

The debate about triglycerides makes the cholesterol controversy seem like an open-and-shut case. High triglyceride levels in the blood are unquestionably associated with increased risk of developing heart and blood vessel diseases. The debate turns on whether triglycerides directly contribute to the artery-clogging disease atherosclerosis or whether they are only an indicator for other factors that do the damage more directly. If they are merely an indicator, then some experts question the need to institute treatment to bring elevated levels to normal. . . .

Triglyceride levels in the blood tend to be high when a person is overweight. In addition, some people are said to be carbohydrate-sensitive: consumption of sugars and refined starches and large amounts of alcohol tend to raise their triglyceride levels. Women who take oral contraceptives may also have raised triglyceride levels. At least one person in 20 is born with a genetic predisposition to developing an elevated level. . . .

As Dr. [William] Castelli [director of the Framingham, Massachusetts, Heart Study] put it, an American with high triglycerides has an increased risk of heart disease if for no other reason than the resulting unfavorable ratio of HDL to LDL. "If you get them to lower their triglycerides by losing weight," he said, "you'll see a lot of favorable changes: a fall in LDL, increase in HDL, and decreases in blood pressure, uric acid, and blood sugar."

He urged that anyone found to have a high triglyceride level also be tested for levels of the various cholesterols. . . .

. . . High triglyceride levels are primarily related to overly fatty, overly sweet, overly caloric American diets. The first step in lowering triglycerides is to lose weight if you are above the ideal. In addition it is wise to reduce consumption of fats, especially saturated fats. . . . For those who are carbohydrate-sensitive, keeping sugar and alcohol intake to a minimum is especially important. Dr. Castelli said that fructose is even more harmful than glucose and ordinary table sugar.

In contrast to the potentially harmful effects of sugars, consumption of unrefined, high-fiber starchy foods can help to lower blood triglyceride levels. . . .

A diet that emphasizes whole grain breads and cereals, dried beans and peas, fruits and vegetables has been shown to lower triglyceride levels dramatically. This is the very diet that is being widely recommended for people who have cholesterol problems and those with diabetes. Indeed, it is the diet that most prevention-oriented nutrition specialists recommend for everyone. Exercise may also help to lower triglycerides, perhaps through its effect on weight loss.

ASK YOURSELF:

To what extent does your present diet emphasize the food described here? Which lipoprotein is most apt to be elevated in blood when blood triglycerides are elevated?

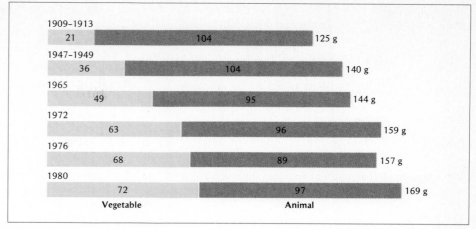

FIGURE 4-21. Changes in availability of fat from animal and vegetable sources since 1909 in the United States. [Sources (1) Friend, B., L. Page, and R. Marston, "Food Consumption Patterns in the United States: 1909–13 to 1976," in Levy, R., B. Rifkind, B. Dennis, and N. Ernst (eds.), *Nutrition, Lipids and Coronary Heart Disease*, New York: Raven Press, 1979 (p. 505). (2) Welsh, S.O., and R. Marston, "Review of Trends in Food Use in the United States, 1909 to 1980," Reprinted by permission from *Journal of the American Dietetic Association*, 81:120, 1982.]

HOW MUCH FAT IS SUGGESTED?

We have noted so far in this chapter that 2 to 3 percent of the total kilocalories should be in the form of linoleic acid. Moreover, we have learned that about 10 to 15 percent of the kilocalories as fat is needed for normal absorption of fat-soluble vitamins. Nonetheless, most people probably require at least 15 to 20 percent of the kilocalories as fat to provide a palatable diet with sufficient satiety value.

In Chapter 2 we learned that *Dietary Goals for the United States* recommended that our usual intake of 42 percent of total kilocalories as fat be reduced to 30 percent [13]. In addition, the National Academy of Science's Committee on Diet, Nutrition and Cancer recommended that total fat intake be reduced to 30 percent of total kilocalories to decrease the chances of developing cancer [14].

If you wish to reduce your fat (and cholesterol) intake, some suggestions for doing so are included in *Dietary Guidelines for Americans* (Table 2-2). As a comment on those suggestions, moderate use of eggs is probably about four per week, while a 2-oz serving of liver might be consumed not more than once a week. Some additional suggestions are:

1. By using chiefly fruits for dessert, you can avoid both the fat and sugar in baked products.
2. Learn to eat bread without butter or margarine.
3. Take snacks such as fresh fruit, carrot, green pepper, and celery sticks, bread or crackers with you from home to avoid the fat present in readily available snack items such as potato chips, corn chips, Danish pastries, doughnuts, and ice cream.

4. Cook fresh vegetables just to the crisp stage to preserve the flavor so that no fat is needed for added flavor.
5. Use skim or 1 percent milk in place of whole milk.
6. Substitute yogurt for sour cream.
7. Substitute whole milk or even skim milk in a recipe calling for cream.
8. Restrict your use of meats such as sausage, salami, frankfurters, and liverwurst, all of which are high in fat.

SUMMARY

1 Important lipids in nutrition include triglycerides (fats), cholesterol, and phospholipids, including lecithin.
2 The fatty acids of triglycerides may be saturated, monounsaturated, or polyunsaturated. Saturated fatty acids may be of short-, medium- or long-chain lengths, while unsaturated fatty acids are of long-chain lengths.
3 Cholesterol is an important structural component of cellular membranes and nervous tissue, including the brain. The catabolism of cholesterol in the liver produces bile salts which are essential for fat digestion and absorption. The body is able to synthesize all the cholesterol it needs and does not require it in the diet.
4 Digestion of triglycerides requires bile salts from the liver to aid in digestion. Pancreatic lipase is the most important enzyme for digesting triglycerides.
5 The route of absorption of fat-soluble substances is the lymphatic route.
6 Triglyercides are an important energy source. To obtain energy from them, the body first breaks them down to glycerol and fatty acids. Fatty acids are then catabolized to acetyl CoA, which is oxidized to produce CO_2, water, and energy in the form of ATP.
7 Ketosis exists when high levels of ketones accumulate in the blood and are excreted in the urine. This occurs whenever large amounts of triglyceride are catabolized in the absence of carbohydrates.
8 Lipids are transported in the blood by lipoproteins which are soluble in the blood because of their protein coating. Scientists have long been interested in the relationship of blood lipoproteins to coronary heart disease.
9 In the United States since 1909, the availability of total fat in the diet has steadily increased. Various official groups have recommended a decrease in fat intake in attempts to lower the risks of heart disease and cancer.

FOR DISCUSSION AND APPLICATION

1 Using techniques described in the *For Discussion and Application* section of Chapter 3,
   a. Review how the kilocalories that came from fat compared with recommendations in *Dietary Goals for the United States* (Chapter 2).
   b. Calculate the percentage of total kilocalories that came from saturated fat and from linoleic acid (polyunsaturated fat). How did this compare with the dietary goals? What foods contributed most of the saturated fat in your intake? The polyunsaturated fat intake?
   c. Calculate the P/S ratio using figures for linoleic acid for polyunsaturated fat. How does this ratio compare with that recommended? If the diet is high in polyunsaturated fats and low in saturated ones, is the P/S ratio high or low?
2 Use Appendix F to determine the amount of cholesterol in your daily intake. How does this amount compare with the Dietary Goals? What foods contributed most of the cholesterol in your diet?
3 Assuming your record is typical of your usual diet, what changes, if any, should you make in your diet relative to fat and cholesterol? Why?
4 Suppose Barry, described at the beginning of the chapter, is your friend. His diet contains between 5 and 10 percent of the kilocalories as fat. In view of the benefits of fats discussed in this chapter, do you believe he might eventually develop any nutritional problems if he continues on such a low-fat diet? Why or why not?
5 What advice would you give a friend who is told by her physician that she has unusually high blood cholesterol levels? She ignores her physician's advice about means to lower the levels, and instead begins to take lecithin capsules. What advice would you give her? Could taking lecithin be harmful? Helpful?

SUGGESTED READINGS

Deutsch, R. M., *The Fat Counter Guide*, Palo Alto, Calif.: Bull Publishing Co., 1978. A simple guide, emphasizing fats as a source of kilocalories.

American Heart Association Cookbook (3d ed.), New York: David McKay Co., 1979. There are over 500 low-calorie, low-fat, low-cholesterol recipes in this classic cookbook.

Stare, F. J. (ed.), *Atherosclerosis,* CPC International, Best Foods Division, Englewood Cliffs, N.J., 1974.

Bennett, I., *The Prudent Diet,* David White, New York, 1973.

Mayer, J., *Fats, Diet, and Your Heart,* Newspaperbooks, Norwood, N.J., 1976.

5 LIPIDS, CARBOHYDRATES, AND DISEASE

What comes to mind when you think of malnutrition? Tiny, spindly-armed children with swollen bellies and little to eat? Undernutrition, or lack of food and nutrients, is only one side of the malnutrition coin. Another challenge faces the populations of industrialized countries—the challenge of overnutrition, or consumption of too much food. Overnutrition as well as undernutrition may be a serious health hazard.

Overnutrition is not limited to high kilocalorie intakes and consequent obesity. High intakes of fats, other lipids, and sugars may also contribute to health problems. Some investigators have associated high levels of dietary fat and cholesterol with coronary heart disease and cancer. Others have studied the possible relationship between highly refined carbohydrate and dental caries, diabetes, and coronary heart disease. Researchers have also examined the relationship of low-fiber diets to many diseases, including cancer, since highly refined diets tend to be low in dietary fiber.

This chapter reviews the relationships of dietary fat, refined carbohydrate, and dietary fiber to some of the so-called "diseases of civilization." One aim is to help you appreciate the challenges of sound scientific research, the dangers of jumping to conclusions without sufficient evidence, and the importance of carefully evaluating research findings. Another objective is to help you understand why controversy exists among scientists regarding advice that should be given the public about diet and disease prevention. Even though much of the research dealing with the relationship of diet to disease is inconclusive, following a sound, nutritious diet is essential for maintenance of health. This chapter emphasizes principles such as moderation in eating and variety of food choices to help you in planning a reasonable, nutritious diet.

DIETARY LIPIDS AND CORONARY HEART DISEASE (CHD)

For more than 40 years diseases of the heart and blood vessels have been the leading cause of death in the United States. *Cardiovascular disease (CVD)* is an overall term referring to all diseases affecting the heart and blood vessels. *Coronary heart disease (CHD)* specifically refers to damage to the heart muscle due to inadequate blood supply from the coronary arteries. Eventually, when the damage is severe enough, an individual has a heart attack. At present, heart attacks cause two-thirds of all deaths from CVD [1], and almost one-third of deaths from all causes in individuals aged 35 to 64 years [2]. In 1979, 4 million Americans suffered from symptoms of CHD. Investigators estimate that more than 1.25 million people suffer heart attacks each year in the United States, and 20 to 25 percent of these die before medical personnel reach them [2].

Since much of the research directed toward diet relates specifically to CHD rather than to other forms of CVD, this chapter explores possible causes of CHD, and in particular examines the relationship of diet to CHD.

Atherosclerosis and Coronary Heart Disease (CHD)

The most common reason for inadequate blood supply to the heart muscle is atherosclerosis of the *coronary arteries*—those that nourish the heart muscle. The normal smooth flow of blood throughout the body can be impeded when arteries thicken, harden, and become inelastic, a disorder referred to as *arteriosclerosis* or hardening of the arteries. *Atherosclerosis* is a specific type of hardening of the arteries characterized by a buildup of fatty deposits, called *plaques*, in the artery walls. These fatty deposits are high in cholesterol, but also contain phospholipid, triglyceride, connective tissue, *fibrin* (the clotting substance of the blood), and an increased number of smooth muscle cells (those cells normally making up the innermost lining of the arteries). As plaques build up in the artery walls, they tend to narrow the lumen through which blood flows. The surfaces of the plaques frequently become rough, causing blood platelets to clump together, which in turn leads to the formation of a clot that can completely block the blood flow (Figure 5-1). When this occurs in a coronary artery a heart attack or *myocardial infarction* results. Partial blockage of a coronary artery may result in chest pain, especially when a person exercises. This condition is called *angina pectoris*.

Atherosclerosis may also cause weakening in an artery wall, resulting in an *aneurysm* or "ballooning out" of the artery. In this condition, a break in the artery wall may occur, resulting in a stroke if the defect is in a small artery in the brain, or in death if the defect is in a large artery such as the *aorta*.

Atherosclerosis develops slowly over a 20-to-40-year period, but may

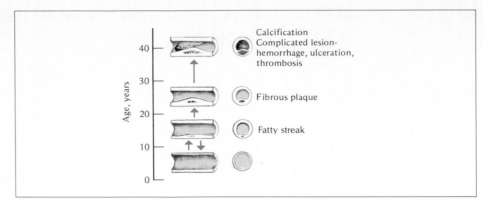

FIGURE 5-1. Steps in development of atherosclerosis.

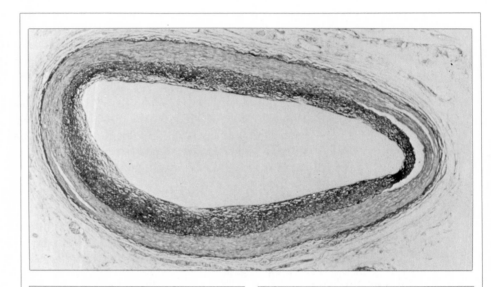

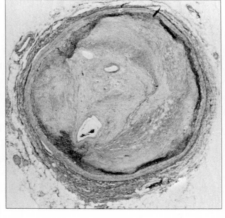

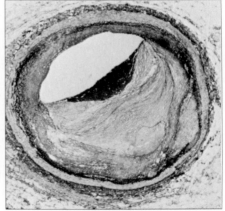

Coronary arteries may remain free of atherosclerosis throughout life, illustrated here by a cross section of an artery from a 100-year-old woman (a) yet in many individuals heart attacks result from blockage of a coronary artery by atherosclerotic placques (b) or by a blood clot forming on placques (c). *(National Heart, Lung, and Blood Institute; National Institutes of Health)*

produce no symptoms until the sudden occurrence of heart attack, stroke, angina, or sudden death. It appears to begin in childhood or adolescence. In affluent, industrialized countries the extent of atherosclerosis is substantial in males by age 25, and symptoms of CHD are seen in many by the age of 40.

Many factors, including diet, have been implicated as possible causes of CHD. Some experts believe that the causes are embedded in the lifestyles of individuals living in affluent countries under stressful conditions, indulging in cigarette smoking and having an abundant food supply high in kilocalories and rich in fat, cholesterol, and sugar. Assessing risk factors pertaining to coronary heart disease reinforces the likelihood that our way of life is involved.

Risk Factors and Coronary Heart Disease (CHD)

Factors or characteristics which have been shown in population studies (studies of groups of individuals living in their usual way) to be associated with a high incidence of CHD are called *risk factors*. Risk factors are determined by measuring various characteristics, such as smoking or food consumption patterns, in a large population over a long time period to observe which ones are statistically associated with the development of heart attacks, angina, or stroke. Having a risk factor for CHD does not mean that one inevitably will develop the disease, but that one's *chances* or *risks* are greater than for an individual who has no risk factors. Moreover, individuals with more than one risk factor run a greater chance of developing the disease than if they have only one.

In a population study, two or more variables which increase or decrease at the same time are said to be statistically positively correlated. (*Variables* are simply factors that can change—that is, increase or decrease.) For example, if over a period of 5 years the death rate from heart attacks in a population increases at the same time that the incidence of high blood pressure increases, these two variables are positively associated, or correlated. On the other hand, if one variable increases while another decreases, the two are said to be negatively correlated. Whether the correlation is positive or negative, there is a statistical association between variables when the extent of change is greater than would be expected by chance alone. A statistical correlation does not *prove* that one variable is *causing* the other to occur, however. For example, the fact that the incidence of high blood pressure increased in a population at the same time that deaths from heart attacks increased does not *prove* that high blood pressure caused the heart attacks. The heart attacks may have increased because the age of the population increased, for example. This may or may not be related to the increased incidence of high blood pressure. Thus, additional studies would be needed to prove cause and effect.

Probably the best known study of risk factors related to CHD in the United States is the Framingham study in which more than 5000 men and women living in Framingham, Massachusetts, have been studied since 1949 [3]. Measurements have included, among others, body weight, blood levels of cholesterol, triglycerides, glucose, high-density lipoproteins (HDL), and low-density lipoproteins (LDL) (see Chapter 4 for a review of the lipoproteins). In addition, blood pressure, urinary glucose, smoking habits, and dietary intakes of cholesterol, fat, saturated fat, and kilocalories, have been documented. The investigators studied (and continue to study) the possible statistical relationships between different variables (e.g., blood levels of cholesterol or specific lipoproteins) and occurrence of heart attacks, angina, or stroke. From such a study, major (or primary) as well as secondary risk factors have been determined. Primary risk factors are directly associated with disease occurrence, while secondary factors are indirectly associated.

The Framingham study shows that among those who eventually develop CHD, the four major risk factors are (1) elevated blood cholesterol levels (particularly if LDL levels are elevated and HDL levels are decreased), (2) hypertension (high blood pressure), (3) diabetes, and (4) cigarette smoking. Secondary risk factors include obesity, high blood triglyceride levels, lack of physical exercise, and excessive amounts of stress. Men are clearly at greater risk

TABLE 5-1. RISK FACTORS FOR CORONARY HEART DISEASE (CHD)

RISK FACTORS	COMMENTS
THOSE THAT CANNOT BE CHANGED	
Sex	Men are at greater risk than women until menopause, after which risk for women is as great as for men.
Age	Risk increases with age for both men and women.
Family history	Occurrence of CHD or stroke in close relatives increases one's chances of developing these disorders.
MAJOR FACTORS THAT CAN BE CONTROLLED	
Elevated blood cholesterol levels	Elevated blood levels of either total cholesterol or LDL (low-density lipoproteins) increase risk for CHD. Low levels of HDL (high-density lipoproteins) also increase risk.
Hypertension (high blood pressure)	Chances of developing CHD or stroke are greatly increased with hypertension.
Diabetes	Diabetes doubles one's chances of developing CHD. Women with diabetes have the same risk as men of the same age who are free of diabetes.
Cigarette smoking	The heavy cigarette smoker is much more likely to develop CHD or stroke than the nonsmoker. Risks decrease significantly soon after a person stops smoking.
SECONDARY FACTORS THAT CAN BE CONTROLLED	
Obesity	Obesity alone does not increase risks, but in many people weight gains are accompanied by elevation in blood lipids, in blood pressure, and in a tendency to develop diabetes, each of which increases risk for CHD.
Lack of physical exercise	The Framingham study showed that deaths from CHD were higher among those who were least active physically.
Elevated blood triglyceride levels	Increases risks only when accompanied by increased blood cholesterol levels [4].
Oral contraceptives	Use of oral contraceptives by women over 40 years of age increases risks for CHD, particularly if they also smoke cigarettes [5].
Stress related to personality type	Some investigators believe that risk is greater for individuals who are aggressively ambitious, highly competitive, and constantly working against deadlines—in other words, they are subject to a particular kind of stress [5].

than women until women pass the menopause. Risk factors are discussed in greater detail in Table 5-1. The risk factors we will be focusing on in this chapter are elevated blood cholesterol levels and high blood triglyceride levels. The discussion will center upon how diet may affect these risk factors, and, in turn, affect coronary heart disease.

THE DIET–HEART HYPOTHESIS

Many nutrition researchers promote the diet–heart hypothesis. This hypothesis suggests that high blood lipid levels induce the formation of atherosclerotic plaques in the artery walls, and that lowering blood lipid levels by diet will decrease these plaques and, consequently, decrease chances of developing CHD (Figure 5-2). The specific dietary changes recommended include decreasing intakes of kilocalories, total fat, saturated fat, and cholesterol, and increasing slightly the intake of polyunsaturated fats.

Scientists and physicians disagree about whether the general public should modify their diets to try to prevent CHD. Some authorities contend that there is no harm in adopting a diet designed to lower blood lipid levels, and that doing so will in all likelihood lower the risks for CHD. Others believe that it is premature to advise the public in this way, and that only those with already developed risk factors should make dietary changes. It is worthwhile to look at the kinds of evidence available on this question.

The data relating dietary fat and cholesterol to the development of atherosclerosis and CHD come from several kinds of studies. For the most part, results are not conclusive, but instead point the way toward additional research. It is important to interpret the results of these studies cautiously. Box 5-1 discusses several types of studies used to define the relationship between diet and disease, including CHD, and some of the cautions needed in interpreting these studies.

FIGURE 5-2. Stages in development of coronary heart disease according to the diet–heart hypothesis. This diagram illustrates the sequence of events hypothesized to relate diet to the development of coronary heart disease.

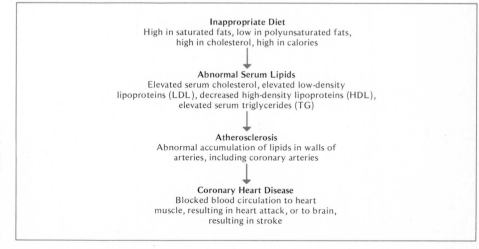

Inappropriate Diet
High in saturated fats, low in polyunsaturated fats, high in cholesterol, high in calories

↓

Abnormal Serum Lipids
Elevated serum cholesterol, elevated low-density lipoproteins (LDL), decreased high-density lipoproteins (HDL), elevated serum triglycerides (TG)

↓

Atherosclerosis
Abnormal accumulation of lipids in walls of arteries, including coronary arteries

↓

Coronary Heart Disease
Blocked blood circulation to heart muscle, resulting in heart attack, or to brain, resulting in stroke

Epidemiological Studies

Epidemiological studies contribute important evidence that diet is related to CHD. These are studies in which the incidence or occurrence of disease in large populations is documented along with factors that might be potential causes. The Framingham study is an example of such a study. Epidemiological studies are of great value in providing clues as to which factors are *possible* causes. These factors must be studied further by other methods to determine the real cause or causes. Over more than a half century, epidemiological studies have indicated the following about diet and CHD:

1. Comparisons of countries with very different dietary habits reveal that most groups with lower intakes of saturated fat and cholesterol tend to have lower blood cholesterol levels and lower incidence of CHD. The highest incidence of CHD and high blood cholesterol levels occurs in countries with high intakes of these lipids. [6,7].
2. Persons from countries with low blood cholesterol levels who migrate to countries with high levels soon acquire high levels as they adapt to the diet of the new country [6].
3. Even in countries with high blood cholesterol levels and high incidence of CHD, persons with markedly different dietary habits, such as vegetarians, who have low intakes of saturated fat and cholesterol, also have lower blood cholesterol levels and lower incidence of CHD than the general public [6,7].
4. Since 1950 in the United States there has been a gradual decline in dietary cholesterol and saturated fat intake and an increase in polyunsaturated fat intake, increasing the P/S ratio of the diet. Since 1958, the average serum cholesterol level has decreased, and a decline in the death rate from CHD began in about 1965 and continues to decline. Improved methods of providing emergency care and treatment of heart attacks may account in part for this improvement, as well as wider and more effective treatment of hypertension. But lifestyle changes may also be important factors because the number of cigarette smokers has declined since 1965, and the above-mentioned dietary changes have occurred [1,2,8].

Although we cannot *prove* that the observed dietary changes *caused* the decline in serum cholesterol levels and deaths from heart attacks, these statistics nevertheless lend support to the diet–heart hypothesis [8].

Since the associations found in epidemiological studies indicated that dietary fat and cholesterol *might* be factors in causing CHD, scientists began to perform carefully controlled metabolic studies with human subjects to study the effects of diet on blood lipids.

Metabolic Studies

Studies using controlled diets under laboratory conditions are called *metabolic studies* because they permit investigation of how the body is metabolizing nutrients, in this case fat and cholesterol (Box 5-1). In these studies, the exact food

5-1 BOX

Research in Nutrition

Magazines, newspapers, TV talk shows, and advertisements today abound with nutrition claims—so much so that many people are confused about what or whom to believe. Does vitamin E prevent heart attacks? Does too much fat cause heart attacks? Or cancer of the colon? Should you decrease the amount of saturated fat and cholesterol in your diet? Nutrition researchers engage in experimentation to help provide answers to questions such as these. An understanding of how nutrition research is conducted with animal and human subjects should help you to decide whether or not a claim made about nutrition is probably factual, fictitious, or unproven.

The Research Process The research process involves examining relationships among specified variables. For example, a blood cholesterol value constitutes a variable. Variables are often dependent on other variables. Blood cholesterol levels, for example, tend to decrease with an increase in consumption of polyunsaturated fats, and increase as saturated fat consumption increases. Blood cholesterol levels are therefore *dependent* on the relative amounts of saturated and polyunsaturated fats in the diet. But researchers had to do many painstaking studies to establish this fact. Generally, a researcher tries to control or keep constant all the variables that might affect the one under study (here, blood cholesterol), except for one which the experimenter varies. To study the influence of the degree of saturation of dietary fat on blood cholesterol levels, for example, a researcher might undertake a *metabolic study* using human subjects. In such a study, subjects consume a carefully measured or weighed diet and their metabolic responses are determined by measuring specified components of urine and blood or other tissues. In the study in question,

the researcher might feed subjects a purified diet made up of starch, sugar, casein (a purified protein), and vitamin and mineral pills. She might divide the study into three different time periods, feeding a different source of fat in each period (e.g., coconut oil, high in saturated fat; olive oil, high in monounsaturated fat; and safflower oil, high in polyunsaturated fat). She would then observe how the blood cholesterol levels vary with each dietary fat. To be certain that the *order* in which subjects consumed the oils would not affect the results, she would randomize the order in which individual subjects consumed the oils. In other words, one subject might receive olive oil in period 1, safflower oil in period 2, and coconut oil in period 3. The order in which subjects received the oils should include all possible combinations. In this research design, each subject is his or her own *control*, since he or she will consume each of the three oils at different times.

The results of a metabolic study apply only to the specific diet fed to the subjects, which may differ in important ways from the diets consumed in everyday, nonexperimental situations. For example, the above researcher would find that coconut oil raises while safflower oil lowers blood cholesterol levels. But she would not be able to apply her results directly to a population consuming a mixture of traditional foods, including dietary fiber and a mixture of fats, many of which she would not have studied.

Metabolic studies generally last only a short time (from about 4 to 24 weeks) because they are expensive and require subjects to lead highly regimented lives. They therefore are generally not used to determine the effects of a given diet over extended time periods.

Another example of a study design, called an *intervention trial*, makes clear the need for an adequate control group. If a researcher wished to study the effects of vitamin C on colds, for example, he would divide a large group of people into an *experimental* and a *control group*. The experimental group would receive vitamin C tablets, while the control group would receive a placebo—tablets that look and taste like vitamin C, but which are made up of some substance known to have no effect on colds. The two groups of subjects would be instructed to take their tablets in exactly the same way for the same period of time, while recording any signs of colds. Neither the subjects nor investigators should know which subject is in which group. Such an experiment is said to be "double blind" since both the subjects and experimenters are "blind" as to which group the subjects are in. The placebo is used because human beings can be easily influenced by the attitudes and suggestions of investigators, or by their own notions about diet. Suppose, for example, that a subject is firmly convinced that vitamin C prevents colds. Knowing that he or she is taking vitamin C tablets, the subject may unconsciously fail to recognize cold symptoms. Whenever possible, then, a placebo should be administered to a control group.

Often, intervention trials study dietary variables that are very difficult to disguise, however. Those trials in which the experimental diet included low intakes of total fat, saturated fat, and cholesterol and high intake of polyunsaturated fats generally have not been conducted in double-blind fashion.

Experimental and control groups should be alike in all factors apt to affect results. If sex and age of the subjects make a difference, for example, there should be the same number of subjects in each group of a given sex and age. The two groups should also be alike in their susceptibility to whatever is being studied; colds, for example. The study should be conducted over a long enough period of time to observe expected changes. Furthermore, the number of subjects per group should be large enough to rule out chance variation. Suppose an investigator wished to study whether or not large doses of

vitamin C caused cancer patients to feel better able to perform everyday activities. Suppose, too, that one cancer patient improved in her ability to perform daily tasks because of some chance occurrence, such as a sudden psychological burst of energy. If she were one of only six subjects in a group, the results for the whole group would be greatly affected by the chance occurrence that influenced her performance. If she were one of 75 subjects, however, her chance occurrence would have little effect on the group results.

Checking to see whether or not a study meets the many criteria described will aid you in deciding whether or not the study was well designed, and whether or not it is likely that the investigators' conclusions are valid.

Animal Studies Several kinds of studies can be conducted using human subjects, but since investigators must be certain that humans won't be harmed by an experiment, animals are frequently used instead to provide clues to important factors to study in humans. Moreover, animals can be used to study effects of diet that cannot ethically be determined using human subjects. For example, scientists can study development of atherosclerosis in animals by sacrificing them and studying their arteries, whereas only recently is there promise that physicians may soon be able to detect atherosclerosis in living humans [1]. Another reason for using animals is that their short life spans allow studies to be completed in a short time, using several generations. The major drawback to animal research is that results can almost never be applied *directly* to human subjects because humans do not necessarily absorb or metabolize a nutrient or substance exactly as an animal does. A special case is that of substances that may be toxic or harmful to human subjects. Because these substances cannot ethically be given to human subjects, detection of their harmful effects in animals is taken to indicate that they should not be permitted in human diets. In cases other than those related to safety in the food supply, it is therefore prudent to question the advocacy of following a dietary practice based solely on animal studies.

Scientists are human and therefore susceptible to making errors, misinterpreting data, or allowing their biases to creep into their studies. Before accepting the results of a specific study, the scientific community therefore generally waits until the same results are obtained by a different group of scientists working in a different laboratory or with different subjects. Keep this in mind the next time you hear on the radio or read a newspaper account of a "new discovery" in nutrition. Remain skeptical until the results are replicated by another properly executed study.

The attitude of the wise consumer should be that of the good scientist—that is, the attitude of open-minded skepticism. Open-mindedness encourages one to examine new ideas even when they conflict with one's preconceived notions, while skepticism protects one from accepting proposals that are inadequately supported by sound scientific evidence. Increasing your knowledge of what constitutes sound evidence is a good way to cultivate healthy skepticism.

intake of subjects is known. Many such studies have corroborated the diet–heart hypothesis. Generally, they show that the amount of dietary cholesterol and the ratio of dietary saturated to polyunsaturated fat influence blood cholesterol levels.

Results of metabolic studies show that dietary cholesterol increases blood cholesterol in a stepwise fashion as the cholesterol intake is increased from less than 200 mg/day to 1000 mg or over [9]. Metabolic studies also demonstrate that dietary saturated fat elevates blood cholesterol levels, while dietary polyunsaturated fat lowers them [10,11,12].

The public may be confused by publicity about studies reporting no changes in blood cholesterol levels when subjects were told to add one or two eggs per day (as cholesterol sources) to their usual diets [13,14]. Since these studies were not controlled metabolic studies, however, the investigators could not be certain of the actual food intake of their subjects. In other words it was impossible to determine the variations in total fat and saturated or polyunsaturated fats that could have influenced blood cholesterol levels. A recent study with a different research design reported opposite findings [9]. In this study subjects were asked to continue consuming their usual diets with the daily addition of either whole eggs containing approximately 500 mg of cholesterol or an egg substitute that was free of cholesterol. The eggs and egg substitute were distributed to subjects in a double-blind design. The egg substitute represented the placebo, and subjects were their own controls (see Box 5-1). Under these circumstances, blood cholesterol levels were significantly higher when subjects added whole egg to their diets than when they added the egg substitute.

Metabolic studies have shown that the human body has a threshold for dietary cholesterol; therefore, intakes above 500 to 600 mg/day frequently do not further increase blood cholesterol levels [15]. This explains why some studies reported no elevation of blood cholesterol when subjects added one or two additional eggs to their usual diet; their usual diets already contained amounts of cholesterol over the threshold level [16].

Although metabolic studies have established that high dietary cholesterol and saturated fat tend to elevate blood cholesterol levels, while polyunsaturated fats tend to lower them, the question of whether or not lowering blood cholesterol levels by dietary means will prevent CHD cannot be answered using metabolic studies. It is impossible to keep a large enough group of subjects on metabolic studies for the 20-or-30-year period required to provide such answers.

Animal Experiments

Animal experiments add to scientific knowledge about diet and atherosclerosis, even though the results cannot be applied directly to human beings (see Box 5-1). The important fact that investigators have gleaned from over 60 years of animal experimentation is that dietary fat and cholesterol are unquestionably related to the production of atherosclerosis [16]. Furthermore, when the blood cholesterol level of animals is lowered significantly by feeding a diet free of cholesterol, atherosclerosis is reversed [16]. The extent to which this might happen in humans, however, is yet to be determined.

Intervention Trials

Another method used to study diet and CHD is to modify the diet of a large group of people and follow them for a period of several years to assess whether or not they develop signs of CHD when compared with a comparable group of people who continue on their usual diets. This kind of study is called an *intervention trial* (Box 5-1). Several such trials have shown that a low saturated fat, low cholesterol, high polyunsaturated fat diet lowers blood cholesterol levels by 8 to 15 percent [8]. Nevertheless, these trials have failed so far to clearly demonstrate that the incidence of heart disease is decreased by these changes This may be because insufficient numbers of subjects have been used, or because atherosclerosis was already so advanced that reversal could not be achieved [6]. Moreover, making sure that all subjects closely adhere to the diet prescribed is exceedingly difficult in these studies.

An intervention trial [17] reported in 1981 may come close to providing convincing evidence of the effectiveness of dietary change, but awaits evaluation by the scientific community. This study began in Oslo, Norway, in 1972. Men aged 40 to 49 years who had high blood cholesterol levels, but no other known risk factors for CHD except that more than 75 percent smoked cigarettes, were selected. They were then assigned randomly to two groups. One group (the control) continued with their usual diet and smoking habits, while the other received individual counseling about diet and means to stop or decrease smoking. The diet recommended was lower in total fat, saturated fat, and cholesterol, and higher in polyunsaturated fat than the usual diet. After 5 years those who adhered closest to the experimental diet had the largest decrease in blood cholesterol levels, and, most importantly, had a 47 percent lower occurrence of heart attacks than the control group. The investigators estimated that changes in blood cholesterol levels accounted for 60 percent of the reduction in the rate of heart attacks, while decreased cigarette smoking accounted for about 25 percent. Careful evaluation of this study by scientists is needed before we can assume that these results are applicable to the general public.

In 1982, results of the Multiple Risk Factor Intervention Trial (MRFIT) were reported [18]. This study, sponsored by the National Heart, Lung and Blood Institute (NHLBI), recruited 12,866 men aged 35 to 57 years who were at high risk for CHD because they had high blood pressure, elevated blood cholesterol, and were cigarette smokers. The men were randomly assigned to the control group who received "usual care" from their personal physicians, or to the experimental group who participated in a special program aimed at cessation of smoking, lowering blood cholesterol levels by diet, and lowering blood pressure by weight reduction and/or drugs. The study continued for 7 years. Although risk factors were lowered by the special intervention program in the experimental group, they were also lowered in the control group, but not to the same extent. But the death rate from CHD was not significantly less in the experimental group, contrary to expectations. The investigators believe these unexpected results may be explained partly by the widespread use of diet by physicians to lower blood cholesterol levels at the time the study began (1972). This resulted in men in the control group receiving similar dietary treatment to those in the experimental group. More importantly, the investigators suspect that the drugs used to treat hypertension were damaging to some of the men who had specific heart abnormalities. Except for this group of men, the study indicated lower mortality rates from CHD among the men in the experimental group [18]. This study demonstrates the complexities of designing and executing intervention trials in human subjects.

The kind of study that would convince all critics that a diet lower in total fat, saturated fat, and cholesterol and higher in polyunsaturated fats than the current diet would decrease the occurrence of CHD would require a very large number of male subjects, beginning in adolescence. The subjects would be divided into two groups: One group would receive the modified diet while the other would follow the usual diet. Factors other than diet such as smoking and high blood pressure would have to be controlled. The study would need to last for 25 to 30 years or longer, because the objective would be to determine whether or not diet alone could prevent atherosclerosis and heart disease. Clearly a study of such magnitude is too expensive and too unwieldy to be properly executed. Consequently, we are left with less than perfect methods of experimentation on this question.

Despite decades of research, then, the diet–heart hypothesis has yet to be proved. So far, most investigators agree that: (1) blood cholesterol levels tend to be high in adults who later suffer heart attacks; (2) blood cholesterol levels can be lowered significantly by decreasing dietary saturated fat and cholesterol, while also increasing polyunsaturated fat intake; but (3) conclusive evidence currently is lacking that such dietary modifications will reduce or prevent the incidence of coronary heart disease in a population.

It is important to keep in mind that CHD has many causes, of which diet is only one possible cause. Furthermore, nutrients other than lipids may be involved in promoting CHD. Among nutrients currently under study for their involvement in CHD are protein [19], sucrose vs. starch [20], dietary fiber (discussion follows), sodium and potassium due to their relationship to hypertension (see Chapter 12,) magnesium [21], zinc and copper [11], calcium [23,24], chromium [25], fluoride [26], vitamin E (see Chapter 11), vitamin C (see Chapter 9), and niacin (see Chapter 10). Although a great body of research has focused attention on dietary lipids, investigators in the field have long speculated that nutrient interrelationships are involved in the production of atherosclerosis and CHD.

Recently, scientists began to realize that total blood cholesterol levels may be less important in understanding CHD than the distribution of cholesterol between low-density and high-density lipoproteins (see Chapter 4). Future research in this area may yield important insights into the relationship between diet and CHD.

Diet Strategy

Dietary Goals for the United States, promulgated by the Senate Select Committee on Nutrition and Human Needs [27], recommended that *all* Americans should modify their diets in a manner suggested by the American Heart Association. According to these goals, Americans should decrease their total fat intake from 40 to 30 percent of the kilocalorie intake. They should also reduce saturated fat and increase polyunsaturated fats to 10 percent of the kilocalories each, using monounsaturated fats to make up the remaining 10 percent. Cholesterol intake should be reduced, according to these goals, to 300 mg/day or less, and kilocalorie consumption should be reduced to avoid overweight. *Dietary Guidelines for Americans* also suggests avoiding too much dietary fat, saturated fat, and cholesterol [28].

These recommendations have generated controversy among physicians, nutritionists, and food industry representatives. Some of the arguments and counterarguments are noted in Table 5-2. Obviously, more research is needed before we have clear answers to many of our questions about dietary fat and cholesterol as causative agents in CHD.

At this stage of our scientific knowledge, what dietary recommendations make sense? First, keeping one's weight within the normal range is recommended for overall good health. One way to decrease kilocalorie intake without jeopardizing the nutritive value of the diet is to decrease the total intake of fat and sugar. Second, practicing moderation in diet is always a sensible guide to follow. Many nutritionists consider a diet containing 40 to 45 percent of total kilocalories as fat and more than 500 mg of cholesterol to be an excessively rich diet. According to this view, a more moderate choice is a diet containing less fat, saturated fat, and cholesterol. Third, choosing a wide variety of foods, most of which are nutrient-dense foods, increases one's chances of obtaining all the nutrients needed. Generally, this means varying the kinds of foods one chooses for a given meal. In other words, having the same food daily for breakfast or lunch greatly restricts the variety of foods in the diet. For many people, such dietary changes would improve the overall nutritional value of their diets.

TABLE 5-2. DIETARY GOAL RECOMMENDATIONS FOR CHANGES IN LIPID CONSUMPTION: ARGUMENTS AND COUNTERARGUMENTS

	PRESENT AMERICAN DIET, %	DIETARY GOALS, %
Total fat (% of total kcal)	40	30
Saturated fat (% of total kcal)	16	10
Polyunsaturated fat (% of total kcal)	7	10
Monounsaturated fat (% of total kcal)	19	10
Cholesterol, mg/day	600 mg	300 mg

ARGUMENTS AGAINST RECOMMENDATIONS	ARGUMENTS IN SUPPORT OF RECOMMENDATIONS
1. We lack proof that following the dietary goals will, in fact, prevent CHD [29].	1. It is impossible to conduct the definitive experiment; at present, evidence indicates high probability that incidence of CHD would be lowered by dietary changes [30,31].
2. Since we lack clear evidence that dietary changes will prevent CHD, we should instead find those people who have either symptoms of CHD or high-risk factors and treat them [29].	2. CHD develops over 20–40 years. By the time symptoms appear, extensive atherosclerosis has developed, which can be reversed only slightly by treatment. Attempting to prevent atherosclerosis is therefore a preferable approach [32].
3. Risk is highest among people with serum cholesterol levels higher than 250 mg/100 mL (about one-third of middle-aged Americans). We need to find these people and treat them instead of changing everyone's diet [33].	3. There is evidence that the risk for CHD increases linearly above 180 mg/100 mL of serum cholesterol. Finding individuals with blood levels above this level would be difficult and expensive. Overall dietary change would be a more practical way to lower blood cholesterol levels [16].
4. We cannot anticipate the consequences of increasing intakes of polyunsaturated fatty acids, since some evidence indicates the possibility of increased incidence of cancer [34] and gallstones [35] from high intakes.	4. While some studies suggest increased risk, others indicate no increased risk of cancer [36] when diets are high in polyunsaturates. In any event, the recommended intake is only a small increase over present intakes of polyunsaturates. Furthermore, recent evidence indicates that polyunsaturated fats may aid in preventing blood clots [32].

Some scientists who want evidence to be "solid as a rock" before they recommend dietary changes for the general public oppose the dietary goals. Others, who believe that current evidence is sufficient to make recommendations to the public, support the goals.

DIETARY FAT AND CANCER

Cancer is an abnormal overgrowth or tumor of the cells, having no useful function. It grows at the expense of healthy tissue and, unless arrested, spreads and eventually becomes fatal.

The second leading cause of death in the United States, cancer is among the most dreaded of diseases. In women, the leading cause of cancer death is breast cancer, closely followed by lung cancer, while in men colon cancer ranks second to lung cancer [37]. Risk factors related to the occurrence of cancer in this country include environmental factors such as cigarette smoking and exposure to industrial chemicals, and diet. Research on possible links between diet and cancer is just beginning, in contrast to the more extensive investigation undertaken to study the relationship between diet and heart disease. Diet is thought to influence the development of cancer in a variety of ways. Specific cancer-causing agents such as saccharin or aflatoxins (see Chapter 17) may be found in certain foods. The composition of the diet may also affect the development of cancer by altering metabolic factors that influence tumor formation, or that promote tumor growth. So far, the evidence for possible relationships between fat or cholesterol intake and cancer stems chiefly from epidemiological studies and animal experimentation.

Epidemiological Studies

Epidemiological studies show that countries with the highest total fat intake, such as the United States and countries in northern Europe, have high mortality rates from breast (Figure 5-3) and colon cancer (Figure 5-4), while those with low fat intake (Thailand, Japan, Chile) have low mortality rates from these diseases. Some studies suggest that high meat intake is associated with high mortality rates from breast and colon cancer [38], but it is unclear at this time whether this is due to the fat contributed by meat, to the production of possible carcinogens (cancer-causing agents) in the broiling or frying of meat, or to some other factor [39].

Some hypotheses have been offered as to how high fat intakes may be a

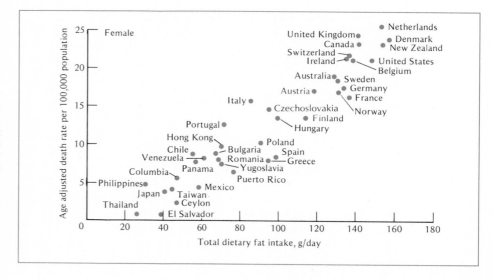

FIGURE 5-3. Correlation between fat consumption and mortality from breast cancer in different countries. As total dietary fat intake increases, so does mortality from breast cancer. These data merely suggest a relationship between these two variables; they do not mean that high dietary fat intake *causes* breast cancer mortality.

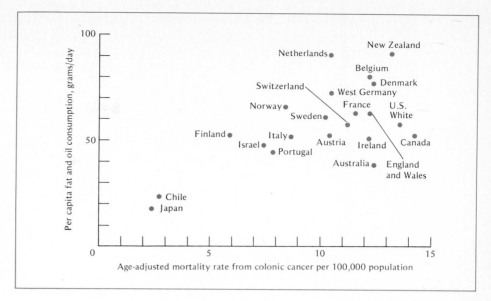

FIGURE 5-4. Correlation between fat consumption and mortality from colon cancer in different countries. While there is a relationship between per capita fat consumption and colon cancer, this does not mean that high fat intake causes colon cancer.

factor in colon cancer. Investigators have postulated that high intakes of dietary fat induce high secretions of bile acids, which might influence development of colon cancer [39]. Bile acids are required for the digestion and absorption of fats, after which they move on to the ileum where some are reabsorbed and the remainder are attacked by intestinal bacteria in the colon, producing modified bile acids. Several investigators have worked on the hypothesis that fecal bile acids or modified bile acids may function as tumor promoters in the colon [39]. No one has yet been able to isolate from either human or animal feces *carcinogens* (cancer-causing substances) derived from bile acids, however.

For many years scientists have known that high intakes of fat increase the incidence of breast cancer in animals. Current research in women centers around trying to find out whether or not a high fat diet modifies certain hormones in the body, which may be involved in the production of breast cancer [39]. As noted earlier, although some studies have suggested that diets high in polyunsaturated fatty acids may be related to increased incidence of cancer [34], others have found no basis for this fear [36].

Confusion recently arose because some, but not all, epidemiological studies suggest that unusually low blood cholesterol levels are associated with high incidence of colon cancer in men, but not in women [40]. Factors responsible for this relationship are uncertain, but the studies do not indicate that low blood cholesterol levels *cause* colon cancer [40]. The unusually low blood cholesterol levels may be the result of metabolic changes due to the cancer. Genetic factors also may be involved. Experts in CHD believe that evidence from these studies in no way changes the recommendation that individuals who have high blood cholesterol levels should lower them through diet [41]. Obviously, more research is needed in this important area.

Diet Strategy

In June 1980, the National Cancer Institute asked the National Research Council of the National Academy of Sciences to review current scientific information regarding the relationship of diet to cancer, and to develop recommendations concerning diet for the general public. The committee concluded that the evidence currently is stronger for a causal relationship between high fat consumption and cancer of the colon and breast than for any other dietary component studied [42]. The report recommends that total fat intake be reduced from the present 40 percent to 30 percent of total kilocalories, or lower, and recommends a reduction in both saturated and unsaturated fats.

The full dietary recommendations of this report are discussed in Chapter 2. Some industry groups, particularly the meat industry, have protested that too little evidence implicates fat as a causative factor in cancer, so that controversy can be expected regarding these dietary suggestions.

A CLOSER LOOK

You may be confused and frustrated to read that increased polyunsaturated fats in the diet may be protective against heart disease, but possibly harmful in terms of cancer. The report, *Diet, Nutrition and Cancer*, from the National Academy of Sciences [42] notes that in animals, when total fat intake is low (approximately 10 percent of total kilocalories), polyunsaturated fats are more carcinogenic than saturated fats. This is not the case at higher levels of fat intake, however. Furthermore, the report observes that evidence in humans is insufficient to draw any conclusions about the carcinogenesis of different kinds of fats.

Although this report recommends that total fat, saturated and unsaturated, be decreased, remember that unsaturated fats include monounsaturated and polyunsaturated fats. *Dietary Goals for the United States* noted that the current intake of monounsaturated fat represents 19 percent and saturated fat 16 percent of total kilocalories. It recommends that each of these be reduced to 10 percent of total kilocalories. On the other hand, these goals found the polyunsaturated fat intake to be 7 percent of total kilocalories, and recommended a modest increase to 10 percent. This amount of polyunsaturated fat in the diet represents a moderate, not a high, level. Most experts believe it is prudent not to exceed this amount in view of the fact that the long-term consequences of a diet unusually high in polyunsaturates are unknown. The recommendations of the *Dietary Goals for the United States* regarding fat are therefore in line with those of the Committee on Diet, Nutrition and Cancer.

CARBOHYDRATES AND DISEASE

Sugars and Tooth Decay

Simple, refined carbohydrates are more conducive to tooth decay than are complex carbohydrates. Thus, this section will focus largely on the influence of sugars on tooth decay. Although sucrose appears to be the most *cariogenic* (decay-causing) sugar, fructose, glucose, and maltose also can be cariogenic.

As pointed out in Chapter 3, our consumption of sugar has greatly increased during the twentieth century. At the same time, dental caries (tooth decay), diabetes, obesity, heart disease, cancer, and other diseases have increased among Americans. Is there a relationship? Can we say that increased sugar consumption causes some of these diseases?

By far the most certain harmful effect of sugar is its relationship to tooth decay. Virtually no one in the United States is untouched by tooth decay; it affects an estimated 98 percent of the population. The National Institute of Dental Research reports that we spend more than $2 billion yearly to repair tooth decay problems, an expenditure that meets only a small part of the need for dental care in the United States. To repair all the damage due to dental caries in this country would require an estimated $8 billion more than we are currently spending [43]. Before exploring how sugars can cause tooth decay, take a few minutes to study the structure of the tooth in Figure 5-5.

Factors Contributing to Tooth Decay The word *caries* is derived from a Greek word meaning "rottenness." Dental caries is actually an infectious disease. It is produced by specific microorganisms that live on the tooth and produce acid from sugars. The acid attacks the hard enamel of the tooth, allowing penetration of bacteria that eventually destroy parts or all of the tooth.

A pregnant woman's nutritional status can influence the structural development of her unborn child's teeth; improperly developed teeth are more susceptible to dental caries. It is interesting to note here that tooth development starts as early as the sixth week of life in the embryo as the tooth buds begin to differentiate.

Age influences susceptibility to dental caries. The tooth is at greatest risk for caries development in the first years after it has erupted, before its surface is

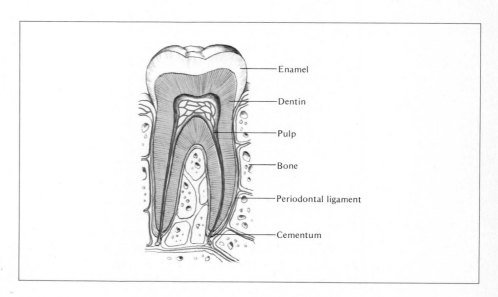

FIGURE 5-5. Diagram of tooth structure.

Enamel

Dentin

Pulp

Bone

Periodontal ligament

Cementum

completely hardened. This explains, in part, why young children whose primary teeth are newly erupted are so prone to dental caries.

Many environmental factors influence the development of dental caries [44]. The type and form of carbohydrate eaten, other kinds of food eaten, frequency of food intake, amount of money available to children to purchase high-sugar snacks, quality of dental hygiene, and extent of professional dental care are all important environmental influences on the development of dental caries. Factors which influence food habits such as social, cultural, economic, and physical factors are indirect influences on the development of dental caries [45].

How Does Sugar Cause Tooth Decay?   Dietary sugars play a central role in tooth decay by acting as the substrate for acid production, which in turn causes the tooth to demineralize and decay [46]. Sugars also play an important part in the development of *dental plaque* and hence dental decay. Dental plaque is a sticky white, gray, or yellow film produced by oral microorganisms from sugars. The plaque adheres firmly to the teeth if proper brushing and flossing do not remove it. Oral bacteria multiply rapidly in the plaque, fermenting dietary sugars to produce acids which, in turn, cause the enamel of the teeth to demineralize and decay.

Research Evidence

Human remains from cultures that consumed little sugar show very little evidence of dental caries. Modern problems with dental caries began to occur around the middle of the nineteenth century, at the same time that sugar consumption rose dramatically. Many populations who changed their patterns of consumption from a traditional diet of starchy, complex carbohydrate foods to increasing levels of sugar demonstrated corresponding increases in dental caries [47].

Russell reported that 20-to-24-year-old civilians living in Near and Far Eastern countries whose usual annual sugar consumption was 6 to 19 kg (13.2 to 41.8 lb) per person experienced a tooth decay rate of 0.6 to 5.0 teeth per person annually [47]. In contrast, among South American natives where sugar consumption varied from 23 to 44 kg (50.6 to 98.8 lb) per person annually, decay rates ranged from 8.4 to 12.6 teeth [47]. Sugar consumption in the United States is now about 130 lb per person per year. Decay rates in the United States parallel this high sugar consumption. The average American 15-year-old has 10 decayed, missing, or filled teeth [48].

A number of surveys have demonstrated significantly increased dental caries in Eskimos and African tribesmen who changed from their traditional food patterns that were low in sugar content to modern refined foods, high in sugars. In 1938 the diets of the natives of Tristan da Cunha, a group of islands in the South Atlantic, were noted to consist of potatoes and fish, but no refined sugar. Not one cavity in a first permanent molar was found in individuals under the age of 20. By 1962, however, when the average consumption of sugar was a pound per week per person, individuals under the age of 20 exhibited a 50 percent rate of caries in first permanent molars [49]. There are groups of people, however, such as those of Easter Island, who consume diets very low in sugar and sweets, and still demonstrate a high prevalence of dental caries [50]. Obviously, sugar intake alone is not the only factor influencing development of dental caries. Heredity, the nutritional quality of the diet during tooth formation, dental hygiene, and dietary components other than sugar might account for these results.

An important study, the Vipeholm Dental Caries Study, involved feeding a controlled diet to a group of subjects [51]. Adults living in a mental institution who were fed a low-sugar diet of good nutritional quality with few between-meal snacks were observed to have very little dental decay. Then, over a 5-year period, these adults were fed sugar in breads, drinks, and candies such as caramels, toffees, and chocolates. The bread and sugar drinks were given with meals, but candies were given between meals. Results indicated that the sugar in the bread and drinks was not responsible for any great increase in dental caries, but that the candies resulted in significant increases in dental caries. The authors of the study concluded that sugar is most likely to cause dental caries if it is in a sticky form, and if it is eaten frequently between meals. In this form, the sugar tends to be retained on the surfaces of the teeth. When these foods are removed from the diet, the teeth are less susceptible to caries. The authors also observed that individuals in their study differed greatly in their susceptibility to caries, perhaps due to hereditary factors [51].

It is important to consider the ethical implications of this type of study. By giving these subjects sugar in the second phase of the study, the researchers were placing them at risk from the standpoint of health. Furthermore, one wonders how capable these mental patients were of giving informed consent. Today, because of strict guidelines governing the kind of research permitted on human subjects, it is unlikely that a study of this type could be conducted.

Some investigators believe the frequency with which sugary foods are eaten may be more important than the total amount of sugar consumed daily. For example, Sweeney [45] offers the example that if you eat five cough drops in 15 minutes the resulting acid might be in contact with your teeth for about 35 minutes. But if you eat the cough drops one every 15 minutes, the teeth might be in contact with acid for 100 minutes. The longer the tooth is in contact with acid, the greater the likelihood of decay. Other investigators point out, however, that taken together the data indicate that the total amount of sugar consumed is as important as the frequency [52].

Diet Strategy

Practical applications of our knowledge concerning sugars and tooth decay lead us to conclude that sugar and high-sugar foods, especially those that are sticky and/or dissolve slowly, should be restricted between meals. If there is a choice between sugar in solid vs. liquid form, it makes sense to select the liquid, since it is less likely to stick to the teeth and cause caries. If sweets are eaten, whether with or between meals, care should be taken to brush, floss, and rinse the teeth immediately after eating. Foods high in sugar eaten at mealtime are more apt to be washed away from the tooth surface by liquids and other food than if the same foods are consumed alone between meals.

Relatively safe between-meal snacks include fresh fruits or fruits canned in juice, rather than heavy syrup. Raw vegetables and raw fibrous fruits often serve as cleansing agents and help to remove other foods from the teeth surface. In addition, chewing such foods can stimulate the flow of saliva, which not only washes sugar from the tooth surface, but also causes an increase in salivary bicarbonate, and consequently a decrease in oral acidity.

Although raw fruits and vegetables contain sugars, they are far less cariogenic than sucrose, perhaps because the sugar is not highly concentrated, or because these foods are quickly cleared from the mouth and do not stick to the teeth.

Remember that sucrose is of extremely low nutrient density, as are most high-sugar foods. One cannot therefore recommend high sugar intakes for this reason alone.

Sugar and Diabetes

The relationship between a high proportion of sucrose in the diet and dental caries is relatively well established. Charges have also been made that high sucrose intakes lead to diabetes and coronary heart disease, but there are conflicting opinions among investigators about any causative relationships.

Diabetes is a general term referring to metabolic disorders in which there is excessive excretion of urine. In diabetes mellitus, the disorder we are discussing here, the individual has difficulty metabolizing carbohydrates, usually because of either too little production of insulin or the inability to properly utilize insulin. As a consequence, blood glucose levels become abnormally high because insulin is essential for promoting removal of glucose from the blood. Diabetes appears to develop chiefly in people who have a genetic predisposition to the disease.

In the early 1960s, researchers reported that people such as Eskimos and African tribesmen who moved from their native lands, where the incidence of diabetes was low, to western countries developed a higher incidence of diabetes on the westernized diet. The dietary factor involved was thought by some to be the high sugar level common in western diets [53], but there could also have been a decrease in the intake of dietary fiber. Furthermore, the total kilocalorie intake also may have increased, and the amount of exercise decreased, leading to obesity, which increases one's chances of developing diabetes.

In laboratory rats sucrose feeding has been shown to increase fasting insulin levels and decrease the body's ability to use insulin [54], both of which are conditions found in mild diabetes occurring in humans in adulthood. In genetically susceptible rats, investigators have been able to produce practically all the symptoms of diabetes, including kidney and retinal damage, by feeding sucrose, whereas feeding the same amount of starch did not produce these symptoms [55].

These results with animals cannot be applied directly to humans, as noted earlier. So far, studies with human subjects fail to answer the question of whether sucrose intake *causes* diabetes. The old notion that high or frequent intakes of sucrose can exhaust the ability of the pancreatic cells to produce insulin in individuals having the genetic predisposition to diabetes has been abandoned, however [56]. We now know that sugars are not unique in stimulating insulin production, since amino acids also have this function.

The evidence is clear that obesity greatly increases the *risk* of developing diabetes. If sugar intake is a cause of excessive kilocalorie consumption for an individual, then it plays an indirect role in increasing the risk of developing diabetes for those who have the genetic potential.

Although in the past diabetic patients have been told to avoid sugar and sweets to guard against elevated blood glucose levels, recent research indicates that after a meal blood glucose levels depend not only on how rapidly the meal's carbohydrates are absorbed, but also on the amount of fat and protein in the meal. Consequently, some investigators say that diabetics can safely consume sugars in meals, but others believe that more research is needed, since a meal's influence on as yet unstudied factors, such as blood insulin levels, may be equally important. In view of this uncertainty and because high sugar diets are low in nutrient density, the prudent diabetic will continue to avoid sugary foods.

Sugar and Coronary Heart Disease

The proposal that high sugar consumption may be related to CHD arose from the possibility that certain sugars may elevate blood cholesterol or triglyceride levels, thereby increasing the risk for CHD. Although high blood triglyceride levels alone do not increase the risk for CHD, they add to the risk if they occur along with elevated blood cholesterol levels.

Yudkin reported that high sucrose consumption in 15 countries over a period of years was associated with high death rates from CHD [57], but Grande [58] pointed out that many other countries with high sucrose intake have low death rates from CHD. In addition, there is a high correlation between high sucrose and high saturated fat consumption in countries mentioned by Yudkin. Thus, the high saturated fat rather than the high sucrose intake may be the culprit in CHD [58,59].

Metabolic studies with normal human subjects show that high sucrose intakes do not produce higher blood cholesterol or triglyceride levels than starch *if* the amount of sugar fed is no more than in the usual western diet, and *if* the subjects are kept at normal weight [58]. Some investigators estimate, however, that about 9 percent of the adult population in the United States is "carbohydrate-sensitive," meaning that if they consume large amounts of carbohydrates, their blood triglycerides become abnormally high [60]. Ordinarily, treatment of such patients includes restriction of sucrose as well as weight control [61].

At present, then, the evidence fails to support the contention that high sucrose intakes directly *cause* CHD. Many investigators believe that high intakes of carbohydrates may aid in decreasing the risk of CHD simply because such a diet tends to be lower in fat, including saturated fat, than the usual diet [59]. Generally, nutritionists discourage high sucrose diets, but for reasons other than any possible relationship to CHD.

Diet Strategy

What is the place of sucrose and other sweeteners in our diets, then? It seems clear that sucrose is not the toxin it has sometimes been made out to be, but a diet is likely to provide more nutrients and dietary fiber if most of the carbohydrate comes from minimally processed complex carbohydrates and those sugars that occur naturally in fruits. In an ideal diet, sucrose, honey, jams, jellies, and syrups would be used for occasional sweetness, as minor components of the diet. Moderation is a good rule to follow in nutrition, and intakes of sucrose as high as 20 to 30 percent of total kilocalories are probably immoderately high.

Dietary Fiber

Ten years ago nutrition textbooks devoted practically no space to dietary fiber. Authorities believed that since it could not be absorbed, it was of little use to the body except to avoid constipation. Now there is an upsurge of interest in the benefits of including adequate dietary fiber in the human diet. Some investigators have related diets low in fiber to gastrointestinal disorders as well as to cancer of the colon, heart disease, and diabetes [62].

Dietary fiber was defined in Chapter 3 as those components of the plant cell wall and other plant polysaccharides that resist digestion in the upper intestinal tract. Foods that contribute dietary fiber to our diet include whole grains, legumes, seeds, vegetables, and fruits. The proportion of the different components of dietary fiber (cellulose, hemicelluloses, pectins, lignin, and gums) varies from one food to another. At present, most food composition tables do not include values for dietary fiber because analytical methods do not yet permit accurate analysis. Instead, such tables may list crude fiber, the plant residue remaining after treatment with acid and alkali. Table 3-3 (Chapter 3) compares total dietary fiber with crude fiber figures for certain foods.

Physicians have long known that dietary fiber or "roughage" relieves and prevents constipation. Fiber appears to have this efffect because of its ability to swell in water, and to hold water to its surface, referred to as bulking capacity. The bulky, soft mass accumulating in the colon stimulates nerve endings in the colon and rectum to move the bowel contents without strain. Dietary fiber has other important properties, however, each of which is discussed in relationship to diseases postulated to be related to fiber.

Research Evidence   There is a considerable amount of research supporting as well as questioning the hypothesized relationship between dietary fiber and diseases. In the 1960s, Dr. Denis Burkitt and Dr. Hugh Trowell [62], working independently as physicians in Africa, publicized their observations that a long list of diseases including diverticular disease, coronary heart disease, diabetes, and cancer of the colon were very common in western industrialized countries, but were rare or unknown among Africans living in rural communities on their traditional, unrefined diets. In studying the differences between the traditional and the westernized diets, these investigators hypothesized that the natural high-fiber content of traditional African diets might be protective against these diseases. This kind of evidence does not *prove*, of course, that low intakes of dietary fiber actually cause any of these diseases. Other dietary as well as nondietary factors may be culprits. Let us look at the current state of knowledge regarding the relationship of dietary fiber to these diseases.

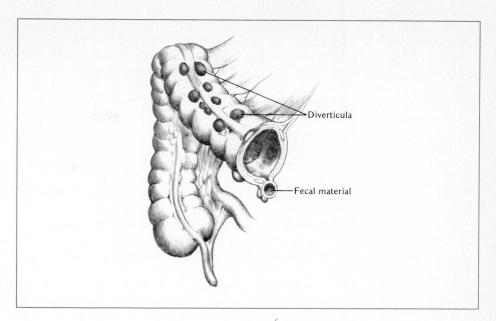

Diverticula

Fecal material

FIGURE 5-6. Diverticular disease. Diverticula or small sacs or pouches form along the colon.

In diverticular disease, small distended pouches or sacs (diverticula) form along the colon (Figure 5-6). The sacs are thought to result from pressure inside the colon, which causes small sections of the colon to "blow-out" at points of weakness to form the pouches or diverticula. If feces stagnate in the pouches, infection develops, resulting in pain and discomfort. Sometimes a diverticulum bursts, requiring surgical repair.

One study in Britain indicated that diverticular disease was higher among groups consuming low amounts of dietary fiber [63]. Moreover, many physicians currently treat diverticular disease by prescribing diets high in dietary fiber plus extra wheat bran, and some investigators conclude that individuals who consume low-fiber diets are more apt to develop diverticular disease [64]. Nevertheless, additional carefully controlled studies are needed before we can be certain that lack of dietary fiber actually causes this disorder, or that dietary fiber is effective in its treatment [65]. Of all the postulated effects of dietary fiber, its relationship to "the development or relief of symptoms of diverticular disease is probably the one that is more generally accepted [66]."

Some components of dietary fiber, namely pectins, guar gum, and oat bran have been shown to lower serum cholesterol levels in human subjects, thus decreasing a risk factor for heart disease [67,68]. Pectins and guar gum are water-soluble, and oat bran also contains a higher percentage of water-soluble than insoluble polysaccharides [69]. Insoluble components of dietary fiber do not seem to affect blood cholesterol levels. Exactly how soluble fiber components lower blood cholesterol levels is uncertain, but one possibility is that they bind bile acids in the intestinal lumen, increasing their fecal excretion. As a result, the liver must break down more cholesterol to form bile acids required for digestion of fats in food. This process could decrease blood cholesterol levels.

Although there is interest in the possible relationships between low-fiber diets and colon cancer, there is presently too little evidence to demonstrate such relationships [42,66]. Several hypotheses have been proposed to explain how fiber might prevent colon cancer. These include:

1. Fiber may promote the growth of those types of colon bacteria that cannot form carcinogens from bile salts.
2. The concentration of carcinogens might be effectively diluted by dietary fiber because of its water-holding properties.
3. Carcinogens might stay in the colon a shorter time if fiber decreases transit times.
4. Dietary fiber may bind tightly to carcinogens, promoting their removal from the intestinal tract.
5. Bacterial action on dietary fiber in the colon produces fatty acids which can increase the acidity of the colon contents. This situation lowers the concentration of colonic ammonia which otherwise may promote cancer [66].

To date, none of these hypotheses has ben fully investigated.

Some researchers are studying the possibility that dietary fiber may aid in preventing and possibly treating obesity. This hypothesis is described in Chapter 8, but so far studies on use of high-fiber diets for weight control are lacking [70].

Recently, much research has focused on high-fiber diets in patients with diabetes mellitus. These studies show less elevation of blood glucose in diabetic patients after high-fiber meals than after fiber-free meals [71]. Furthermore, soluble fibers such as pectins and guar gum are most effective [71], and the effect is greater if fiber is fed as a part of a high- rather than a low-carbohydrate diet [72]. This effect of soluble fibers on blood glucose levels means that insulin dosages can be decreased or even discontinued in some patients [71]. The reasons why fiber influences blood glucose levels are uncertain, but investigators propose that soluble fibers may slow emptying of the stomach, or slow the rate of absorption of carbohydrates. Another possibility is that hormonal activities in the intestines or pancreas may be altered by soluble fibers to produce the effects observed [71].

At this point, we do not know to what extent low-fiber diets may cause diabetes to develop in individuals prone to this disease, but high-fiber diets may be useful in treating some diabetics [73].

In evaluating research studies which attempt to relate dietary fiber to disease, several concepts need to be kept in mind. Dietary fiber occurring in its natural state in plants has a complex structure. Scientists have isolated different components of dietary fiber and studied each separately. This allows for control of all factors except the one component of dietary fiber under study. Unfortunately, however, isolation of fiber components disrupts the plant cell wall and may change the physical and chemical properties so that they no longer resemble those occurring in the natural state.

Equally important is the recognition that adding an isolated source of dietary fiber such as bran to the typical western diet in no way parallels the kind of diets described in epidemiological studies in Africa in which high-fiber intakes were

NUTRITION IN THE NEWS

PERSONAL HEALTH. A NEW DIET FOR DIABETICS MAY OFFER NUTRITION BENEFITS FOR ALL

Jane E. Brody, *The New York Times*, February 18, 1982

Sunday breakfast is a sliced orange, Spanish omelet, two pieces of whole-wheat toast with margarine and a glass of skim milk. Monday dinner is roast beef with mashed potatoes, corn, green beans and spinach, rye bread with margarine and grapes. . . .

This may not sound like a "diet," but it is. These meals were selected from a 1,500-calorie high-carbohydrate, high-fiber diet plan that has helped many diabetics reduce or eliminate their dependence on insulin and at the same time achieve better control of their blood sugar. . . .

Diabetics are not the only ones who can benefit from the low-fat, low-sugar menu, which emphasizes starchy foods like whole-grain cereals, beans, rice, potatoes and bread, along with fruits and vegetables.

The American Diabetes Association has recommended it for nearly all Americans "interested in good health and nutrition." For research has shown that the high-carbohydrate, high-fiber diet also lowers blood levels of cholesterol and triglycerides (and thus may help prevent heart disease), helps people lose weight without going hungry, counters constipation, controls the symptoms of hypoglycemia and may even prevent diverticulitis and cancer of the colon.

For diabetics, the diet may help ward off some of the most debilitating complications of their disease, including clogged blood vessels and nerve damage. The old diabetic diets were high in animal protein and fat and low in carbohydrates, and seemed to encourage the development of clogged arteries and heart disease, which cause 75 percent of the deaths among diabetics.

The new diet has been used successfully in the treatment of more than a thousand patients with adult-onset diabetes by Dr. James W. Anderson, diabetologist at the University of Kentucky in Lexington. . . .

. . . A number of studies in Europe using related diets have shown similar improvements in blood sugar control among diabetics. . . .

. . . In a recent interview, Dr. Anderson explained how the diet works. "Fiber smooths out the ups and downs of blood sugar," he noted.

Even in healthy people, he explained, a low-fiber meal prompts a precipitous rise in blood sugar, which is followed by the release of insulin to clear the blood of excess sugar. The blood sugar then falls below fasting level, often producing symptoms of irritability and hunger. With a high-fiber diet, however, the blood sugar rise after meals is more modest (which means less of a need for insulin) and the drop afterward not as extreme.

This is beneficial to diabetics, who have difficulty maintaining a stable blood sugar level. . . .

The main drawback of the high-carbohydrate, high-fiber diet Dr. Anderson and others prescribe is increased flatulence. However, . . . initial bloating experienced when dietary fiber is increased substantially usually subsides in a few weeks as the body adapts to the new menu.

ASK YOURSELF:

Which foods in the Exchange List in Appendix B are high in starch, but relatively low in fat? Which starchy foods are high in dietary fiber? Which meats are lowest in fat, and therefore apt to be emphasized in this diet? In your present living conditions, how could you increase the amount of vegetables and fruits in your diet? Should a diabetic attempt to follow this diet without his or her physician's advice?

observed to be correlated with low incidences of the diseases discussed above [62]. The African diets included yams, cassava, okra, and a wide variety of seeds, fruits, and leafy vegetables [74]. Dietary fibers from these foods have yet to be carefully studied in human subjects. Additionally, these African diets tend to be high in plant foods and low in animal foods, just the opposite of the situation in western countries. African diets therefore tend to be lower in fat and higher in carbohydrates than western diets. Some of the relationships of the African diets to lower incidence of many diseases may be due to interactions of several components of the diet and not to dietary fiber alone [66]. Furthermore, it is difficult to be sure that certain diseases do *not* exist in isolated rural parts of Africa. In addition, people in western countries generally live longer than rural Africans. Therefore, diseases associated with older ages would be expected to be more prevalent in western countries.

Can Too Much Dietary Fiber Be Harmful?

Many people believe that if a little of something is good, a lot more is better, and some people may be applying this generalization to · dietary fiber. There is evidence, however, that dietary fiber decreases fat, protein, and mineral absorption, and while the losses of protein and fat are not large enough to be considered serious, mineral losses may be important, especially in people who have low amounts of minerals in their diets [75]. Further study is required to find out whether, after a period of time on a high-fiber diet, the body adapts and so loses fewer minerals.

Diet Strategy

Most nutritionists believe that human beings require some dietary fiber, since our digestive systems function best in its presence. The optimal amount needed and the exact benefits one can expect are presently unknown, however. On the other hand, we know that different components of dietary fiber have different properties. For example, purified cellulose has few of the properties of dietary fiber. Bran does not absorb nearly as much water as many vegetable fibers do. In fact, the properties of isolated components of dietary fiber may be changed by the isolation process. It seems sensible, therefore, to consume dietary fiber as it occurs *in foods* rather than to add a highly purified form, such as cellulose or bran, to a highly refined diet. Such a decision would mean substituting whole-grain breads and cereals for highly refined ones, and increasing the intake of legumes, nuts, seeds, fruits, and vegetables.

It is a good idea to change gradually from a highly refined diet to one containing more of the above foods, and to keep in mind that one person may be able to tolerate, without symptoms, a higher fiber diet than another. Too much fiber can cause diarrhea, abdominal cramps, and excessive gas.

In conclusion, it is important to note that there is a need for further research before we can thoroughly understand the relationships among carbohydrates, lipids, and disease. In the meantime, we must be careful to critically evaluate available research before jumping to quick conclusions about the possibility of preventing diseases by dietary means.

The evidence to date has prompted many nutrition scientists to recommend that the American public should eat less fat, especially saturated fat, and less cholesterol, sugar, and salt. They also encourage Americans to maintain ideal body weight, since obesity is linked to high blood pressure and diabetes, and therefore to heart disease and stroke. Avoiding high intakes of fat and sugar should aid in controlling body weight.

The Committee on Diet, Nutrition and Cancer of the National Academy of Sciences recommends that dietary fats be decreased to 30 percent of total kilocalories or less to decrease the risk of cancer, particularly of the breast and colon [42]. Although some scientists protest that recommendations of decreased fat and cholesterol intake may not decrease the incidence of heart disease, and therefore may anger or frustrate the public, others have maintained that the dietary recommendations are the "prudent consensus" of most scientists today, and are not "hard and fast" rules. The dual concepts of moderation and variety in planning diets are reasonable and practical.

SUMMARY

1 Causes of cardiovascular disease are many, but it seems likely that diet and lifestyle figure prominently.
2 The four major risk factors among individuals who develop CHD include: elevated blood cholesterol levels, hypertension, diabetes, and cigarette smoking. Secondary risk factors include obesity, elevated blood triglycerides, lack of physical activity, stress, and family history of CHD.
3 According to the diet–heart hypothesis accepted by many investigators, a diet high in kilocalories, saturated fat, and cholesterol and low in polyunsaturated fats increases blood cholesterol levels. High blood cholesterol levels increase one's chances of developing atherosclerosis, which leads to heart attacks.
4 Studies show that blood cholesterol levels tend to be high in adults who later have heart attacks. These levels can be lowered by decreasing dietary saturated fat and cholesterol while increasing polyunsaturated fat intake. However, we lack firm evidence to assure that such a diet will reduce the incidence of CHD in a population.
5 Epidemiological and experimental evidence strongly suggests that high fat intakes are causally related to cancer of the breast and colon.
6 Eating sugar and high-sugar foods, especially in a sticky form, greatly increases the risk of developing dental caries.
7 We lack evidence to say that a high sucrose intake

causes diabetes, but evidence is clear that obesity greatly increases the risk of developing diabetes.
8 There is insufficient evidence that sucrose directly causes CHD, but individuals with elevated blood triglycerides should restrict sucrose intakes.
9 Lack of dietary fiber has been postulated to be related to the development of diseases such as coronary heart disease, diverticular disease, diabetes, and colon cancer. Evidence to date is strongest that dietary fiber may be beneficial in treating diverticular disease. Most nutritionists believe that the human body requires some dietary fiber.

FOR DISCUSSION AND APPLICATION

1 Compare the diet strategies suggested for preventing these diseases: coronary heart disease, cancer, diabetes, and dental caries. What are the common threads running through the various diet strategies? Are there any contradictions in the diets suggested for preventing these disorders?
2 Many people have become disillusioned with scientists who constantly report newly discovered links between the development of cancer and various things in the environment. Their attitude is "Why bother? Almost everything causes cancer." What would you suggest to these people about food and nutrition? How would you approach them in trying to convince them of the importance of eating a moderate, varied diet?

3 In the very near future there may be a pill or a vaccine that will prevent dental caries. If such a prevention technique is available, people may feel justified in eating sticky, sweet foods because, they may feel, the pill will prevent tooth decay. Would you agree with them? What are flaws in their logic? How would you approach them in suggesting that diet is still important for healthy teeth?

4 Many of the general public are very concerned about eating the best diet possible to prevent heart disease. Write an article that might appear in your local newspaper. Explain, in a way that the public would understand, the relationship between diet and heart disease. Make recommendations about diet as part of your article.

SUGGESTED READINGS

Cavaiani, Mabel, *Low Cholesterol Cuisine,* Chicago: Contemporary Books, Inc., 1981. This is a recipe book appropriate for the lay public. In addition to cholesterol, the author also covers sodium content of the recipes.

Eighth Report of the National Health, Lung, and Blood Advisory Council, NIH Publication No. 80–2104, Publications Section, Office of Information, NHLBI, Bethesda, Md., 20205. This report describes recent achievements made in the attack on cardiovascular disease and high blood pressure.

Healthy People: The Surgeon General's Report on Health Promotion and Disease Prevention, U.S. Department of Health, Education and Welfare, 1979. This report discusses the general state of health in the United States and spells out health goals and strategies to improve health.

6

PROTEINS

There is no life without protein. This discovery by Mulder in 1838 launched an era of research into the mysteries of this nutrient. The word *protein* means "to come first" or "to take first place." In recent years some nutritionists and the general public appear to have regarded protein as *the* most important nutrient, producing what some critics have called "the protein mystique" [1]. One manifestation of this "mystique" is the heavy promotion of protein supplements, as if the American diet could not provide enough protein.

Claire is the basketball coach for the women's team at a major university. She hears much talk among coaches at meetings and tournaments about athletes requiring high protein intakes. She also receives a great deal of literature promoting protein supplements for athletes. Because of her training in physiology and biochemistry, she questions the claim that athletes need unusually high amounts of dietary protein. She therefore decides to consult faculty members in

153

the nutrition department at her university on this question. What does she find out?

Elliott, a college sophomore, has just joined a group which follows vegetarian diets for two reasons: (1) it believes that such diets are healthier than the typical American diet, and (2) it believes that production of foods for vegetarian diets is less wasteful of the earth's food production resources than diets containing meat. Some members of the group eat eggs, milk, and cheese, while others consume no foods of animal origin. Elliott wants to know whether either one of these diets is apt to be low in protein. What are the facts about protein in vegetarian diets?

This chapter not only provides answers to these questions, but also describes the variety of important roles that proteins fulfill in the body. In addition, it considers how the body uses protein, the consequences of insufficient protein intake, how much protein the body needs, and combinations of foods that can meet those needs. Finally, after completing this chapter, the student should be able to place claims made for protein and protein supplements into a reasonable perspective.

WHAT ARE PROTEINS?

Although protein, carbohydrates, and fats all contain carbon, hydrogen, and oxygen, proteins are distinctive in that they also contain nitrogen (N). The nitrogen in proteins is present in the amino acids that are the basic units making up the protein molecule.

Nitrogen gets into plant and animal proteins by a circuitous route. The atmosphere contains large amounts of nitrogen gas (N_2), but neither plants nor animals by themselves can utilize this form of nitrogen. Instead, nitrogen-fixing bacteria in the root nodules of legumes participate in a cycle in which they convert nitrogen from the air to nitrates in the soil (Figure 6-1). Plants use the nitrates to synthesize amino acids and proteins. Animals obtain the amino acids they need by consuming plants or other animals. Nitrogen-containing wastes from animal bodies, corpses, and decayed plants are converted to nitrates by soil bacterial action. The cycle is completed when specific denitrifying bacteria convert soil nitrates to atmospheric nitrogen.

Life as we know it would be impossible if this cycle did not exist, for neither proteins nor DNA and RNA could be formed. DNA (deoxyribonucleic acid) constitutes the hereditary material of the cells, and contains the "blueprint" for making all the different proteins the cells need. RNA (ribonucleic acid) participates in protein synthesis, to be discussed later in this chapter.

PROTEIN STRUCTURE

Amino acids are so named because each one contains an amino group (containing nitrogen) and an acid group (Figure 6-2). Food and body tissue proteins contain about 22 different amino acids, but a given protein may contain from 8 to

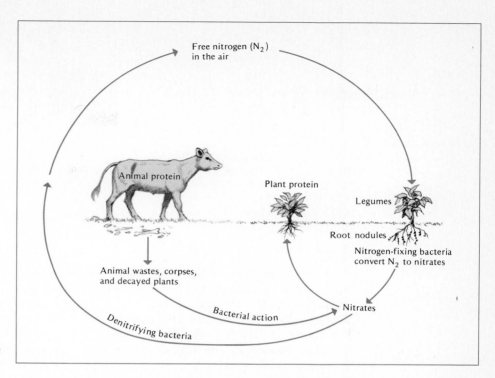

FIGURE 6-1. The nitrogen cycle.

18 of them. Body cells manufacture all the hundreds of different proteins the body needs. To synthesize a protein, the cell must have available all the amino acids that are in that protein, and must be able to link them together in the proper sequence. The linkage between amino acids is a *peptide bond*, shown in Figure 6-3. Two amino acids linked by a peptide bond form a *dipeptide*; a *tripeptide* contains three amino acid residues and two peptide bonds; a *polypeptide* contains 10 or more amino acid residues. The number of amino acids in proteins varies from about 50 in very small proteins, such as insulin, to as many as 400,000 in very large proteins. Notice that as amino acids link together to form either peptides or proteins, one end of the molecule has a free amino group, while the opposite end has a free carboxyl group (Figure 6-3).

FIGURE 6-2. Chemical structure of amino acids. Each amino acid contains an amino group and an acid (carboxyl) group arranged as shown. The composition of the R group distinguishes one amino acid from the other. All R groups for all amino acids contain carbon and hydrogen, and some also contain oxygen, additional nitrogen, and sulfur.

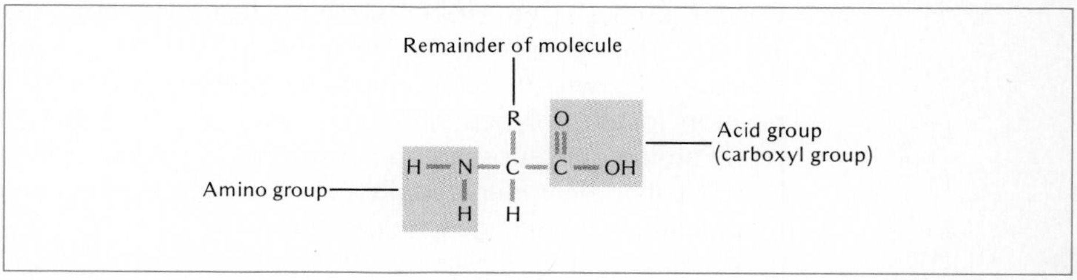

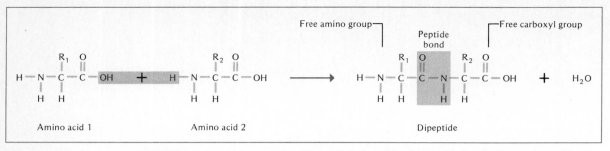

FIGURE 6-3. In proteins, amino acids are linked together by peptide bonds. Two amino acids are represented, showing their amino and acid groups. The remainders of their molecules are

represented by R_1 and R_2, respectively. As a peptide bond forms, the acid group ($-\overset{\overset{\text{O}}{\|}}{\text{C}}-\text{OH}$) of one joins to the amino group ($\text{H}-\underset{\underset{\text{H}}{|}}{\text{N}}-$) of the other, splitting out water in the process.

Linking the proper amino acids together in the required sequence is merely the first step in synthesizing proteins. Next, the polypeptide chain coils in a specific manner, and finally arranges itself into the shape characteristic of the protein in question. Not until it has achieved the three-dimensional conformation or shape at which it is most stable will the protein become biologically active.

Many proteins assume fibrous shapes while others are globular. *Collagen* of bones and tendons, *elastin* of stretchable tissues such as blood vessels, and *keratin* of hair and nails are all fibrous proteins. In fibrous proteins, the polypeptide chains, coiled in a specific manner, are arranged so as to form a long fiber. Globular proteins, on the other hand, consist of coiled polypeptide chains compactly folded into a more or less spherical shape. Enzymes, antibodies, many transport proteins, and protein hormones are globular proteins and are water-soluble. The tough, fibrous proteins such as collagen, elastin, and keratin are insoluble in water. Some fibrous proteins, on the other hand, such as myosin of muscle and fibrinogen (required in the blood for normal clotting) are soluble in water.

The exact amino acid sequence in a given protein differs from one species to another. The hemoglobin in your body, for example, differs somewhat in amino acid sequence from that in a dog or cat. Species differences in proteins are due to the fact that, at conception, each individual receives DNA codes that are unique for the species. As a consequence, hemoglobin, insulin, and other proteins in human beings differ slightly in amino acid sequence from those in other animals.

Within the human species, genetic differences account for certain errors in protein synthesis and explain some medical disorders. An example is sickle cell anemia. This anemia occurs in individuals whose genetic code directs bone marrow cells, when synthesizing hemoglobin, to place the amino acid valine in a position in the polypeptide chains normally occupied by glutamic acid. This single amino acid substitution causes the red blood cells to "sickle" or become crescent-shaped under certain conditions, impeding blood circulation in an individual having this genetic disorder.

ESSENTIAL AND NONESSENTIAL AMINO ACIDS

Although body cells can synthesize most of the proteins needed for cellular functions, some cells synthesize proteins that are used throughout the body. Hemoglobin, for example, is synthesized by bone marrow cells. Bone marrow cells need to have on hand 574 amino acid molecules to synthesize one molecule of hemoglobin. The correct number of molecules of each specific amino acid in hemoglobin must be among the total 574 amino acids. Some of the amino acids needed for hemoglobin synthesis can be manufactured by body cells while others must be obtained from food. Those the cells can manufacture in sufficient amounts are classified as *nonessential*, or *dispensable*, *amino acids*, while those that must be supplied in the diet are *essential*, or *indispensable*, *amino acids*. The amino acids belonging in these two categories are listed in Table 6-1. Two of the essential amino acids, methionine and phenylalanine, are "spared" if certain nonessential amino acids are in the diet. Specifically, cystine and cysteine are synthesized in the body from methionine, while tyrosine is synthesized from phenylalanine. If cystine and tyrosine are in the diet, they "spare" methionine and phenylalanine, respectively, for other uses.

The nonessential amino acids are just as necessary as the essential ones for protein synthesis. If the cells became unable to synthesize, let us say, aspartic acid and none was circulating in the blood for bone marrow cells to use, hemoglobin synthesis would stop.

Recall from the Introduction and Chapter 4 that only those nutrients that the body cannot synthesize in the amounts needed are called essential nutrients. So far, you have learned that one fatty acid, linoleic acid, and nine amino acids are

TABLE 6-1.   ESSENTIAL AND NONESSENTIAL AMINO ACIDS

ESSENTIAL AMINO ACIDS	NONESSENTIAL AMINO ACIDS
Histidine	Alanine
Isoleucine	Arginine
Leucine	Asparagine
Lysine	Aspartic acid
Methionine*	Cysteine* (and cystine*†)
Phenylalanine	Glutamic acid
Threonine	Glutamine
Tryptophan	Glycine
Valine	Hydroxylysine
	Hydroxyproline
	Proline
	Serine
	Tyrosine‡

*Methionine, cysteine, and cystine contain sulfur, and are frequently designated "the sulfur-containing amino acids."
†Cystine is made up of two cysteine molecules linked together.
‡Tyrosine is synthesized in the body from phenylalanine.

essential in the diet. No specific carbohydrates are required in the diet since the body can synthesize those needed. Later you will see that vitamins, minerals, and water are also essential in the diet.

FUNCTIONS OF BODY PROTEINS

Proteins are involved in the biological processes of all plants and animals. A large variety of uses are made of proteins in the human body. Some of these are highly specialized, while others are more general, affecting the entire body.

Structural Proteins

Many proteins are integral structural components of body tissues. For example, muscle proteins include the structural proteins *myosin* and *actin*. The hardest tissue in the body, the enamel of the teeth, is made up basically of a very strong protein similar to keratin into which fine crystals of calcium phosphate are embedded; this protein is highly resistant to corrosion by acids or other agents. As noted earlier, collagen and keratin are important structural proteins.

Enzymes

Among the most important proteins in the body are enzymes. Enzymes are protein catalysts formed by the living cell. As noted in the Introduction to this book, most chemical reactions in the body would occur very, very slowly if enzymes were not present to speed up the reactions. Each enzyme in the body catalyzes only one, or at best only a few, different chemical reactions, and most chemical reactions in the body require enzymes. You can imagine, then, that the number of enzymes in the body must be exceedingly large, and that is the case.

Since enzymes are proteins, they are large molecules, frequently larger than the molecules they act upon. Enzymes tend also to be specific for certain compounds. The enzyme molecule seeks out and attaches itself to the substrate molecule (the substance acted upon), and catalyzes a specific chemical reaction, but the enzyme is not used up or changed in the reaction (review Figure 0-2 in the Introduction). Almost every body function involves enzyme activity.

Hormones

Many hormones are proteins, including insulin, thyroid hormones, parathyroid hormone, calcitonin, and glucagon. Briefly, some of the functions of protein hormones follow. Insulin lowers blood sugar, while glucagon raises it. Parathyroid hormone raises the calcium level in the blood while calcitonin prevents such an increase. Thyroid hormones regulate the rate at which cells oxidize food for energy.

Antibodies

Antibodies are proteins synthesized by tissues of the lymph nodes, the gastrointestinal tract, and the spleen. Antibodies protect the body from illness due to viruses, bacteria, and foreign animal cells. Although occasionally we do become ill with bacterial or viral infections, we are unaware of the many occasion in which antibodies ward off infections.

Blood Clotting

When you cut your finger, normally a clot rapidly forms. Proteins play an important part in blood clotting. The trauma of the cut vessel triggers the conversion of a plasma protein, *prothrombin*, to thrombin, an enzyme. Thrombin, in turn, acts upon another plasma protein, *fibrinogen*, to produce fibrin. A network of fibrin threads forms a clot, which plugs the wound and stops the bleeding. Prothrombin and fibrinogen are both manufactured by the liver; normally blood levels of these proteins are maintained high enough to result in rapid clotting if an injury occurs.

Protein Carriers

Carrying Nutrients Into Cells Chapter 4 indicated that protein carriers are needed to transport sugars from the intestinal lumen across the membrane into the mucosal cell. In the same way, protein carriers in cell membranes transport certain nutrients from the blood into individual body cells. These carriers remain in the membrane of the cell, carrying a nutrient into the cell, then going back for more. Some of these proteins are specific for only one nutrient. For example, calcium-binding protein transports calcium across the membrane of the intestinal cell, and therefore is essential for calcium absorption. On the other hand, a single protein carrier may transport several different amino acids from the intestinal lumen to the mucosal cell.

Carrying Substances in the Blood Many protein carriers are used to transport substances in the blood. Lipoproteins, which carry triglycerides and cholesterol, were discussed in Chapters 4 and 5. Serum iron travels in the blood attached to a protein called *transferrin*; serum copper travels attached to *ceruloplasmin*, another protein. Vitamin A is transported in blood attached to *retinol-binding protein*. Inability to synthesize retinol-binding protein in some cases of protein malnutrition results in inability to use vitamin A stored in the liver, and vitamin A deficiency sometimes results. *Hemoglobin* is a protein containing iron which carries oxygen from the lungs to the tissues, and picks up carbon dioxide from the tissues and carries it to the lungs, where it is breathed off. Transport proteins obviously benefit the entire body.

Maintenance of Fluid Balance

Blood proteins help to maintain the normal distribution of water in the body. A man of average weight (70 kg, 154 lb) has about 40 liters (L) of water in his body. About 25 L are inside the trillions of cells in the body, and is called the *intracellular* fluid. All the fluid outside the cells is called the *extracellular* fluid, and amounts to about 15 L in a 70-kg man. The extracellular fluid includes that between cells (*interstitial* fluid) and that in the blood (blood *plasma*).

For the body to operate normally, this distribution of fluids must be maintained. For example, a sudden decrease in blood volume can result in shock and death. Normally the body uses several mechanisms to maintain the plasma volume, but one of the most important mechanisms involves plasma proteins. Plasma proteins are so large that they cannot leak out through the pores of the blood vessel walls; in addition, they attract water (they are hydrophilic or "water-loving"). Maintaining normal levels of plasma proteins, then, helps keep water inside the blood vessels, and prevents it from leaking out into the interstitial fluid. The most important blood protein having this effect is *albumin*, but globulins and fibrinogen have some effect. If blood proteins, particularly albumin, become significantly diminished in concentration, the result is *edema*, or abnormal accumulation of interstitial fluid, accompanied by a decrease in plasma volume (Figure 6-4). This condition accounts for the edema observed in kwashiorkor, discussed later in this chapter. When edema occurs, the affected parts of the body (feet, legs, face, hands, or abdomen) become puffy and swollen.

Acid-Base Balance

FIGURE 6-4. Blood proteins aid in maintaining normal fluid distribution between the blood plasma and the interstitial fluid.

Normally the body keeps the blood in a slightly alkaline state—between a pH of 7.35 and 7.45. In so doing, it maintains acid-base balance. In the pH system, a pH between 0 and 6.9 is acidic; the lower the number the greater the acidity. A pH of 7 indicates neutrality, while a pH above 7.0 indicates alkalinity. The higher the number the greater the alkalinity. Acidity increases as the concentration of hydrogen ions (H^+) increases in a solution, while alkalinity increases as their

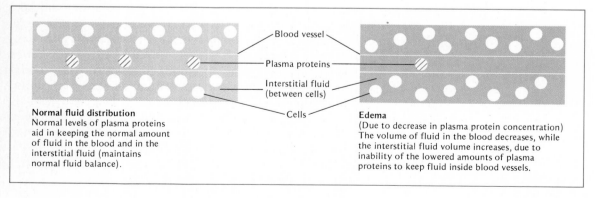

Normal fluid distribution
Normal levels of plasma proteins aid in keeping the normal amount of fluid in the blood and in the interstitial fluid (maintains normal fluid balance).

Blood vessel

Plasma proteins

Interstitial fluid (between cells)

Cells

Edema
(Due to decrease in plasma protein concentration)
The volume of fluid in the blood decreases, while the interstitial fluid volume increases, due to inability of the lowered amounts of plasma proteins to keep fluid inside blood vessels.

concentration decreases. [The H^+ forms when the hydrogen atom loses one electron.]

A drastic change in the degree of acidity or alkalinity of the blood can prove fatal; consequently, the body uses several different mechanisms to regulate the blood pH. One important method is the use of buffers. Buffers operate by either releasing H^+ or removing them from a solution as needed to prevent pH changes. Proteins have the ability to act as buffers, aiding the body in maintenance of acid-base balance.

Use of Protein for Energy

Although the body can obtain energy from either food or body protein, as discussed in Chapter 3, it is wasteful and expensive to use protein for energy. Foods high in protein are among the most expensive foods available, and are more economically used for their unique role of providing amino acids for body protein synthesis. If the individual is not consuming an adequate kilocalorie intake, however, some food protein will be used for energy and cannot then be used for protein synthesis. The most efficient system is to provide sufficient kilocalories from dietary carbohydrate and fat, while consuming sufficient protein for synthesis of body proteins.

From this brief survey of the functions of body proteins, it is clear that proteins play exceedingly important roles in the body. Let's turn now to proteins in foods.

FOOD SOURCES OF PROTEIN

Many people equate meat with protein. Is meat the best source of protein? We can think about the food sources of protein in several ways: how concentrated the protein is on (1) a weight basis, (2) a serving basis, or (3) in relation to the kilocalories furnished by the food. In addition, we can also look at how expensive the protein source is. Figure 6-5 indicates that among our most concentrated protein foods on a weight basis are poultry, fish, meats, peanuts, wheat germ, and cheddar cheese. Milk is 3 to 3.5 percent protein, while cereals such as rice and oatmeal, and potatoes are only about 2 percent protein. Foods low in protein concentration nevertheless are important protein sources when substantial quantities are eaten. Vegetables and fruits in general have a low concentration of protein.

Since 100 g (3 ½ oz) of meat, poultry, or fish constitutes a usual serving, Figure 6-5 also indicates the amount of protein in a serving of these foods. But one serving of cheddar cheese is usually 1 oz, less than one-third the amount shown in Figure 6-5. Appendix C presents the protein in usual servings of food. In studying your own diet, you will consider the amount of nutrients in serving size portions of food, rather than on a weight basis.

In terms of the best low-kilocalorie sources of protein, Figure 6-6 indicates that chicken (not fried), lean meat, and fish, cottage cheese, and skim milk are

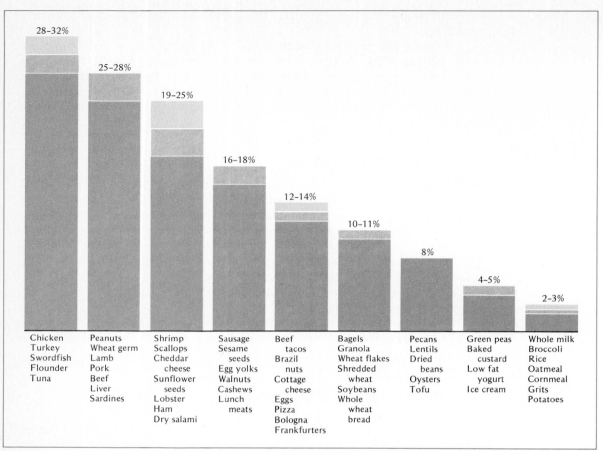

FIGURE 6-5. Percentage by weight of protein in foods.

among the best low-kilocalorie sources. Notice that broccoli contributes about 10 g of protein per 100 kcal; however, you would need to consume 2½ cups of cut-up broccoli to obtain 100 kcal. Among high-kilocalorie protein sources are bologna, frankfurters, peanuts, bacon, breads, cereals, and ice cream.

Costs of foods have been increasing sharply recently, and foods highly concentrated in protein are usually among the more expensive foods. Table 6-2 shows the cost calculated by the authors of 15 grams of protein from a few representative foods.

By far the cheapest protein source is dried beans, but these require supplementation with other foods to form high-quality protein, discussed later in this chapter. The least expensive brands of nonfat dry milk have been the cheapest protein source among animal foods for a number of years. Today, however, chicken is often priced low enough that it is an equally inexpensive source.

Meats generally are among the most expensive protein sources. One way to cut down on the costs of protein foods is to decrease meat consumption by

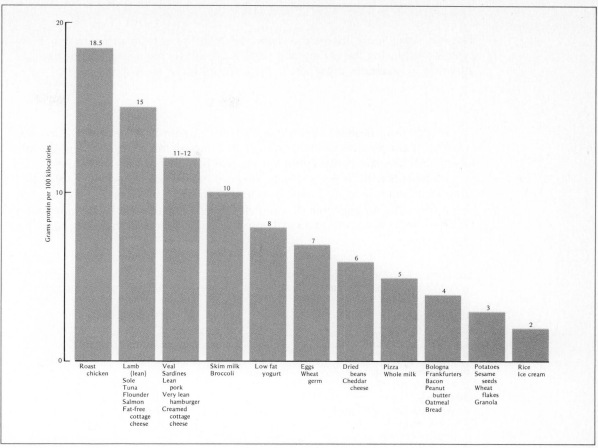

FIGURE 6-6. Number of grams of protein per 100 kilocalories furnished by an assortment of foods.

diluting it with pasta or grains in casserole dishes, and by consuming more meals containing no meat.

Changes in Protein Sources

The amount of protein available in the American food supply is almost the same today as it was in 1909, according to the U.S. Department of Agriculture; that is, it was 102 g per person per day in 1909 and 104 g in 1980 [2]. Protein availability has remained at 12 percent of total kilocalories since 1909. Our sources of protein have changed, however, since that time. In 1909 about 52 percent of our dietary protein came from animal sources, while today 70 percent comes from animal sources, as Figure 6-7 indicates. Notice that our consumption of flour and cereal products has greatly diminished over the years. Meat, fish, and poultry now furnish approximately 42 percent of our protein, and dairy products supply approximately 21 percent, compared with approximately 30 percent and 16 percent, respectively, in 1909.

THE BODY'S USE OF PROTEIN

To understand more thoroughly how the body turns food proteins into body proteins displaying the variety of functions previously mentioned, let us turn our attention to digestion, absorption, and metabolism of protein.

Digestion

The objective of protein digestion is to break protein molecules down to their constituent amino acids or dipeptides. To accomplish this, enzymes must be able to establish intimate contact with the peptide bonds of protein molecules.

Proteins that have been *denatured* are more easily attacked by digestive enzymes than those as they exist in nature. *Denaturation* refers to the change in shape or spatial arrangement of a protein molecule without breaking any of the peptide bonds. A protein that has been tightly folded into a compact space, for

TABLE 6-2. COST OF 15 g OF PROTEIN (ONE-THIRD OF THE RDA FOR THE ADULT WOMAN) AT PRICES IN THE GREATER WASHINGTON, D.C. AREA IN OCTOBER 1982.

FOOD	WHERE PURCHASED	PRICE PER LB (EXCEPT AS NOTED)	COST OF 15 g PROTEIN
Soybeans	Food co-op	0.36	$0.035
Pinto beans	Food co-op	0.31	0.04
Black beans	Food co-op	0.39	0.06
Red beans	Food co-op	0.43	0.06
Milk, nonfat dry, reconstituted	Supermarket	0.31 qt	0.11
Chicken, mixed fryer parts	Supermarket	0.49	0.11
Chicken, fryer (not cut up)	Supermarket	0.69	0.15
Bread, white, enriched	Supermarket	0.46	0.17
Bread, whole wheat	Supermarket	0.50	0.18
Milk, fluid skim	Supermarket	0.45 qt	0.20
Eggs, large	Supermarket	1.09 doz	0.21
Rice, brown	Food co-op	0.49	0.22
Milk, dried skim (brand for drinking)	Supermarket	0.49 qt	0.23
Cottage cheese, 4% fat	Supermarket	0.88	0.23
Rice, white enriched	Supermarket	0.49	0.24
Cottage cheese, 1% fat	Supermarket	1.00	0.27
Cheddar cheese	Food co-op	2.01	0.27
Rice, brown	Supermarket	0.68	0.30
Beef, regular ground	Supermarket	1.69	0.31
Beef, very lean ground	Supermarket	1.99	0.32
Cheddar cheese	Supermarket	2.89	0.38
Frankfurters	Supermarket	1.58	0.42
Beef, rump roast	Supermarket	2.39	0.54
Beef, flank steak	Supermarket	3.99	0.61

Supermarket foods priced were chiefly store brands. Dried beans, brown rice, and cheddar cheese were less expensive at the food co-op than at the supermarket.

Values for protein obtained from 1. Adams, C. F., *Nutritive Value of American Foods,* Agriculture Handbook No. 456, Washington, D.C.: USDA, 1975; and 2. Robertson, L., C. Flinders, and B. Godfrey, *Laurel's Kitchen,* Petaluma, Calif.: Nilgiri Press, 1976.

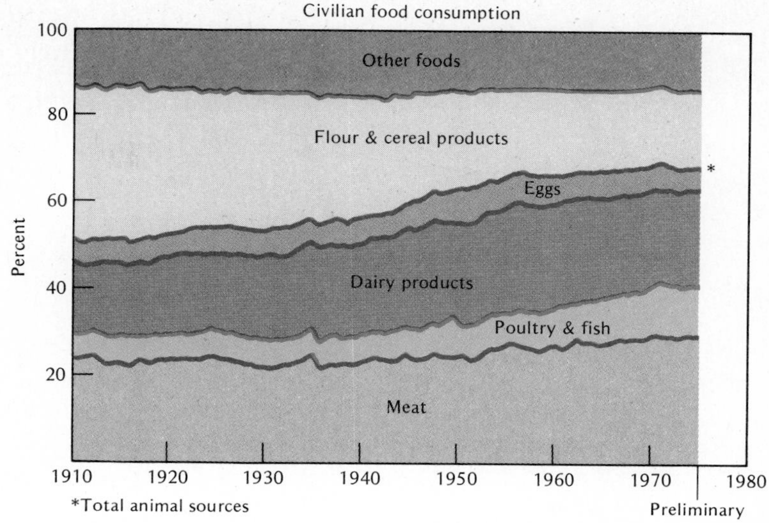

Civilian food consumption

Other foods

Flour & cereal products

Eggs

Dairy products

Poultry & fish

Meat

*Total animal sources

Preliminary

FIGURE 6-7. Changes in sources of protein in the U.S. diet since 1910. Total animal sources of protein increased since 1910, while flour and cereal products greatly declined. (Source: USDA.)

example, spreads out and loosens up when it is denatured. Proteins can be denatured by exposing them to heat or by changing the pH or salt concentration of the environment. When you cook meats, poultry, fish, eggs, legumes (dried beans), cereal grains, or other foods containing proteins, you denature the proteins. The acid in sour milk or yogurt, or in a marinade used on meats or fish also denatures the proteins. Stomach acid denatures food proteins, including the enzymes you consume in raw foods, such as fruits and vegetables.

Heating foods does not invariably result in greater digestibility of the proteins. Since food proteins often exist in close association with carbohydrates, heating may cause a reaction between the protein and carbohydrates, decreasing the digestibility of the protein. For example, experimental rats digest evaporated milk less well than fresh whole milk because the heat processing of evaporated milk causes the protein to react with lactose [3]. Furthermore, exposing foods to dry heat for long periods may cause extra linkages to form between neighboring amino acids in the polypeptide chains as they lie side by side. Digestive enzymes may be unable to break these linkages. The digestibility of proteins in breakfast cereals, for example, is diminished somewhat by toasting or puffing [4]. In a practical sense, lessened digestibility of proteins due to methods of food processing or preparation is of concern only in circumstances in which the amount of protein in the total diet is low. This is not a problem in countries with an abundance of food proteins.

A CLOSER LOOK

Beware of claims in the popular media that a food or supplement will provide your body with needed enzymes! Normal individuals synthesize all the enzymes

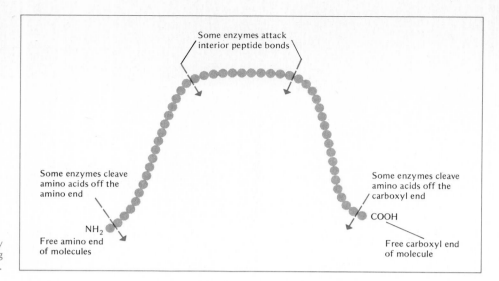

FIGURE 6-8. Specificity of protein-digesting enzymes.

needed in the body. Any enzymes in a food you eat (and raw foods *do* contain enzymes) will be denatured and their ability to function destroyed by your stomach acid, or by the alkaline pH of the intestinal tract. (Enzymes operate best at a specific pH, and are denatured by a markedly higher or lower pH.) Your body then will simply digest the denatured enzymes. Enzymes in food are not absorbed as such and therefore cannot get into the blood and body cells.

Several different enzymes are involved in protein digestion. Some are specific for peptide bonds in the interior of the protein, while others are specific for bonds at either the amino or the carboxyl end of the protein or polypeptide chain (Figure 6-8). Protein-digesting enzymes are also specific for peptide bonds involving particular amino acids.

Pepsin in the stomach begins protein digestion, breaking large protein molecules into very large polypeptides. These large polypeptides are then subjected to the action of pancreatic and intestinal enzymes, resulting finally in chiefly amino acids. A small amount of dipeptides also are end products of protein digestion. In the absence of pepsin, as when the stomach has been surgically removed, pancreatic enzymes digest proteins just as well as they do large polypeptides. Protein digestion is summarized in Table 6-3.

All enzymes exhibit optimal activity at a pH specific for each enzyme. Pepsin is most active at the acid pH which occurs in the stomach during and after a meal. The other protein-digesting enzymes are most active at the alkaline pH of the duodenum and jejunum.

Proteins generally are digested rapidly in the upper intestinal tract. This is the case partly because the stomach, especially after a high-protein meal, allows the acid chyme to enter the small intestines slowly. The slow rate of stomach emptying prevents overloading the intestines with substrate which could overwhelm the enzymes.

TABLE 6-3. SUMMARY OF PROTEIN DIGESTION

ORIGIN OF ENZYME	ENZYME	SUBSTRATE	END PRODUCTS OR ACTION
Stomach	Pepsin (attacks interior peptide bonds)	Proteins	Very large polypeptides
	Rennin (in infants)	Casein of milk	Clots milk proteins
Pancreas	Trypsin (attacks interior peptide bonds)	Proteins Large polypeptides	Small polypeptides Some dipeptides
	Chymotrypsin (attacks interior peptide bonds)	Proteins Large polypeptides	Small polypeptides Some dipeptides
	Carboxypeptidase (cleaves amino acids off carboxyl end of chain)	Polypeptides	Free amino acids, and some dipeptides
Small intestines	Aminopeptidase (cleaves amino acids off amino end of chain)	Polypeptides	Free amino acids, and some dipeptides
	Dipeptidases	Dipeptides	Free amino acids

The final end products of protein digestion are chiefly amino acids, with some dipeptides.

Much of the protein in the intestinal lumen after a meal originates from the body itself, and consists of digestive enzymes and sloughed-off epithelial cells from the intestinal mucosa. Such proteins are called *endogenous* proteins because they originally were synthesized within the body. While dietary proteins appear to be digested chiefly in the duodenum and jejunum, endogenous proteins, including "spent" enzymes, are digested in the lower half of the intestinal tract [5]. Although the body absorbs amino acids from digestion of endogenous proteins, the body must resynthesize these proteins, so the process simply amounts to a recycling of the amino acids. One should not consider endogenous proteins to be a new source of amino acids for the body as are food proteins.

Absorption

The amino acids resulting from protein digestion are absorbed by active transport. This mechanism requires the expenditure of energy and the use of specific carriers to transport specific amino acids from the intestinal lumen across the membrane of the intestinal mucosal cell. There is some competition among amino acids for transport carriers, depending in part upon the amount of amino acids present to be absorbed. This competition rarely, if ever, results in poor absorption of amino acids in normal individuals, however, because the large absorptive surface of the

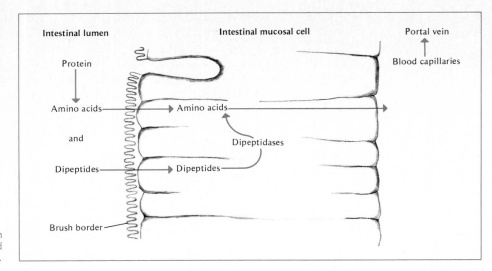

Intestinal lumen   Intestinal mucosal cell   Portal vein

Blood capillaries

Protein

Amino acids —————→ Amino acids ———————→

and

Dipeptidases

Dipeptides ————→ Dipeptides —

Brush border —

FIGURE 6-9. Absorption of amino acids and dipeptides.

intestinal mucosa coupled with the measured release of acid chyme from the stomach assures efficient absorption.

Amino acids are not the sole products of protein digestion, since some small peptides, particularly dipeptides, are absorbed across the mucosal cell membrane. As dipeptides enter the intestinal mucosal cells, dipeptidases present either in the microvilli or in the fluids of the mucosal cell immediately break them down to amino acids (Figure 6-9). Amino acids are absorbed into the portal blood and carried to the liver.

Metabolism

Dietary proteins are unique in their capacity to furnish the body with amino acids required for body protein synthesis. Carbohydrates and fats cannot perform this function. On the other hand, dietary protein can be used, if necessary, to provide the body with energy, or excessive intakes can be converted to body fat. Let us look a little closer at how the body metabolizes protein.

After a meal containing protein there is an influx of amino acids to the liver from the portal blood. The liver removes those amino acids it needs for synthesis of liver and blood proteins (albumin and fibrinogen, for example). The liver also monitors the amino acids needs of other parts of the body [5]. For example, it synthesizes many of the nonessential amino acids and puts them in the circulating blood for use by other tissues. Directly after a meal containing protein there is a surge of amino acids from the liver into the circulating blood.

To obtain an overall view of protein metabolism, let us use Fig 6-10 as a guide for our discussion. Each body cell can synthesize its own protein providing it can obtain *sufficient energy* and the *right assortment and amount of amino acids*. These amino acids do not all necessarily come from food but may come from body tissues. To understand protein metabolism more thoroughly, let's begin with step 1, Figure 6-10.

The Metabolic Pool of Amino Acids   Those amino acids that are circulating in the blood and lymph, and are held as free amino acids in organs, especially the liver and muscles, are referred to as the "metabolic amino acid pool." Figure 6-10 indicates that the amino acids in this pool may have originated either from the diet (step 1), or from the catabolism of body proteins (step 3). The origin of the amino acid makes no difference to the tissue cell when it is ready to synthesize the many proteins it needs for normal function. The free amino acids in the metabolic pool consist chiefly of nonessential amino acids, however, since the body keeps a limited inventory of essential amino acids.

The Dynamic State of Body Proteins   Proteins in the body are in a dynamic state; that is, they are constantly being broken down and replaced, indicated by steps 2 and 3 in Figure 6-10. As a protein breaks down, it adds amino acids to the metabolic pool which are mixed with those from the diet. The cell then takes up the amino acids it needs from the pool to resynthesize the protein in question. The time required for this cycle of breakdown and resynthesis of specific proteins is called the *turnover rate*. Some proteins have a much higher turnover rate than others. For example, collagen in the adult has a very long turnover rate—a matter of years—while the turnover rate of proteins in intestinal mucosal epithelial cells is very rapid—3 to 4 days. Muscle and brain proteins have a slower turnover rate than many other proteins. The ability to use amino acids from the breakdown of body proteins has survival value in times of food deprivation because it allows the body to synthesize proteins in organs that are essential for life, such as the heart, liver, and kidneys, using amino acids from the catabolism of less essential proteins, such as those of muscles.

FIGURE 6-10. Scheme indicating general aspects of protein metabolism.

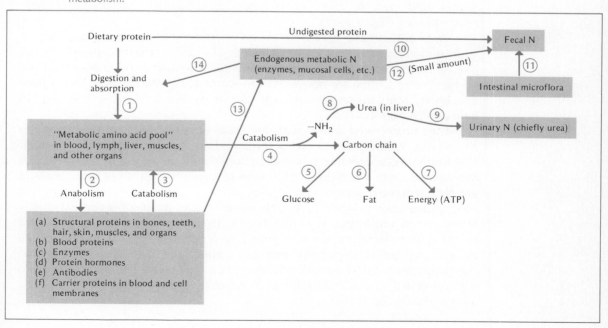

Catabolism of Amino Acids   Amino acids are not stored in the body in the sense that fat or glycogen is stored. As the protein intake increases above the amount needed to synthesize new proteins during growth or to maintain (replace wornout) proteins, the excess amino acids are catabolized (step 4, Figure 6-10). The first step in catabolism of amino acids is deamination—the removal of the amino groups (—NH_2). The remaining carbon chain may be used to synthesize glucose (step 5) or fat (step 6) or it may be used for energy (step 7), depending upon the body's needs at the moment.

When amino acids are catabolized, the liver converts the amino groups to *urea*, the major nitrogen-containing end product of protein catabolism (step 8). Urea is then sent in the blood from the liver to the kidneys for excretion in the urine (step 9). A small amount of urinary nitrogen is in the form of creatinine from muscle metabolism and uric acid, from nucleic acid (DNA) catabolism.

The liver is the chief site of catabolism of essential amino acids, except for the so-called branched-chain amino acids (valine, leucine, and isoleucine). These are catabolized in muscles and the kidneys. When a larger quantity of essential amino acids is consumed than the body needs, the liver and muscles catabolize most of the excess.

Conversion of Amino Acids to Fat, Glucose, or Energy   The fate of excessively high protein intakes beyond amounts needed to synthesize body proteins depends upon the total kilocalorie intake. If the kilocalorie intake is higher than needed to maintain body weight, excessive amino acids are converted to body fat. If the kilocalorie intake is lower than needed, much of the amino acids from dietary protein will be oxidized for energy.

In case of near-starvation, the body needs blood glucose for brain function. Amino acids will be used to form glucose (gluconeogenesis) under these circumstances (Figure 6-11).

Figure 6-11 shows that before excessive amino acids can be used for any of these purposes, they must be deaminated. The amino groups removed in this process are excreted in the urine as urea. If the deaminated amino acids are used for fat synthesis, they are converted first to pyruvate, then to acetyl CoA from which fatty acids are synthesized. The fatty acids then combine with glycerol to form fat (Chapter 4).

If the deaminated amino acids are used for energy, they are converted to Krebs cycle intermediates at one of several points, specific for each amino acid. The Krebs cycle intermediates are carbohydrates, as noted in Chapter 3. If deaminated amino acids are used to form glucose, they must first form pyruvate and then glucose (Figure 6-11).

Turning again to Figure 6-10, notice that nitrogen in the feces consists chiefly of undigested protein from food (step 10), but some comes from intestinal bacteria (step 11), and a small amount from endogenous nitrogen (step 12). As pointed out earlier, endogenous metabolic nitrogen comes from digestive enzymes and sloughed-off intestinal mucosal cells (step 13). A high percentage of these proteins is digested in the lower half of the small intestines (step 14) and their amino acids are absorbed (step 1).

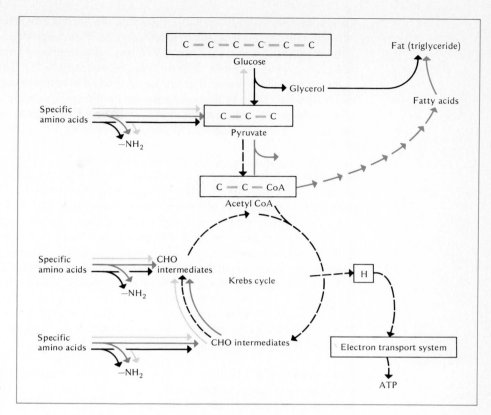

FIGURE 6-11.
Conversion of amino
acids to fat, glucose, or
energy.

Adaptation to Protein Intake A remarkable characteristic of animals is the ability to maintain a relatively constant environment in the blood and body fluids despite external changes that tend to alter it. This phenomenon is called *homeostasis*, mentioned in the Introduction to this textbook. One mechanism for maintaining homeostasis is adaptation. The body can adapt to a fairly wide range of protein intakes.

If the intake of protein increases sufficiently to exceed the ability of the body to catabolize excessive amino acids, the level of blood amino acids continues to rise, temporarily, and the liver (which forms urea) and kidneys (which excrete urea) enlarge. The enlargement is accompanied by increased ability to catabolize amino acids. In this way the body adapts to the higher level of protein intake without storing amino acids. A sign of the greater catabolism of amino acids is a high urinary excretion of urea.

If, on the other hand, the protein intake is low, but kilocalorie intake is adequate, the catabolism of amino acids diminishes markedly, allowing the body to conserve essential amino acids. The turnover rate of body proteins also slows down, saving amino acids. The urinary excretion of urea will be low under these conditions.

The case of starvation is quite different. In starvation, the body's first need is for glucose to maintain activity of the nervous system. The body cannot convert fatty acids from body fat stores to glucose, so it forms glucose from amino acids. The adaptation in this instance is not toward conserving amino acids, because preserving nervous system activity takes higher priority [5]. The excretion of urea in this case will be higher than in the case of a low-protein, adequate-kilocalorie intake. As starvation or protein depletion continues, the body catabolizes muscle proteins to supply amino acids to maintain the visceral organs that are vital to life. Eventually, the body's ability to adapt is exceeded, however, and the individual dies.

When an individual who has become adapted to a low-protein but adequate kilocalorie intake is placed on a high-protein diet, his or her body will retain protein for a time while becoming adapted to the new diet. This is explained as follows. Scientists have observed in normal animals that initially, upon consuming a low-protein diet or starving, there is a rapid loss of certain body proteins, especially from the liver and gastrointestinal wall. These proteins have been called "protein reserves" or "labile body proteins," but they are not stores or reserves in the sense that adipose tissue represents stored fat, or that liver and muscle glycogen represent ready glucose stores. Once adaptation has taken place, the liver and intestinal wall no longer release these proteins. When this individual again consumes adequate protein, these proteins are resynthesized. During this time of resynthesis, the individual will be in *positive nitrogen balance*. What is meant by nitrogen balance?

Nitrogen Balance (N Balance)   Nitrogen balance is a technique used to study the circumstances under which amino acids are kept within the body for protein synthesis, on the one hand, or are catabolized with overall losses of body protein, on the other hand. In using this technique, investigators determine the *nitrogen* content of food consumed and of the urine and feces during a specified time period. They then study the difference between intake and excretion. Nitrogen is chosen as the means of assessing amounts of protein because it is easily determined in the laboratory. Since proteins generally are about 16 percent nitrogen, the protein content is calculated by multiplying grams of nitrogen by the factor 6.25 ($^{100}/_{16}$).

Suppose you were a subject on a nitrogen balance study. You would have to agree to consume all your meals under the supervision of the research staff in a laboratory. You would be served weighed portions of food, the nitrogen content of which would be determined by chemical analysis of representative samples of the food. You would have to agree to avoid eating or drinking anything other than food or drink supplied (except for water). During specific periods of the study, you would have to collect all urine and feces and turn these into the laboratory for analysis of the nitrogen content. Losses of nitrogen from your body via sweat, hair losses and sloughed-off skin cells would not be measured because of the difficulty in doing so. Usually, in short balance studies, these losses can be ignored.

The investigators would compare your intake of nitrogen with the excretion, and would find that during the study your body was either in nitrogen *equilibrium* (zero balance), in *positive* nitrogen balance, or in *negative* nitrogen balance. When in nitrogen equilibrium, the intake and excretion of nitrogen is the same.

When in positive balance, the excretion is less than the intake; in negative balance, the excretion is more than the intake.

If you are a normal adult, the investigators would find that you were in *nitrogen equilibrium* during the study if the diet they fed you was adequate in kilocalories and furnished about the amount of protein of good quality that you were accustomed to consuming. (The *quality* of protein is determined by its amino acid composition, discussed later in this chapter.) The human body adjusts its excretion of nitrogen to the intake of protein, within certain limits. As noted earlier if you customarily consume a high-protein diet, you will excrete relatively large amounts of nitrogen in the urine. If, on the other hand, you usually consume a low-protein diet, your excretion of urinary nitrogen will be relatively low on your customary diet. However, if the investigators fed you a higher protein diet than your body was adjusted to, your body would retain some nitrogen for a time (you would be in positive nitrogen balance). As noted earlier, this nitrogen is used to synthesize certain enzymes and other proteins in larger amounts than you maintained on a lower protein intake. Because of this tendency to adjust to the protein intake, investigators usually feed adult subjects either a low-protein or a

TABLE 6-4. CONDITIONS RESULTING IN DIFFERENT STATES OF NITROGEN (N) BALANCE

STATE OF N BALANCE	CONDITIONS RESULTING IN STATE OF N BALANCE
A. N equilibrium (no gain or loss of N) Example: Intake 10 g N Excretion 10 g N Difference 0	1. Normal, nonpregnant adult, consuming a diet adequate in amount and quality of protein and adequate in kilocalories.
B. Positive N balance (gain of N in body) Example: Intake 10 g N Excretion 8 g N Difference +2 g N	1. Growth (in an infant, child, adolescent, or pregnant woman). 2. Recovery period after protein losses from surgery, injury, high fever, or severe emotional stress. Lost proteins are built up again upon recovery. 3. The diet fed during the balance study was higher in protein than subject was accustomed to (short balance study).
C. Negative N balance (loss of N from body) Example: Intake 10 g N Excretion 12 g N Difference −2 g N	1. Period of trauma such as surgery, injury, high fever, or severe emotional stress. 2. Starvation. 3. Low kilocalorie diet resulting in weight loss. 4. Lack of an essential amino acid in diet. 5. Protein intake lower than absolute requirement for individual. 6. Diet fed during study was lower in protein than subject had been accustomed to (short balance study). 7. Complete immobilization of body, as in enforced bed rest.

protein-free diet for a few days prior to a study so that all subjects are closer to the same plane of protein metabolism when the study begins.

Conditions that might result in either positive or negative nitrogen balance are noted in Table 6-4. Losses of nitrogen from the body occur (and the person is in negative nitrogen balance) during periods of trauma, starvation, or immobilization, or if the diet is too low in kilocalories, in one or more essential amino acids, or in total protein. The kilocalorie level of the diet is important because dietary protein will be catabolized for energy and therefore cannot be used for protein synthesis whenever the kilocalorie intake is lower than body needs.

From Table 6-4 it should be apparent that dietary protein needs increase during periods of growth or recovery from trauma or diseases that have resulted in nitrogen loss. Usually it is impossible to feed a person enough protein *during* periods of trauma or stress to prevent nitrogen losses, but during the recovery period extra protein beyond the needs of the normal healthy person should be provided to aid in the rehabilitative process. Notice that immobilizing the body results in negative nitrogen balance, hence the practice in hospitals of getting patients up and about as soon as possible.

Nitrogen balance studies allow investigators to observe the *overall* state of protein metabolism (whether your body is gaining or losing nitrogen, or just holding its own), but allows no assessment of whether or not one organ or part of the body is losing nitrogen to support the needs of another.

Synthesis of Nonessential Amino Acids   Body cells cannot synthesize essential amino acids because they lack the proper enzymes to form the carbon chains of those amino acids. As noted previously, the body synthesizes tyrosine from phenylalanine, and cysteine and cystine from methionine. The other nonessential amino acids are synthesized from certain carbohydrate derivatives (pyruvate, or others) or from other nonessential amino acids. Once the cell obtains the appropriate carbon chain, it adds an amino group, usually obtained from other nonessential amino acids. It is important for the diet to contain not only all of the essential amino acids in the amounts needed, but it must furnish enough total protein to supply the amino groups for synthesis of nonessential amino acids.

Synthesis of Body Protein   Scientists began to understand the remarkable process by which body cells synthesize proteins only about 20 years ago. A simplified description of this process is given in Figure 6-12. The process involves DNA, deoxyribonucleic acid, the genetic material in the cell nucleus, and RNA, ribonucleic acid. The process is presented here to emphasize the necessity for each amino acid to be present at the site of synthesis if a protein is to be successfully produced. While studying Figure 6-12, review the diagram of a cell, Figure 0-1, in the Introduction to this book.

HOW MUCH PROTEIN DO WE NEED?

The amount of protein recommended in the diet to meet body needs for normal, healthy people in the population has been set by the Food and Nutrition Board of

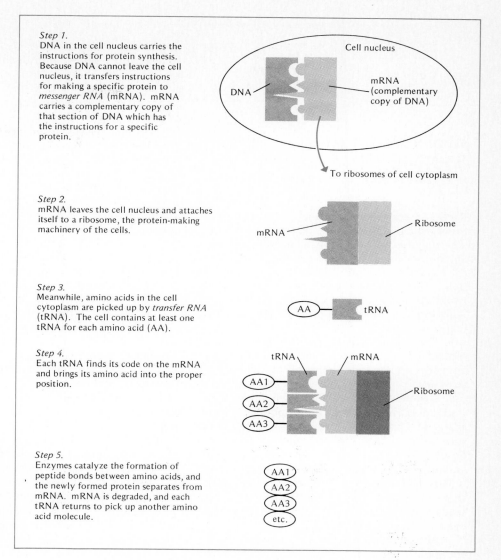

Step 1.
DNA in the cell nucleus carries the instructions for protein synthesis. Because DNA cannot leave the cell nucleus, it transfers instructions for making a specific protein to *messenger RNA* (mRNA). mRNA carries a complementary copy of that section of DNA which has the instructions for a specific protein.

Step 2.
mRNA leaves the cell nucleus and attaches itself to a ribosome, the protein-making machinery of the cells.

Step 3.
Meanwhile, amino acids in the cell cytoplasm are picked up by *transfer RNA* (tRNA). The cell contains at least one tRNA for each amino acid (AA).

Step 4.
Each tRNA finds its code on the mRNA and brings its amino acid into the proper position.

Step 5.
Enzymes catalyze the formation of peptide bonds between amino acids, and the newly formed protein separates from mRNA. mRNA is degraded, and each tRNA returns to pick up another amino acid molecule.

FIGURE 6-12. The system of protein synthesis, simplified. Each amino acid needed for synthesis of a specific protein must be present in the cell at the time of synthesis for this system to work.

the National Research Council, National Academy of Sciences. These are the Recommended Dietary Allowances (RDA) for protein (Appendix A). The amount recommended for the adult is 0.8 g per kilogram of ideal body weight. Let us see what this means.

Your ideal body weight refers to the weight considered to be normal for an individual of your sex and height. The protein need is related largely to the lean tissue in your body. If your weight is unusually high because of excessive body fat, you do not need more dietary protein than you would if your weight were ideal. Look up your ideal body weight in Appendix I. If your current weight is within the range given in the table for your sex and height, convert your current

NUTRITION IN THE NEWS

STUDIES SUGGEST A HARMFUL SHIFT IN TODAY'S MENU

Jane E. Brody, *The New York Times,* May 15, 1979

Recent investigations into the dietary habits of prehistoric peoples and their primate predecessors suggest that heavy meat-eating by modern affluent societies may be exceeding the biological capacities evolution built into the human body. The result may be a host of diet-related health problems, such as diabetes, obesity, high blood pressure, coronary heart disease and some cancers.

The studies challenge the notion that human beings evolved as aggressive hunting animals who depended primarily upon meat for survival.

The new view—coming from findings in such fields as archeology, anthropology, primatology and comparative anatomy—instead portrays early humans and their forebears more as herbivores than carnivores. According to these studies, the prehistoric table for at least the last million and a half years was probably set with three times more plant than animal foods, the reverse of what the average American currently eats. . . .

According to Dr. John R.K. Robson, professor of nutrition at the University of South Carolina, the development of agriculture some 10,000 years ago led to a steady narrowing of food choices, possibly to man's nutritional detriment because it limited sources of dietary fiber, vitamins, minerals and trace elements. The amount of saturated animal fat and cholesterol in the diet was significantly increased by the domestication of animals and resulting consumption of dairy products, eggs and fat-laden meats. Wild game is much leaner than domestic animals. . . .

The popular portrait of man as a rapacious and successful hunter who ate little else but the kill he brought home for his family and community to share arose largely from discoveries of archeological sites laden with fossilized bones of large prey. . . .

Within the last decade, however, archeologists have begun to look for and find microscopic evidence of plant foods, such as the presence of pollen grains and plant crystals in fossilized human feces, or coprolites. . . . As recently as 3,000 years ago, the inhabitants of rock shelters in southwestern Texas consumed (except for grasshoppers) a limited amount of animal protein, according to coprolite analyses by Dr. Vaughn M. Bryant, Jr., anthropologist at Texas A.&M. University in College Station.

Dr. Glynn Isaac, an anthropologist at the University of California at Berkeley . . . points out, however, that the fossil evidence does not tell what proportion of the diet may have been meat. . . .

But if the hunt, a high-risk and low-yield activity, had to have been the primary source of food for protohumans, Dr. Adrienne Zihlman, anthropologist at the University of California at Santa Cruz, believes the human species . . . would have undoubtedly died out, since there would have been inadequate supplies of food for the women, children and nonhunting men who remained at the home base.

Further, the digestive tract of the carnivore is designed for quick processing of food and rapid excretion of wastes before they putrify and poison the animal. The carnivore's digestive tract is short (only about three times the length of its torso), smooth and straight. The herbivore has a very long small intestine and long, smooth large intestine designed for processing bulky foods that take a long time to digest.

The human intestinal tract, while not as long as the herbivore's, is much longer than the carnivore's (about 12 times the length of the torso) and the surface area is further increased by puckering. Food takes a long time to be digested and wastes are eliminated slowly, a design more suitable to a diet high in plant matter than meat. And while the carnivore has weight in pounds to kilograms by dividing by 2.2 (there are 2.2 lb in 1 kg). If your weight is above or below the range, use the average figure given as your *ideal weight*, and convert it to kilograms. Now, multiply 0.8 g by your own weight, if normal, or your ideal body weight to find the protein RDA for persons of your sex and weight.

The adult male listed in the RDA table weighs 70 kg while the adult female weighs 55 kg. The male therefore has an RDA of 70 kg × 0.8 kg = 56 g of protein per day, while the female has an RDA of 55 kg × 0.8 g = 44 g of protein per day [6]. Does this mean that if the man consumes only 50 g/day that he will become protein-deficient? Review the discussion of the RDAs in Chapter 2 to be certain that you can answer this question correctly.

During periods of growth the protein need *per kilogram of body weight* is greater than for the nonpregnant adult. The RDA in infancy, childhood, adolescence, pregnancy, and lactation exceeds 0.8 g per kilogram. Nevertheless, infants and small children do not require large quantities of protein because of their small body size. The protein needs in pregnancy and lactation and in infancy, childhood, and adolescence are discussed in Chapters 14 and 15. Protein needs of the elderly are considered in Chapter 16.

Many athletes believe they have unusually high protein requirements. Box 6-1 addresses the athlete's need for protein.

Quality of Dietary Protein

The RDA for protein assumes that the *quality* of dietary protein is fairly high. A protein of high quality provides all the essential amino acids in a relatively small amount of protein. Since protein quality influences the amount of protein needed, let's look further into this topic by considering the amino acid *pattern* of proteins.

Amino Acid Pattern of Proteins Proteins that are best utilized by the body are those whose patterns of essential amino acids are like those of body proteins. By a

Do Athletes Have High Protein Requirements?

Many coaches and athletes believe that very high protein intakes are necessary to support large muscle mass and to improve performance. A survey of 75 athletic trainers and coaches reported that 51 percent thought that protein was more important than any other factor in increasing muscle mass [7]. The notion that protein is an essential fuel for exercise dates back to the chemist, J. von Liebig, in 1851 [8]. We now know, however, that the fuel for muscle exercise comes from carbohydrate and fat (Chapter 3).

During the time when a person is changing from a sedentary lifestyle to one of great physical activity—whether it be as an athlete or in a work situation requiring hard physical exertion—the muscle mass will increase. The time required for the phase of active muscle building varies with the intensity of the exercise, the time devoted to it daily, and the proportion of body muscles involved. The point is that the active phase of muscle building is limited. During this limited time, additional dietary protein is needed to support the increment in muscle mass, but the increased need is rather small.

Durnin estimated the protein requirements

Although this woman has developed her muscles through windsurfing, she will not need a high protein diet to maintain them. *(Christopher Brown/Stock, Boston, Inc.)*

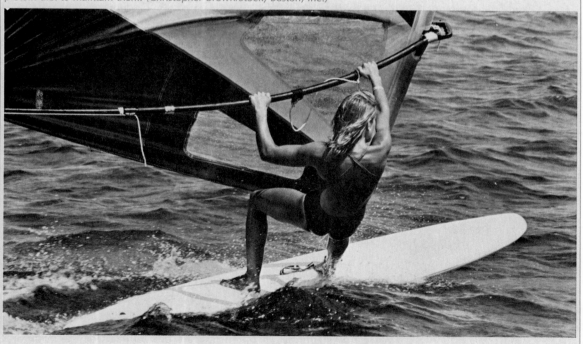

for a male athlete weighing 70 kg (154 lb) who is in the active phase of muscle building [9](Table 6-5). The total protein need, even when accumulating new muscle mass, amounts only to 47 g of protein. This amount of protein can be obtained from a variety of foods. Examples are:

	g PROTEIN		g PROTEIN
2.8 oz chicken	26	1 c navy beans	15
2 c milk	16	1 egg	6
1 oz cheddar	7	2 c milk	16
cheese	49 g	4 slices bread	12
			49 g

Athletes generally consume considerably more protein than this amount. Most athletes consume between 10 and 15 percent of their kilocalorie intake as protein, while expending 3000 kcal or more per day. One can calculate that at 10 percent of 3000-kcal intake, 300 kcal would be consumed as protein ÷ 4 kcal/gm = 75 g of protein. At 15 percent of 3000 kcal as protein, 113 g of protein would be consumed. This amount is two or three times the estimated requirement [9]. Some investigators recommend that athletes consume no more than 15 percent of their total kilocalories as protein [10].

Athletes who, while engaging in prolonged, intensive exercise, excrete hemoglobin or other protein in the urine may need a higher protein intake than estimated by Durnin [11]. Even then, a diet supplying 10 to 15 percent of the kilocalories as protein will easily cover this additional need.

Do high-protein intakes improve physical performance? Studies indicate that they do not. One study indicated that a protein intake of 2.8 g per kilogram of body weight per day did not improve physiological work performance when compared with an intake of 1.4 g per kilogram of body weight per day [12]. Another study showed that men in Marine Officer Candidate School who were given a protein supplement did no better in physical performance than those not receiving the supplement [13].

Claire, the basketball coach mentioned at

TABLE 6-5. ESTIMATION OF DAILY PROTEIN REQUIREMENT FOR A 70-kg MALE ATHLETE IN THE PHASE OF MUSCLE MASS DEVELOPMENT

EXPLANATION OF NEED	g N NEEDED	g PROTEIN NEEDED (g N × 6.25)
For increasing muscle mass.	1	7.0
To replace N in sweat losses during 4 hours of strenuous exercise.	1.2	7.5
To replace N lost in urine, feces, and skin (average losses).	3.92	25.0 (rounded)
To provide 30% more protein to cover individual differences in need (25 g × 0.3 = 7.5 g).	—	7.5
Total		47.0 g

These values are based upon reports in the scientific literature. All individuals lose nitrogen in urine, feces, and skin, and heavy exercise appears not to increase this loss. There is individual variation, however, in the amount lost, but estimating 30% more protein than the average should cover needs of all but 2.5% of population. The extra intake required to cover needs for muscle building is small—only 7.0 g/day.

SOURCE: Durnin, J. V. G. A., "Protein Requirements and Physical Activity," in Parizkova, J., and V.A. Rogozkin (eds.), Nutrition, Physical Fitness and Health, International Series on Sports Sciences, vol. 7, Baltimore: University Park Press, 1978.

pattern of amino acids we mean the amounts of amino acids present in the protein relative to one another. Table 6-6 shows the essential amino acid pattern for high-quality proteins (those utilized best) for human beings. Notice that the amino acid present in smallest amounts in this pattern is tryptophan, while threonine occurs at about three times, and leucine and the aromatic amino acids at a little more than six times the level of tryptophan.

TABLE 6-6.   ESTIMATED AMINO ACID REQUIREMENTS OF HUMANS

AMINO ACID	REQUIREMENT mg/kg BODY WEIGHT/DAY			AMINO ACID PATTERN FOR HIGH-QUALITY PROTEINS mg/g OF PROTEIN
	INFANT* (4–6 MONTHS)	CHILD (10–12 YEARS)	ADULT	
Histidine	33	?	?	17
Isoleucine	83	28	12	42
Leucine	135	42	16	70
Lysine	99	44	12	51
Total S-containing amino acids (methionine and cystine)	49	22	10	26
Total aromatic amino acids (phenylalanine and tyrosine)	141	22	16	73
Threonine	68	28	8	35
Tryptophan	21	4	3	11
Valine	92	25	14	48

Based upon amino acid requirements for humans, the amino acid pattern for high-quality proteins is given in column 5 (in milligrams of amino acid per gram of protein). This pattern indicates that in order to synthesize needed proteins, the body must obtain from the diet, for example, about three times as much threonine and tryptophan, and a little more than six times as much leucine as tryptophan.

*Two grams per kilogram of body weight per day of protein of the quality listed in column 5 would meet amino acid needs of the infant.

SOURCE: *Improvement of Protein Nutriture,* Food and Nutrition Board, National Research Council, National Academy of Sciences, Washington, D.C., 1975.

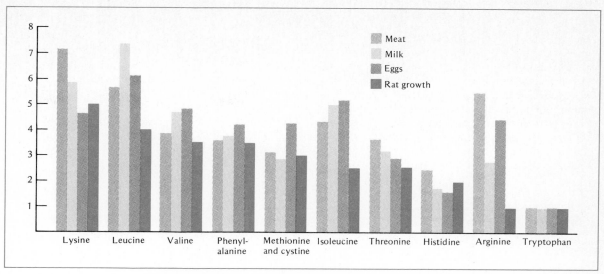

FIGURE 6-13. The amino acid pattern of high-quality proteins (meat, milk, and eggs) compared with the pattern needed for rat growth. The amino acid proportions are calculated on the basis that tryptophan = 1.0. (Arginine is required for rat, but not human, growth.) (Source: Redrawn from Flodin, N.W., "Amino Acids and Protein. Their Place in Human Nutrition Problems," *Journal of Agricultural and Food Chemistry,* 1:222, 1953.)

If we assign tryptophan the value of 1.0, we can easily compare the amino acid pattern of one protein with another. For example in Figure 6-13, we see that the highest quality proteins such as those from eggs, milk, and meat have patterns of amino acids similar to the one required for mammalian growth (in this case, the laboratory rat). There tends neither to be a marked deficit nor an excessive amount of any amino acid. On the other hand, comparing the amino acid pattern of wheat protein with that required by the growing rat (Figure 6-14), we see that wheat is low in lysine and relatively high in leucine and arginine. Rice, oats, barley, rye, and millet are also low in lysine relative to the needs of the growing rat, as well as to the needs of the human being.

The Limiting Amino Acids Imagine for a moment a child making a string of beads, using pop beads that snap into place. The cell's synthesis of protein can be thought of as occurring in the same way, with each amino acid, represented by a specific color of bead, being hooked onto the next one in its proper sequence. The amino acids yet to be incorporated into the protein can be thought of as piled up, waiting, like a pile of beads. The amount of protein the cell can synthesize is limited by the amino acid "bead" present in the smallest amount relative to the amount needed. If the cell has to rely entirely upon wheat protein for its amino acids, for example, *lysine* will be the *limiting amino acid*. This means that the amount of lysine present in the pile of beads will be low relative to the amount needed to make body protein. The cell would begin to make the protein in question, but when all the lysine was used up, synthesis of that protein would

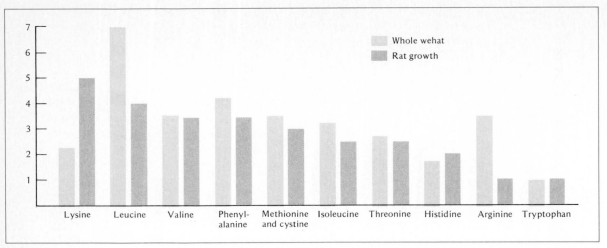

FIGURE 6-14. The amino acid pattern of a lower quality protein (whole wheat) compared with the pattern needed for rat growth. The amino acid proportions are calculated on the basis that tryptophan = 1.0. (Source: Redrawn from Flodin, N.W., "Amino Acids and Protein. Their Place in Human Nutrition Problems," *Journal of Agricultural and Food Chemistry,* 1:222, 1953.)

stop. The rest of the amino acids from the wheat would be mostly catabolized, and the nitrogen excreted as urea, representing a waste of protein.

In general, animal foods such as eggs, milk, cheese, meats, fish, and poultry contain high-quality proteins. Small amounts of these proteins supply all the essential amino acids in the proportions needed by growing as well as by adult human beings. Plant proteins tend to be low in one or more essential amino acids. Although it is *possible* for an adult to eat enough of a single plant protein source (in most cases) to obtain enough of the limiting amino acid, the protein is utilized inefficiently. Again, this means that the amino acids other than the limiting one will have been consumed in *much* higher amounts than needed, and will be catabolized, resulting in inefficient utilization of nitrogen from the protein. Since protein is the only source of the amino acids needed to make body protein, we do not wish to waste it needlessly.

Complementing Proteins   Fortunately, the amino acids from plant sources need not be wasted as just described. By combining a plant source low in one amino acid with another supplying that amino acid, we can *complement* or *mutually supplement* proteins. Figure 6-15 shows that the pattern of dry peas and beans, compared with the pattern needed by the growing rat, is high in lysine, but is low in sulfur-containing amino acids (methionine and cystine). However, grains, represented by wheat (Figure 6-14), supply methionine and cystine, and the *combination* of grains and beans in the proper proportion represent higher quality protein than either consumed alone. Vegetarians should use complementary protein combinations in planning their diets (Box 6-2).

Assessment of Dietary Protein Quality   Scientists have used various methods to assess protein quality, some of which appear in Appendix M. These methods have been used chiefly to study the quality of individual sources of protein, but we really need to know the quality of the *complex diet* that humans actually consume.

One cannot use the values obtained from individual proteins to predict what the quality of a mixed diet containing all the individual proteins will be. There are two reasons this is not possible. One is that there may or may not be proper complementarity of the dietary proteins in the total diet. The second is related to a peculiarity of the *efficiency* with which the body uses (utilizes) proteins. The body utilizes food proteins most efficiently if they are fed at levels *lower* than those needed by the body. Apparently this is an effort by nature to protect the body in dire circumstances when little protein is available. As the amount of protein fed nears the levels actually required by the body, the efficiency of utilization decreases, and the body wastes some of the protein. Consequently, an *additional* amount of the protein must be fed to cover the poorer efficiency of utilization.

The RDA allows for this decrease in efficiency of utilization as the dietary protein intake approaches the amount required. For example, egg protein is fully utilized at intakes below the requirement, but loses 30 percent in efficiency of utilization when it is fed at requirement levels. In addition, the mixture of proteins in the American diet is judged to be about 75 percent as well utilized as egg protein. The RDA takes *both* of these into account, so that the 0.8 g per kilogram of body weight recommended is sufficient to meet the increase in need brought about by both these situations.

Are some groups in the United States consuming low-protein diets? The Health and Nutrition Examination Survey (HANES) of 1971–1974 indicated that

FIGURE 6-15. The amino acid pattern of peas and beans compared with the pattern needed for rat growth. Here, the pattern is calculated based upon threonine = 2.5. (Source: Redrawn from Flodin, N.W., "Amino Acids and Protein. Their Place in Human Nutrition Problems," *Journal of Agricultural and Food Chemistry*, 1:222, 1953.)

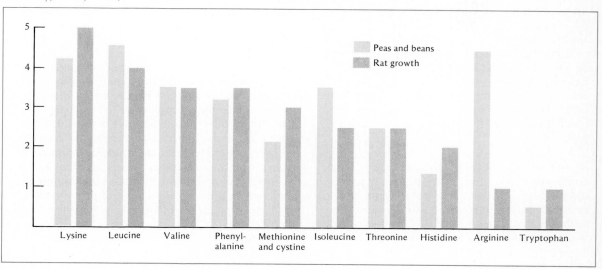

6-2 BOX

Vegetarian Diets

In recent years, many people in affluent countries, particularly in the United States, have become interested in vegetarian diets upon realizing that meat production as currently practiced uses up an excessive amount of the earth's resources compared to nonflesh foods. Throughout history, however, many groups have practiced vegetarianism through economic necessity, or because of religious or philosophical convictions.

Vegetarian organizations usually define vegetarianism as abstaining from consumption of flesh foods (meat, poultry, and fish), but many individuals call themselves vegetarians even though they eat poultry or fish, and abstain only from "red" meats (beef, pork, and lamb). From the point of view of nutrition, it is convenient to divide vegetarians into *lacto-* or *lacto-ovo-vegetarians*, who consume milk or milk and eggs, respectively, and *total vegetarians* ("pure" or "strict" vegetarians) who consume no foods of animal origin. *Vegans* make up a special group of total vegetarians who use no products of animals, including silk, wool, leather, etc.

The basic foods in a well-planned vegetarian diet consist of grains (cereals), breads, pasta, beans, peas, nuts, seeds, vegetables, and fruits and, if the person is a lacto-ovo-vegetarian, milk, cheese, and eggs. Usually small amounts of oil, butter, honey, molasses, or sugar also are used.

Misconceptions Several misconceptions exist about vegetarian diets. One is that it is very difficult to obtain enough protein of good quality, but this is far from true. It was demonstrated long ago that if one consumes a large enough amount of *a wide variety* of minimally processed vegetarian foods to support normal weight in adults, the protein intake will be adequate in both quantity and quality [14]. It is important, then, not to restrict food choices to a few foods. Elliott, whose concern about the protein intake on vegetarian diets was mentioned at the beginning of the chapter, need only remember to maintain normal weight while choosing a wide variety of vegetarian foods.

Another misconception is that vegetarian diets are starchy and therfore fattening. Although vegetarian diets tend to be higher in carbohydrates than the usual American omnivorous (containing meat) diet, vegetarian diets generally are lower in fat content [15,16]. Whether or not a diet is "fattening" depends upon whether its kilocalorie level is high relative to the needs of the individual in question. Many people lose weight when they first change from an omnivorous to a vegetarian diet, apparently because the greater bulkiness of the diet results in their "feeling full" at a lower kilocalorie intake than they had been accustomed to. Although obesity is less common among vegetarians than among omnivores, it still exists, and vegetarianism is obviously not a solution to the problem of obesity.

Complementing Proteins Groups of people throughout the ages have used complementary protein combinations in their customary diets. Examples are the combination of garbanzo beans (chick peas) and sesame seeds in Middle Eastern hummus, and rice and beans or corn and beans in many parts of Central and South America and the Caribbean islands.

Investigators believe it is best to consume good quality protein (either animal protein or supplementary plant–plant or plant–animal combinations) in each meal rather than only once or twice a day. This is based upon research with young women who were in nitrogen equilibrium if they consumed a moderate amount of

TABLE 6-7. MUTUAL SUPPLEMENTARY RELATIONS BETWEEN DIFFERENT VEGETABLE PROTEINS

PROTEIN FOOD*	PROTEIN EFFICIENCY RATIO†
Sesame (10%)	1.7
Peanut (10%)	1.6
Sesame (5%) + peanut (5%)	2.0
Chickpea (10%)	1.5
Chickpea (5%) + sesame (5%)	2.2
Soya bean (10%)	2.1
Soya bean (6%) + sesame (4%)	2.4
Rice (6%) + red gram (3%) + amaranth (1%)	2.5
Wheat (6%) + red gram (3%) + amaranth (1%)	2.4
Pearl millet (6%) + red gram (3%) + amaranth (1%)	2.3
Sorghum (6%) + red gram (3%) + amaranth (1%)	2.5
Skim milk (10%)	2.6

*Protein contributed by each of the protein foods is given in parentheses.
†Level of protein 10%; duration of feeding 4 weeks. The protein quality of each of these foods or food combinations was assessed using PER (protein efficiency ratio), described in Appendix M. Protein quality improves as the PER increases.
SOURCE: Rao, M.N., and M. Swaninathan, "Plant Proteins in the Amelioration of Protein Deficiency States," *World Review of Nutrition and Dietetics,* 11:106, 1969.

high-quality protein divided into three meals a day, but were in negative nitrogen balance if they consumed the same amount of high-quality protein at only two of the three meals [17].

Table 6-7 indicates that a mixture of soy and sesame seed proteins has a nutritive value very close to that of milk proteins. Legumes (beans), including soybeans, supplement the amino acid content of cereals well, since cereals tend to be low in lysine, while beans supply lysine but are low in methionine, which cereals supply. Peanut protein also supplements cereals such as oats, wheat, rice, and corn well.

Some vegetarians choose to use products called *meat analogs,* manufactured from soybeans and other plants. These resemble beef, pork, poultry, sausage, and shellfish in texture and flavor. They are easy to use in menu planning because they can be substituted for meat; furthermore, they are free of cholesterol and may be lower than meat in fat. However, they tend to be expensive, very high in sodium, and are not comparable to meats in vitamin and mineral content.

Nutrients Requiring Attention Lacto-ovovegetarians who consume a wide variety of foods need not be concerned about having an adequate diet as long as they consume enough kilocalories to maintain normal body weight in adults and normal growth in children. Total vegetarian diets, on the other hand, are apt to be low in certain nutrients unless special plans are made to include them. These nutrients are *calcium, riboflavin,* and *vitamin B$_{12}$,* and for children and pregnant women, *vitamin D.* In addition, absorption of iron and zinc may be less than in omnivores. The best source of calcium in the American diet is milk and milk products, so if milk products are not consumed, rather large quantities of cooked turnip, mustard or collard greens, tofu (soybean curd), almonds, and unhulled sesame seeds (preferably finely ground) would need to be consumed. Riboflavin also might be low because, again, milk is the best source, but cooked greens and whole or enriched grains can be consumed in large enough amounts to reach the RDA.

Vitamin B_{12} is of special concern because this vitamin occurs only in animal foods, having been formed by bacteria in the rumen of cattle and sheep, and in the intestinal tract of other animals. Although some popular writers claim that fermented soybean products are sources of vitamin B_{12}, they are not reliable sources. Since vitamin B_{12} deficiency can eventually result in severe damage to the nervous system, all total vegetarians should consume a food, such as soy milk, that has been fortified with vitamin B_{12}. A recipe for homemade soy milk that is fortified with both vitamin B_{12} and calcium is offered by Robertson et al. [18]. Several recent reports in the medical literature make it clear that the infant of a total vegetarian mother whose diet is unsupplemented with vitamin B_{12} is at high risk for vitamin B_{12} deficiency if fed only breast milk.

Vitamin D does not occur in plant foods, and infants, children, and pregnant women consuming a total vegetarian diet should receive a supplement of this vitamin. Vitamin D-fortified soy milk or a vitamin D tablet may be used.

The well-chosen vegetarian diet is usually higher in iron than the usual American diet, but iron from plant sources is not as well absorbed as that from meat. However, it has recently been demonstrated that a source of vitamin C consumed with plant foods markedly increases the absorption of iron, so the practice of including a source of vitamin C in each meal is recommended.

Weaning an infant to a total vegetarian diet, or feeding a 1- or 2-year-old such a diet presents certain problems, the chief of which is that the bulkiness of the diet prevents the infant or small child from consuming much food at one feeding. One risks the possibility that poor growth will result if the total kilocalorie intake is too low. Whenever possible, it is recommended that infants and small children be fed milk in addition to plant foods. Otherwise, soy milk fortified with sufficient calcium, vitamin B_{12}, and vitamin D so that the child receives the RDA daily is recommended. Frequent feeding of small children is necessary, and complementary protein sources should be fed.

Food guides for meal planning are shown in Table 6-8 and 6-9. Well-planned vegetarian diets can be nutritionally adequate and may have health advantages [19].

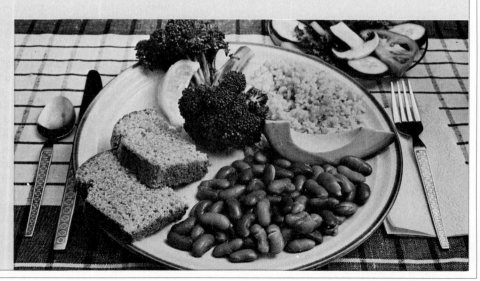

To obtain high-quality protein, vegetarians can complement protein sources, indicated here by the rice and bean combination. (Randy Matusow)

TABLE 6-8. FOOD GUIDE FOR LACTO-OVO-VEGETARIAN ADULTS

GROUP	NO. OF SERVINGS	SERVING SIZE AND EXCHANGE
1. Legumes, nuts, seeds	1 serving legumes or meat analogs or soybean curd 1 serving nuts or seeds	1 c cooked legumes (beans) 2–3 oz meat analogs 20–30 g dry textured vegetable protein 1½ oz or 3 tbsp nuts or seeds 4 oz soybean curd
2. Bread, grains, pasta	4–6 servings	1 slice bread ½–¾ c rice, millet, whole wheat, berries, cracked wheat, oats 1 c dry breakfast cereal ½–¾ c noodles, macaroni, spaghetti
3. Fruits and vegetables	4 or more (a source of vitamin C in each meal) At least one dark leafy vegetable. Serve dark yellow vegetables often	1 c raw vegetables ½ c cooked vegetables or fruits 1 piece fruit
4. Milk or cheese	2 servings	1 c milk (fluid) ⅓ c dried skim milk 1⅓ oz cheddar cheese ½ c cottage cheese 1 c soybean milk (fortified) 1 c yogurt
5. Eggs and fat	3–4 eggs a week 1 serving oil a day 1 serving margarine a day	1 egg 1 tsp oil 1 tsp soft margarine

Additional kilocalories should come chiefly from these foods. Relatively small amounts of sugars, honey, and syrups should be used. Some additional fat may be used, but avoid large intakes. Use a wide variety of different foods in groups 1, 2, and 3.

TABLE 6-9. FOOD GUIDE FOR TOTAL VEGETARIANS (ADULTS)

GROUP	NO. OF SERVINGS	SERVING SIZE AND EXCHANGES
1. Legumes (beans)	1¼ serving legumes (plus calcium and vitamin B_{12} from other sources) or ⅓ serving legumes and 2 servings fortified soybean milk	1 c cooked beans 1 c soybean milk (fortified with vitamin B_{12}, calcium, and vitamin D)
2. Grains	4 servings bread 3–5 servings grains and 1 serving nuts or seeds	1 slice bread ½–¾ c cooked grains 1½ oz or 3 tbsp nuts or seeds
3. Vegetables	4 servings (include 3 servings dark green leafy vegetables* and include a source of vitamin C in each meal)	1 c raw vegetable ¾ c cooked vegetable
4. Fruits	1–4 servings (include a source of vitamin C in each meal)	4–6 oz juice 1 piece fruit

*Greens should be those low in oxalate such as mustard, turnip, and collard greens.
SOURCE: Robertson, L., C. Flinders, and B. Godfrey, *Laurel's Kitchen*, Petaluma, Calif.: Nilgiri Press, 1976.

the average protein consumption in this country was 78 g/day, but the same study indicated that a little more than 20 percent of women in income groups below the poverty level had protein intakes below two-thirds of the RDA. Because of the margin of safety built into the RDAs, we cannot say these women were not consuming enough protein to meet their needs; however, it is not surprising to find that *women* were the ones reported to consume less protein than the RDA because many women consume low-kilocalorie diets, thereby lessening the possibility of obtaining all the nutrients recommended.

The importance of the kilocalorie intake in maintaining nitrogen equilibrium was demonstrated many years ago in a group of women whose ages varied from 30 to 85 [20]. Both protein and kilocalorie intakes declined with age, but at any age women were shown to be in negative nitrogen balance if the kilocalorie intake was less than 1500 kcal/day. Remember that if the kilocalorie intake is too low, protein will be catabolized to supply energy. Our sedentary lifestyle causes women to decrease their kilocalorie intake to avoid gaining weight, but it appears that a deliberate effort to build increased physical activity into one's lifestyle would be beneficial, allowing one to consume more food, and a more nutritious diet.

Many people in the United States doubtless consume high-protein intakes (over 15 percent of their total kilocalorie intake). Might there be any harm in such a practice? We have observed that individuals with normal liver and kidney function adapt to a high-protein intake with no obvious signs of harm. Yet much of the protein in such a diet is simply being torn down and its nitrogen excreted. Since dietary protein sources are among our most expensive, this represents a monetary waste. In the sense that only food proteins can furnish the essential amino acids needed for body protein synthesis, this practice also represents a real waste of resources required to produce protein foods. Furthermore, there is a possibility that high-protein intakes may modify the body's metabolism of calcium (see the osteoporosis discussion in Chapter 16).

A CLOSER LOOK

If your protein intake is higher than 15 percent of total kilocalories, how can you cut it back to a reasonable level? Here are a list of possible changes you could make.

- Decrease portion sizes of meat, poultry or fish to 2 oz.
- Consume meat, poultry, or fish "diluted" in mixed dishes with pasta, grains, or bread.
- Consume more vegetarian meals, using complementary protein combinations.
- Avoid adding cheese or eggs to meat or poultry dishes.
- Snack on popcorn, fruit, or vegetable sticks rather than on cheese, meat, or other high-protein foods.

Infants and small children require a higher amount of protein, of essential amino acids, and of kilocalories per kilogram of body weight than adults. Breast milk usually provides these needs during the first 6 months of life. After 6 months, weaning foods adequate in kilocalories, protein, vitamins, and minerals need to be added to the breast milk diet for normal growth to continue.

The disease called protein-calorie malnutrition (PCM) is most prevalent among infants and small children in many countries of the Far East, Middle East, Africa, and Central and South America. The mortality rate from birth to 4 years of age may be used as an index of the general nutritional condition of the population. The death rate for infants from birth to 1 year of age was reported in 1976 to be 250 per 1000 in Zambia and Bolivia, 140 per 1000 in India and Pakistan, and 95 per 1000 in Brazil, compared with 19 per 1000 in the United States [21].

PCM does not occur among segments of the population that can afford to purchase enough food to satisfy their hunger. But even among the poorer people in the population, not everyone develops severe manifestations of PCM, although in a country such as Guatemala as many as 8 percent of the adults hospitalized have been reported to suffer from moderate to severe PCM [22].

In countries where PCM is rampant, children typically do not grow at the rate observed in well-nourished populations and may be said to have mild-to-moderate PCM. At a given age, the children are shorter and lighter in weight than those in the same country with the same genetic potential who are well-fed. Although this appears to be an adaptive mechanism, allowing the children to survive, these children are retarded in bone development, and in normal development of lean as well as adipose tissue. There is concern, also, that mental development may not be completely normal, and that productivity in adulthood may be curtailed [22].

A certain percentage of the children do, however, develop signs of severe PCM, manifested by *marasmus* (a chronic, severe wasting of the body tissues), in which no edema occurs, at one end of the continuum and *kwashiorkor*, in which edema occurs, at the other end. One of these forms may be seen more frequently in some parts of the world than others; for example, kwashiorkor has been the more prevalent form in parts of Africa, while marasmus has occurred more frequently in the Middle East. The child with marasmus usually is emaciated ("skin and bones"), has no signs of fatty liver or of dermatitis (skin scaliness), and usually has serum albumin levels within normal limits. The child with kwashiorkor has more body fat (but it is flabby), shows edema (sometimes chiefly in the legs, but often also in the abdomen and face), has a typical peeling dermatitis ("flaky-paint"), has an enlarged and fatty liver, and low serum albumin levels. Growth retardation is typical of each of these forms of PCM. In general, marasmus is seen in younger children (3 months to 3 years), while kwashiorkor occurs more frequently from 1 to 5 years. However, many children do not have signs of clear-cut marasmus or kwashiorkor, but have various combinations of symptoms of each.

Experimentally, symptoms similar to kwashiorkor have been produced by feeding animals diets adequate in kilocalories but deficient in protein, while marasmus has been produced by feeding low-calorie–low-protein diets. In many parts of the world it appears that kwashiorkor results from feeding the child, upon weaning from the breast, a diet almost adequate in kilocalories but high in starch or sugar and low in protein, while marasmus results from feeding a diet low in both kilocalories and protein. However, Gopalan observed in India that marasmus and kwashiorkor appear among children fed the same diet [23]. It may be that under these circumstances, the child who develops marasmus has been able to adapt better to the poor diet, while the development of kwashiorkor, with its more severe symptoms, may be due to a failure of the hormonal system to adapt. Nevertheless, whenever fullblown kwashiorkor or marasmus develops, the child is seriously ill and cannot survive without proper care.

PCM is complicated by poor sanitary conditions resulting in frequent infections during which the need for protein increases. Frequently the child eats poorly when sick, or else the custom in the culture may deprive a child of nourishing food during illness. A vicious cycle develops in which the increased protein need fails to be met by the diet until a depleted protein state lowers the child's resistance to infection. Episodes of infection become more and more frequent until the child eventually develops PCM. A dramatic illustration of the effect of malnutrition on infection is the mortality rate from measles among children in countries affected by PCM. In Mexico, the mortality rate from measles has been reported to be 180 times higher than in the United States [24].

The treatment of severe forms of PCM requires skilled care, usually in a hospital. Once the child is out of danger, a diet supplying sufficient kilocalories and protein, plus all other needed nutrients, to promote "catch-up" growth is recommended, along with a program of supervised physical activity and psychosocial stimulation. The latter aspect of the program is an attempt to overcome the lag in learning during the illness which usually prevents a child from exploring his or her environment and responding to stimuli.

Although PCM could be prevented by changes in the economic situation in countries that would result in more equitable distribution of food to people, less revolutionary programs involve:

1. Encouraging breast feeding and discouraging bottle feeding (because of the danger of illness from contaminated water and bottles).
2. Educating mothers in adequate methods of supplementing breast milk and feeding children after weaning.
3. Improving sanitary conditions to diminish episodes of infection.

Successful programs have been established in rehabilitation centers located in villages, often called "Mothercraft Centers [25]. In successful centers, the cooperation of families with small children is obtained, and a center equipped for cooking exactly as the village homes are equipped is constructed. Mothers bring small children to the center and leave them all day, but agree to spend a certain amount of time themselves in the center to learn about proper feeding of small children and sanitary practices. The children are fed an adequate diet obtained from foods commonly available in the area. Their growth rate is carefully recorded to impress upon the mothers the importance of proper feeding. The most successful of these programs also include immunization of the children as an integral part of the program. Dr. Bengoa, an expert on these programs, concludes that these programs can drastically reduce the incidence of severe forms of PCM, but mild-to-moderate forms can be solved only by reorganization of economic and political systems [25].

SUMMARY

1 Proteins are large molecules made up of basic units called amino acids linked together by peptide bonds. They perform a variety of functions in the body.

2 Proteins are digested by a series of digestive enzymes to amino acids and dipeptides. The dipeptides are broken down to amino acids in intestinal mucosal cells so that only amino acids reach the portal blood and are transported to the liver.

3 The specific amino acids used by the body to synthesize a given protein may come either from food or from catabolized body protein, since there is a constant cycle of synthesis and catabolism of most body proteins.

4 When amino acids are catabolized, the amino group is removed, converted to urea in the liver, and excreted by the kidneys. The remaining carbon chain may be converted to glucose, fat, or energy as needed.

5 The body can adapt to a range of low- or high-protein intakes. Nitrogen balance may be used to study this adaptation, as well as to examine circumstances that influence the body to gain or lose nitrogen.

6 To synthesize body protein, cells need to have at the site of synthesis all the essential amino acids, and must be able to synthesize the unessential amino acids. In addition, sufficient kilocalorie sources must be available.

7 The quality of dietary protein depends upon its amino acid pattern relative to that of body proteins. Most animal foods in small amounts furnish a pattern of amino acids like that of the body. Plant proteins tend to be low in one or more essential amino acids. Nevertheless, they can be combined with one another or with animal proteins in such a way as to produce high-quality protein, furnishing the amino acid pattern needed.

8 Vegetarian diets can be planned so that they are nutritionally adequate. Guides are given for planning vegetarian diets.

9 Protein-calorie malnutrition (PCM) is a disease affecting young children in many countries. It often occurs in circumstances in which the child suffers many episodes of infection, compounded by a diet too low in kilocalories, protein, or both to meet the child's needs. Efforts to combat this disorder are discussed.

FOR DISCUSSION AND APPLICATION

1 From your dietary record, compare the percentage of your total kilocalories that came from protein with *Dietary Goals for the United States*. If your diet was high in protein, was it also high in fat? For those students in the class who had high intakes (over 15 percent of kilocalories), what kind of diet was consumed? How many of these were diets for weight control? How many of the diets that were high in protein were also high in fat? What choices of food accounted for this?

2 If your diet contributed more protein than the RDA, how would you modify it to just meet the RDA? What are the arguments for and against a high-protein intake?

3 Jocelyn has decided to follow a lacto-ovo-vegetarian diet. Her parents object on the grounds that she might become malnourished. What arguments can you marshal to help Jocelyn strengthen her case?

SUGGESTED READINGS

Robertson, L., C. Flinders, and B. Godfrey, *Laurel's Kitchen: A Handbook for Vegetarian Cookery and Nutrition*, Petaluma, Calif.: Nilgiri Press, 1976. This is a sound, well-written book about vegetarianism. Many recipes are included.

Lappé, F. M., *Diet for a Small Planet*, New York: Ballantine Books, 1982. This is a revision of the classic book about use of complementary protein sources.

Osman, J. D., *Thin from Within: Vegetarian Edition*, Washington, D.C.: Review & Herald Publishing Co., 1981. Advice for the vegetarian who has difficulty achieving desirable weight.

7 ENERGY BALANCE

While you are reading this book, your body is using energy to move your eyes across the page, and to contract skeletal muscles to hold your body in position as you read. At the same time, energy is being used to support breathing, the heart beat, blood circulation, and activities of the liver and kidneys. In addition, body cells are using energy to synthesize needed compounds such as proteins, phospholipids, and hormones. Energy is also being used to transport sodium, potassium, and other minerals across cell membranes. If you have recently had a meal, energy is being used to transport glucose and amino acids into intestinal mucosal cells. Your body cells constantly need energy—they never take a vacation.

In the preceding chapters, we emphasized that the body's primary need is for energy. If energy intake is too low, the body consumes its own tissues to sustain vital body functions. What is meant by energy? How much does a person need? What factors affect the need? Do foods high in energy make you feel more energetic? How can you estimate your own energy need? How can you estimate the energy needs of a group of people? Does it matter how an athlete meets his or her energy needs? Which foods are high and which low in energy value? These questions will be addressed in this chapter.

ENERGY: WHAT IS IT?

The sun's energy supplies power for all life. Green plants, through photosynthesis, change the energy from sunlight to chemical energy, locked in the chemical bonds of starch, sugars, proteins, and fats. Human beings receive chemical energy when consuming plants or animals that have consumed plants. Energy cannot be recycled, therefore all living organisms require constant input of the sun's energy (Figure 7-1). Energy is not a substance you can feel or taste or see. It has no mass. Yet body cells die within a few minutes of being deprived of energy.

  Energy is defined as the ability to do work. In nutrition we are concerned with the human body's ability to do *biological work*—those kinds of activities described at the beginning of this chapter. Previous chapters made clear that the body obtains chemical energy from carbohydrates, fats, and proteins by a stepwise oxidative process in which useful energy is captured in the form of ATP (adenosine *tri*phosphate). When cells require energy, they break the high energy bonds of ATP molecules and use some of the released energy for such vital processes as (1) the synthesis of new compounds, (2) mechanical or muscular work, and (3) transport of substances across membranes. Some of these activities are illustrated in Table 7-1.

  We can measure the energy needs of the body simply by measuring heat given off. Let's see why this is so. The body captures in the form of ATP only about 40 percent of the energy in carbohydrates, fats, and protein—the remaining energy is lost as heat. When body cells use ATP to synthesize compounds or for

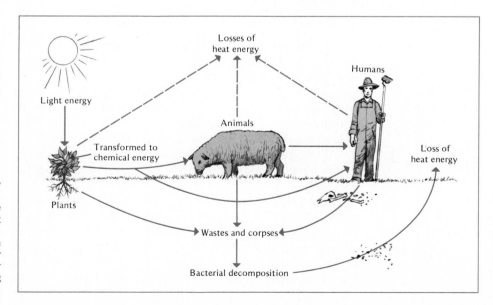

FIGURE 7-1. Energy flow through the biosphere. The energy flow is in one direction and does not return to the source. Heat lost in this system cannot be used for energy by plants or animals, including human beings.

TABLE 7-1. EXAMPLES OF BODY ACTIVITIES REQUIRING ENERGY

BIOLOGICAL WORK	EXAMPLES	COMMENTS
Synthesis of compounds	Structural proteins (myosin, actin, etc.) Blood proteins (hemoglobin, albumin, etc.) Antibodies Hormones (both protein and steroid) Cholesterol Liproproteins Glycogen Triglycerides Phospholipids	During growth some cells use as much as 75% of their ATP for synthesis of new compounds.

Mechanical work	Muscle contractions:
	    Skeletal muscles
	    Heart muscle
	    Walls of intestines
		Efficiency with which chemical energy is converted into muscular work is less than 20–25%. The rest is lost as heat.

Active transport across membranes	Intestinal cells during absorption (amino acids, glucose, galactose, sodium). Kidney tubules (amino acids, glucose, sodium, potassium). Transport in or out of other body cells (sodium, potassium, calcium, iodine in thyroid cells).	Cells in kidney tubules use as much as 80% of their ATP for transport purposes.

muscle contractions, only 20 to 35 percent of the ATP energy is used—the rest is lost as heat. Eventually, almost all this captured energy also is transformed to heat. For example, in Chapter 6 we discussed the continuous turnover of body proteins. Energy from ATP is placed in the peptide bonds that form between amino acids as proteins are synthesized, but when proteins are broken down, this energy is released as heat. Furthermore, the work of body organs is converted to heat. For example, the friction of blood flowing in the vessels, and the movement of muscles when, for example, you move your arms or legs, causes friction which produces heat. Therefore, practically all the energy expended by the body is eventually transformed to heat.

The laws of thermodynamics apply to the human body as well as to other parts of the universe. The fact that energy cannot be created or destroyed during ordinary physical or chemical processes, but is only converted from one form to another, is called the *Law of Conservation of Energy*, or the *First Law of Thermodynamics*. What does this law mean to nutrition scientists? It means that although the human body ultimately converts the chemical energy in food to heat, which is then lost from the body, *that* heat nevertheless can be accounted for in the environment surrounding the person. It is not lost from the point of view of the universe. If a person consumes more food energy than his or her body expends, the excess can be accounted for in the synthesis of body fat or other tissues and through heat loss.

On the other hand, an individual who uses up more energy than he or she consumes in food must burn up some body tissues. By studying the amount of energy entering the body, that residing in the body, and that expended by the body, scientists can account for all the energy in the system. This means that there is no magical, mysterious way of losing body fat, despite claims often made in the popular media. Body fat will be oxidized for energy whenever the kilocalorie intake is less than the body expends.

Two types of energy are important in the body: (1) active or kinetic energy, and (2) potential energy. *Active or kinetic energy* is involved in performing work for internal processes or those activities involving muscular work, noted in Table 7-1. Kinetic energy is supplied when high-energy bonds in ATP and other high-energy compounds are broken within the cells. *Potential energy* is energy that is stored or inactive, such as that residing in glycogen or body fat. Potential energy serves as an important emergency source when food is scarce. ATP is a source of potential energy, but the amount stored in the tissues at any one time is small.

The unit most often used by nutritionists to measure energy is a unit of heat, the *kilocalorie* (kcal). As pointed out earlier, a kilocalorie is the amount of heat required to raise the temperature of 1 kilogram (1000 grams) of water 1° Celsius or centigrade (C). It is a larger unit than the gram-calorie used in physics and chemistry, which is the amount of heat required to raise the temperature of 1 g of water 1°C. Generally, nutritionists as well as the general public refer to the kilocalorie simply as the calorie, understood to be the larger kilogram calorie.

The *kilojoule* (kJ) is the unit for measuring energy in the metric system, which is rapidly becoming the system of weights and measures used throughout the world. Since 1 kcal equals 4.184 kJ, any discussion of energy values will involve considerably larger numbers if kilojoules are used. Nutrition organizations are gradually moving toward adoption of the kilojoule, but the general public will doubtless be slow in feeling at home with the term. We shall continue to use the kilocalorie in this book, but will show kilojoule equivalents when appropriate. Table 7-2 shows the relationship between kilocalories and kilojoules.

HOW MUCH ENERGY DOES THE BODY NEED?

The answer to this question sounds simple: The body needs enough food energy to equal the daily expenditure, or loss, of energy, assuming that the body has a moderate store of body fat. (A healthy body needs to have *some* fat stores.) Another way of saying this is that a person needs to consume the amount of food energy that allows for maintenance of desirable body weight (see Chapter 8). Many people in the world encounter difficulty in achieving this goal because of their inability to obtain enough food; therefore, their body weights tend to be lower than desirable (see Chapter 18). On the other hand, many people in affluent countries, where vast quantities of food are readily available, tend to consume more food energy than needed; therefore, their body weights tend to be higher than desirable. Surprisingly, a great many people in affluent countries nevertheless maintain desirable body weight without thinking about how to do it.

TABLE 7-2.   RELATIONSHIP BETWEEN KILOCALORIES AND KILOJOULES

1 kilocalorie (kcal) = 4.184 kilojoules (kJ)
= 4184 joules (J)
= 1000 "small" calories
1 kilojoule (kJ) = 0.24 kilocalories (kcal)
= 1000 joules (J)
1 megajoule (MJ) = 240 kilocalories (kcal)
= 1,000,000 joules (J)

For quick computations, if a high degree of accuracy is not needed, one can convert kcal to kJ by multiplying number of kcal by 4.2 (rather than by 4.184).

Energy balance is an overall term used in relationship to energy metabolism in the same sense that nitrogen balance is used in protein metabolism (Chapter 6). *Energy balance* is the relationship of energy consumed to that used up or stored by the body. Most people are interested in this relationship because it affects their body weight. For those adults who maintain normal body weight day after day with little change, the energy intake equals the expenditure, and they are at equilibrium. It is important to notice, however, that obese or underweight people frequently maintain the same body weight for long periods, and consequently are also at equilibrium during those periods.

Energy intake greater than the expenditure is positive energy balance. It results in increased body mass, which is appropriate in periods of growth in children and pregnant women, and during periods of recovery from wasting diseases or trauma. In these circumstances, the increased body weight is normally due to lean body tissues, bone mass (in the case of children), and some fat stores. For the athlete who is in the active phase of building larger muscles, the extra kilocalorie intake accounting for positive energy balance may be used chiefly to build lean tissues. Since muscles increase in a finite manner, the athlete will be in positive energy balance for this purpose for only a limited time. Positive energy balance frequently results in increased and unwanted accumulations of body fat for many people. Negative energy balance, when intake is less than the expenditure, is the desired state when one is losing excessive body fat. It is undesirable, however, when it results in emaciation of the body, as in anorexia nervosa (see Chapter 8).

Clearly, then, we can estimate the number of kilocalories needed daily by estimating the energy expenditure, assuming that one needs neither to gain nor lose fat stores.

How do we estimate energy expenditure? What is energy expended *for*? In answering these questions it is useful to categorize uses for which the body expends energy: (1) *basal metabolism*, (2) *the effect of food*, and (3) *physical activity*.

Basal Metabolism

Energy expended for basal metabolism is used for all the vital functions of the body when the body is at rest, and not digesting food. *Basal metabolism* refers to the energy required to support the vital functions of the body while at physical, mental, and emotional rest in a room of comfortable temperature, 12 to 18 hours after eating. It encompasses energy used for breathing; beating of the heart; circulation of the blood; action of the liver, kidneys, and other organs; and transmission of nerve impulses and other vital functions. It excludes energy needed for physical activity or for digestion and absorption of food. The *rate* at which body tissues metabolize the fuel nutrients for energy under these conditions is called the *basal metabolic rate* or *BMR*. These terms are frequently used interchangeably with the term *basal metabolism*.

Several factors determine whether or not one individual expends more energy than another for basal metabolism. Body size is an important factor: A larger person expends more energy for BMR than a small one. The component of the body size that is most influential appears to be the amount of lean tissue in the body.

Lean Body Mass Investigators have established that energy used for basal metabolism resides in the lean body mass [1,2]. Lean body mass (LBM) consists of the total body weight minus the weight of body fat. Metabolic activities do not take place in body fat since it is simply an inactive storage form of potential energy. Technically, LBM is made up of two components: the body cell mass and the extracellular mass (Figure 7-2). The extracellular mass consists of bone, connective tissue, and body fluids, each of which has extremely low metabolism which, for our discussion, can be ignored. The metabolism of LBM is due, therefore, almost entirely to skeletal muscles, the vital organs (liver, heart, lungs, kidneys, brain, and nerves), and to the protoplasm of adipose tissues (Figure 7-3). Since fat stores make up a high percentage of body weight in some people, the protoplasm of their fat cells contributes to the BMR, but the stored fat does not.

Individuals having a high percentage of their body weight as lean tissue have a higher BMR than those with a lower percentage. Males generally have a higher

FIGURE 7-2. Division of the body composition of a reference male and female into four compartments. (Source: Cunningham, J. J., ''Body Composition and Resting Metabolic Rate: The Myth of Feminine Metabolism,'' *American Journal of Clinical Nutrition,* 36:721, 1982.)

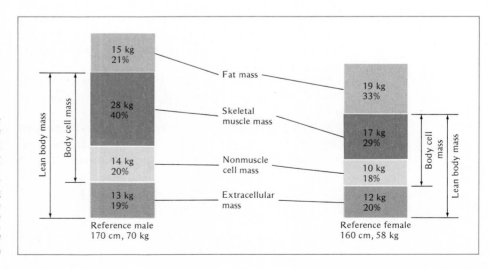

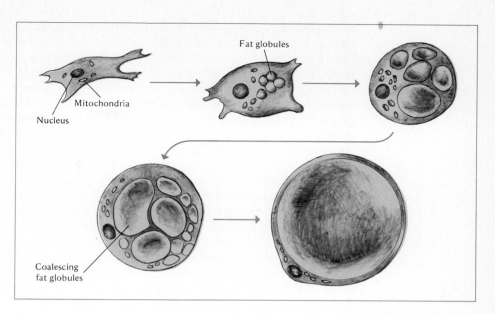

FIGURE 7-3. The fat or adipose tissue cell. As more and more fat is stored in a cell, fat droplets fuse until finally a giant fat drop takes up most of the room in the cell. The nucleus and cytoplasm of the cell are pushed to the periphery. Metabolism takes place only in the cytoplasm of the fat cell. (Source: Dabis, P. W., and E. P. Solomon, *The World of Biology*, 2d ed., New York: McGraw-Hill Book Co., 1979, p. 266.)

Labels in figure: Fat globules, Mitochondria, Nucleus, Coalescing fat globules

BMR than females of the same height, weight, and age, due to greater proportion of lean body mass in males. Female sex hormones appear to favor the deposition of body fat, while male hormones do not. Note that in Figure 7-2 the reference female has 33 percent of her body weight as fat, while the reference male has only 21 percent. Furthermore, the largest difference between them in body cell mass is that his skeletal muscle mass is much greater than hers. Athletic training in women can significantly increase their proportion of lean body mass and decrease body fat [3]. Athletes should realize, however, that reducing body weight (and body fat) below certain limits is incompatible with good health. For a 154-lb (70-kg) man, minimal weight compatible with health is 136 lb (61.8 kg), with 3 percent of the body weight as fat. For a woman originally weighing 125 lb (56 kg), minimal weight is 107 lb (48.6 kg) with 12 percent of the body weight as fat [10].

The basal metabolic rate decreases gradually from early adulthood to old age, due chiefly to a decline in lean body mass [1]. The aging process entails excessive loss or destruction of body cells and their replacement with fat and connective tissue. This results in the increase in the proportion of fat tissue in the body [1,4]. Even individuals who weigh exactly the same at age 75 as at 25 will have a significantly higher percentage of body weight as fat at age 75 than at age 25.

Investigators have observed, however, that not all cells, organs, or tissues that contribute to the lean body mass have the same rate of metabolism per unit of mass. Table 7-3 indicates that for the adult man the brain and liver together account for 53 percent of the BMR, although these organs make up only about 4 percent of the body weight. (1.4 kg + 1.6 kg ÷ 70 kg × 100). In the infant the brain and liver account for 64 percent of the BMR, while these organs comprise about 12 percent of the infant weight (0.92 kg + 0.30 kg ÷ 10 kg × 100). The "all other" category consists of skeletal muscles and the lean or active metabolizing part of adipose tissue. Although skeletal muscles are at rest under basal conditions, they nevertheless maintain tonus, or a steady contraction that keeps them firm. Energy needed to maintain muscle tone and the lean portions of adipose tissue is therefore an important part of that needed for BMR. Simply stated, the significance of the differences in metabolic rate among tissues making up the lean body mass is that, although the total BMR increases as lean body mass increases, the relationship is not a linear one. This means that the BMR does not increase by a set amount for each unit increase in lean body mass.

The BMR in terms of kilocalories per kilogram of body weight is highest during the first few months after birth. This is explained by the fact that in the infant a high proportion of the body weight is due to organs having high rates of metabolism (15 percent of body weight) compared with the adult (6 percent of body weight). In addition, the rapid growth rate immediately after birth increases the BMR, since energy is required to grow new tissues. After early infancy the BMR per kilogram of weight declines gradually until adolescence, when a slight increase occurs during the pubertal growth spurt. A decline then occurs until adulthood is reached.

Classic studies of body responses to chronic kilocalorie deprivation (starvation) similar to conditions commonly occurring in war-torn countries have demonstrated that the BMR declines at a faster rate under these circumstances than can be explained by the decrease in total body weight [5,6]. This phenomenon has been explained as follows: Since the BMR measures the *average* metabolic rate of all the cells contributing to the lean body mass, it is possible for the BMR to decrease due to disproportionately large losses of lean tissue from certain parts of the body such as the liver, for example [1]. These changes can decrease the average BMR, but are insufficient to markedly lower the total body

TABLE 7-3. PERCENTAGE OF BMR DUE TO FIVE ORGANS AND REMAINDER OF THE BODY IN AN INFANT AND AN ADULT

ORGAN	10-kg (22-lb) INFANT BMR = 540 kcal/day			70-kg (154-lb) MAN BMR = 1780 kcal/day		
	ORGAN WEIGHT,	ORGAN METABOLISM		ORGAN WEIGHT,	ORGAN METABOLISM	
	kg	kcal/day	% of BMR	kg	kcal/day	% of BMR
Brain	0.92	240	45	1.4	365	21
Liver	0.30	105	19	1.6	560	32
Heart	0.05	30	6	0.3	180	10
Kidney	0.07	28	5	0.3	120	7
Lung	0.12	24	4	0.8	160	9
Total of above	1.46	427	79	4.4	1385	79
All other	8.64	113	21	65.6	395	21

SOURCE: Holliday, M.A., D. Potter, A. Jarrah, and S. Bearg, "The Relation of Metabolic Rate to Body Weight and Organ Size." *Pediatric Research*, 1:185, 1967.

weight. Long-term studies of undernutrition in which male volunteers were fed about one-half the number of kilocalories they were accustomed to (comparable to diets common in northern Europe during times of famine in World War II) revealed that after these subjects had consumed the diet for 6 months, their average BMR was significantly lower than at the outset. The lower BMR was found to be due chiefly to loss of lean body mass, but, in addition, a lower rate of metabolism *within* active metabolizing tissues played an important role. In other words, under long-term kilocalorie deprivation, the body cells adjust so as to use energy to maintain functions vital to life, a mechanism which increases the chances of surviving periods of undernutrition. This is another example of the body's ability to maintain *homeostasis*, an internal steady state, by coordinating physiological processes (see Chapter 6).

Hormonal Secretions   Several hormones affect the BMR, but none as directly as those of the thyroid gland, *thyroxine* and *triiodothyronine*. These hormones regulate the rate at which the body cells oxidize carbohydrates, protein, and fat for energy. Abnormally high thyroid secretions result in an unusually high BMR, requiring a person to maintain a diet high in kilocalories to prevent weight loss. Unusually low thyroid secretions, on the other hand, result in a low BMR, causing weight gain if food intake is not drastically reduced.

Secretions from the adrenal and pituitary glands can also affect basal metabolism. Adrenal hormones, released as a result of strong emotions such as fright, fear, or anger, increase the BMR for a short period of time. Increased adrenal secretions cause the heart to beat more rapidly, and prepare the muscles for immediate "fight or flight." A surge of energy expenditure as a result of fright, fear, or anger therefore enables the body to respond to an emergency situation.

The pituitary gland affects the BMR indirectly by secreting thyroid-stimulating hormone, which causes the thyroid gland to release its hormones. Failure of the pituitary gland to perform this function results in a low BMR.

Other Factors   Elevation of the body temperature above normal, either due to feverish illness or because environmental circumstances prevent heat loss from the body, increases the BMR. By definition, the normal BMR occurs at normal body temperature, 98.6°F. Increasing the body temperature results in an increased rate of metabolism because all enzymatically catalyzed reactions increase their rate of reaction as body temperature rises. One investigator calculated that every degree Fahrenheit elevation of the body temperature results in an increase in energy expenditure of 7.2 percent [7]. The old adage "feed a cold and starve a fever" is incorrect if one wishes to prevent a person from losing body weight during a feverish illness.

Under conditions of extreme heat, an individual's BMR increases because extra energy is required to cool the body. In these circumstances, the heart and the sweat glands must perform extra work [8].

If the body becomes chilled from swimming in cold water, a prolonged cold shower, or exposure to a cold environment with insufficient clothing to prevent heat losses, the BMR will increase because extra kilocalories must be expended to maintain normal body temperature. If cooling is severe enough, involuntary muscular contractions (or shivering) occur, which markedly increase heat production. Shivering also triggers the release of adrenal hormones, which increase heat production as previously noted. Living in a cold climate will increase the BMR, however, only if housing, modes of transportation, and clothing are unable to prevent the body from becoming frequently chilled. Rarely is this the case in the United States [9].

Pregnancy results in an increased basal metabolism because the mother synthesizes new maternal tissues as well as those of the placenta and fetus. The practical implications of a higher BMR during pregnancy are discussed in Chapter 14. The BMR per kilogram of body weight is higher during all periods of childhood than in adulthood because of the energy required for growth.

Measuring Basal Metabolism   The major reason physicians measure the BMR is to exclude thyroid gland activity as a source of a patient's symptoms. If the patient's BMR is within the normal range, thyroid activity is judged to be normal. *Hyperthyroidism*—due to an overly active thyroid gland—results in an abnormally high BMR, with symptoms of nervousness and underweight. *Hypothyroidism*—due to an underactive thyroid gland—results in a low BMR, with symptoms of obesity and sometimes slow mental activity. Normal ranges for BMR are 1100 to 1500 kcal (4200 to 6000 kJ) for women, and 1600 to 1900 kcal (6500 to 8000 kJ) for men. Although most physicians today probably use blood tests to determine thyroid activity, described later, these are indirect indicators of the BMR.

When the BMR is determined in laboratory studies, subjects must be under *basal conditions*. The individual is lying in bed, and is awake but relaxed physically, mentally, and emotionally. He or she has had no food during the previous 12 to 18 hours. The room temperature must be comfortable so that the individual need not shiver to stay warm, nor sweat to cool the body. The test ideally is done soon after the subject awakens in the morning after a restful night's sleep.

How do scientists measure energy expended for BMR? We have noted that energy needs can be determined by measuring heat given off. But how can scientists measure the heat given off by an individual under basal conditions? He or she would have to be placed in a specially insulated room called a *room calorimeter*. The room must be large enough to accommodate the subject lying in bed. Insulation must prevent escape of heat and entry of heat or cold. Heat given off by the body is measured by observing the difference in temperature of a known volume of water flowing through copper tubing in the room. Heat eliminated by the evaporation of water from the skin and lungs is also measured. Either outdoor air or oxygen may be introduced as needed, and carbon dioxide removed. This method is expensive and few of these calorimeters exist today.

Methods in which heat production is measured are classified as *direct calorimetry*. Past research established that the same results obtained by direct calorimetry can be obtained by the simpler, less expensive method of measuring oxygen consumption or carbon dioxide production. Why is this an alternative?

You will recall from previous chapters that the oxidation in the body of

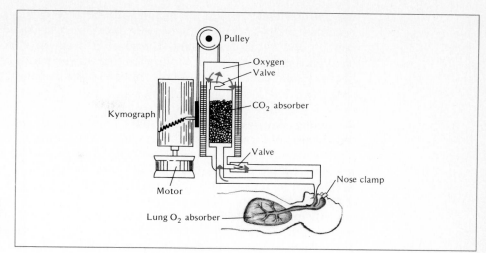

FIGURE 7-4. The Benedict portable respiration apparatus, used to determine BMR.

carbodydrates, protein, and fat for energy uses up oxygen and produces carbon dioxide while releasing energy. In other words, carbon atoms in these compounds combine with oxygen to form carbon dioxide, while hydrogen atoms combine with oxygen to form water. Scientists therefore can measure *oxygen consumed* or *carbon dioxide produced* as an indirect indicator of the amount of energy produced. Methods measuring either oxygen consumption or carbon dioxide production, or both, are classified as *indirect calorimetry*.

Researchers are likely to use indirect calorimetry when determining the BMR. An instrument used for this purpose is diagrammed in Figure 7-4. The subject, under basal conditions, breathes oxygen through the mouth for a 6-min period. The amount of oxygen consumed is recorded in the process. From a standard table one finds that the kilocalorie value of 1 L of oxygen used up under basal conditions is 4.825 kcal. From the amount of oxygen consumed during the test, one calculates how much would be consumed in 24 h. For example, a subject who consumed 1.08 L in 6 min would consume $1.08 \times 10 = 10.8$ L in 1 h and $10.8 \times 24 = 259.2$ L in 24 h. This individual's BMR, therefore, is $259.2 \times 4.825 = 1250$ kcal.

Other instruments allow a subject to breathe room air (through the mouth with the nose clamped) while the exhaled air is collected within a specified time. The volume of air exhaled is also monitored. The concentrations of oxygen and carbon dioxide in the expired air are measured and compared with the known composition of the room air. In this way the amount of oxygen consumed and carbon dioxide produced during the test period are determined. One then calculates the BMR from the oxygen consumption as already described. Standard tables give the kilocalorie value per liter of carbon dioxide produced under basal conditions, so the calculation can also be made using the carbon dioxide values.

These techniques for measuring BMR are difficult to carry out and interpret, however. Subjects or patients need to be trained to relax while in the awkward state of breathing through the mouth with the nose clamped shut. If a subject becomes anxious and hyperventilates (breathes more rapidly or deeper than normal), the results are invalid. The method is almost impossible to use with children. Furthermore, it is very difficult for subjects to meet basal conditions because these conditions exist only in the first few minutes before arising in the morning.

Predicting Basal Metabolism Is there any way to predict or estimate an individual's BMR without actually measuring it? Since BMR is proportional to LBM, it would be easy to calculate BMR if we knew an individual's LBM. But scientists cannot *directly* measure LBM, and indirect methods for determining LBM, such as underwater weighing (a method of assessing body density), are expensive and often difficult.

Alternatively, physicians tend to use charts in which BMR is calculated from the individual's *body surface area*, expressed in square meters. How is surface area related to BMR? Investigators observed many years ago that heat produced for BMR by small animals is greater per unit of body weight than that produced by

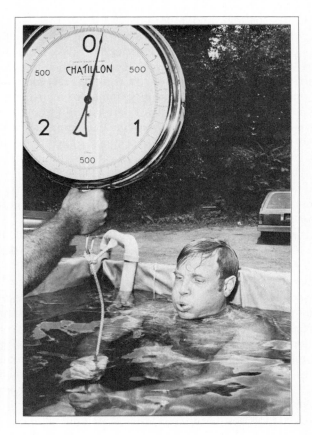

Preparing to measure body volume by the water displacement technique. Upon expelling the air in his lungs, this man's weight will be recorded after his entire body is submerged under water. The percentage of his body weight that is fat and lean tissue can be calculated from his body density which is Weight in air ÷ (weight in air − weight in water). *(Michael Lennahan)*

larger animals. The apparent reason is that, because the surface area of smaller animals is greater in proportion to body weight than that of larger animals, heat loss is greater—therefore heat production must be greater. For example, imagine two men, A and B, weighing 150 lb each, but A is 5 ft tall, while B is 6 ft tall. B has the larger surface area and therefore requires more kilocalories for BMR.

But a practical problem also arises with this concept. How can one measure an individual's surface area? Early in this century an investigator, Dr. E. F. DuBois, actually measured the surface area of a large number of subjects who dressed in thin, close-fitting garments that completely covered their bodies. The researcher then obtained a complete mold of each body by pasting strips over this foundation. From the molds, he determined the surface area for each subject. Using these data, DuBois developed a chart for determining body surface area from height and weight [11]. Other investigators used DuBois' data to develop a nomogram (a chart showing relationships among variables) that physicians frequently use to estimate or predict BMR (Figure 7-5).

Although some scientists have questioned the validity of reporting BMR in relation to surface area [12,13,14], others maintain that, when used for individuals of a single sex, body surface area is as good an estimate of BMR as is LBM [3]. Body surface area is easily estimated from height and weight (Figure 7-5), while LBM can be determined only in the laboratory. Even then, various methods for estimating LBM give different results. One should remember that, when using body surface area, different expected standards apply to males and females. *Physiologically*, however, the fact is that BMR is directly related to LBM. The difference in BMR between men and women of the same height and weight is due to the higher amount of LBM in the male, and not due to a basic sex difference. In other words, on the basis of kilograms of LBM, heat production for BMR is the same for men and women [3].

Energy Expended for Eating: The Effect of Food

If a person maintains basal conditions except that he or she eats some food, extra energy will be expended beyond the basal level within minutes afterwards. This extra energy is used to digest and absorb the food and to support certain metabolic processes that occur in the cells. In effect, then, there is a small energy cost due to food consumption.

When the usual mixed diet containing carbohydrates, protein, and fat is consumed, the energy cost of food consumption amounts to about 6 to 10 percent of the energy needed for basal metabolism plus that for physical activity. If a young man needs 1400 kilocalories for basal metabolism and 1000 kilocalories for physical activity, his energy need to cover the effect of food is about 240 kilocalories (10 percent of 2400 kilocalories).

This effect of food has been called in the past the *specific dynamic action* (SDA) of food, but is preferably termed the *calorigenic effect* or *dietary thermogenesis*. The greatest elevation in energy expenditure occurs about 1 to 2 hours after a meal and returns to basal levels by 3 to 4 hours after the meal.

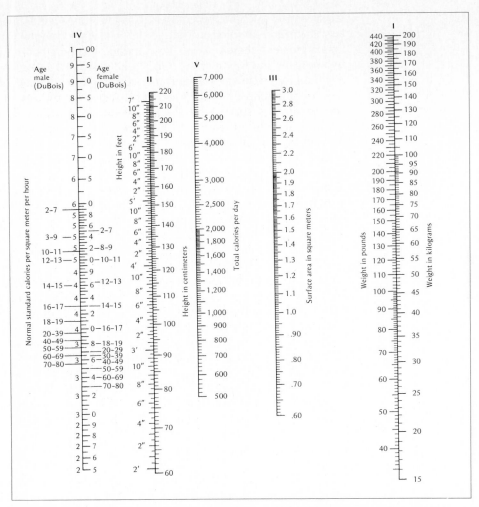

FIGURE 7-5. Nomogram for derivation of kilocalories expended for basal metabolism (Scale V, labeled Total Calories per Day). The nomogram is meant to be used only for people of normal weight for height. (1) Locate weight on Scale I and height on Scale II. Stick a pin at the point where a ruler intersects Scale III. This point represents the individual's surface area. (2) Locate age and sex on Scale IV. Place a ruler at this point and at the point of the individual's surface area. (3) Place a pin at the point where the ruler intersects Scale V and read off the basal energy requirement in kilocalories (kcal). (4) To convert kcal to kJ, multiply by 4.184. [Source: Nomogram of Boothby and Sandiford (1936), adapted by the Mayo Clinic and reprinted with their permission in Briggs, G. M., and D. H. Calloway, *Bogert's Nutrition and Physical Fitness,* Philadelphia: W.B. Saunders Co., CBS College Publishing, 1979, p. 29.]

Resting Metabolic Rate (RMR)

Since basal conditions exist naturally only in the few minutes after waking in the morning before getting out of bed, and since attainment of basal conditions is otherwise inconvenient for the subject, determining the *resting metabolic rate*

(RMR) or *resting metabolism* is now more common than determining the BMR. RMR "includes the specific dynamic action of meals and is an average minimal metabolism for the night and the periods of the day when there is no exercise and no exposure to cold" [9]. RMR represents, therefore, the metabolism of an individual living in his or her usual way while at rest and at comfortable room temperature. The same instruments may be used for determining the RMR as for BMR, but the subject is not in a fasting state. If measurements are made 4 h after a meal, however, results can be very close to those for the BMR [14].

Physicians today rarely use instruments that measure oxygen consumption or carbon dioxide expenditure to determine basal or resting metabolism, but instead tend to favor blood tests. These tests constitute an indirect assessment of resting metabolism, since they measure whether or not the thyroid gland secretes normal amounts of the hormones that govern the rate of metabolism in body tissues. The most reliable of these tests determines the concentration of free (unbound to protein) thyroxine (T_4) in the blood. The test requires only that the subject give a blood sample, but does not require basal conditions. An abnormally high amount of T_4 in the blood indicates that a person has an unusually high resting metabolism, while a low amount signifies low resting metabolism.

Energy Expended for Physical Activity

Both basal metabolism and resting metabolism exclude energy expenditure for physical activity. Any muscular activity increases the energy needs above basal requirements. The extent of energy expenditure for physical activity depends upon the intensity of the activity (how many muscles are involved and how much exertion is required of them), and how long the activity continues. For example,

A CLOSER LOOK

Some popular reducing diets claim that protein has a much larger calorigenic effect than carboydrates or fat, and that high-protein diets aid in weight loss because one has to use more kilocalories to utilize the protein. This idea originated with Professor Max Rubner in 1902 who noted that when he fed meat to a dog as the sole food source, the calorigenic effect was markedly larger than if only sugar or only lard was fed. Several studies have attempted to determine the effect of protein on the calorigenic effect in human subjects. Since human beings cannot survive on meat alone, we are interested in the effects of high-protein *mixed diets* versus low-protein mixed diets, and not in the effect of protein alone. A very carefully executed study at Pennsylvania State University, using young male subjects, indicated that consumption of a high-protein diet (129 g/day) resulted in only about 5 percent greater energy production than did consumption of a diet containing 38 g of protein/day [15]. It appears, then, that claims of loss of large amounts of energy and consequent weight loss due to high-protein diets are greatly exaggerated. When next you are favorably disposed to a claim about diet which cites research evidence, ask yourself: Am I moved to accept the claim *because* research studies are cited? Is the evidence cited from animal studies alone? Is it possible that the research studies are misinterpreted, misquoted, poorly designed, poorly executed, or outdated?

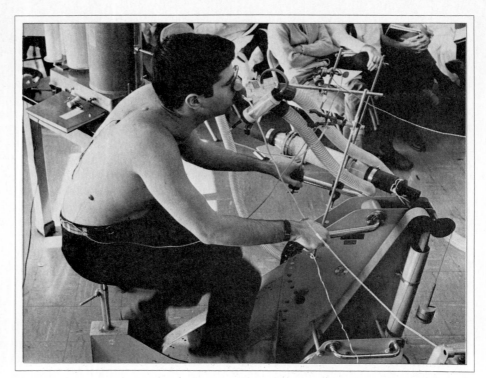

Energy expenditure for physical activity can be determined by measuring oxygen consumption while exercise is performed. The work of the heart is also being monitored here. *(Hugh Rogers/Monkmeyer)*

the energy cost for physical activity is least when one is lying down (about 0.1 kcal/kg body weight per hour), while it is slightly higher when one sits quietly, since muscles must be used to hold the body erect (0.4 kcal/kg/h). When knitting, one is using a small number of muscles and expends about 0.7 kcal/kg/h, while activities using a larger number of muscles, such as walking at 3 mph, require about 2.0 kcal/kg/h. An activity using an even greater number of muscles, such as rowing, requires about 9.8 kcal/kg/h, while rowing in a race, when there is maximum exertion, requires about 16 kcal/kg/h [16]. For physical activities which entail moving the body through space, the energy expenditure is greater for moving a heavier than a lighter body the same distance at the same rate. A 110-lb woman expends less energy walking up a flight of stairs at a standard rate than does a woman who weighs 150 lb.

Unfortunately for students and professors, mental activity does not greatly increase energy expenditure over RMR unless the effort results in extensive nervous contraction of muscles. The brain functions constantly and contributes much to the energy expenditure of the RMR, but the extra energy needed to support 1 h of strenuous mental activity can be supplied by one-half a peanut [15]. The desire to eat while studying for exams is usually psychological in origin, and not due to any physiological need to replace energy lost in mental activity.

Most Americans are considered to be either sedentary or primarily engaged in only light physical activity. In such cases, resting metabolic needs require by far the largest energy expenditure while less energy is used for physical activity.

For example, a woman 25 years old who is 5 ft 3 in tall and weighs 110 lb might have a RMR expenditure of 1200 kcal/day, but if she is sendentary she will require only 500 to 600 kcal/day for physical activity. In other words, her resting energy needs account for approximately two-thirds of her daily energy requirement. People who routinely engage in vigorous physical activity 8 h or so per day will, on the other hand, expend more energy to support physical activity than for resting metabolism. Many Americans have recently become athletes. Box 7-1 discusses the energy needs of athletes.

MEASURING THE BODY'S TOTAL ENERGY NEEDS

We can estimate the body's total energy need by combining our estimate of the energy needed for resting metabolism with that needed for physical activity. We shall discuss ways to estimate energy requirements for specific *groups* of people, and shall then describe a method more suitable for estimating *individual* needs.

Estimating Average or Group Needs

For young adults, a rough approximation of the resting metabolism is 1 kcal (4.2 kJ) per kilogram of body weight per hour for men, and 0.9 kcal (3.8 kJ) for women. (Divide the body weight in pounds by 2.2 to obtain kilograms.) Therefore, a young man weighing 70 kg (154 lb) would require $1 \times 70 \times 24$ h = 1680 kcal/day for resting metabolism. A woman weighing 58 kg (128 lb) would require $0.9 \times 58 \times 24$ h = 1250 kcal (rounded). For adults over age 50, a general estimate is 0.9 kcal (3.8 kJ) per kilogram for men and 0.8 kcal (3.3 kJ) for women.

TABLE 7-4.   **ESTIMATING KILOCALORIES NEEDED FOR PHYSICAL ACTIVITY**

TYPE OF DAY'S ACTIVITY	kcal per kg per h
Very light activity: sitting most of the day; about 2 h of walking slowly or standing.	0.6
Light activity: typing, teaching, shop work, laboratory work, some walking but no strenuous exercise.	0.8
Moderate activity: little sitting; housecleaning, gardening, carpentry, light industry, walking.	1.1
Strenuous activity: little sitting; outdoor work involving continuous activity such as unskilled labor or forestry; prolonged exercise such as skating or dancing.	1.7
Very strenuous activity: little sitting; heavy physical work such as lumbering; prolonged exercise such as tennis, swimming, basketball, football, or running.	2.4

Directions:
1. Determine body weight in kg by dividing weight in pounds by 2.2.
2. Determine number of waking hours by subtracting number of hours of sleep from 24 hours.
3. Choose the type of activity that most closely describes your usual level of activity (the activities you spend the most time performing).
4. Multiply the kilocalories for that type of activity by your body weight in kilograms and by the number of waking hours.

SOURCE: Adapted from Taylor, C. M., and O. F. Pye, *Foundations of Nutrition*, 6th ed., New York: The Macmillan Co., 1966, p. 48.

Energy Needs of the Athlete

Athletes generally need higher intakes of kilocalories than their sedentary peers. The number of kilocalories needed depends upon the amount of body fat desired, the weight and height of the individual, and the energy costs of training. A larger amount of body fat may be desirable for a swimmer, for example, than for a marathon runner. Usually, athletes can rely on their appetite to guide them in amounts of food needed [17].

Weight loss is sometimes desirable for those who wish to qualify for such sports as wrestling. The maximal rate of weight loss should be 2 lb per week and should be achieved at a kilocalorie intake of no less than 1800 to 2000 kcal. Use of starvation or semi-starvation results in loss of lean tissue, dehydration, and fatigue, and should never be used (Chapter 8). Weight control diets should be similar to those recommended in Chapter 8.

We noted in Chapter 6 that protein is not a major fuel for muscle work. Instead, muscles obtain energy from fat and carbohydrates. The intensity of exercise coupled with the athlete's *maximal oxygen consumption* determines the proportion of energy that the body derives from carbohydrates or fat [10]. Maximal oxygen consumption is that point at which the exercise becomes increasingly difficult, but the athlete is unable to deliver more oxygen to his or her muscles. Maximal oxygen consumption is significantly greater in trained than in untrained athletes, allowing them to sustain high-intensity exercise for longer periods.

The largest amount of energy reaching body cells results from reactions of the Krebs cycle, which, you will remember, oxidizes carbohydrates and fats. The Krebs cycle operates under *aerobic* conditions—meaning that oxygen is required. When the body is at rest, or during prolonged light exercise, fatty acids are the primary energy source, requiring the muscles to utilize oxygen.

Once an athlete reaches his or her maximal oxygen consumption, exercise beyond that point must be supplied by energy from *anaerobic* reactions—those that operate in the absence of oxygen. The breakdown of stored muscle glycogen to glucose and then to pyruvic acid occurs in the absence of oxygen, and supplies a small amount of ATP. This is the source of the burst of energy, shown by an athlete in the last part of a 1- or 2-mile race. Energy from anaerobic breakdown of glycogen also supports an athlete engaged in high-intensity sports of short duration, such as a 100-yard swim, or short sprints during soccer or basketball.

Two types of muscle fibers play crucial roles in energy metabolism during exercise. *Fast-twitch muscle fibers* are used during high-intensity, short-term activities and depend on anaerobic metabolism of glycogen for energy. Any activity resulting in breathlessness uses these muscle fibers, which utilize glucose anaerobically. *Slow-twitch muscle fibers* are used during endurance activities, and depend on aerobic metabolism of carbohydrates and fats. Sports such as swimming, field hockey, soccer, middle-distance running, and basketball require that the athlete use both types of muscle fibers. Proper training improves the efficiency of each of these types of muscle fibers.

The dietary sources of energy for the athlete during training need not be different from those recommended for the nonathlete. An appropriate diet provides 15 percent of total kilocalories from protein, 30 percent from fat, and the remainder from complex carbohydrate [17]. Choosing a wide variety of food from the food groups listed in the Exchange System (Appendix B) will increase one's chances of obtaining all the needed nutrients.

What and when should the athlete eat before an event? Most sports physicians recommend eating at least 3 h prior to an event to allow for gastric emptying. Both pre-event excitement and high amounts of dietary fat can slow stomach emptying. High-fat foods are apt to remain in the stomach about 5 h, while starchy foods remain about 2 h. Meats and other high-protein foods remain about 3 h. These emptying rates should be taken into account in planning pre-event meals. Some athletes favor liquid pre-event meals since these are easily tolerated despite nervous tension.

For events of short duration, the composition of the pre-event meal does not affect performance. It is important for psychological reasons that athletes choose foods they believe from past experience allow them to feel most comfortable during the event.

For events of long duration, advantages seem to result if the pre-event meal is high in carbohydrates. This is probably because prolonged exercise is supported by aerobic metabolism, and aerobic metabolism of carbohydrate is highly efficient because less oxygen is required to oxidize a given amount of carbohydrate than of fat. The concept of glycogen loading for endurance sports is discussed in Chapter 3.

Proper training and an adequate diet work together in allowing athletes to perform at maximal levels. There are no magical or "wonder" foods that give an athlete an extra boost toward achieving his or her performance goals.

To the resting metabolism one needs to add the energy needed for physical activity. A rough way to estimate this is to categorize one's usual type of day's activities as in Table 7-4. Let's say that the woman described above who weighs 58 kg (and is 25 years old), decides that the category marked *light activity* describes her usual day. She ususally sleeps 8 h. She would calculate her energy expenditure for physical activity as follws: 0.8 kcal × 58 kg × 16 h = 742 kcal (740 kcal rounded). Since her resting metabolism was roughly estimated earlier to be 1250 kcal, her total kcal estimate therefore totals 1990 kcal (1250 + 740 = 1990, or 2000 kcal rounded).

Estimations of energy needs by this rough method may or may not suit a specific individual. If the woman described above finds that upon consuming 2000 kcal/day she gains weight, then obviously the estimate is erroneous. Either her estimate of activity is too high, or her resting metabolism is lower than estimated, or a combination of these is at work. It is impossible to know at what point the estimate is wrong. Rough approximations of this sort are best used to estimate the energy needs of a particular group of people rather than of individuals.

Estimating Individual Needs

Energy needed for resting metabolism of young adults may be estimated from Table 7-5 in which the percentage of body fat is included. Notice that a thin woman has a higher percentage of body fat than the average man. The percentage of body weight that is fat can be determined accurately only by the use of specialized, expensive equipment, and is done only in research studies, but

TABLE 7-5. NORMAL VALUES FOR THE RESTING RATE OF ENERGY EXPENDITURE OF ADULTS

		BODY FAT	WEIGHT, kg							
MEN	WOMEN	PERCENTAGE	45	50	55	60	65	70	75	80
Thin		5		0.99	1.06	1.12	1.19	1.26	1.32	1.39
Average		10		0.94	1.01	1.08	1.14	1.21	1.28	1.34
Plump	Thin	15	0.82	0.89	0.96	1.03	1.09	1.16	1.23	1.30
Fat	Average	20	0.78	0.84	0.91	0.98	1.05	1.11	1.18	1.25
	Plump	25		0.80	0.86	0.93	1.00	1.07	1.13	1.20
	Fat	30			0.81	0.88	0.95	1.02	1.08	1.15

To use this table, one needs first to decide whether one is thin, average, plump, or fat. There is no readily available guide for deciding this, except those described in Chapter 8 for judging obesity or fatness. Theoretically, the figure nearest your weight in kilograms and degree of body fatness for sex, multiplied by 1440 (the number of minutes in 24 h) is your RMR. This table can also be used to estimate your energy expenditure for sleep by simply multiplying the appropriate figure for weight, sex, and degree of body fatness by number of minutes spent in sleep.

SOURCE: Durnin, J.V.G.A., and R. Passmore, *Energy, Work and Leisure,* London: Heinemann Educational Books, Ltd., 1967.

skinfold measurements are frequently used to estimate body fatness (Chapter 8).

Estimates of the energy needs for physical activity can be determined more accurately than the method described for groups by keeping a record of the amount of time spent at specific activities throughout a 24-h period. Using a table of energy costs of different activities, such as the one in Appendix H, calculate the energy expenditure. To use this table, multiply the kcal/min by the number of minutes spent in a specific activity, then multiply by your body weight in kilograms. For example, a woman weighing 56 kg (123 lb) who swam a slow crawl for 30 min would expend 215 kcal (0.128 × 30 × 56). If she spent 30 min playing a flute, her expenditure would be 59 kcal (0.035 × 30 × 56). It should be noted that figures in Appendix H *include* the RMR; therefore, to calculate *total* energy need one calculates the expenditure for sleep from Table 7-4 and adds to that the energy expenditures for all activities during the waking hours.

Tables showing the energy costs of physical activities all have their limitations. Figures in such tables are ususaly based on only a few actual determinations, consequently they should not be considered exact. All activities in which the body is moved through space such as walking, climbing, or swimming involve expenditures of energy directly proportional to body weight. Energy expenditure for other activities, such as playing musical instruments or playing cards, is not directly related to body size. In Appendix H, however, expenditure for all activities is given in terms of body weight. Another limitation is that people vary in their efficiency at performing physical tasks or activities. Athletes, for example, expend less energy performing a specified activity for which they are trained than a novice. This means that not everyone can be expected to expend the exact amount recorded in the table when performing a given activity. Despite limitations, however, Appendix H indicates the wide variations in energy expenditure that exists due to the intensity of activities.

One may use this table to estimate one's total energy expenditure by keeping a detailed diary of physical activity for a 24-h period, including time spent sleeping. The diary should be kept in minutes, and should account for every minute—1440 min in 24 h. Table 7-6 shows a calculation of a total day's activities for a husband and wife, both students. He is currently writing his master's thesis, and is home most of the day, attending only one seminar at school. He does most of the cooking, but is remarkably inactive, driving to school and walking a minimal amount. She also spends a great part of her time in sedentary activities, sitting in class and studying. But she is quite active physically, walking to and from school and engaging in such activities as dancing, swimming, and running. Her total kilocalorie need is consequently greater than his, although he is considerably heavier than she. If she were as inactive as he is, however, her total kilocalorie need would be less than his. It may be the case, too, that this was an atypical day for each person. Keeping a daily record for a week often provides a better estimate of usual physical activity.

TABLE 7-6. CALCULATION OF TOTAL ENERGY NEEDS OF TWO COLLEGE STUDENTS, ONE 70-kg MALE AND ONE 55-kg FEMALE. EACH PERSON RECORDED ACTIVITIES THROUGHOUT 24 h, ACCOUNTING FOR EACH MINUTE.

| | NO. OF MIN | | kcal/min | ENERGY COST min × kcal/min | |
ACTIVITY	MALE	FEMALE	(FROM APPENDIX H)	MALE	FEMALE
Dressing, showering, etc.	30	70	0.035	1.05	2.45
Cooking	45	15	0.045	2.03	0.68
Eating	75	95	0.023	1.73	2.19
Light housework, washing dishes, etc.	40	35	0.045	1.80	1.58
Sitting, writing	595	465	0.029	17.26	13.49
Sitting quietly	70	30	0.021	1.47	0.63
Driving car	20	—	0.022	0.44	—
Walking 3 mph	40	130	0.066	2.64	8.58
Sitting, talking	45	45	0.029	1.31	1.31
Running (9 min/mi)	—	30	0.193	—	5.79
Swimming (slow crawl)	—	45	0.128	—	5.76
Vigorous dancing	—	60	0.168	—	10.08
TOTAL:	960	1020		29.73	52.54
No. of min sleeping	480	420			
Total no. of min	1440	1440			

His energy need:
   For physical activity: 29.73 kcal × 70 kg = 2081 kcal
   For sleep (Table 7-5): 480 min × 1.21 = 581
         (average fatness)   2662 or 2660 kcal

Her energy need:
   For physical activity: 52.54 kcal × 55 = 2890 kcal
   For sleep (Table 7-5): 420 min × 0.91 = 382
         (average fatness)   3272 or 3270 kcal

Researchers measure energy used for specific physical activities by using special lightweight instruments that can be worn on the back while the subject performs the task. The expired air is metered so the exact amount is recorded. Samples are collected and analyzed for oxygen and carbon dioxide. By using standard tables the researcher can calculate the kilocalorie value of the gases exchanged. Since respiration equipment requires subjects to breathe through the mouth while wearing a nose clip that prevents escape of breath through the nose and requires them to carry a piece of equipment on their back, it is quite possible that under these circumstances their energy expenditure may differ from that when the task is performed without the equipment.

Some Americans, particularly some women, may be existing on a diet *too low* in kilocalories for optimal health. Let's take as an example Marguerite, a 20-year-old college student 5 ft tall weighing 99 lb. She has never been physically active, even during adolescence. A record of her physical activity, calculated in the manner shown in Table 7-6, indicated that her energy expenditure for physical activity (including RMR) was 1136 kcal, and her energy expenditure during 8 h of sleep was 374 (Table 7-5). Her estimated energy need is therefore 1136 + 374 = 1510 or 1500 kcal (rounded). When given this estimate, Marguerite exclaimed, "I would really get fat if I ate that much! I watch my calories very closely and I'm sure I maintain my weight on 900 to 1000 kilocalories per day." Let's assume that she is correct—that her intake is 900 to 1000 kcal/day. The table in Appendix I indicates that her weight is within the normal range for her height and sex. Why the discrepancy between her estimated needs and the number of kilocalories she usually consumes? Why isn't she losing weight if her body needs 1500 kcal, but she only consumes 1000 kcal?

More than likely the explanation is that, although Marguerite's weight is within the normal range, she has a higher percentage of fat in her body and a lower percentage of lean tissue than those subjects whose values were used in setting up Table 7-5 and Appendix H. Probaby this difference in body composition is due to her lack of physical activity. Although she has maintained normal body weight, she is obese. (Obesity exists when there is excessive body fat.)

Is there any reason to be concerned about this situation—one that is not uncommon among women in the United States? Yes, there are several reasons. One is that an individual is unlikely to obtain all the essential nutrients, particularly minerals, when the kilocalorie intake is so low. Another is that protein cannot be efficiently utilized when the kilocalorie intake is too low. Furthermore, obesity is apt to lead to complications such as diabetes or gallstones.

Marguerite would profit from a routine exercise program, thereby increasing the proportion of lean tissue and decreasing the proportion of fat tissue in her body. Her RMR would increase with her lean tissue, and she would be able to maintain normal body weight at a higher kilocalorie intake. The chances would increase that her diet would be adequate nutritionally, particularly if she followed criteria of dietary planning set out in previous chapters. In addition, she would probably notice a new feeling of well-being that usually accompanies a regular exercise program.

To recap, total energy needs can be estimated by adding the energy needed for physical activity to that required for resting metabolism. An alternative method involves using a table in which resting metabolism is included in the figures for physical activity. One calculates the energy used for physical activity using such a table, then adds kilocalories expended during sleep. The amount of energy expended for physical activity is a function of how strenuous the activity is and how long one engages in it. Those activities requiring moving the body expend greater expenditure the heavier the body. In the final analysis maintaining energy balance so as to maintain desirable weight should be one's goal. To achieve this objective requires one to balance energy intake with expenditure, a subject discussed in greater detail in Chapter 8.

Comparing Actual Energy Need with the RDA

Recommended Dietary Allowances are set for kilocalories (or energy) without regard for whether those kilocalories come from carbohydrates or fats. This is because a kilocalorie derived from the metabolism of carbohydrate is the same as one derived from fat metabolism. The important consideration is the total kilocalorie intake in relation to an individual's expenditure.

The RDAs for kilocalories, unlike those for protein, vitamins, and minerals, are set at levels judged to meet the needs of *average* persons within each sex and age group. Recall that for protein and other nutrients, the RDAs are sufficiently high to meet the needs of about 98 percent of the population, and are therefore higher than the needs of the average person. Setting kilocalorie recommendations in a similar fashion would encourage obesity, since excessive kilocalories are stored in the body as fat.

Appendix A shows the recommended range of energy intakes (RDAs) for males and females in different age groups. In adults, notice that the male is 70 in tall and weighs 70 kg (154 lb), while the female is 64 in tall and weighs 55 kg (120). Light activity is assumed for adults who live at comfortable temperatures, with no need to produce extra energy to keep warm or cool. The energy RDAs are greater for males than for females of the same age after age 11, and an increased energy allowance is recommended during pregnancy and lactation.

These recommendations are of greatest value for planning diets to meet the energy needs of large groups of people. Individuals frequently find that the recommendation for a specific age and sex is inappropriate for them because they differ in body size or in levels of physical activity from the persons described in the table.

For these reasons it is incorrect to assume that a person has either an inadequate or excessive kilocalorie intake if his or her usual intake is observed to differ from the RDA. One needs to assess an individual's energy need in relation to desirable body weight. If a person's body weight is significantly higher than desirable, and the excess can be attributed to fat rather than lean tissue, one can assume that the kilocalorie intake is higher than desirable. Consequently, the individual needs to either decrease the energy intake or increase the expenditure through exercise, or both, to achieve desirable body weight (see Chapter 8).

ENERGY VALUE OF FOODS

In order to balance energy intake with expenditure, one must take into account the energy value of foods. In a practical sense, one needs to know the extent to which kilocalories in foods are actually available to the body. Some of the energy value of foods is unavailable to the body for two reasons: (1) foods are incompletely digested and absorbed, and (2) digested and absorbed proteins are incompletely metabolized, resulting in loss of urea in the urine.

That portion of the energy present per gram of carbohydrates, fat, and protein in foods that is available for use in the body is called the *physiological fuel value*. *General* values you have learned for physiological fuel values are 4 kcal/g of carbohydrates, 9 kcal/g of fats, 4 kcal/g of protein, and 7 kcal/g of alcohol. How did scientists obtain these figures? How are these figures used?

The amount of energy locked within the chemical bonds of carbohydrates, fat, or protein in foods can be determined in the research laboratory by burning a sample in a bomb calorimeter (Figure 7-6). The values obtained are called *heats of combustion*. The digestibility of the carbohydrate, protein, or fat in a food is estimated by measuring the amounts of these nutrients that appear in the feces under standard experimental conditions. The amount unaccounted for is assumed to have been digested and absorbed, and is usually reported in percentage. The general physiological fuel values of 4, 9, and 4 kcal per g for carbohydrates, fats, and proteins, respectively, were derived early in this century by determinations of heats of combustion and of digestibility of the typical mixed diet in the United States. Commonly accepted values are shown in Table 7-7.

Physiological fuel values can be used to estimate the number of kilocalories in a food if one knows the number of *grams* of carbohydrate, fat, protein, or alcohol in the food. Tables of food composition in terms of 100-g portions give this information. To demonstrate this estimation, we find in such a table that 100 g

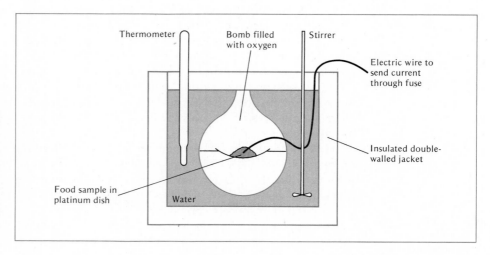

FIGURE 7-6. Sketch of a bomb calorimeter. The dried food is placed in the bomb and ignited with an electrical spark. The food burns in an atmosphere of oxygen. The kilocalorie value is calculated from the rise in the temperature of the water surrounding the bomb.

TABLE 7-7. METHOD OF ESTIMATING PHYSIOLOGICAL FUEL VALUES IN GENERAL USE.

ENERGY SOURCE	HEAT OF COMBUSTION (a) kcal/g	DIGESTIBILITY (b) %	ENERGY LOSS (c) kcal/g	PHYSIOLOGICAL FUEL VALUES (a − c) × b kcal/g	ROUNDED kcal/g	kJ
Carbohydrate	4.1	98	0	4.01	4.0	17
Fat	9.45	95	0	8.98	9.0	38
Protein	5.65	92	1.25 (in urine)	4.05	4.0	17
Alcohol	7.1	100	0.1 (in breath)	7.0	7.0	29

The physiological fuel value is derived by multiplying the heat of combustion figure by the percentage digestibility. For protein and alcohol, a correction for energy loss during metabolism is made before multiplying by percentage digestibility.

These are general values derived from a diet in which about 70 percent of protein comes from animal sources and 30 percent from plant sources. They are not appropriate for diets having markedly different compositions. Both heats of combustion and digestibility vary rather widely within food sources of each of these energy sources. It should be understood that these values are for *pure* carbohydrate, fat, protein, and alcohol.

of cheddar cheese contains 25 g of protein, 32 g of fat, and only 2 g of carbohydrate. Using the values 4, 9, and 4, we find:

25 g protein   × 4 kcal/g = 100 kcal from protein
32 g fat   × 9 kcal/g = 288 kcal from fat
 2 g carbohydrate × 4 kcal/g =   8 kcal from carbohydrate
                                           ———
                                           396 kcal

Of course 100 g (3.5 oz) of cheese is a large amount; one serving is more apt to be about 1 oz. So 396 kcal ÷ 3.5 = 113 kcal per 1 oz serving.

The concentration of kilocalories in foods tends to be high in those foods that are high in fat or refined carbohydrates, and low in those high in water. Table 7-8 shows the kilocalorie contribution of representative foods. As was pointed out in Chapter 2, many high-kilocalorie foods are also low in nutrient density, meaning that they supply relatively low amounts of protein, vitamins, and minerals for the kilocalories they furnish. The terms *energy* and *kilocalories* are used synonymously in nutrition—yet misunderstandings about the term *energy* often arise. These are addressed in Box 7-2.

LOOKING AHEAD

All nutritionists agree that maintenance of normal body weight is important for health. We have seen that balancing energy intake with energy expenditure is necessary to maintain normal weight. In the following chapter we will consider why many people appear to have problems maintaining ideal body weight, and which diets for weight control make sense. In addition, practical suggestions for controlling food intake and increasing energy expenditure will be offered.

NEW HOPE FOR FIGHTING FAT.

M. Marks, *The Washington Post*, April 15, 1982

At least three U.S. drug companies are making a high-stakes effort to develop a drug that would slim down dangerously obese adults by burning off excess weight—thereby inducing a slight fever.

The compounds under study . . . do not attack fatness by the usual route of suppressing the appetite.

Instead, they mimic the metabolic effects of exercise by burning up fat, a principle called thermogenesis. . . .

A drug that will burn off fat regardless of diet may be pie in the sky and could produce serious side effects. Diet experts generally agree that the only safe, reliable way to lose weight is to eat less and, for people who can do so safely, to exercise more. The researchers themselves caution that their testing has been confined to animals—rats, mice and beagles.

But the effort the companies are making indicates that they see a large potential market.

"This is really big, really serious stuff . . . , potentially 30 to 40 million dollars a year," said an industry source who asked not to be identified, "and you're not going to take a chance on losing a patent on something like that." . . .

Any human tests in this country would get serious FDA scrutiny for potential side effects, weighing them against the drug's expected benefits.

William Grigg, an FDA spokesman, said he could not speculate on approval for an untested drug, but he noted that many approved drugs have unwanted side effects because "nothing is 200 percent safe."

"If a drug showed great promise, I would think there would be a good possibility of [a slight fever] being overlooked" for approval, he said.

An industry source said that there was no question that the drugs would have some side effects, but that the developers would be seeking to minimize these so that anything other than fat cells would be affected only by extremely large dosages.

An obese person would take the drug for a week or two without seeing a change, then would lose weight gradually while experiencing a slight fever. When he or she got down to the proper body weight, the drug would cease to have an effect and the supervising doctor would stop treatment. . . .

Dr. Walter N. Shaw, who headed the Lilly project, conceded that an obese person using the drug could lose weight while eating too much and later regain the weight. But, he said, the hope is that people would use the time they are on the drug to restructure their eating habits. . . .

The demand for weight-reduction aids is immense. Grigg said that total diet aid sales in 1980 were $311 million, a 50.4 percent increase over the year before. Most of the increase is attributable to a jump from $110 million to $200 million in nonprescription sales. . . .

ASK YOURSELF:

If this drug finally becomes approved by the FDA, is it apt to solve the obesity problem in the United States? What problems or risks might be involved in its use? What kinds of testing should be done to prove its effectiveness and safety?

TABLE 7-8.   COMPARISON OF CONCENTRATION OF KILOCALORIES IN COMMONLY CONSUMED FOODS

	CONCENTRATION (kcal/100 g OF FOOD)	SERVING SIZE, g	kcal PER SERVING
HIGH-kcal-CONCENTRATION FOODS			
Cream (coffee)	211	1 tbsp	30
Cream (whipping)	352	2 tbsp	105
Cheese (cheddar)	398	1 oz	115
Butter	716	1 tsp (1 pat)	35
Margarine	720	1 tsp (1 pat)	35
Salad oil	884	1 tbsp	110
Pie (apple)	256	⅙ of 9 in pie	400
(pecan)	418	⅙ of 9 in pie	580
(lemon meringue)	255	⅙ of 9 in pie	360
Cake (chocolate)	366	2 in sector of 8 in cake	310
(pound)	473	3½ in × 3 in × ½ in	140
(angel food)	259	2 in sector of 10 in cake	105
Candy (fudge)	400	1 oz	120
(peanut brittle)	421	1 oz	120
(milk chocolate)	520	1 oz	140
Ice cream (rich)	222	½ c	175
Doughnuts	391	1 average	160
French fried potatoes	274	20 strips	220
Peanut butter	582	1 tbsp	95
Roasted peanuts	582	1 oz (30 nuts)	65
English walnuts	651	2 tbsp	100
Beef (rib roast)	440	3 oz	380
Bacon (lean)	545	2 strips	140
LOW-kcal-CONCENTRATION FOODS			
Skim milk	36	8 oz (1 c)	90
Apple	58	1 medium	80
Orange	49	1 medium	80
Broccoli (cooked)	26	½ c	20
Raw cabbage	24	1 c	17
Raw carrots	42	1 carrot	30
Celery	17	2 stalks	15
Spinach (cooked)	23	½ c	20
Ice milk	152	½ c	90

SOURCE: Watt, B.K., and A.L. Merrill, *Composition of Food. Raw, Processed and Prepared*, Agriculture Handbook No. 8, Washington, D.C.: U.S. Department of Agriculture, 1963.

7-2
BOX

Misconceptions about Food and Energy

The word "energy" is often used in confusing ways. An example illustrates some of the problems.

Charlotte, a college student, arose one bright Saturday morning, announced that she felt full of "vim and vigor," and after breakfast mowed the lawn and cleaned her room, and later in the day she cooked the family's dinner. When her mother asked: "What happened to give you such a burst of energy?", Charlotte replied: "Oh, I ate a new kind of candy bar I got yesterday. It's high in energy, but low in calories."

Is it likely that the candy bar was responsible for her sudden burst of energy? Can a food be "high in energy, but low in calories"? Let's see if we can find alternate reasons to explain Charlotte's "vim and vigor." Perhaps it was related to the fact that Saturday was the first sunny day after a rainy, gloomy, final-exams week. Or it might have been related to the fact that her new boyfriend was to meet her family that day. In other words, feeling "full of energy" nearly always has a very strong psychological component. On the other hand, real malnutrition can prevent one from feeling vigorous. Anemia, vitamin deficiencies, protein-calorie malnutrition, and starvation can all result in loss of a vigorous feeling of well-being. However, even in cases of malnutrition, high motivation sometimes enables individuals to perform phenomenal feats requiring great physical exertion. Examples are those malnourished prisoners during World War II who tunneled their way out of concentration camps.

Charlotte's remark that her burst of energy came from a candy bar "high in energy, but low in calories" erroneously implies that calories (kilocalories) and energy are different. The fact is that if a food is low in kilocalories, it is also low in energy value, since the energy value of foods is measured in kilocalories. It is misleading to state that such a food is "high in energy," implying that it can make you feel energetic.

Even though *energy* related to food and nutrition properly refers to *kilocalories*, making certain that your body cells have available all the kilocalories needed does not ensure that you will feel energetic or vigorous. Furthermore, we know of no special food that can make you feel vigorous. While your chances of feeling full of vigor and ready to work improve if you are well-nourished (as opposed to malnourished), nevertheless, your psychological state can exert such a negative effect that you can feel exhausted despite being well-nourished.

Some people think that taking vitamin pills gives them "pep" or "energy." Your body uses many of the vitamins in very small amounts to aid the cells in obtaining energy from carbohydrates, fat, and protein, but vitamins *themselves* are not oxidized in the body to produce energy. Furthermore, swallowing large amounts of vitamins so as to increase the amount in the cells over the requirement does not increase the amount of energy you get from carbohydrates, fats, or proteins.

Understanding the influence of emotional and mental states on your feelings of well-being should help you remain skeptical about claims that any food will make you feel suddenly vigorous or energetic.

SUMMARY

1 Energy is defined as the ability to do work. The body requires energy for synthesis of chemical substances, for muscle contractions, to transport nutrients across cell membranes, to produce glandular secretions, and to transmit nerve impulses.

2 All energy used by the body eventually is converted to heat. The body obtains energy it needs by oxidizing carbohydrates, fats, and proteins, using up oxygen and producing carbon dioxide in the process. Therefore, the energy expenditure of the body can be determined by measuring heat or carbon dioxide given off, or oxygen consumed.

3 Energy balance exists when the kilocalorie intake equals the expenditure. Positive energy balance exists when the intake exceeds the expenditure, resulting in weight gain. Negative energy balance, on the other hand, results in weight loss because the intake is less than the expenditure.

4 Basal metabolism or the basal metabolic rate (BMR) indicates the energy used for all the vital functions of the body under conditions of complete physical, mental, and emotional rest after a 12-to-18-h fast. Energy needed for physical activity and to digest and absorb food is excluded from the BMR.

5 If a person under basal conditions eats some food, extra energy is expended by the body within minutes afterwards. This extra energy has been called the *specific dynamic action* (SDA) of food, *dietary thermogenesis*, or the *calorigenic effect* of food. On ordinary diets containing a mixture of carbohydrates, fats, and protein, the calorigenic effect of food amounts to 6 to 10 percent of the kilocalories expended for BMR plus physical activity.

6 Because basal conditions are difficult to achieve, most physicians measure *resting metabolic rate* (RMR) rather than the BMR. When the RMR is measured, the subject should be resting in a comfortable room but need not be in the fasting state.

7 The expenditure of energy for physical activity depends upon the amount of time devoted to an activity, how strenuous the activity is, and, for those activities in which the body is moved, the weight of the body.

8 The kilocalorie value of foods can be determined in research work by burning the food in a bomb calorimeter. The concentration of kilocalories in foods is lowest in those having a high water content and highest in those high in fat or refined carbohydrates.

FOR DISCUSSION AND APPLICATION

1 Record your own activities on a typical day, writing down what you did during 24 h (1440 min). A suggestion for recording follows:

TIME	ACTIVITY	NO. OF MIN
11:00 P.M.–7:00 A.M.	Sleeping	480
7:00 –7:20	Showering, dressing	20
7:20 –7:30	Preparing breakfast	10
7:30 –7:50	Eating breakfast	20
	etc.	

Then use Appendix H to determine the energy cost of activities, as shown in Table 7-6. Determine energy cost for sleep by using Table 7-5. Do you believe your total energy estimate to be a realistic one? Do you usually consume about this number of kilocalories per day?

2 Calculate the kilocalorie value of 50 g of a food that is 2 percent protein, 20 percent carbohydrate, and 10 percent fat.

3 Develop a daily exercise plan to allow you to work off 300 kilocalories daily. Be realistic. Make sure you can follow the plan.

4 Using Table 7-8, determine the amount of each food that will yield 100 kilocalories. This will help you appreciate the relative energy values of these foods.

SUGGESTED READINGS

Vodak, P., *Exercise: The Why and the How*, Palo Alto, Calif.: Bull Publishing Co., 1980. This little book tries to clarify myths relating to exercise. In simple, easy directions the author guides one to incorporate exercise into everyday living.

Ikeda, J., *For Teenagers Only: Change Your Habits to Change Your Shape*, Palo Alto, Calif.: Bull Publishing Co., 1978. An attractively illustrated book allowing adolescents to proceed at their own pace as they learn how to lose weight.

8 ENERGY IMBALANCES: OVERWEIGHT AND UNDERWEIGHT

When people hear that you are studying nutrition, what is the first question they ask you? It is probably one related to how to lose weight. Chapter 7 dealt with concepts of energy balance and imbalance. These subjects provide a basis for understanding the related concepts of obesity and underweight, which are the focus of this chapter. Obesity, defined as excess body fatness, constitutes an enormous problem in affluent countries. Two investigators recently estimated that the present extent of obesity among adults in the United States amounts to 2.3 billion pounds of excess weight. To dramatize the problem, they calculated the total fossil fuel equivalent of the food kilocalories saved if all obese individuals dieted to achieve desirable body weight. They found that the kilocalories saved would be equivalent to 1.3 billion gallons of gasoline, enough to fuel almost 1 million automobiles per year. In terms of electrical energy, the kilocalories saved would be sufficient to supply the cities of Boston, Chicago, San Francisco, and Washington, D.C., for 1 year [1].

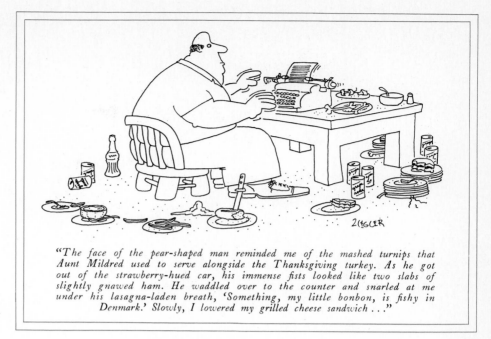

"*The face of the pear-shaped man reminded me of the mashed turnips that Aunt Mildred used to serve alongside the Thanksgiving turkey. As he got out of the strawberry-hued car, his immense fists looked like two slabs of slightly gnawed ham. He waddled over to the counter and snarled at me under his lasagna-laden breath, 'Something, my little bonbon, is fishy in Denmark.' Slowly, I lowered my grilled cheese sandwich ...*"

Paradoxically, in recent years a problem of extreme underweight, called *anorexia nervosa*, has emerged in affluent countries, particularly among adolescent girls and young women. (The term *anorexia* means lack of appetite, while *nervosa* refers to mental disorders.) In this chapter, we will discuss the nature and extent of these problems, their health hazards, possible causes, and methods of prevention and treatment.

OBESITY: HOW EXTENSIVE IS IT?

Throughout human history, the majority of people have been able to barely obtain enough food to survive; only the wealthy or prosperous were privileged to consume rich or even adequate diets. Because such diets were available primarily to the elite, obesity was often (and still is in some cultures) regarded as a status symbol. In ancient Rome, the imposing size and stature of the wealthy senator won him the esteem of the hungry masses. Today in Nepal obesity is regarded with favor, so much so that it would be impolitic for political leaders, who might generally be considered overweight in our society, to even consider losing weight [2].

In western industrialized nations, however, where food is usually much more readily available, many individuals have come to view obesity as a scourge. Our society often views obesity as a sign of gluttony, and leanness as a much sought after, but often unattainable, goal.

An estimated 25 to 45 percent of the U.S. adult population is considered to

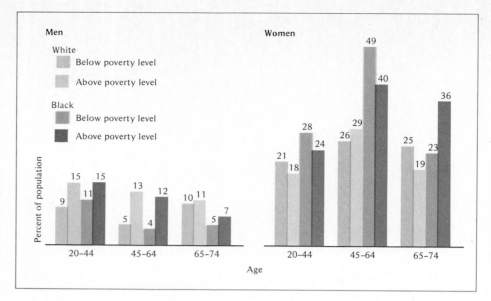

FIGURE 8-1. U. S. adults classified as obese, 1971–1974. (Source: *Health United States, 1976–77. Chartbook.* Department of Health, Education and Welfare. DHEW Publication No. (HRA) 77-1233, 1977.)

be obese [3]. Furthermore, about 3.5 to 10 percent of women and 3.5 to 6.5 percent of men are classified as *severely* obese; the percentages vary with different age groups [4]. The prevalence of adult obesity in the United States is illustrated in Figure 8-1. This figure indicates that a higher proportion of women than men were found to be obese. Black women were more often obese than white women, but black men and white men were equally likely to be obese. Males with higher incomes were more often obese than those with lower incomes.

Obesity has often been considered synonymous with the condition of "overweight," but these conditions are not identical and the terms should not be used interchangeably. While obesity indicates excessive body fatness, overweight means simply that a person's weight is greater than the standards for height and sex (Appendix I). Excessive weight is not necessarily due to fat since muscles, fat, fluid, and bones all contribute to body weight. For example, a football player may have a relatively small amount of body fat, but may be overweight due to a large proportion of lean tissue. He is overweight but not obese. On the other hand, a person of normal weight may have an excessive amount of body fat due to sedentary living. Such a person is obese. Usually, a person who is obese is overweight; however, not all overweight individuals are obese.

HOW DO WE ASSESS OVERWEIGHT AND OBESITY?

An individual is often considered to be overweight if he or she weighs 10 percent or more above his or her desirable weight, and obese if he or she weighs 20 percent or more than desirable weight. The most commonly used method of determining desirable weight is the use of height-weight tables (Appendix I).

These tables are based on the premise that once adults attain their full height there is no need for them to gain additional weight as they grow older; the healthiest individuals do not weigh more with age than they did in their early twenties. Physicians or researchers may also use the *body mass index*, which is weight divided by height squared (wt/ht^2).

Since body weight does not necessarily indicate fatness or obesity, other methods of assessing obesity are of interest. A quick way to assess whether or not you are obese is to simply inspect your nude body before a mirror. Do you look obese? Do you have rolls of fat around the waist or abdomen? Are your hips bulging? Does your abdomen protrude far beyond your chest? You can confirm your impressions by the pinch test. Take a fold of skin and its underlying fat and lift it from the side of your lower chest or the back of your upper arm, and pinch it. If the pinch measures more than an inch of skin and tissue, you are probably obese.

Other simple tests are sometimes used to indicate fatness. The ruler test requires that you lie flat on your back and relax; in this position the surface of the abdomen between the ribs and the pubic area will be either flat or concave if your body fat is not excessive. If you place a ruler on the abdomen, parallel with the vertical axis, it should rest on the breast and pubic bone and should not balance precariously on the crest of a "hill" formed by abdominal fat.

Clinicians and researchers may use one of several rather sophisticated techniques for estimating body fatness. These include procedures which evaluate body density, total body water, or whole body potassium. Such studies find that about 14 percent of the body weight is fat in normal-weight young males, while about 22 percent is fat in normal-weight young females. Percent of body fat greater than 25 percent of body weight for males and 30 percent for females indicates obesity [5].

Physicians may use calipers to obtain a more precise measurement of skinfold thickness than the pinch test described earlier. Skinfold calipers measure the thickness of a double layer of skin and fat. Because about half the body fat in persons younger than 50 years is located directly beneath the skin, skinfold measurements provide an index of body fatness. The sites most often measured are in the triceps area (on the back of the upper arm, halfway between the elbow and shoulder bone), and in the subcapsular area (below the shoulder blade).

HAZARDS OF OBESITY

In our society being thin is "in." The desired look for women is thin, sleek, willowy. Men desire to be muscular, but trim. Because fatness is considered unattractive, the obese individual may suffer discrimination when seeking employment. In fact, one personnel placement professional in New York City estimated that for each pound of overweight a person bears, he or she may lose approximately $1000 a year in income [6]. Social and psychological pressures, lack of acceptance, peer criticism, and difficulty in finding suitable clothes are just a few of the many problems which may lead the obese person to develop a poor self-concept, personality disturbances, and social adjustment difficulties.

In addition to emotional and psychological burdens, other health hazards are associated with obesity. Experts in this field classify obesity as *mild or moderate* (10 to 30 percent above desirable weight), *severe* (30 to 100 percent above desirable weight), and *massive or morbid obesity* (more than 100 percent above desirable weight) [7]. Massively obese people die at younger ages than nonobese people. They are more prone to liver, kidney, and blood-clotting disorders, respiratory difficulties, and are at greater risk for developing heart disease, especially if middle-aged or older [8].

While moderate obesity alone does not increase the risk for developing heart disease, moderately obese people who also have hypertension (high blood pressure), diabetes, or high blood cholesterol levels are more prone to develop heart disease [8]. In addition, one's chances of developing diabetes and hypertension are greater if one is obese. Both gallbladder disease and gout (deposition of uric acid crystals in joints) occur to a greater extent in the obese than nonobese. Obesity complicates arthritis because the joints must bear extra weight. Obese women have a higher than normal occurrence of menstrual disorders and pregnancy complications. Recurrence of breast cancer and decreased survival rate from this disease has also been reported to be greater among obese than nonobese women [9]. Both severely and massively obese people are more prone to accidents because of reduced physical agility, and face greater risks when anesthesia or surgery is needed. Medical, esthetic, and social concerns all focus our attention on the problem of obesity.

WHAT CAUSES OBESITY?

Twenty or thirty years ago physicians typically believed that persons who ate too much became obese as a consequence of various emotional problems such as depression, anxiety, personality disturbances, or lack of self-confidence. The obese were frequently castigated for lacking will-power or self-control. Today, health professionals realize that this view was an oversimplified and often erroneous perception of the cause of obesity. While many of the proposed causes of obesity are in fact only hypotheses, we now know that obesity may be caused by a number of different and often complex disturbances and situations. In fact, different individuals are apparently obese for different reasons; it is actually more correct to speak, not of "obesity," but of "obesities."

Stated simply, obesity develops when more kilocalories are consumed than are used; if *kilocalorie input* is greater than *output*, the body will gain weight. In other words, the basic cause of obesity is positive energy balance. Many people experience great difficulty, however, in balancing input with output in such a way as to avoid obesity. Why is this the case?

Hereditary and Environmental Factors

Research clearly demonstrates that obesity can be inherited in animals. Investigators have produced strains of obese rats, mice, dogs, and chickens. Assessing the relative influence of heredity versus environment on the development of obesity

FOR HEALTHIER, LONGER LIFE, DON'T THINK TOO THIN

Philip J. Hilts, *The Washington Post*, December 27, 1980

The "desirable weight" charts in doctor's offices all over the country are about to be revised—possibly pushing desirable weights up by 15 pounds—and if we want to live longer, we all should revise our ideas about fat and health, according to Dr. Reubin Andres, a professor at Johns Hopkins and clinical director of the National Institute on Aging.

Popular belief says that thin people live longer and fat people will be brought down sooner by their weight. But that belief, though it is hawked by scores of diet books and even doctors, may be flat wrong. In fact, skinny people may be the ones who die sooner, according to some studies reviewed by Andres.

Andres, whose field is obesity and aging, has reviewed more than 40 studies of weight and longevity, covering some 6 million people. The studies ranged from Helsinki policemen and Italian villagers to 750,000 Americans by the American Cancer Society and 5 million people by American insurance companies.

"The populations were extremely diverse, but what's important is that the results all point in the same direction—the desirable weight if you want to live longer has been underestimated. The current chart on doctors' walls, and our own ideas of desirable weight fixed by a sense of esthetics, are not desirable if you want to live longer," Dr. Andres said.

Among the surprises in studies that Andres looked at were these:

- Highest longevity among middle-aged workers at a Chicago utility company occurred in men who were 25 to 32 percent over their "desirable" weight.
- There was minimal mortality among 70-year-old Californians who were 10 to 20 percent "overweight."
- Lowest mortality among San Francisco longshoremen was found in the group that was 30 percent overweight.

In a long-term study of residents of Framingham, Mass., men in similar age groups were found with lowest mortality toward the heaviest end of the scale. Among women in the same town, longevity was greatest in a broad range of middle weights—including some previously thought to be overweight—and mortality highest among the very thinnest and fattest women.

Andres offers two explanations for longer life at somewhat higher weights: heavier people can better tolerate chemotherapy for cancer, and their extra weight may also help them fight diseases that leave others emaciated. . . .

A recent article in Johns Hopkins Magazine surveying the new results in weight and health quotes Dr. David Levitsky, associate professor of psychology and of nutrition at Cornell University.

He says that perhaps half the people who are overweight will suffer ill health effects from it, and half will not. "I'm not saying it's okay to be fat. If you are fat you have to look out for certain pathologies. . . ." But if you don't suffer from any of the obesity-exacerbated diseases, he says, then fat is not necessarily bad and losing weight probably will not gain you a longer life.

ASK YOURSELF:

What are desirable weights based on? (See Appendix I.) Do these studies showing highest longevity among those over their "desirable" weight mean that weighing more will cause an individual to live longer? How might this type of news article be interpreted by the lay public? Might it have any harmful effects? Are reporters always accurate in reporting a scientist's statements?

in human populations is difficult, however. Although knowledge of parental weight trends has sometimes proven useful in predicting whether a child will become overweight in later years [10], determining whether this is due to genetics or to family food habits is difficult. The problem is that obese parents may have obese children, not because of inheritance, but because all family members are exposed to the same environmental influences. If these include exposure to large amounts of foods with encouragement to consume them, obesity is apt to result. The observation that obese people often have obese pets illustrates that eating and exercise patterns rather than heredity may be the culprits.

To learn more about the influence of genetics on obesity, researchers have studied identical twins (because their genetic makeup is the same) who were separated at birth and brought up in different environments. If one twin lived in a normal-weight family and grew into an adult of normal weight, while the other lived in a family of overweight people, and became overweight, we could conclude that environmental influences rather than heredity play a major role in determining one's weight. Other studies have looked at adopted children to determine if their patterns of weight gain resembled those of the family they lived with. Meyer reviewed both types of studies and concluded that inheritance does play an important role in obesity [11]. However, there is no question that the environment promotes or hinders the development of obesity no matter what genetic potential exists.

Many obese people apparently fail to respond to internal or biological *hunger* or *satiety* signals (signals that the person has had enough) and respond instead to external cues. The time of day ("it's 6 o'clock, time for dinner"); a certain activity ("I always snack when I watch television"); the availability of food ("I can't resist fudge when it's in the house"); the smell of food ("whenever I smell the doughnuts in a shop, I have to stop and have one") all trigger *appetite*, the psychological desire to eat. The obese person apparently experiences a greater response to these cues than does the normal-weight person who is more apt to respond to internal (physiological) cues which signal hunger and satiety.

A number of experiments have illustrated receptivity to internal and external cues. In one type of experiment, obese and nonobese subjects were placed on a very bland liquid diet for a period of time. There was little pleasure associated with the food visually or with regard to taste. In addition, each individual ate alone in a hospital room, accompanied only by the machine that delivered the formula. Obese persons drastically reduced their kilocalorie intake and lost weight under these circumstances. On the other hand, normal-weight subjects ate enough to maintain their normal weight. The study demonstrated that when the food was dull and there were few environmental or external cues to stimulate eating or make it pleasurable, the obese ate very little [12].

Dr. Theodore Van Itallie summed up his experience as a researcher on environmental factors and obesity as follows:

> In the U.S., where food is ubiquitous, usually highly palatable, and always readily available from vending machines, the household refrigerator, neighborhood super-markets, and fast-food restaurants, human beings may . . . succumb to environmental influences. There may not be anything basically wrong with most obese people.

The problem simply may lie in the fact that human beings have had to store fat in order to survive. When it becomes easy rather than difficult to obtain extra calories from the environment, obesity is the natural outcome [12].

Many environmental factors are responsible for the lifestyles assumed by people. Because of the habit of driving everywhere in an automobile, many people fail to consider that walking or riding a bicycle rather than driving would result in significantly greater energy expenditure. Labor-saving devices at home make housekeeping a much less arduous task than was the case early in this century. Both our overconsumption of palatable food and our tendency to avoid exerting ourselves doubtless explain much of the obesity in the United States.

Do Obese Children Become Obese Adults?   Years ago, adults typically viewed the plump baby as a happy, healthy baby. If the baby becomes a fat child, parents hoped that the child would outgrow it. Today, however, childhood obesity is regarded as a special health problem.

Although we are uncertain of exactly how many children are obese, the Ten State Nutrition Survey of 1968–1970 [13] found that among 12- to 13-year-olds 17 percent of white and 9 percent of black males, and 12 percent of white and 11 percent of black females were obese. Among older teenagers even higher percentages were obese. A recent study in New York City of nursery school children 3 to 6 years of age showed that 12 percent were more than 20 percent over desirable weight, while almost 5 percent were more than 30 percent over desirable weight [14].

Will a fat child become a fat adult? Some investigators believe the chances are very great that this will happen [10,15,16], while others have found that obese infants do not always become obese children, and obese children do not necessarily become obese adults [17,18]

Psychological Factors

Some obese people may have learned to use food to satisfy various emotional needs rather than merely to satisfy hunger. Inability to recognize and express such emotions as anger, fear, or anxiety may lead to disturbed eating patterns such as binge eating (eating huge amounts at one time) in some people [19]. A typical pattern of eating among many obese people is called "the night-eating syndrome." Such individuals eat very little during the day, but begin to eat in the evening and continue for several hours, while often experiencing feelings of agitation, and later insomnia. This pattern is considered a response to stress [19]. Cases in which obesity results from basic psychological disorders can sometimes, but not always, be successfully treated with appropriate psychotherapy [20]. No specific personality type has been found to characterize obese people, however.

Experimental obesity has been produced in animals by punishing them. Overeating as a result of punishment in such animals continues even after punishment ceases [11]. Comparable cases are unknown in humans, but many people overeat during times of extreme emotional stress. What happens to your own eating pattern when you experience a high degree of pressure before exams?

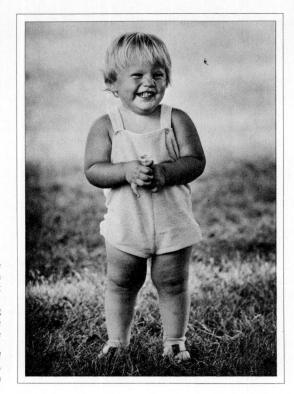

Will this obese 1-year-old become an obese adult? We can't tell for this individual, but habits of overeating and of engaging in little physical activity may be established early in life. *(© Michael Hayman/Photo Researchers, Inc.)*

Are you likely to eat more than usual? Responses to emotional stress vary. Some individuals are unable to eat while others are unable to stop eating.

Lack of Physical Activity

In a classic study using a motion picture technique, obese and nonobese adolescent girls were observed while playing various sports. The normal-weight girls spent 90 percent of their tennis playing time in motion, compared to the obese girls who spent only 50 percent of their playing time in actual motion. The obese girls swam one-third less when they were in the water than did the normal-weight girls [21]. This study failed to document the amount of physical activity engaged in before the girls became obese, so it does not make clear whether lack of activity *caused* the obesity. Lack of physical activity appears to be a significant factor in maintaining obesity, however, once it has developed.

Exercise is important because it aids in regulating the physiological appetite mechanism so that the appetite conforms to internal hunger signals, rather than to environmental signals [22]. When a person is very sedentary, the physiological hunger-satiety mechanism does not gear itself low enough, and obesity may result.

Fat Cell Hypothesis

In the early 1970s, a group of investigators proposed that obesity developing in infancy or childhood leads to lifetime obesity because such individuals have a larger than normal number of fat cells, which can never be diminished. These researchers distinguish between hyperplasia, or increased number of fat cells, and hypertrophy, or increased size of fat cells. Obesity beginning in adulthood, according to this hypothesis, is associated with hypertrophy but not with hyperplasia of fat cells [23]. These investigators believe that an increase in fat cell number is likely to occur in the first 5 years of life and during adolescence [24]. Concern for the influence of infant and child feeding practices on future obesity developed as a result of this hypothesis.

Soon, however, other studies challenged the validity of the fat cell hypothesis. An increase in the number of fat cells was observed to occur in some who became obese in adulthood [25,26], and in normal-weight adults with aging [27]. In addition scientists realized that methods used to determine the number of fat cells may fail to give a true picture because (1) methods used to estimate the total amount of body fat may be inaccurate, and (2) "empty" fat cells (not yet filled with fat) are undetected by the methods commonly used [28]. In fact, one should refer not to the number of fat cells, but to the number filled with fat.

Even though there are methodological problems, studies show that those obese individuals who have an unusually large number of adipocytes (fat cells) filled with fat lose weight by decreasing the size, but not the number, of fat cells. Furthermore, they tend, when placed on weight-gaining or weight-losing diets, to gain or lose weight more rapidly than individuals with a normal number of cells filled with fat [28]. There is as yet no convincing proof, however, that obesity develops as a result of having a large number of fat cells [29].

The fat cell hypothesis, although it has generated much important research, remains unsubstantiated at present. An outgrowth of this hypothesis is the tentative proposal that when an individual is neither gaining nor losing body fat, the number of fat cells remains constant due to an equal rate of building up and tearing down of fat cells [30]. According to this proposal, one does not keep the same fat cells, but there is gradual turnover, as is the case with other body cells. Obesity thus could develop due either to a slow rate of tearing down, or to excessively rapid replication and maturation (building up) of fat cells. Genetic, nutritional, or hormonal factors might all be involved in changing the rate of building up or tearing down of fat cells [30]. Further research doubtless will modify the fat cell hypothesis, and perhaps will lead to more productive ways to prevent or treat obesity.

Faulty Food Intake Regulation Mechanisms

Obesity may result from a defect in the way the body regulates food intake. In the normal individual, food intake is regulated to meet energy output needs. Few people consume exactly the same number of kilocalories each day, or expend the same number. Most of us vary our kilocalorie intake and our level of exercise from day to day; yet our body weights remain remarkably constant. The body must therefore possess some innate mechanisms for regulating food intake. An appreciation of the difference between hunger and appetite can enhance our understanding of these mechanisms.

Hunger and *appetite* represent two different conditions. Hunger is an innate, often unpleasant sensation that one experiences when there is a physiological need for food. A hungry individual may have stomach pains and feel irritable, light-headed, or weak. Appetite, on the other hand, refers to a learned desire for food even when one isn't hungry in a physiological sense.

Some people may be *hungry*, but not have the *appetite* to eat. "I know I should eat—I haven't had anything all day, but I just don't feel like eating." On the other hand, many people eat when they aren't hungry. How often have you had a snack an hour after a meal, even though you were full? Have you ever stopped by a bakery to sample some wonderful-smelling cookie or cake, in spite of having just had dinner? Do you ever have a craving for a specific food, such as your mother's fried chicken or chocolate cake, when you're not really hungry? These are all examples of appetite, not of hunger. Both hunger and appetite play a role in food intake regulation, but the concern is that many obese individuals frequently respond to appetite cues, eating when they are not actually hungry.

Satiety is also an important component of food intake regulation. Satiety exists when one stops eating because of the feeling of "having had enough" or of being satisfied. What mechanisms tell us that we've had enough, causing us to stop eating? Many obese people report, "Once I start eating, I can't stop." Do some people have defective satiety mechanisms?

Although there is as yet no well-integrated theory of how the normal body regulates food intake, several mechanisms are known to play some role in the process. Two aspects of the physiological mechanisms governing food intake have been noted: A short-term mechanism balances energy intake against output on a daily basis; a long-term mechanism helps the body maintain constant weight week after week by correcting "errors" in daily energy intake [31].

The brain is thought to play a major role in regulating food intake, but other parts of the body are also clearly involved. In the early 1950s, investigators believed that two brain centers formed an important part of the mechanism for controlling hunger and satiety. The hypothalamus, a part of the brain that regulates many basic body functions, is foremost in this hypothesis. Animal studies show that if areas located in the central portion of the hypothalamus are destroyed, the animals overeat and become obese. If, on the other hand, areas located on either side of the central portion are destroyed, the animals refuse to eat; unless they are force-fed, they will starve to death. In the first instance, the *satiety center* was destroyed, causing the animals to overeat; in the second one the *feeding center* was destroyed, resulting in their refusal to eat. This hypothesis remains an important one today even though we now know that destruction of the central portion of the hypothalamus does not abolish satiety completely [32]. According to this hypothesis, then, the feeding center signals us to eat when we are hungry, while the satiety center tells us to stop eating when we have had enough.

What signals does the feeding center receive that trigger its activity? We are not sure. The *glucostatic hypothesis* suggests that receptors in both the feeding center and satiety center are sensitive to glucose. It is hypothesized that hunger occurs when the rate of uptake or utilization of glucose by body cells, including those of the feeding center, is low and that satiety occurs when the rate of utilization of glucose by the cells is high. The satiety center shuts off the feeding center when the rate of utilization of glucose reaches a certain level [31]. Mayer believes that this may be an important short-term mechanism for regulating food intake. Other investigators believe, however, that a drop in the utilization of all fuel-producing substances (carbohydrates, fats, and proteins) results in hunger. Some investigators believe that the regulating system involves not only the brain but other organs, too, such as the liver [32].

Most of us recognize hunger pangs resulting from stomach contractions as important signs of hunger, but investigators still do not understand exactly what triggers these contractions. They understand a little more about what stops them, however. Animal studies show that stimulation of nerves in the nose, mouth, and throat areas by food odors, flavors, and textures work in concert with intestinal hormones to produce satiety [32]. The hormone, *enterogastrone*, released by the duodenum upon entry of food into the duodenum, causes gastric motility to diminish, contributing to satiety. In addition, the duodenum is unusually sensitive to the concentration of dissolved substances in the acid chyme as it flows in from the stomach. The more concentrated the dissolved substances, the more dehydrated the wall of the duodenum becomes as fluid is drawn in to dilute the dissolved substances, and the greater the satiety effect [32]. Some obese individuals may have basic defects in one or more of the mechanisms that control hunger and satiety.

The *thermostatic hypothesis*, proposed many years ago, states that an animal eats to produce heat to maintain its body temperature, and stops eating as its temperature begins to rise above normal [32]. This hypothesis was based in part on the observation that warm-blooded animals eat more in cold than in warm environments. Many obese people are highly resistant to physical exercise, perhaps because the body heat generated tends to elevate the body temperature. Although scientists have yet to prove that some part of the brain that governs food intake is sensitive to slight changes in body temperature, most authorities believe that body temperature is a part of the complex system that controls food intake [31,32].

Long-term regulation of food intake may involve total body fat or adipose tissue. Many obese as well as normal-weight people reach a plateau in body weight after which they do not continue to gain. The *lipostatic hypothesis*, so called because of the tendency for body fat or *lipid* to remain *static* or unchanged, suggests that in the long run, some kind of signal causes the body fat stores to stabilize at a certain level for each person. According to this hypothesis, when an obese person resumes eating his or her usual diet after losing weight by dieting, the body sends out some kind of signal that results in the individual's eating enough to regain the lost body fat [33]. The person seems unable to eat only enough to maintain this new, lower weight. We are not certain what this signal is, but some investigators propose that free fatty acids and prostaglandins (hormonelike substances that profoundly affect a variety of body processes) may reach the brain from the fat stores, conveying the message [32]. If this hypothesis proves to be true, it will support the position that weight loss should take place *slowly* rather than rapidly to allow the "lipostat" or mechanism that governs the level of body fat to set itself at a lower level [33]. Theoretically, then, some people may be "biologically programmed to be obese" [7]; that is, their "lipostat" may be set too high, or some other biological mechanism controlling food intake may work improperly.

Dietary Thermogenesis

Who hasn't observed with amazement the tall, thin young man who eats very large amounts of food at every meal, and never gains weight? Who isn't also familiar with the middle-aged man who complains that he gains weight "just by looking at food?" Several investigators are currently engaged in research attempting to establish whether or not the thin young man who eats so much has inherited metabolic mechanisms that cause his body to waste kilocalories from food as heat (thermogenesis) instead of converting them to fat. Recall from Chapter 7 that the increase in heat production over the basal metabolism soon after food is consumed is called *dietary thermogenesis* or the calorigenic effect of food. Perhaps, compared with the thin individual, the plump one is much more efficient at converting food energy to body fat. This research area is currently attracting the interest of both scientists and the general public.

One question posed by researchers is whether or not dietary thermogenesis (the conversion of food kilocalories to body heat rather than to fat) occurs in a special form of fat, called brown fat. Brown fat is unusual in that it produces large amounts of heat. It is widely distributed throughout the body in infancy and early childhood, apparently because the body heat-regulating mechanism is immature during those years [34]. In adulthood, it disappears from most subcutaneous areas and is found chiefly around organs such as the kidneys and adrenals. Researchers want to know whether or not obese people have less brown fat, or whether their brown fat is less able to produce heat than that of lean people [35].

Several mechanisms other than brown fat may result in inefficient conversion of excess kilocalories to fat, and consequent loss of energy as heat [36]. One group of researchers, for example, studied the *sodium pump mechanism*, which normally keeps the mineral sodium outside the cells and the mineral potassium inside the cells. The pumping mechanism uses up energy, representing a substantial proportion of the energy required for basal metabolism. Some obese patients were shown to have reduced activity of this mechanism, implying that they might need less total body energy than normal people [37].

Whether or not dietary thermogenesis actually occurs in human beings has not been clearly established. Although some investigators claim they have documented that lean individuals lose more body heat after eating than obese individuals, others have not obtained these results [38]. Obviously, much more research is needed on this question.

What Conclusions Can Be Drawn?

Despite the thousands of research studies which have investigated the causes of obesity, we still have much to learn. Our ability to pinpoint the cause or causes in individual cases will improve as research continues. Although we currently lack techniques to determine the exact causes of most cases of obesity, treatment is still possible. Because many obese people have been unable in the past to maintain weight loss after a weight-reducing program, however, *preventing* obesity appears to be a more promising approach than attempting to treat it.

PREVENTING AND TREATING OBESITY

The obese person faces huge hurdles in trying to lose weight, and even more difficulty in maintaining weight loss. Individuals who are 50 lb overweight and trying to lose 2 lb per week need to spend a lengthy time—at least 25 weeks—to reach their goal. Most individuals experience plateaus in body weight during a weight loss program. These plateaus may last for varying lengths of time before weight loss resumes, and generally are times of great frustration. Often additional kilocalorie restriction is required before weight loss takes place after a plateau is reached. Once desired weight loss is finally achieved, the most difficult challenge remains—that of maintaining the new, lower weight. Up to 70 percent of all those who are successful in losing weight merely regain it. This high failure rate has been termed the "yo-yo" syndrome—the constant, and for some people, the lifelong process of losing, gaining, losing, and regaining weight. One obesity expert has suggested that if we think of treatment goals in terms of 5-year cures, "People who are obese have a smaller probability of 'cure' than people with cancer" [39].

How then can obesity be prevented? Prevention of childhood obesity is best accomplished by involving the whole family in forming sound eating and exercise habits. Beginning with infant feeding, breast feeding is recommended because the infant controls the amount of food consumed, while with bottle feeding the adult may encourage overfeeding by urging that the bottle be emptied. Even the breast-fed infant can become overweight, however, especially if the mother uses the breast as a pacifier. If every time the baby cries, he or she is offered the breast, overeating can result. Delaying the introduction of solid foods until the infant is between 4 and 6 months of age is also generally recommended to prevent overeating, although clearly there are cases in which an infant requires additional food earlier. While it is reasonable to believe that these measures will help in preventing early obesity, proof is lacking at present. Nevertheless, these measures *may* help and can also be recommended for other reasons which are discussed in Chapter 15.

To encourage young children to develop sound eating habits, parents need to set a good example, as children are great imitators. Children who observe parents or older siblings regularly enjoying high-kilocalorie, low-nutrient-density foods learn to value such foods highly. Parents should be aware of how their attitudes toward eating influence a child's beliefs and understandings. Insisting that children always "clean their plates" may teach them to routinely eat more than the satiety mechanism indicates is needed. "Finish your broccoli, then you can have dessert" places great value on dessert, and may also promote a dislike of broccoli. Offering children food to relieve depression, boredom, or anxiety or to "quiet them down" may set the pattern for eating for reasons other than to satisfy biological hunger. On the other hand, the practice of serving unsweetened fruit for dessert most of the time, and limiting or excluding fried foods and other foods high in fat and sugar from the family diet will aid in establishing the habit of consuming mostly high- rather than low-nutrient-density foods. A nutritious family diet adequate but not excessive in kilocalories can include a wide and interesting variety of foods and can form the basis of pleasurable as well as healthful mealtime experiences.

Children should also be taught to appreciate the importance of physical activity. Normally, small children enjoy being physically active. Parents can encourage such activity and, in addition, can plan for year-round physical activity for each member of the family. Making physical exercise a part of the way of living in the family will aid each child in establishing lifelong habits of physical activity. The importance of consciously incorporating planned physical activity into one's lifestyle cannot be overemphasized in a society which encourages sedentary living.

Young adults need to be aware that obesity frequently begins when there is a drastic change in lifestyle—the change from home to dormitory living at college; from college life to a job; from single life to married life; the changes occurring after pregnancy—all these are times when weight gain frequently begins. Knowing that weight gain may occur allows one to be more conscious of the possibilities and to monitor one's eating and exercise habits so as to avoid weight gain.

Once individuals are obese, how can they be helped to lose and keep off excess weight, in view of our uncertainty of the causes? For people who gain weight easily, the problem is usually lifelong. The solution, then, is to gradually change one's entire lifestyle. Usually this entails increasing physical activity, consuming a nutritionally well-balanced but low-kilocalorie diet, and learning to control external factors that influence eating. Many people look for an easy, effortless way to control weight—alas, a fruitless search. Such people resist changing their entire way of living, but few people achieve permanent weight loss without doing so.

Many strategies have been used to treat obesity. Some of these approaches involve drastic measures, promote short-term weight loss only, and may be harmful in the long run, while others are more sensible. Many such treatments are summarized in Table 8-1.

The public is inundated with information on weight-reduction schemes. In August 1978, a survey of four women's magazines reported that on the average each issue contained three articles on dieting, nutrition, and planning low-kilocalorie meals [53]. Many people who try to lose weight choose a method that

TABLE 8-1. ASSESSMENT OF SEVERAL TREATMENT STRATEGIES FOR OBESITY

TREATMENT	DETAILS OF TREATMENT	COMMENTS
DRUGS 1. Amphetamines	Prescribed to diminish appetite.	Effectiveness diminishes over time. Nervousness and insomnia are side effects. Serious danger of addiction.
2. Thyroid hormones	Prescribed to increase rate of metabolism, which often decreases in individuals who have dieted over long periods.	Effectiveness diminishes over time. May result in loss of lean tissue, and may have adverse effects on heart and skeleton [40].
3. HCG (Human chorionic gonadotropin, a hormone obtained from urine of pregnant women). Simeons Treatment.	Given by injection along with 400–500 kcal diet.	Controlled studies indicate no effect of HCG on weight loss, although of course the low kcal diet is effective [41,42]. Claims that HCG suppresses appetite have not been substantiated [41].
4. Diuretics	May be part of some weight control "plans." Some physicians may also prescribe them. Causes water loss through the urine.	Any weight loss is due to water and not fat loss. Long-term use can cause potassium deficiency since this drug promotes potassium excretion.
FASTING	Usually used for massively obese in hospital setting. Patient is permitted only noncaloric fluids, vitamins, and mineral supplements.	Brings about rapid weight loss at first, but rate declines somewhat as BMR decreases. Individual apt to gain rapidly upon resuming eating because method fails to teach new food behavior patterns to sustain new, low weight. Loss of lean tissue and ketosis occurs. Hair falls out during long fasts. Depression often develops.
PROTEIN-SPARING MODIFIED FAST (PSMF)	Patient fasts, except that 350–600 kcal/day permitted as high-protein foods or as special liquid preparations. These may consist of hydrolyzed proteins (amino acids and peptides) or mixtures of carbohydrate, protein, and fat (the Cambridge Diet). Mineral and vitamin supplements are needed, and are sometimes supplied in the liquid preparation.	Brings about rapid weight loss, but with less loss of lean tissue than fasting alone. Several deaths from heart aberrations occurred even among patients under physicians' care [43]. Fasting of any sort should never be done except under close supervision of a well-qualified physician who monitors metabolic effects. Patient apt to regain weight quickly after PSMF.
INTESTINAL BYPASS SURGERY	Surgical removal or tying off a large portion of the small intestines to diminish the absorption of food.	Used only in patients who are 100 lb or more overweight, and who have serious health problems requiring weight loss. Diarrhea, gastrointestinal bleeding, obstruction of the in- Continued on next page.

TREATMENT	DETAILS OF TREATMENT	COMMENTS
		testines, liver disease, arthritis, kidney stones, and malnutrition all have resulted from this treatment [41]. Yet improved self-esteem and reduced blood pressure, serum lipids, and need for insulin by diabetics also have resulted [41].
LOW-CARBOHYDRATE DIETS [44–49]	Diet contains 50–60 g carbohydrate or less, while protein and fat content is high. A diet this low in carbohydrate causes ketosis (see Chapter 4). Kilocalorie intake is usually less than 1000 kcal/day, even when urged to eat all of allowed foods desired, because ketosis decreases the appetite.	Results in weakness, fatigue, sometimes nausea, dizziness due to sudden fall in blood pressure when one rises from a reclining position, high blood uric acid levels (a danger for an individual predisposed to gout), and bad breath [50]. These diets are often high in saturated fat and cholesterol. The diet fails to teach people how to change food habits so as to control weight. Individuals find the diet attractive at first because they lose weight rapidly during the first week, but this loss is chiefly water [51]. Some proponents claim loss of large amounts of weight despite very high kilocalorie intakes, but this has been disproved [51].
HIGH-FIBER DIETS	Include large amounts of foods high in dietary fiber. Rationale is that this might (1) slow the rate of eating since more chewing is required; (2) increase satiety due to expansion of the intestines; (3) dilute the number of kilocalories in a given volume of food, and somewhat diminish the absorption of fuel nutrients [52].	There is as yet no scientific proof of effectiveness [52]. Research is needed.
FORMULA DIETS	Liquid formula, usually in skim milk, containing 900 kcal/day. Formula contains vitamins and minerals.	Soon becomes monotonous and boring. Low in dietary fiber. Fails to retrain eating habits so as to maintain weight lost.
WEIGHT WATCHERS	Individual pays to attend weekly meetings. Diet advocated is nutritionally sound. Some behavior modification techniques are taught.	Weight loss is slow, considered by nutritionists to be desirable. Individual follows fairly rigid meal plan which may not take into account personal preferences, but many obese are better able to follow a rigid plan. Group support is helpful to many.

is scientifically unsound and often dangerous. Individuals who resist basic changes in eating and exercise patterns are easy prey to promises of quick, painless ways to lose weight. How can you avoid being taken in by unsound diets for losing weight? Suggestions are offered in Box 8-1.

Since many popular weight-reduction programs have serious flaws, what kind of plan for weight control makes sense?

Planning a Reasonable Weight Control Program

Most people who are excessively fat will have the problem of combating adiposity all their lives. A successful weight control program is one that allows significant reduction in body fatness while keeping the body well nourished, followed by maintenance of the new, lower body weight. Contrary to the hopes and wishes of most people, there is no miracle diet, no quick or easy scheme. The

---

8-1 BOX — Recognizing Unsound Claims about Weight-Reducing Diets

Be wary if the diet:

- Promises ease and comfort, with little or no effort on your part. Successful dieting is usually *not* easy or else more people would experience success at losing weight and maintaining the loss.
- Promises extremely rapid weight loss, such as 5 to 8 lb per week. Only starvation or an imbalanced diet very low in carbohydrates can produce such rapid loss, and then only for the first week, usually. The early weight loss is chiefly water, not fat, and the *rate* of loss diminishes the longer one remains on such a diet.
- Includes only a few foods, or uses one food a great deal (for example, grapefruit in each meal). Such limited choices of food result in inadequate nutrient intakes, and many result in unusually high intake of some substances (such as cholesterol on an "egg diet"). The monotony of these diets also results in boredom and quick abandonment of the diet.
- Requires you to purchase vitamins, or other unusual or special substances such as lecithin or kelp. There is no evidence that any vitamins, minerals, or substances such as the ones mentioned enhance weight loss.
- Promises fantastic improvement in beauty, glamor, strength, or sexual prowess. One proponent claimed that following her diet would result in moving fat from the hips to the breasts, if one wanted this to happen! You do not need to be a physiologist to know that this cannot occur. Use your common sense.
- Is published in a book or magazine, as a result of which you find yourself thinking all the claims made must be true. In a free society, anyone can publish anything he wishes, true or not, if he can find someone who will publish it. In the same way, anyone can say anything she likes on TV if she can persuade a producer to allow it. Don't believe everything you read or hear!
- Rapidly gains popularity, and then disappears from the media with equal rapidity. If a diet really worked, it would not lose favor so rapidly.

authors believe that a reasonable weight control program has three aspects: (1) increased physical activity, to increase expenditure of energy, to strengthen muscles, and to condition the heart and vascular system; (2) behavior modification to help one gain control over external or environmental stimuli to eating; and (3) a diet that allows one to maintain good nutrition while losing weight and while maintaining permanent weight loss. These will be considered in turn. But first, some general observations.

People who need to lose more than 5 or 10 lb should obtain a complete physical examination from their physician to ascertain that they are fit enough to embark upon a program which will include weight reduction and exercise.

Generally, slow weight loss is preferable to rapid loss because one is more likely to keep the weight off if the loss has occurred slowly. A loss of ½ to 1 lb per week is a preferable rate, but the loss should never be greater than 2 lb per week. A kilocalorie deficit of 500 kcal per day (3500 kcal per week) is usually assumed to result in a loss of 1 lb per week, since 1 lb of fat contains about 3500 kcal. As we have pointed out, however, early weight loss on almost any reducing diet, or in starvation, is due chiefly to water and not to fat. Therefore, loss of *weight* does not necessarily signify loss of body *fat*. Nevertheless, the calculation that a weekly deficit of 3500 kcal will result in weight loss of 1 lb per week is useful, and is used by most nutritionists and physicians.

Increasing Physical Activity Most people gain weight after age 30 because of the gradual decline in BMR and the usual decline in physical activity. Such gain can be avoided if one continues to be physically active, while cutting back somewhat on food intake, as needed. Physical exercise is beneficial in weight control programs, for many reasons. Increasing energy expenditure through exercise allows weight reduction to occur at a higher kilocalorie intake than is possible otherwise. This is beneficial for at least two reasons: (1) It increases the likelihood that the diet will be adequate in minerals and vitamins because more food can be consumed, and (2) it allows for more efficient utilization of protein for growth and maintenance. You'll recall that if the kilocalorie intake is too low, protein in the diet will be used for energy and not for protein synthesis (see Chapters 6 and 7). In addition, proper exercises can strengthen specific muscles, improve blood circulation to specific parts of the body, and condition the heart and lungs. Psychological benefits accrue, too, as a person often experiences feelings of greater relaxation and physical strength due to exercise.

A widely held myth is that exercise does little to help lose weight. Exercise critics enjoy pointing out that one must perform calisthenics for 22 h or chop wood for 10 h or play golf for 20 h to lose a single pound of fat. But there is another way to look at the energy cost of exercise. Playing golf 2 h (at an energy expenditure of 175 kcal/h) twice a week (700 kcal altogether) could result in a loss of 1 lb of fat after only 5 weeks. If one followed such a program year round, a loss of 10 lb would result [54]. One investigator studied 11 obese women who walked rapidly at least 30 min per day for a year *without dieting* [55]. Their weight loss paralleled the amount of time spent walking. When weight loss stabilized, these

In almost any weight-loss program involving kilocalorie restriction, weight loss is more rapid in the first few days than it is later. This initial weight loss is due primarily to oxidation of glycogen stores, resulting in some water loss, since glycogen is stored with water. Ketogenic diets result in additional water loss due to the excretion of ketones. Continuing on a weight-reducing program for 1 or 2 months results in less water loss and greater losses of body fat.

women lost more weight if they proceeded to increase the amount of walking. Another study, in which elderly volunteers made no dietary changes but progressed from rapid walking to jogging for periods up to 1 year, resulted in a decrease in average skinfold measurements of 17 percent, indicating body fat loss [56]. There is no doubt, then, that exercise alone is beneficial in achieving weight loss, and that incorporating both exercise and diet in a weight control plan is even more effective.

Another common myth maintains that exercise increases the appetite, preventing a negative energy balance by increasing food intake. This is true only if one engages in strenuous, prolonged exercise resulting in large energy expenditures, as is the case for lumberjacks, farm workers, and athletes who exercise about 8 h per day. Studies show, however, that vigorous exercise of moderate duration such as running, swimming, or performing calisthenics for 1 h per day does not result in increased appetite [54]. Frequently, one finds that walking vigorously for 30 min to an hour actually diminishes the appetite.

Some people are interested in reducing the fat accumulated in only one area of the body. Usually genetic factors govern the distribution of fat in the body, except for some unusual hormonal disorders. Generally, fat distribution over the body cannot be effectively changed by "spot" exercises. A person who inherits large hips, for example, will not be able to transform this measurement except through *general* weight loss. Specifically exercising the hips or going on a special diet will be ineffective. In fact, it has been demonstrated that although the circumference of the racquet-holding arm in professional tennis players was larger than the other arm due to increase in amount of muscle tissue, there was no difference in the amount of fat on the two arms. Therefore, greater exercise of the more active arm did not result in decreased fat deposits on that arm [57]. Nevertheless, exercising specific parts of the body can tighten muscles and make one feel trimmer.

Many kinds of exercise are effective in weight loss. It is most important to choose a form of exercise that can be built into the daily lifestyle. Preferably, exercise should employ large muscle groups and should be rhythmical. Routine walking, bicycling, or jogging to work and back every day is ideal because it establishes a habit and is done purposefully. Engaging in a sport or form of exercise one enjoys ensures continuation of the exercise over a long period. The contribution of exercise to weight loss or maintenance of a new, lower body weight is greater the more intense the physical exertion and the longer the time spent doing it. The minimum amount of exercise shown to be effective in

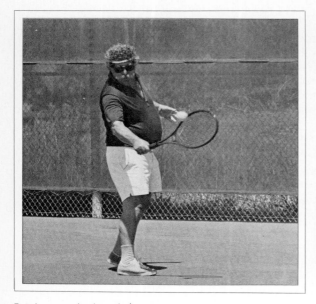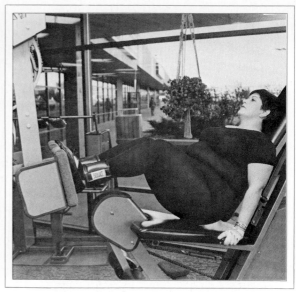

Routine exercise is a vital component of a successful plan to lose weight and maintain the loss. (A, © Phyllis Greenberg/Photo Researchers, Inc.; B, © Michael Gamer/Black Star)

contributing to weight reduction is an expenditure of 300 or more kilocalories per session, consisting of 20 to 30 min of continuous exercise at least three times per week. Exercising only 1 or 2 days a week is ineffective. If frequency of exercising is increased to four or more times per week, less intense exercise than 300 kcal per session may effectively add to weight loss [58]. Directions were given in Chapter 7 for use of Appendix H to estimate energy expenditure during physical activity.

It is a good idea to begin an exercise program slowly, choosing the kind of exercise you can keep doing under your circumstances of living. By setting aside a certain time each day for exercise, one can establish a habit, making it less likely that other factors will interfere. Exercising with a friend or group may be more enjoyable than exercising alone.

Konishi [59] dramatized the relationship between the kilocalorie value of foods and exercise by calculating the amount of exercise required to burn up kilocalories in food (Table 8-2). For example, 12 min riding a bicycle at the rate specified is required to oxidize one large apple, while 31 min of bicycle riding gets rid of the kilocalories in an ice cream soda.

Behavior Modification Behavior modification focuses on changing specific observable behaviors, and has been successfully used in weight-loss programs. Obese people often believe they have no control over eating—that they are somehow driven to eat and eat and eat. The basis of behavior modification in weight control is the observation that, for many obese people, eating behavior is a *learned* response to environmental stimuli. In other words, the obese person has learned to associate environmental or *external* cues with eating, instead of his or her physiological hunger-satiety mechanism. Because such behavior is learned, it can also be unlearned.

**TABLE 8-2. ACTIVITY NEEDED TO BURN UP KILOCALORIES IN FOOD ENERGY
EQUIVALENTS OF FOOD KILOCALORIES EXPRESSED IN MINUTES OF ACTIVITY**

FOOD	kcal	WALKING[a] (min)	RIDING BICYCLE[b] (min)	SWIMMING[c] (min)	RUNNING[d] (min)	RECLINING[e] (min)
Apple, large	101	19	12	9	5	78
Bacon, 2 strips	96	18	12	9	5	74
Banana, small	88	17	11	8	4	68
Beans, green, 1 c	27	5	3	2	1	21
Beer, 1 glass	114	22	14	10	6	88
Bread and butter	78	15	10	7	4	60
Cake, 1/12, two-layer	356	68	43	32	18	274
Carbonated beverage, 1 glass	106	20	13	9	5	82
Carrot, raw	42	8	5	4	2	32
Cereal, dry, 1/2 c, with milk and sugar	200	38	24	18	10	154
Cheese, cottage, 1 tbsp	27	5	3	2	1	21
Cheese, cheddar, 1 oz	111	21	14	10	6	85
Chicken, fried, 1/2 breast	232	45	28	21	12	178
Chicken, TV dinner	542	104	66	48	28	417
Cookie, plain, 148/lb	15	3	2	1	1	12
Cookie, chocolate chip	51	10	6	5	3	39
Doughnut	151	29	18	13	8	116
Egg, fried	110	21	13	10	6	85
Egg, boiled	77	15	9	7	4	59
French dressing, 1 tbsp	59	11	7	5	3	45
Halibut steak, 1/4 lb	205	39	25	18	11	158
Ham, 2 slices	167	32	20	15	9	128
Ice cream, 1/6 qt	193	37	24	17	10	148
Ice-cream soda	255	49	31	23	13	196
Ice milk, 1/6 qt	144	28	18	13	7	111
Gelatin, with cream	117	23	14	10	6	90
Malted milk shake	502	97	61	45	26	386
Mayonnaise, 1 tbsp	92	18	11	8	5	71
Milk, 1 glass	166	32	20	15	9	128
Milk, skim, 1 glass	81	16	10	7	4	62
Milk shake	421	81	51	38	22	324
Orange, medium	68	13	8	6	4	52
Orange juice, 1 glass	120	23	15	11	6	92
Pancake with syrup	124	24	15	11	6	95
Peach, medium	46	9	6	4	2	35
Peas, green, 1/2 c	56	11	7	5	3	43
Pie, apple, 1/6	377	73	46	34	19	290
Pie, raisin, 1/6	437	84	53	39	23	336
Pizza, cheese, 1/8	180	35	22	16	9	138

Continued on next page.

TABLE 8-2. ACTIVITY NEEDED TO BURN UP KILOCALORIES IN FOOD ENERGY EQUIV-
ALENTS OF FOOD KILOCALORIES EXPRESSED IN MINUTES OF ACTIVITY *(Continued.)*

FOOD	kcal	WALKING[a] (min)	RIDING BICYCLE[b] (min)	SWIMMING[c] (min)	RUNNING[d] (min)	RECLINING[e] (min)
Pork chop, loin	314	60	38	28	16	242
Potato chips, 1 serving	108	21	13	10	6	83
Sandwiches						
Club	590	113	72	53	30	454
Hamburger	350	67	43	31	18	269
Roast beef with gravy	430	83	52	38	22	331
Tuna fish salad	278	53	34	25	14	214
Sherbet, ⅙ qt	177	34	22	16	9	136
Shrimp, french-fried	180	35	22	16	9	138
Spaghetti, 1 serving	396	76	48	35	20	305
Steak, T-bone	235	45	29	21	12	181
Strawberry shortcake	400	77	49	36	21	308

[a]Energy cost of walking for 70-kg individual = 5.2 kilocalories per minute at 3.5 mph.
[b]Energy cost of riding bicycle = 8.2 kcal/min.
[c]Energy cost of swimming = 11.2 kcal/min.
[d]Energy cost of running = 19.4 kcal/min.
[e]Energy cost of reclining = 1.3 kcal/min.
This table allows you to calculate the amount of different types of physical activity needed to burn up kilocalories in specific foods.
SOURCE: Konishi, F., "Food and Energy Equivalents of Various Activities," *Journal American Dietetic Association,* 46:187, 1965.

The first step in utilizing behavior modification techniques to control eating is to find out what prompts the individual to eat. What external cues trigger eating? Is it the time of day? An activity such as watching television? What kinds of food are eaten? How much? With whom? When? What emotional responses are associated with eating? To answer these questions, it is necessary for the individual involved to keep a diary of all food eaten and of the factors associated with eating.

Using information furnished by the diary, in formal behavior modification programs a trained therapist helps the individual identify factors that trigger eating. The outcome of work with the therapist (or without a therapist if one follows one of many available books) is the gradual evolution of a new eating pattern by teaching the person small but significant changes in eating behavior. For example, if having fudge brownies in the house results in relentless consumption of brownies until they are all gone, a goal of refraining from buying brownies and bringing them into the house can be set. If the individual eats every time he watches television, a goal might be to limit eating to a room in the house where there is no television. Other strategies to help individuals develop control over their eating environment include:

- Slowing the rate of eating by putting the fork down on the plate between bites of food, or by swallowing the food in the mouth before putting more food on the fork.

- Keeping food out of sight ("out of sight—out of mind").
- Avoiding placing bowls of food on the table, which increases the urge to "finish it up."
- Eating only when sitting in a specified place with the table completely set.
- Avoiding combining any other activity, such as reading or television viewing, with eating. Instead, the focus becomes the enjoyment of the food itself.

An important part of any behavior modification program provides reinforcement for "appropriate behavior." One can do this by setting up a "contingency contract," or promising to reward oneself with something of value, contingent on carrying out the specified behaviors. For example, if an obese person follows the plan to eat only at the dining room table with her place fully set with china and silverware, she might reward herself with a movie she has been wanting to see. The reward must be something the individual prizes or enjoys doing.

Many studies indicate that people frequently experience positive energy balance, not because they eat unusually large amounts of food but because they exercise so little [54]. Behavior modification techniques can be used to change from habitual sedentary practices to those requiring greater energy expenditure. The first step is to keep a record of daily physical activities as described in Chapter 7, noting for each activity whether it is classified as light (under 150 kcal/h), moderate (150 to 250 kcal/h), or heavy (over 250 kcal/h). One then totals the number of minutes per day spent at each level of activity. If the majority of the time is devoted to light activity, change is indicated. Using the diary, one can decide what changes are practical ones. Among possible changes are:

- Walking short distances in preference to riding.
- Climbing stairs in preference to taking the elevator.
- Replacing coffee breaks with exercise breaks.
- Getting off the bus or subway 8 to 10 blocks before your stop, and walking the rest of the way.
- Routinely parking a distance from your place of work or school, and walking the remaining distance.
- Running in place or doing calisthenics during TV programs or commercials.
- Riding a stationary exercise bike while watching TV programs.

Rewarding oneself for reaching set exercise goals is helpful, just as it is in relationship to eating behavior [54].

The goal of behavior modification is to help a person gain control over circumstances that govern input and output of energy. A great many studies have been done on the effectiveness of this technique in bringing about weight loss. Generally, results have been encouraging, although there is some question about the ability of patients to continue weight loss on their own after cessation of work with a therapist [60].

Planning A Reasonable Weight-Reducing Diet   Diet constitutes the third part of the exercise–behavior modification–diet triad. The first step in planning the diet is to set a realistic goal about how much weight one should lose. Unfortunately, the

American idea that women should by sylphlike means that many women are desperately unhappy about their weight even though they are not over standard weight for their height [61]. This view is frequently encountered among college students, and points out that parents, teachers, and public health personnel need to work with children and teenagers to help them attain a realistic assessment of their body size. For people who really do need to lose weight, however, a physician who specializes in weight control or a dietitian or nutritionist can help the person set a reasonable goal. It may be not only unrealistic but also unreasonable to expect the massively obese or those who have been obese since childhood to reach weights as low as those specified in standard weight tables (Appendix I).

Once a decision is made about how much weight is to be lost, the kilocalorie level of the diet can be set according to the extent of energy expenditure projected from increase in exercise, and the rate of loss one hopes to attain. Generally, a deficit of 3500 kcal per week is expected to result in a loss of 1 lb per week, as previously noted, and a loss between ½ to 2 lb per week is recommended. Dietitians and nutritionists generally recommend that women consume between 1200 and 1500 kcal/day on a weight-reducing diet, and that men consume between 1500 and 1800 kcal/day. Patients are then counseled to weigh themselves once a week in the nude before breakfast and after voiding. The weight record allows the individual to ascertain whether the combination of diet and exercise is resulting in the rate of weight loss desired.

Characteristics of a reasonable weight-reducing diet are outlined in Box 8-2. This information helps one evaluate the reasonableness of diets that come and go in the popular media.

As noted in Chapter 2, the Exchange System is a good method to use to ensure variety and balance in the diet. Table 8-3 uses the Exchange System to plan 1000-, 1200-, and 1500-kcal diets in which about 54 percent of the kilocalories

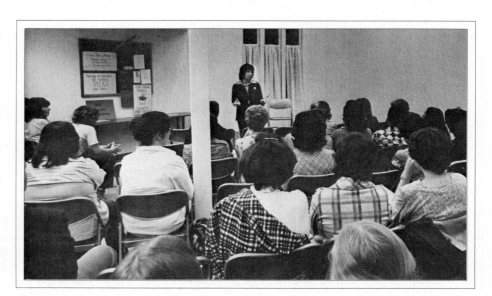

Many overweight people find that groups provide positive support as they attempt to lose weight. (© Josephus Daniels/Photo Researchers, Inc.)

The reasonable weight-reducing diet:

- Is a part of a total program which encourages changes in lifestyle incorporating, in addition to the diet, greater physical activity and measures to gain control over one's eating behavior. Physical activity should be increased sufficiently to allow weight loss on a diet of at least 1000 kcal/day.

- Is one that an individual can adhere to for the rest of his or her life, adapting the kilocalorie intake to allow maintenance of the new, reduced weight. This rules out the liquid-protein fast, liquid formula diets, "the grapefruit diet," the "egg diet," and very low carbohydrate diets, all of which one can follow only a short time.

- Should allow for a wide variety of food choices. This allows the diet to be "tailored to the individual" and increases likelihood of nutritional adequacy. Such a diet accommodates ethnic food preferences, and allows people to incorporate some of their favorite foods.

- Is low enough in kilocalories to allow one to lose from ½ to 2 lb per week, not more. Slow weight loss is clearly preferable to rapid loss, since rapid loss too frequently is followed by rapid regaining of the lost weight, and often more.

- Is nutritionally adequate, providing recommended amounts of vitamins, minerals, and proteins without being excessively high in fat or sugar. In other words, the diet consists chiefly of high-nutrient-density foods. Following the guide of moderation, the diet should not be too high in saturated fat, sugar, cholesterol, alcohol, or salt, and should supply a moderate amount of dietary fiber. A diet that uses the Exchange System is apt to include a wide variety of foods, increasing the chances of having a nutritionally adequate diet (Chapter 2).

- Has fairly good satiety value. Although there is nearly always some hunger while on a weight-reducing diet, individuals cannot adhere to the diet if they are constantly hungry. Diets extremely low in kilocalories (less than 1000 kcal) are not likely to have good satiety value. Diets with moderate amounts of dietary fiber, fat, and protein are most apt to have good satiety value.

come from carbohydrates, 20 percent from proteins, and 26 percent from fat. The diets are based upon the Exchange Lists, Appendix B.

If individuals on a weight-loss program reach a point at which weight loss becomes much slower than desired, they should plan to increase exercise and perhaps lower their kilocalorie intake somewhat. Generally, a diet of less than 1000 kilocalories is not recommended because it is unlikely to be nutritionally adequate. Again, the alternative is to increase physical activity.

Alcohol consumption contributes a significant number of kilocalories to the diet of many Americans. About 10 percent of the kilocalories consumed in the United States, on the average, are estimated to come from alcohol. Generally, the practice of consuming cocktails before dinner tends to increase rather than diminish kilocalorie intake [7]. It is important for individuals who are attempting

TABLE 8-3.   EXCHANGES FOR 1000-, 1200-, and 1500-kcal WEIGHT REDUCING DIETS (54% OF kcal FROM CARBOHYDRATE, 20% FROM PROTEIN AND 26% FROM FAT)

FOOD AND LIST NO.*	NO. OF EXCHANGES		
	1000 kcal	1200 kcal	1500 kcal
Milk, skim, list 1	2	2	2
Vegetables, list 2	3	3	4
Fruit, list 3	3	4	5
Bread, list 4	4	6	7
Meat, lean, list 5	4	4	5
Fat, list 6	3	4	6

SAMPLE MENU, 1200-kcal DIET

MEAL	FOOD	EXCHANGES
Breakfast	½ c orange juice	1 fruit
	½ c bran flakes	1 bread
	1 slice whole wheat toast	1 bread
	½ tsp margarine	½ fat
	1 c skim milk	1 milk
Snack	1 medium peach	1 fruit
Lunch	2 slices whole wheat bread	2 bread
	1 oz mozzarella cheese	1 medium fat meat (omit ½ fat exchange)
	3 slices tomato	1 vegetable
	½ raw green pepper	1 vegetable
	1 c plain yogurt (2% milk fat)	1 low-fat milk (omit 1 fat exchange)
	1 small apple	1 fruit
Dinner	2 oz chicken (skin removed)	2 meat (lean)
	1 tsp oil used in cooking	1 fat
	½ c green peas	1 bread
	½ c carrots	1 vegetable
	lettuce salad	free
	1 tsp oil (vinegar or lemon juice, free)	1 fat
	1 small pear	1 fruit
Snack	¼ c 2% fat cottage cheese	1 lean meat
	4 soda crackers	1 bread

*The Exchange Lists are in Appendix B.
Selecting foods, or exchanges, from each of the six exchange lists allows one to plan meals to meet nutrient needs and keep within a given daily kilocalorie diet.

weight loss to appreciate not only the kilocalorie contribution of alcohol, but that alcoholic beverages generally are of low nutrient density. Appendix C lists the kilocalorie value of commonly consumed forms of alcohol and indicates their low nutritive value.

UNDERWEIGHT

The public generally fails to perceive underweight as a problem in this country; in fact, people often consider it to be a desirable state. Underweight, defined as having a body weight 15 to 20 percent below the weight standards, usually indicates that something is wrong and should be brought to medical attention. Persons who are underweight have decreased resistance to infection, tend to become easily fatigued, and are often sensitive to a cold environment. Underweight results, of course, from a kilocalorie intake too low to maintain normal weight, but diverse reasons may account for the poor intake. Disorders of the intestinal mucosa, such as sprue or celiac disease, may prevent normal absorption of food, or diseases that increase the metabolic rate, such as tuberculosis or hyperthyroidism, may greatly increase the amount of food needed. Psychological or emotional problems may seriously decrease the appetite and food intake in some people.

Long-term undernutrition results in many hormonal changes; women, for example, cease menstruation when a certain proportion of body weight is lost. Successful treatment of underweight depends upon finding the basic cause and removing it. Then methods can be devised to increase the kilocalorie intake by increasing the number of feedings per day and the kilocalorie concentration of the food.

Anorexia Nervosa

Juanita, a 15-year-old, pushed back her plate and heaved a sigh—"I'm stuffed." But her dinner, consisting of small portions of meat, vegetables, and salad, had hardly been touched. Juanita, who is 5'4', has been dieting to lose weight, and now weighs 90 lb after losing 15 lb over the past 2 months. Her goal was always to lose "just 3 more pounds," but each time she achieved this goal, she set a new one.

Juanita is suffering from a condition known as *anorexia nervosa*, a state of emaciation resulting from self-starvation. First identified by physicians more than a century ago, anorexia nervosa now affects thousands of American and European girls, and in rare instances boys, in their teens and early twenties. Although it can be triggered by an initial preoccupation with overweight, the causes are far more complex than overzealous dieting alone would suggest.

The basic cause of anorexia nervosa is as yet uncertain. Some authorities believe it to be primarily a psychological disorder, while others think it originates from disturbances of the hypothalamus or of the pituitary gland in the brain [62]. Although hypothalamic-pituitary disorders exist in the disease, it is not yet known whether these are triggered by psychological stress, or whether they simply result from the state of starvation that develops. More research is currently in progress on this question.

Psychologically, anorexics perceive distortions of body image; in other words, they seem unaware of their extreme thinness and instead view themselves as "fat." Although they actually suffer painful hunger pangs, they very effectively

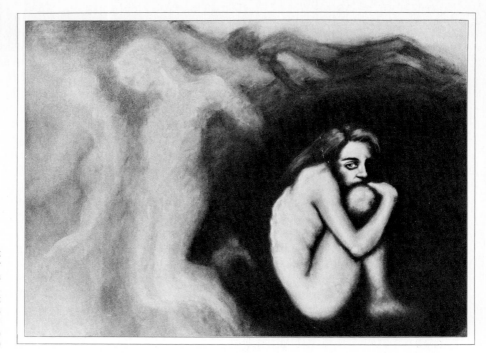

This painting by a patient undergoing treatment for anorexia nervosa expresses the loneliness, isolation, and fear that many of these patients experience. (© 1982 Susan Rosenberg/Photo Researchers, Inc.)

deny these because of an enormous fear of losing control over eating. "If I take just one bite I'm afraid I won't be able to stop" is a typical expression of this fear [63]. They are constantly preoccupied with food, often cooking large amounts and insisting that other people eat while they watch.

Some victims of the disease alternate periods of abstinence from food with huge eating binges, followed by self-induced vomiting or use of laxatives. They often feel guilty or depressed after eating [63]. The most obvious characteristic of the patient is severe weight loss (25 percent or more loss of body weight), resulting in a "skin and bones" appearance. Menstruation stops, muscle tissue wastes away, the skin becomes dry and yellowish, hair becomes stringy, and the basal metabolic rate drops as does blood pressure and pulse. Subnormal body temperature, anemia, and sleep disturbance often result. Because she feels cold, generally the patient covers herself so completely with clothing, even in warm weather, that the extent of her emaciation may not be immediately obvious. Anorexia nervosa is a very serious disease, since 15 to 20 percent of patients die from it.

Typically, anorexics engage in a great deal of physical activity, always denying that they feel any fatigue as a result. They are usually good students, preoccupied with excelling academically. They appear to be self-assertive, but in fact psychologically feel themselves to be completely ineffective, always acting as a puppet of other people. Generally, the anorexic was a "perfect child," giving her parents no problems because of constant compliance to their wishes. The disorder appears in adolescence, a time when children normally learn to become more independent of their parents. During their treatment, many anorexics learn that starving themselves was their way of asserting control over their own bodies, thereby hurting their parents [20].

Treatment is often difficult and prolonged. Nutritional rehabilitation must be instituted immediately, and psychotherapy for the individual as well as her family should begin as soon as possible. Hospitalization is frequently required to establish a good treatment program. Such a hospital program might include the following plans and rationales. Since the patient suffers from a paralyzing lack of a sense of control over anything (except refusal to eat), the physician and nurses explain to her that they will take over for her, and will help her to eat, and to face and solve her problems. If she does not eat the food on her tray, chosen by a dietitian after consulting the patient about her food preferences, she knows that she will be given a liquid formula to drink. If she refuses that, she knows she will be tube-fed. She is given no opportunity to throw food away or induce vomiting or to use laxatives. Generally, this kind of plan is successful in getting the patient to eat and gain weight.

The anorexic's recovery depends primarily on how well she responds to psychotherapy. Behavior modification has been used to induce eating, often by denying the patient physical activity until she gains a specified amount of weight. However, this technique does nothing to change the underlying psychological problems and is not recommended as the sole treatment [63]. Several years of treatment are often required, after which about two-thirds of anorexics recover [64]. Many recovered anorexics report continued struggles with guilt, depression, and other feelings associated with eating, however.

The rapid increase of this disorder in recent years is believed by some authorities to be related to the prevalent social norms of slimness for women in western affluent conditions. In this connection, it is interesting that many seemingly normal female college students report practicing self-induced vomiting as a means of weight control, reflecting the difficulty many feel in balancing food intake and expenditure so as to effectively maintain desirable weight.

The Binge-Purge Syndrome

An eating disorder related to anorexia nervosa, and often found in anorexic patients is binge eating (*bulimia*), followed by purging or vomiting. In bulimia the individual experiences a constant and insatiable craving for food, and as a result goes on eating binges, gorging on huge amounts of food. During an episode of binge eating, an individual may consume several pounds of food at one time, resulting in tremendous physical stress. After an eating binge, the person is consumed with guilt and then purges by vomiting or by taking large amounts of laxatives or enemas.

Bulimia and vomiting are not new. In ancient Rome guests at lavish banquets would feast for hours and then tickle their throats with feathers to vomit so that they could eat again. In Roman society, the practice was common among wealthy men; today bulimia is most common among well-educated women, although some men also suffer from the disorder. Many of these women are depressed, and obsessed with being perfectionists. They feel it is very important to have beautiful

NUTRITION IN THE NEWS

WEIGHT, OBSESSION & DEATH

Sandy Rovner, *The Washington Post*, February 9, 1983

The death last week of singer Karen Carpenter, which may have been linked to her battle with eating disorders, has prompted a flurry of frightened phone calls to area centers where anorexia nervosa and bulimia are treated.

. . . The end result of either syndrome can be weight control, of course, but also cardiac arrest.

Dr. William R. Ayers, medical director of the Georgetown Diet Management Center, which has a special program for eating disorders, explains that there can be two basic ways in which the heart is affected adversely. One, he says, is because "the heart muscle, like all muscles, requires basic nutrition," and when fat reserves are used up the body must convert protein to burn as energy.

The heart, Ayers points out, also has some special requirements that involve electrolyte balance—to keep it beating. The key electrolyte is potassium, interacting with calcium, magnesium and sodium.

. . . If . . . food is vomited before it leaves the stomach, . . . essential amino acids are lost, along with potassium that is highly concentrated in stomach acids. There can be further loss of protein through excessive use of laxatives, which speed the transit time of food through the system. Diuretics, which increase the excretion of fluids, cause dehydration and further loss of electrolytes. Any of these practices can weaken the heart, cause irregular heartbeats or eventually cause the heart to stop beating. Moreover, because stomach acids are lost, the body's acid-to-base ratio is unbalanced which can be a long-term cause of incomplete digestion—and heart muscle damage—even when the abusive eating disorder no longer occurs. . . .

ASK YOURSELF:

Is an article like this one apt to encourage an individual with anorexia nervosa or bulimia to seek help? Why are victims of these disorders prone to be secretive about them?

---

bodies and because they cannot control their impulses to eat, they take care of their loss of self-control by making themselves vomit [65]. Some of these women apparently feel that if they can attain thin, willowy figures, other areas of their lives will work out too. They often become so obsessed with this that bulimia followed by purging becomes a daily activity [66]. Purging is a way to get rid, not only of huge amounts of food, but also of anger, depression, and frustration with life in general.

While the individual may be able to maintain normal weight by this practice, other health problems frequently result. The use of laxatives, enemas, and vomiting can lead to disturbances in electrolyte balance and dehydration. Low blood and tissue levels of potassium can eventually lead to cardiovascular and kidney failure and death, if untreated. The enamel on the teeth may erode because of the frequent vomiting. Menstrual irregularities are common among female bulimics.

Bulimia often becomes a habit, and like most habits, it is difficult to break.

Initially the patient should have a thorough medical evaluation to assess other health problems, including emotional and psychological status. After this, the treatment, if it is to be successful, depends on the cooperation of the individual. The person must acknowledge the problem and summon the motivation to cope with it. Some patients are helped by specific instructions about the kinds and amounts of foods to eat. Gaining self-control is important, and if the individual receives specific guidelines about appropriate eating behavior, this may help. Almost always there are underlying emotional disturbances that need to be treated by psychiatric intervention. Behavior modification techniques, as well as group therapy patterned after the approach used by Alcoholics Anonymous may also be effective. Definitive treatment awaits further research into this disorder.

LOOKING AHEAD

This chapter completes our discussion of the energy nutrients: carbohydrates, fats, and proteins, and problems related to them. The next section presents those nutrients (other than water) that are needed in relatively small amounts, but which are essential to good health—the vitamins and minerals.

SUMMARY

1 Overweight, a term indicating that a person weighs more than the standard for sex and height, differs from obesity, which is defined as a state of having excessive amounts of fat in the body.

2 Genetic factors may be associated with faulty food intake regulatory mechanisms, or with the tendency to be highly efficient in converting food energy to body fat, or with the tendency to have a large number of fat cells. As yet, however, scientists are unable to pinpoint the extent to which these factors actually result in obesity in people.

3 Environmental factors may be the chief reason that many people maintain positive energy balance under conditions in which food is abundant and pervasive, and in which physical activity is minimal.

4 Because studies indicate that obese people experience great difficulty in achieving and *maintaining* normal weight, the importance of preventing obesity is obvious. This is best done by establishing and maintaining healthful eating and exercise habits from early childhood.

5 A reasonable weight-reducing program includes a three-pronged attack: (1) increased physical activity, (2) behavior modification to aid the obese person in gaining control over influential environmental factors, and (3) a diet that ensures good nutrition while losing weight, and, at the same time, teaches the

person how to eat so as to maintain the new, lower weight.

6 Anorexia nervosa has increased recently in western countries among adolescent girls. Current treatment generally involves extensive psychiatric counseling in addition to measures designed to entice the person to consume sufficient food to regain normal weight.

7 Bulimia, the tendency to binge eating, followed by purging with laxatives, enemas, or vomiting has been recently reported, especially among young, well-educated women. This disorder has yet to be thoroughly studied.

FOR DISCUSSION AND APPLICATION

1 Find a weight control diet in a current magazine. Evaluate it according to the criteria presented in Boxes 8-1 and 8-2. Is it a reasonable diet? Why or why not?

2 To what extent are your own eating habits the result of environmental or external cues? Record your own food intake for a day, noting where you eat, other activities associated with eating, with whom you eat, how you feel while eating (depressed, angry, elated, etc.). Is your food intake well chosen accord-

ing to the Basic Four? The *Dietary Guidelines for Americans*? The Exchange System? (Chapter 2.) Can you suggest behavioral techniques that might improve your eating habits?

3 How realistic are you and your friends about your body size? Interview several of your friends. Is their body weight within the standards presented in Appendix I? How many of your friends are dissatisfied with their weight in spite of the fact that it falls within desirable limits? Why are they dissatisfied?

4 How extensive is anorexia nervosa and bulimia among your friends and acquaintances? How many friends or acquaintances know someone who suffers from one of these disorders? What factors appear to account for the occurrence of these disorders?

SUGGESTED READINGS

Exercise and Weight Control. This publication from the President's Council on Physical Fitness and Sports discusses the role of exercise in a weight control program. It can be ordered for $1.75 from the Consumer Information Center, Department 150K, Pueblo, Colo. 81009.

Coffey, K., and M.A. Ferrell, *Fun Foods for Fat Folks*, Child Development Center, University of Tennessee, 1973. Designed to help parents help their children lose weight, this book provides hints, information, and recipes.

Mahoney, M., and K. Mahoney, *Permanent Weight Control: A Total Solution to the Dieter's Dilemma*, New York: W.W. Norton & Co., 1976. This book discusses individualized diet and activity plans to help people lose weight and keep it off. It emphasizes gradual changes in an individual's personal, social, and physical environment.

Weight Control and Obesity, Oakland, Calif.: Society for Nutrition Education, revised October 1981. An annotated bibliography of books, pamphlets, journal articles, and audiovisuals pertaining to weight control and obesity.

Van Itallie, Theodore, and Joyce Margie, *Finding Your Thin Self, New Insights on Weight Control*, Bloomfield, N.J.: HLS Press Inc., 07003, 1981. A booklet summarizing the causes and control of obesity.

Cellulite: Hard to Budge Pudge, Food and Drug Administration. One copy free from Consumer Information Center, Dept. 560K, Pueblo, Colo., 81009. A booklet making the point that cellulite is a myth.

PART III

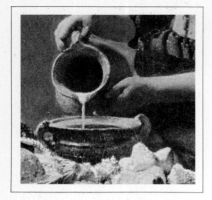

PART III

VITAMINS, MINERALS, AND WATER

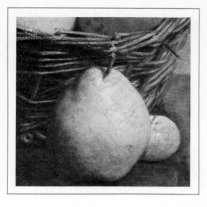

Americans are bombarded with messages urging the consumption of vitamin-mineral pills. According to the supplement merchants, almost everyone needs them, including picky eaters, athletes, business people, students, women taking birth control pills, elderly individuals living on limited funds, and anyone who feels tired. Vitamin-mineral supplements bring their purveyors more than a billion dollars per year, due at least in part to effective advertising.

Do most Americans *need* to take vitamin-mineral supplements? Are foods depleted of these nutrients by the time they reach our supermarkets? Does dependence on highly processed foods and foods from fast-food restaurants mean that one must turn to pills to obtain needed nutrients? *Can* vitamin-mineral pills make up for poor food habits? Do we need to take them daily to protect ourselves against the stress of living in our fast-moving society?

Megadoses (large doses in pill form) of specific vitamins have been advocated by some for prevention or treatment of varying disorders—from the common cold to heart disease. Do specific studies support these claims? Can harm result from megadoses?

Chapters 9, 10, and 11 address these questions as they relate to vitamins, while Chapters 12 and 13 discuss their relevance to minerals and water. To provide a solid basis for evaluating the issues raised by such questions, these chapters examine the important roles played by vitamins, minerals, and water in regulating body processes. Discussions of individual vitamins and minerals focus on specific food sources, results of deficiency, effects of overdosage, and amounts needed in the diets of normal young to middle-aged adults.

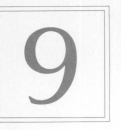

9

WATER-SOLUBLE VITAMINS: VITAMIN C

Vitamin C captured the fancy of many Americans in 1970 when Dr. Linus Pauling, a Nobel Prize-winning chemist, advocated large doses for the prevention of colds [1]. Until that time, interest in this vitamin had waned because scurvy, the deficiency disease associated with lack of vitamin C, ceased to be a public health problem after the mid-1930s. This chapter takes a look at how the body metabolizes vitamin C, how this vitamin functions in body tissues, what happens in a deficiency, controversies about how much is needed, and research on whether or not large doses are useful in preventing or treating colds and other disorders.

What *are* vitamins? *Vitamins* are defined as organic compounds (other than amino acids, fatty acids, or carbohydrates) that are required *in the diet* of animals *in small amounts* for normal growth, maintenance, and development of the body. Vitamins are not sources of energy, but each is indispensable for normal functioning of certain body tissues. The lack of a specific vitamin in tissues produces a specific disorder which is completely corrected by giving the pure vitamin.

Not every animal requires all the known vitamins in the diet. For example, the laboratory rat can synthesize all the vitamin C it needs; thus vitamin C is not a vitamin for the rat.

Those vitamins soluble in water, discussed in this chapter and Chapter 10, include vitamin C and the B vitamins (thiamine, riboflavin, niacin, vitamin B_6, pantothenic acid, folacin, vitamin B_{12}, and biotin). Water-soluble vitamins differ from fat-soluble ones (vitamins A, D, E, and K, discussed in Chapter 11) in that water-soluble vitamins can be lost when cooking water in which they dissolve is discarded. They also differ in that they do not require bile for absorption, they are absorbed via the portal vein, they are not stored in body tissues (except for vitamin B_{12}), and excessive intakes are excreted in the urine. Fat-soluble vitamins, on the other hand, do not dissolve in cooking water, they require bile for absorption, they are absorbed via the lymphatic system and are stored in the body, and they are not excreted in the urine.

Some popular writings claim, erroneously, that certain other substances are vitamins (see Box 9-1). No substance is considered to be a vitamin until an essential function is established for it in animal tissues. In addition, some animal must require it in the diet.

VITAMIN C (ASCORBIC ACID)

Scurvy, the disease resulting from lack of vitamin C, is known to have existed as far back as 1500 B.C. [7]. In the severest form of scurvy, the body seems to literally "fall apart" as degeneration of blood vessel walls, bones, skin, muscle tissues, gums, and teeth occur. Hemorrhaging develops and death ensues if vitamin C is not given in time. James Lind, a physician in the British navy, performed one of the earliest controlled experiments in human nutrition when he divided 12 sailors suffering from scurvy into six groups of two each. Each pair received a different dietary supplement, except for a control group that received none. Those fed oranges or lemons recovered dramatically, while the condition of the remaining subjects continued to deteriorate [8]. Lind's study, published in 1753, contributed to a body of knowledge that enabled Captain James Cook to keep his sailors free of scurvy during his historic voyages of 1772–1775. At every port, Cook ordered his men to bring on board green vegetables and local fruits [9]. Tragically, this information failed to become widely recognized; as late as 1912 all members of a team of explorers headed by Captain Robert Scott died at the South Pole from scurvy [10].

By 1912, scientists referred to the scurvy-preventing substance in fruits and vegetables as "antiscorbutin" or the "scurvy vitamine" [11], and in 1918 this substance was called, for the first time, vitamin C. Little was known about the characteristics of the substance, however, until Albert Szent-Györgyi, working in Hungary, isolated a substance from the adrenal glands of oxen which he called hexuronic acid. By 1932, Szent-Györgyi proved that hexuronic acid was "antiscorbutin" and, soon after, he named the substance *ascorbic acid*, from "anti*scorbutic* factor" [12]. Szent-Györgyi later received the Nobel Prize for his discovery of vitamin C, although Waugh and King in the United States simultaneously proved that a substance they had isolated from lemon juice was "antiscorbutin" [13].

9-1 BOX False Vitamins

Popular books and articles sometimes extol the virtues of "vitamin B_{17}," "vitamin B_{15}," and "vitamin P." Let's examine some of the claims along with the scientific findings regarding these substances.

Laetrile ("Vitamin B_{17}") Laetrile, proposed as a cancer cure, has been the source of much controversy. Several states have legalized it for cancer treatment even though its safety and usefulness have never been proved. Laetrile (amygdalin), obtained from apricot pits and other stone fruits, is made up of glucose, benzaldehyde, and cyanide [2]. Its advocates claim that laetrile attacks only cancer cells, and that normal cells detoxify the poisonous cyanide, which is then excreted by the kidneys. However, a carefully executed study of laetrile treatment in 178 cancer patients recently reported no cures, improvement, or stabilization of cancer and no extension of the life span in cancer patients [3]. Patients in this study did show evidence of cyanide poisoning, contrary to the claims made by proponents, indicating the inability of body cells to detoxify cyanide. This confirms previous reports of laetrile poisoning [2,3].

The medical profession views laetrile as a "fake cancer cure [2]." In no sense can this substance be considered a vitamin, even though one of its proponents has called it "vitamin B_{17}." Bona fide medical and nutrition scientists recognize no "vitamin B_{17}." The controversy about laetrile use for cancer treatment pits those who believe individuals should be able to choose any form of treatment—even if not proved effective—against those who believe that public health is protected by prohibiting forms of treatment until their effectiveness and lack of harmful side effects have been demonstrated.

Pangamic Acid ("Vitamin B_{15}") Pangamic acid has been lauded "as a possible cure for everything short of a transit strike [4]." Its proponents claim that it promotes the supply of oxygen to tissues, stimulates the glands and nervous system, and is useful in treating cancer, circulatory diseases, asthma, rheumatism, aging, diabetes, schizophrenia, and alcoholism! Yet pangamic acid is a substance for which no accepted scientific evidence establishes that it plays any role at all in the body. In fact, there is no definite chemical substance that *is* pangamic acid, for a number of products of variable composition have been called by that name [4]. A recent report indicates that some of the pangamic acids may cause genetic mutations, thereby increasing the chances of inherited disorders that may lead to serious disability or death in future generations [5]. The Food and Drug Administration has declared it illegal to sell pangamic acid as a dietary supplement or as a drug [4].

Bioflavonoids ("Vitamin P") Bioflavonoids, including rutin, hesperidin, citrin, and quercetin, unlike pangamic acid and laetrile, are substances that *do* participate in normal metabolism. They have some antioxidant effects, protecting vitamin C and other plant substances from oxidative destruction [6]. However, although claims have been made that these substances are useful in treatment of heart or circulatory diseases, rheumatic fever, cancer, and arthritis, no accepted scientific evidence establishes any therapeutic role for bioflavonoids. Bioflavonoids are not considered to be vitamins because *there is no evidence that they are required in the diet.* (The body synthesizes all that is needed.) The term "vitamin P" was officially withdrawn in 1950 when scientists agreed that these substances are not vitamins [6].

Certain other substances are known to be growth factors for bacteria and other lower forms of life, but are not required in human diets because the body synthesizes them. These include *coenzyme Q* (ubiquinone), *para-aminobenzoic acid*, and *carnitine*. The only known use the body has for *para*-aminobenzoic acid is as an essential component of folacin, one of the B vitamins. The human body cannot synthesize folacin even if a great deal of *para*-aminobenzoic acid is consumed, therefore no known benefit accrues from consuming this substance. Claims that it prevents gray hair in humans have not been substantiated. It is an ingredient of some sunscreens that are applied to the skin surface, but does not act as a vitamin in these preparations.

You have been warned previously that proponents of the newest diets and dietary supplements are usually out to gain financial profits. One should be skeptical of claims that dietary supplements are effective in treating or preventing a long list of disorders. Furthermore, you can begin to use your growing knowledge of nutrition to help you decide how well the scientific evidence supports claims made for a product.

Functions

Although the manifestations of scurvy can be described in great detail, we still do not understand exactly how vitamin C works in body tissues. It is likely that it operates in several different ways. Vitamin C is a small molecule resembling glucose which is active in two forms: ascorbic acid and dehydroascorbic acid (Figure 9-1). (The prefix *dehydro* means absence of hydrogen.) The conversion of one form of active vitamin C to the other is an example of an oxidation-reduction or *redox* reaction. *Oxidation* occurs when an atom or molecule *loses* one or more hydrogens or electrons. *Reduction* occurs when an atom or molecule *gains* one or more hydrogens or electrons. Many functions of vitamin C are believed to be related to its participation in oxidation-reduction reactions in body tissues.

Antioxidant Properties Many substances in foods and in the body are destroyed or damaged if they become oxidized. Frequently, such substances are protected against oxidation by antioxidants. An *antioxidant* is a substance that protects another from oxidation by itself becoming oxidized. Vitamin C, because of its antioxidant properties, is often added to foods to prevent oxidative changes—for

FIGURE 9-1. The two active forms of vitamin C, ascorbic acid and dehydroascorbic acid, are interconvertible. Diketogulonic acid, an inactive form produced by the oxidation of dehydroascorbic acid, cannot be converted to active forms.

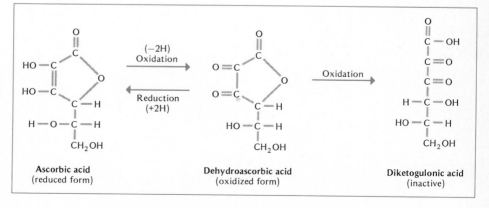

example, it prevents cut fruits such as peaches or apples from darkening when exposed to air. In the body, vitamin C is thought to protect linoleic acid, other polyunsaturated fatty acids, vitamin E, and vitamin A from oxidation [7]. This is an important function because polyunsaturated fatty acids and vitamin E are essential for maintaining the integrity of cellular membranes (see Chapter 4).

Collagen Formation   The most important function of vitamin C appears to be in the formation of collagen, a protein found in connective tissue. Connective tissue consists of insoluble collagen fibers embedded in a continuous matrix called ground substance. Connective tissue is found in skin, cartilage, tendons, ligaments, bone, and blood vessels. Scar tissue also is made up of a high proportion of collagen.

Collagen, like other proteins, is made up of amino acids joined together in a specific sequence. This protein is the only one in the body that contains many molecules of the amino acids *hydroxyproline* and *hydroxylysine*. Even more unusual is the fact that the body first puts *proline* and *lysine* into the polypeptide chain, after which specific enzymes add an —OH group (hydroxyl group) to each proline, or to each lysine, forming hydroxyproline and hydroxylysine. Vitamin C is known to play a role in the *hydroxylation* of (addition of an —OH group to) proline and probably also of lysine.

One role played by vitamin C in this important process apparently involves the mineral iron. To understand this role calls for some background concerning ions, particularly those of iron. An *ion* is an atom or group of atoms carrying an electrical charge. Iron (Fe) frequently exists in one of two *ionic* forms: either as Fe^{2+}, the *ferrous* ion, having two positive charges, or as Fe^{3+}, the *ferric* ion, having three positive charges. In the Introduction to this book we pointed out that an atom has the same number of positively charged protons in its nucleus as it has electrons in the orbits around the nucleus. An atom therefore has no charge. The positive charges of the ferrous and ferric ions result from loss of valence electrons as shown in Figure 9-2.

The enzyme that hydroxylates proline during the collagen formation process requires vitamin C to maintain iron in the ferrous form, keeping the enzyme in its active form   [14], as indicated in Figure 9-3. The hydroxylation of lysine to produce hydroxylysine in collagen is believed to occur by a similar process

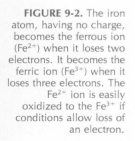

FIGURE 9-2. The iron atom, having no charge, becomes the ferrous ion (Fe^{2+}) when it loses two electrons. It becomes the ferric ion (Fe^{3+}) when it loses three electrons. The Fe^{2+} ion is easily oxidized to the Fe^{3+} if conditions allow loss of an electron.

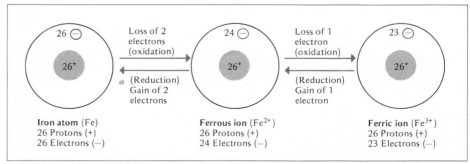

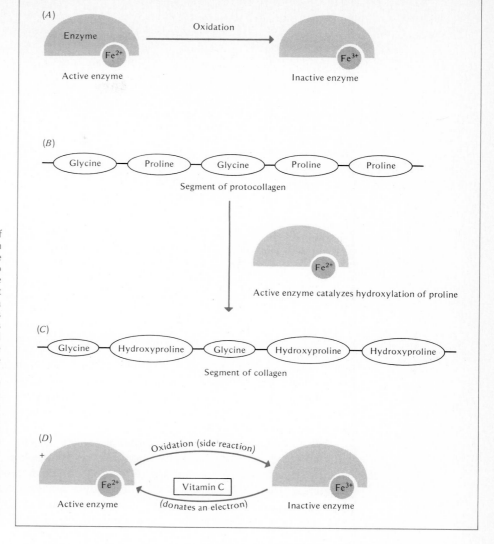

FIGURE 9-3. One role of vitamin C in collagen formation. (*A*) The enzyme needed to hydroxylate proline requires, for activity, that Fe^{2+} be attached at a specific site on its surface. (*B*) Body tissues form the amino acid chain containing large amounts of proline (called protocollagen). (*C*) The active enzyme hydroxylates proline molecules, forming the completed collagen. (*D*) The active enzyme then becomes free, but tissues can easily oxidize Fe^{2+} to Fe^{3+}, inactivating the enzyme. Vitamin C keeps the enzyme active by maintaining iron in the Fe^{2+} state on the enzyme's surface.

requiring ascorbic acid [15]. Vitamin C may play other roles—yet to be elucidated—in collagen formation.

Amino Acid Metabolism   Vitamin C is needed for other important hydroxylation reactions in the body. For example, in the brain vitamin C is required for the hydroxylation of dopamine (formed from the amino acid, tyrosine) to produce norepinephrine (noradrenaline), which can be converted to epinephrine (adrenaline). In addition, it is needed for the hydroxylation of tryptophan to form 5-hydroxytryptophan, the first step in serotonin formation. Both serotonin and norepinephrine are *neurotransmitters*—that is, sustances secreted by nervous

TABLE 9-1. FOOD COMBINATIONS SUPPLYING 250 mg VITAMIN C

	mg
Broccoli, 1 small stalk	126
Green pepper, ½ pod, raw	105
Tomato juice, ½ c	20
Total	251
Cantaloupe, half of a 5-in. diameter melon	90
Brussels sprouts, 4	73
Orange, 1 whole	66
Baked potato	31
Total	260
Collard greens, ½ c	72
Grapefruit (Pink Foster), ½	67
Cauliflower, ½ c, raw	45
Strawberries, ½ c	44
Baked sweet potato	25
Total	253

SOURCE: Adams, C.F., *Nutritive Value of American Foods,* Agriculture Handbook No. 456, Washington, D.C.: U.S. Department of Agriculture, 1975.

tissue which transmit impulses between nerve cells. Norepinephrine and epinephrine are also formed in the adrenal glands by the same process as in the brain. (When secreted by the adrenals, these substances act as hormones.) It isn't yet clear whether or not vitamin C's role in these hydroxylation reactions is the same as in collagen formation.

We frequently associate the hormones of the adrenal medulla (the inner portion of the adrenal glands), epinephrine and norephinephrine, with stress because physical stress or strong emotional states trigger release of these hormones. Their release increases the body's ability to perform strenuous physical activity—"the fight or flight" mechanism. Since vitamin C is required in the synthesis of norepinephrine, stressful situations might be thought to increase the rate at which vitamin C is utilized, increasing the need in the diet. Yet, not all forms of stress seem to increase the need for this vitamin. For example, when soldiers were subjected to the stress of sleeplessness, cold, high-altitude deprivation of oxygen, and vigorous exercise, they did not metabolize vitamin C more rapidly than in normal situations [16,17]. On the other hand, some types of stress such as infections, the trauma of surgery, and severe burns reduce blood and tissue vitamin C levels, increasing the dietary need. Some surgeons routinely prescribe 100 to 250 mg daily before and after surgery. Although the amounts required for normal wound healing after surgery, and the increased need due to infections can be obtained from foods, therapeutic doses of 1 g daily are usually required by burn patients [18]. Table 9-1 indicates that amounts as high as 250 mg/day can easily be obtained from foods. The stresses of daily living in normal,

A CLOSER LOOK

Vitamin C is thought to enhance absorption of inorganic iron by forming a soluble *chelate* with iron, which is then absorbed [19]. Chelating agents are of such a structure that they can bond chemically with a metallic ion, holding it as if in a claw. (The word *chelate* comes from the Greek meaning claw.) Vitamin C chelates iron at the acid pH of the stomach, but the chelate remains soluble—and therefore absorbable—in the alkaline duodenum [19].

One possibility of how vitamin C may chelate inorganic iron is depicted in Figure 9-4. The interaction of vitamin C with iron is but one example of many important interrelationships of vitamins with minerals. Notice in this figure that the form of iron chelated is ferrous iron (FE^{2+}). This form is more easily absorbed than ferric iron (FE^{3+}); and vitamin C, because it readily participates in oxidation-reduction reactions, helps to keep iron in the ferrous state.

healthy individuals have not been demonstrated to increase the dietary need for vitamin C.

Blood Formation and Clotting. Vitamin C is indirectly involved in the formation of red blood cells. Hemoglobin is the iron-containing compound in red blood cells necessary for carrying oxygen to the tissues. Vitamin C enhances the absorption of inorganic iron and therefore indirectly influences the formation of hemoglobin by making iron available for its synthesis [20].

Vitamin C also aids in the formation of the active form of folacin, a B vitamin required for the synthesis of red blood cells (see Chapter 10). In addition, vitamin C may be required for blood clotting, although no mechanism for such action is known. In scurvy, however, clotting is impaired. Another indicator that it is involved in clotting is that large doses counteract the action of drugs such as heparin that are used to prevent blood clotting.

In the 1950s investigators noted that early signs in the blood vessels are similar in both atherosclerosis and scurvy. The suggestion was made that atherosclerosis might be considered a form of "localized scurvy" involving the connective tissue in the artery wall [29]. Despite the fact that conflicting results of studies related to vitamin C and atherosclerosis leave us with no assurance that

FIGURE 9-4. Vitamin C may form a soluble chelate with iron as shown here. When the chelate forms, vitamin C loses hydrogen ions (H^+) [19], leaving electrons with the oxygens, hence the minus charge on each oxygen. Because unlike charges attract one another, the ferrous ion is held between the two oxygens by ionic bonding (electrostatic force). Only a portion of the molecule displays the clawlike properties of a chelate.

generous intakes of this vitamin will result in healthy arteries, this is clearly a research area that merits further attention [29].

Deficiency

Scurvy occurs only among those few animals that are unable to synthesize vitamin C: human beings, monkeys and other primates, and guinea pigs. Early symptoms of deficiency in adults include fatigue, weakness, and listlessness. More severe deficiency results in many small hemorrhages (bleeding) around hair follicles, muscle aches and pains, swollen, painful joints, and swollen, bleeding gums where there are teeth. Eventually teeth loosen, the eyes, mouth, and skin become dry, and hair is lost. Large reddish, bluish, or black spots, similar to large bruises, appear chiefly on the legs and are the result of hemorrhaging. Old scars redden and wounds open again; new wounds fail to heal. Psychological abnormalities, such as depression and hysteria develop, due presumably to derangements in brain neurotransmitters [7]. The disease is fatal if vitamin C is not given in time.

Full-blown scurvy is rarely seen in the United States and other industrialized countries today. The cases occasionally seen in hospitals are chiefly among infants and the elderly. Infants, especially between 6 to 12 months old, may develop the disease if their diets are restricted to milk or milk formulas unsupplemented with fruits, vegetables, or vitamin C. Cases among the elderly occur most frequently in males who live alone. Typically, these men eat restricted diets including very few vegetables and fruits. Meats, breads, cereals, cookies, and cakes contain practically no vitamin C, and subsistence exclusively on such a diet can be expected to result in scurvy in about 3 months.

Absorption and Metabolism

Vitamin C is readily absorbed from the small intestines via the portal vein. It quickly spreads to all the body tissues, but becomes more concentrated in the adrenal glands, the lens of the eye, the pituitary gland, the brain, spleen, and pancreas [21] (Figure 9-5). Presumably the vitamin has some special functions in these tissues, but scientists have little information about those functions, as we have seen.

Body tissues are capable of holding up to a certain "ceiling" amount of vitamin C. Once the ceiling is reached, the tissues are said to be *saturated*. Any additional vitamin C reaching the tissues after saturation is achieved is excreted in the urine.

Levels of vitamin C in the blood may be used as one means of assessing nutritional status (deciding how well-nourished an individual is regarding this vitamin). On a low dietary intake, tissue levels gradually fall, which is reflected in the blood levels. Signs of scurvy develop when blood levels fall to the range of 0.13 to 0.24 mg/100 mL for a period of time [22]. Routine consumption of the RDA of 60 mg/day maintains blood levels at about 0.75 mg/100 mL [23], while routine intakes of 100 to 200 mg/day saturate the tissues and raise blood levels to the ceiling of 1.5 mg/100 mL. Higher intakes than required to saturate the tissues

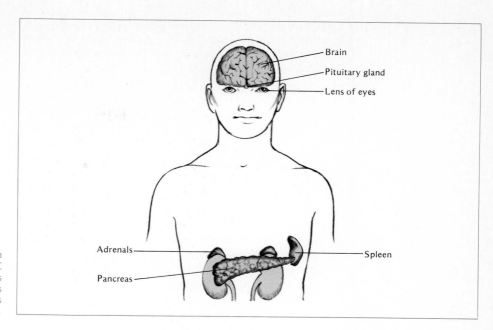

FIGURE 9-5. Upon
absorption, vitamin C
spreads to all the cells
but becomes
concentrated in the areas
shown.

fail to raise blood levels above the ceiling because absorption declines as the intake increases while at the same time the excessive amounts absorbed are readily excreted in the urine. It has been reported that only 70 percent of a 180-mg intake, 50 percent of a 1500-mg dose, and 16 percent of a 12,000-mg dose is absorbed [24].

Urinary excretion of unmetabolized vitamin C falls to low levels as deficiency develops. If deficient individuals are given a single dose of vitamin C, they excrete little of it in the urine because their tissues take it up avidly. In deficiency, vitamin C in the white blood cells falls to a very low level, indicating that little vitamin C remains in body tissues. Thus, vitamin C in the blood, urine, and white blood cells all may be determined when assessing an individual's nutritional status regarding this vitamin. Values indicating deficiency appear in Appendix J.

Two urinary excretion products formed in vitamin C catabolism are oxalic acid and ascorbic acid sulfate. Individuals apparently vary considerably in the amount of oxalic acid they form from vitamin C. These excretion products are usually not helpful in evaluating vitamin C status.

Food Sources

As already indicated, vegetables and fruits are the principal contributors of vitamin C to the diet. Liver is unique among animal foods as a source of vitamin C. A few unusual sources such as acerola cherries have become familiar to health food users in recent years, but use of these sources is expensive and unnecessary, as large amounts can easily be obtained from traditional vegetables and fruits (Table 9-1 and Appendix C).

Cooked vegetables generally are lower in vitamin C than raw ones. Vitamin C is subject to losses not only due to its solubility in water but also from heat, exposure to air, enzyme action, and contact with metals such as copper or iron. Practical suggestions for preserving vitamin C and other vitamins and minerals in preparing and cooking foods at home appear in Box 10-2, Chapter 10. Including some raw vegetables or fruits in the diet each day helps to ensure an adequate intake of vitamin C.

The Need for Vitamin C

Controversy exists over how much vitamin C the body needs. The disagreement centers on differing opinions of the amount that is *optimal*—that amount that is most favorable for good health. Some scientists believe the intake should be high enough to saturate the tissues—100 to 200 mg/day—while others believe that good health is maintained at lower intakes. Still others argue that the amount needed is so large that it can be obtained only in pill form. This section considers the rationale behind the RDAs for vitamin C as well as arguments for recommending higher intakes.

The RDAs The 1980 RDA for adults was set at 60 mg/day, although the 1974 RDA had been 45 mg/day. These amounts are far in excess of the 10 mg/day known to prevent scurvy. Using radioactive ascorbic acid, scientists have been able to study how much of this vitamin is held in body tissues (the body "ascorbate pool") and the rates at which it is metabolized and eliminated. These studies show that a daily intake of 60 mg allows body tissues to maintain an ascorbate pool large enough to protect the body against scurvy for a period of 30 to 45 days. An intake of 60 mg per day is assumed to be 85 percent absorbable. The Food and Nutrition Board justified their recommendation by pointing out that at higher intakes absorption becomes less efficient and the rate of excretion of unmetabolized vitamin C increases [23]. They believe, therefore, that 60 mg of vitamin C is reasonable for normal adults despite the fact that saturation of tissues is not maintained at this intake.

Several factors may increase the need for vitamin C. Cigarette smoking increases the rate at which vitamin C is metabolized, requiring a larger intake to maintain the same body pool as in nonsmokers [25]. Some investigators have reported that blood vitamin C levels are lowered by oral contraceptive drugs, but others have not found this to be the case. It may be that the blood level is lowered only in oral contraceptive users who consume relatively low amounts of the vitamin [26]. Large doses of aspirin, sometimes used in treating arthritis, for example, can increase the loss of vitamin C in the urine and therefore increase the dietary need [27]. Exposure to high temperatures during work also increased the intake needed to prevent a decrease in blood vitamin C levels in mine workers [28]. The increased need in all these cases can be met from dietary sources.

The RDAs for vitamin C at different ages and during pregnancy and lactation are shown in Appendix A. The RDA for the infant is based on the amount present in the breast milk of well-nourished mothers. On a weight basis, children need more vitamin C than adults, as the RDAs reflect. The fetus apparently takes up a rather large amount of vitamin C, especially in the last 6 months of pregnancy, accounting in part for the increased RDA for the mother during pregnancy. The amount of vitamin C in breast milk varies with the mother's dietary intake. The RDA during lactation is high enough to assure adequate levels for the mother and nursing infant [23].

Arguments for Higher Intakes   Some investigators believe that enough vitamin C should be consumed to keep the tissues saturated, since animals that synthesize their own vitamin C maintain a state of saturation [29]. The amount required for this purpose varies from about 100 to 200 mg/day, and is easily obtained from foods.

Contrasted with this view is the contention of Dr. Linus Pauling that optimal daily intakes for adults lie between 1 and 4 g (1000 to 4000 mg) [30]. He bases his recommendation on estimations that those animals that synthesize vitamin C produce about 10 g/day per 70 kg (154 lb) of body weight. Since intakes above 4 g/day tend to increase urinary oxalic acid excretion, escalating the risk for kidney stones, Pauling avoids suggesting more that 4 g daily for the general public [30]. Such large intakes cannot be obtained from food but must be obtained from pills or supplements (called megadosing).

If Pauling's hypothesis is correct, vibrant good health is impossible for people who subsist only on foods, without vitamin supplements, and is attainable only in affluent countries where people can easily obtain large quantities of vitamin C pills. Because it seems important to assess claims that the need is very large, let us examine studies of megadoses of vitamin C on colds and cancer.

Megadosing With Vitamin C

Vitamin C and Colds   Dr. Pauling popularized the notion that megadoses of vitamin C prevent or cure colds, despite the fact that little evidence supported his hypothesis at the time his book was published [1]. Since then, however, several large well-controlled studies have been published, none of which supports Pauling's specific claim that regular consumption of 1000 mg of vitamin C per day results in reduction in the number of colds by 45 percent and reduction in duration by 60 percent [31].

One of the most carefully executed studies was that of T. W. Anderson and colleagues at the University of Toronto [32]. The study was conducted during 14 weeks in the winter of 1972–1973 and included 818 adult volunteers. The subjects were instructed in how to keep a record of illnesses and were assigned randomly to the experimental group (receiving vitamin C) or the control group (receiving a well-disguised placebo). Subjects in the vitamin C group took 1000 mg/day until symptoms of any kind of illness developed, whereupon they took 4000 mg/day during the first 3 days of illness. The experiment was strictly double-blind—neither the investigators nor the subjects were aware of which group an individual belonged to until the study was completed.

Analysis of the results showed no greater incidence of colds in the placebo than in the vitamin C group. The only significant difference was that the vitamin

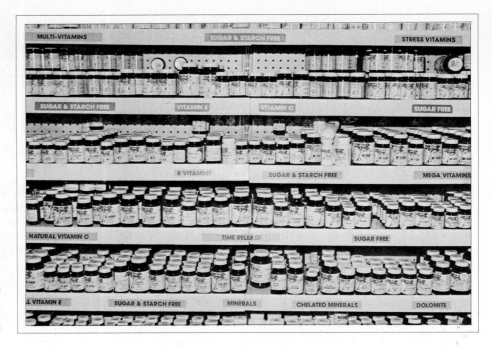

MULTI-VITAMINS   SUGAR & STARCH FREE   STRESS VITAMINS

SUGAR & STARCH FREE   VITAMIN E   VITAMIN C   SUGAR FREE

B VITAMINS   SUGAR & STARCH FREE   MEGA VITAMINS

NATURAL VITAMIN C   TIME RELEASE   SUGAR FREE

L VITAMIN E   SUGAR & STARCH FREE   MINERALS   CHELATED MINERALS   DOLOMITE

The ready availability of vitamin pills in health food stores, supermarkets, and drugstores leads many Americans to think of pills rather than foods as vitamin sources. *(Randy Matusow)*

group recorded 30 percent fewer days "confined to the house" for illness than did the placebo group. The investigators concluded that vitamin C somehow made subjects feel better so they did not miss so much work during illnesses [32].

Further research concerning vitamin C and colds needs to be done in populations with differing initial levels of vitamin C in their body pools [29]. There is evidence that vitamin C deficiency decreases immunity to viruses, and that white blood cells must maintain sufficient concentrations of this vitamin to combat infections [27]. Groups of people having low body ascorbate pools are apt to respond differently to large doses than those initially having an adequate body pool.

Although Dr. Pauling has not conducted studies himself in the area of vitamin C and colds, he should be credited with having generated a great deal of scientific interest and research in the functions and uses of vitamin C.

Vitamin C and Cancer Dr. Pauling aroused interest in a possible relationship of vitamin C to cancer when he published a study in which terminal cancer patients treated with 10 g/day of vitamin C were reported to have survived longer than untreated patients [33]. There was no placebo group in this study, however. In a more carefully controlled study, the vitamin C group showed no greater survival time than the placebo group, and no difference in symptoms, appetite, or weight [34].

There are good reasons to continue research in vitamin C and cancer, however, since most of the patients in the more recent study had received previous therapy which reduced their immunocompetence (ability to combat foreign substances). Vitamin C may play an important role in developing immunocompetence, for in scurvy the body is less able to protect itself against infections and other foreign substances. In addition, tumor tissue avidly takes up vitamin C from the blood, which results in lowered levels in the blood serum and white blood cells [27]. Theoretically, this situation could lead to depletion of vitamin C in normal body tissues, and decrease the ability to combat cancer growth.

Another reason to continue research in vitamin C and cancer is that it is possible that vitamin C may be able to prevent formation of carcinogenic (cancer-causing) substances. For example, nitrosamines are known carcinogens that may be present in some foods, such as cooked bacon, or they may form in the intestinal tract from a reaction between nitrites and amines (see Box 17-2, Chapter 17). Nitrites may be consumed in cured meats, or may be formed in the body from nitrites present in many foods. Amines are also present in many foods and drugs, making it theoretically easy for nitrites to combine with them. Vitamin C appears to prevent the formation of nitrosamines from nitrites and amines [35]. Further work is needed to establish the extent to which routine consumption of vitamin C in foods prevents the formation of nitrosamines and other carcinogens.

Are Large Doses Harmful?   Although many people have consumed 2 g or more of vitamin C daily for long periods without apparent detrimental effects, there are reasons to be concerned about prolonged ingestion of megadoses [36]. Doses above 5000 mg/day frequently result in nausea, vomiting, or diarrhea. Large doses also cause the urine to become acid, circumstances in which uric acid or cystine kidney stones may develop in people who are predisposed to one of these kinds of stones. Since part of the vitamin C catabolized in the body is converted to oxalic acid, large doses also increase the possibility of formation of oxalate kidney stones in susceptible people [37]. Common tests for glucose in the urine, blood in the feces, and diagnosis of gout may be erroneous if large doses of vitamin C are taken [24]. Finally, the body may become conditioned to large doses so that if the dosage is stopped abruptly, the blood levels drop precipitously and some deficiency signs may develop. This situation has been reported in both adults and in newborn infants whose mothers took large doses during pregnancy [38]. Apparently this happens because taking large doses increases the activity of an enzyme that destroys vitamin C. On sudden cessation of the large dosage, the enzyme continues its rapid destruction of the vitamin [24]. Further research is needed in this area, however, since few studies have been reported. It seems advisable when one stops taking large doses to gradually reduce the dosage over a matter of days or weeks to allow the body to adapt to the lower intake.

Although reports that large doses of vitamin C destroy vitamin B_{12} in the body have been disputed [39], a few cases of the anemia characteristic of vitamin B_{12} deficiency have been reported in users of large doses of vitamin C [24]. Further research is needed on this question.

What amount of vitamin C makes sense, then? First, one should realize that megadoses probably act as a drug and not as a vitamin. A safe rule to follow would be to obtain vitamin C from traditional fruits and vegetables. Amounts between 100 to 200 mg/day can be obtained this way if one wishes to keep body tissues saturated. Higher intakes have not been demonstrated to provide clear benefits. During illnesses, one might take about 500 mg/day, but higher doses are not recommended as a routine practice because unforeseen detrimental consequences may result [29].

And what is one to think about the ongoing controversy concerning vitamin C? As one of the investigators in this field, Dr. T. W. Anderson of the University of Toronto points out, one could become extreme either by believing any claim made, or by refusing to believe any of them. Neither position is sensible because the first indicates that one is gullible and uncritical, while the other indicates that one opposes progress in exploring issues. Dr. Anderson's view is a reasonable one: that "we should aim to be open-minded but not naive; skeptical, but not cynical" [29].

SUMMARY

An overview of this vitamin appears in Table 9-2.

1 Vitamin C (ascorbic acid) is the antiscorbutic vitamin (it prevents scurvy).
2 Its functions in the body are incompletely understood, but it appears to participate in oxidation-reduction reactions and act as an antioxidant. It is known to be involved in the formation of collagen, in the absorption of inorganic iron, and in metabolism of certain amino acids.
3 The most important food sources are citrus fruits and certain other fruits and vegetables.
4 Controversy surrounds the intake of vitamin C thought to be optimal for good health. The RDA is less than is required to saturate the tissues, but is well above the amount needed to prevent scurvy. Yet some have argued that megadoses, obtainable only from pills, should be consumed daily.

5 Although megadoses have not been established by carefully executed scientific studies to prevent or cure colds or to be efficacious in cancer treatment, further research is warranted. As a drug (when given in large doses), this vitamin may improve the well-being of patients suffering from certain infections or disabilities. Megadoses in normal healthy individuals appear to be unwarranted.

FOR DISCUSSION AND APPLICATION

1 Make up a questionnaire to determine how many students in your class currently take vitamin pills.
  a. What vitamins at what dosages are in the pills?
  b. How many take only vitamin C and not other vitamins?
  c. What reasons do students give for taking the pills?

TABLE 9-2. AN OVERVIEW OF VITAMIN C

NAME	FOOD SOURCES	FUNCTIONS	DEFICIENCY SYMPTOMS	RDA FOR ADULTS (PER DAY)	ADVERSE EFFECTS (MEGADOSES)
Vitamin C (ascorbic acid)	Broccoli, Brussels sprouts, citrus fruits, tomatoes, strawberries, cabbage, cauliflower, dark green leafy vegetables, melons.	Collagen synthesis, facilitates absorption of inorganic iron, synthesis of neurotransmitters from tyrosine and tryptophan, aids in formation of active form of folacin, acts as an antioxidant.	Hemorrhages under skin, into joints and around teeth; anemia; arrested wound healing; psychological depression. *Scurvy*	60 mg	Diarrhea; risk of kidney stones; obscures some laboratory tests.

d. If someone says: "I haven't had a cold since I started taking vitamin C tablets," does that prove that vitamin C prevents colds? Explain your answer.

2 From your dietary record, compare your intake of vitamin C with the RDA. What were the best sources of this vitamin in your diet?

SUGGESTED READINGS

The Editors of Consumers Guide, *The Vitamin Book*, New York: Simon and Schuster, 1979. A highly readable discussion of vitamins, including information about food sources. Intended for the general reader.

Herbert, V., and S. Barrett, *Vitamins and "Health" Foods: The Great American Hustle*, Philadelphia: George F. Stickley Co., 1981. Written by physician-nutritionists who wish to counteract unsubstantiated claims made about vitamins and certain "health" foods.

Rolman, E., *Is Your Neighborhood Pharmacy Misleading You?* Environmental Nutrition Newsletter 5(3, Supplement): S–2 and S–3, 1982. A registered dietitian found through informal inquiry that pharmacists may give out inaccurate information about vitamin supplements.

10

WATER-SOLUBLE VITAMINS: B VITAMINS

Antonia wonders whether or not she should take vitamin B$_6$ pills, since she is taking an oral contraceptive drug. Ricardo asks whether or not megadoses of B vitamins are useful in schizophrenia. Michelle wants to know if taking vitamin pills will help make up for her haphazard eating habits (she works 30 h a week in addition to being a student). Mei-Ling observes that strict vegetarians she knows never seem to have any obvious signs of vitamin B$_{12}$ deficiency and wonders why. These are all questions posed by students before beginning their study of the B vitamins. These and other questions will be addressed in this chapter.

The B vitamins are those listed in Table 10-1. They enable body tissues to obtain energy from the metabolism of carbohydrates, fats, and proteins, but they are not themselves oxidized to produce energy. Furthermore, some B vitamins are essential in the synthesis of red blood cells which transport oxygen to the cells.

TABLE 10-1. THE B VITAMINS

OFFICIAL NAME*	ALTERNATIVE NAMES
Thiamine	Vitamin B_1, aneurin
Riboflavin	Vitamin B_2, vitamin G (obsolete)
Niacin	Niacinamide, nicotinamide, nicotinic acid
Vitamin B_6	Pyridoxine, pyridoxal, pyridoxamine
Pantothenic acid	Vitamin B_5 (obsolete)
Folacin	Folic acid, folate
Vitamin B_{12}	Cobalamin
Biotin	Vitamin H (obsolete)

*The names for B vitamins used in this text are those agreed upon by the International Union of Nutrition Sciences Committee on Nomenclature. Alternative names are listed here because these frequently appear in journals, books, and magazines.

SOURCE: "Nomenclature Policy: Generic Descriptors and Trivial Names for Vitamins and Related Compounds," *The Journal of Nutrition,* 109:8, 1979.

Since the cells require oxygen for energy production, this is an additional way in which B vitamins are involved in energy metabolism.

If body tissues are *deficient* in B vitamins, they fail to produce sufficient energy and the individual feels tired and listless. If the tissues are already saturated with B vitamins, however, taking additional supplements will not increase the amount of energy one obtains from carbohydrate, fat, or protein oxidation. If individuals report feeling "more energetic" as a result of taking B vitamin supplements, one would need to rule out the placebo effect before believing their assertion (see Box 5-1, Chapter 5). In other words, individuals who *expect* vitamin B supplements to make them feel "more energetic" are apt to report that they do so. Yet, they might report the same effect if they were given a "dummy pill" (a placebo) that they *thought* contained the B vitamins (see Box 7-2, Chapter 7).

How do the B vitamins function in energy metabolism? They act as *coenzymes* which are necessary for activity of many enzymes that catalyze oxidation of carbohydrates, fats, and proteins. Coenzymes are small organic molecules containing as part of their structure one of the B vitamins. Normal body tissues form coenzymes, provided sufficient amounts of the needed vitamins are in the food consumed. Coenzymes bind to the surface of those enzymes that require them, forming active complexes called *holoenzymes* (Figure 10-1). The enzyme itself (the apoenzyme) is inactive without the coenzyme. This chapter discusses specific ways in which coenzymes containing each of the B vitamins function in the metabolism of carbohydrates, fats, and protein. What happens when tissues lack each of the coenzymes is also considered. In addition, amounts needed in the diet, food sources, and adverse effects of large doses are discussed.

How do scientists determine how well-nourished individuals are regarding B vitamins? Originally, vitamins were recognized because deficiency diseases developed in populations receiving too little of them in their diets. In assessing vitamin nutritional status, one needs to realize that deficiency diseases are the end

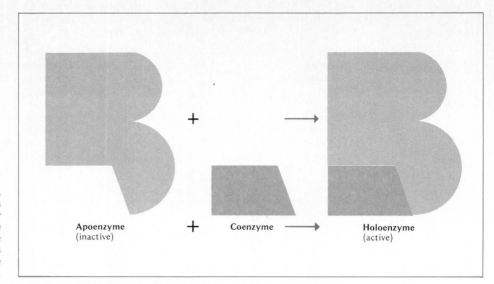

FIGURE 10-1.
B vitamins act as
coenzymes for many
enzymes. The enzyme
is inactive until the
coenzyme combines
with it, forming the
active or holoenzyme.

result of a gradual process of tissue depletion of the nutrient or nutrients in question. In the first stage of deficiency (mild deficiency), the body pool of a vitamin (that amount held in body tissues) becomes depleted (Figure 10-2). In the second stage, changes develop in specific enzyme systems, resulting in improper functioning of some metabolic pathways. This is a state of moderate deficiency and can be detected by biochemical changes in blood or other tissues and by low urinary excretion of the vitamin or its *metabolites* (products formed by metabolism of the vitamin in body tissues). At this stage, symptoms tend to be nonspecific and may include tiredness and irritability. Finally, anatomic changes become visible to the naked eye, and eventually a full-blown deficiency disease such as beriberi (thiamine deficiency) or pellagra (niacin deficiency) develops (Figure 10-2). The time required for a fully developed deficiency disease to manifest itself

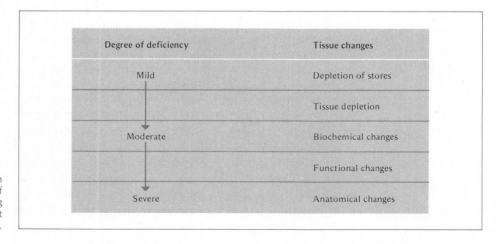

FIGURE 10-2. Stages in
the development of
deficiencies, illustrating
the gradual development
of disease.

depends upon the level of the vitamin originally present in tissues, how much of the vitamin reaches the tissue daily, and the rate at which the vitamin is metabolized and excreted.

It is important to realize that vitamin deficiencies can develop for a variety of reasons. An obvious cause is an inadequate intake, but, less obviously, a low intake can result from ignorance, loss of appetite due to psychological problems or a chronic disease, following food fads, cultural prohibitions (see Chapter 1), or dental problems. Failure to absorb vitamins occurs when the intestinal mucosa is severely damaged by disease (celiac disease, sprue, cystic fibrosis) or when disease or disability results in insufficient secretion of gastric or other digestive juices. Inadequate *utilization* (or usage) of the vitamin by cells may occur as a result of certain diseases (alcoholism results in inadequate utilization of folacin, for example). In addition, periods of rapid growth, presence of infections, or use of certain therapeutic drugs increase the dietary requirement for certain vitamins. Other dietary components or interactions with other vitamins may also influence the utilization of a vitamin. For each of the B vitamins, commonly observed circumstances in which deficiencies develop are discussed in this chapter.

Another important point is that deficiency diseases such as beriberi and pellagra, as they have developed in population groups, are complex deficiencies. In other words, while one can pinpoint a specific vitamin deficiency responsible for many of the manifestations of the disease, other B vitamin deficiencies occurring at the same time account for other signs and symptoms. This occurs because diets that produce deficiency diseases may be inadequate in or entirely lacking a whole food group. Thus, several nutrients are apt to be low in the diet, not just one.

Many people take vitamin supplements "just as insurance." Box 10-1 addresses the question of whether you can depend on pills to make up for a poorly chosen diet.

THIAMINE

Beriberi, the disease now known to result when thiamine is excluded from the diet, was described by the Chinese as long ago as 2600 B.C. [2]. Historically, the disease occurred chiefly in parts of the world where white (polished) rice formed a major part of the diet. White rice has had the bran and germ removed in the milling process. Eijkman, a physician working in the 1890s in the Dutch East Indies, made an important contribution toward solving the mystery of beriberi through his observations that fowls fed white rice developed symptoms resembling beriberi in human beings. He cured these birds by feeding them the rice husks (or bran) removed in the rice-polishing process. Eijkman attributed the disease to a poison in the white rice that could be counteracted by an unknown substance in the rice husks [2]. Scientists at that time lacked the concept that sickness could result from the *absence* of a nutrient in the diet. By 1901, however, another Dutch physician, Grijns, suggested that beriberi was due to the lack of a substance present in rice bran. Researchers attempted to isolate the pure substance from rice bran, and finally succeeded in 1927 [2].

Relatively inexpensive vitamin and mineral supplements have been heavily promoted by manufacturers since the 1940s in western industrialized countries. As a result, many people routinely take a supplement daily "just to be sure," or because, as one stated, "I lead such a hectic life that I don't eat as well as I should, so I take vitamin pills."

Can one rely upon pills to make up for a poor diet? There are many reasons that a poor diet plus vitamin-mineral supplements cannot add up to an adequate diet. First, vitamin and/or mineral supplements fail to contain all those nutrients known to be needed by the human body. Second, it is possible that some nutrients needed by the body are yet to be discovered. Consuming a wide variety of traditional, minimally processed foods is the only way to obtain any such nutrients. Third, a poorly planned diet may be low in dietary fiber or essential nutrients such as linoleic acid or an amino acid. Such deficiencies cannot be remedied by taking vitamin or mineral pills. A person whose lifestyle is so busy that too little time and effort are devoted to obtaining an adequate diet has placed very low priority on food and its relationship to health. The remedy is to reassess one's priorities, allowing sufficient time and effort to nourish oneself by a judicious choice of foods.

A diet based chiefly upon minimally processed, traditional foods is more likely to provide all the nutrients needed than one based on highly processed foods. For example, whole grains contain many B vitamins and minerals that are not present in highly milled white grains, even if enriched (Box 3-1, Chapter 3).

Many people spend large amounts of money for so-called "natural" vitamins. These are supposedly obtained by isolating them from food as opposed to synthesizing them in the laboratory. Most purchasers of "natural" vitamins do not realize that: (1) body tissues cannot tell the difference between synthetic and "natural" vitamins, since chemically they are exactly the same; (2) synthetic vitamins are far less expensive than those isolated from food; and (3) "natural" vitamin supplements contain insignificant amounts of vitamins isolated from foods, but are made up chiefly of synthetic vitamins [1]. The obvious message is that if you insist upon taking vitamin pills, you are probably wasting money if you buy "natural" vitamins.

For those who, for feelings of security, have established the habit of consuming supplements, choosing a multivitamin supplement that supplies not more than 100 percent of the RDA for each nutrient probably can do no harm. But one should not assume that taking pills exonerates one from planning and consuming an adequate diet. A diet based upon a wide variety of traditional, minimally processed foods is by far the superior method for obtaining needed vitamins and minerals.

Functions

Thiamine, after absorption by way of the portal vein, circulates rapidly throughout the fluid compartments of the body, and becomes more concentrated in liver, heart, kidney, brain, and skeletal muscles than in other tissues.

Within the cells, thiamine is converted to its coenzyme forms, the most important of which is thiamine pyrophosphate (TPP). TPP consists of thiamine with two phosphate groups (containing the mineral phosphorus), attached. This coenzyme is needed for the normal function of enzyme systems required for the oxidation of carbohydrates. An example of how TPP functions involves the conversion of pyruvate to acetyl CoA, a necessary step for the entry of acetyl CoA into the Krebs cycle, referred to in Figure 3-18, Chapter 3. Recall from Figure 3-18 that when pyruvate, a 3-carbon compound, is converted to acetyl CoA (containing two carbons), pyruvate loses a molecule of carbon dioxide (CO_2).

Figure 10-3 indicates that TPP is a coenzyme for pyruvate decarboxylase, the enzyme responsible for the removal of CO_2 from pyruvate when it is converted to acetyl CoA. TPP actually attaches itself to pyruvate in this reaction. A molecule of carbon dioxide (CO_2) is then removed from pyruvate, and TPP transfers the resulting 2-carbon compound to a nearby compound called lipoic acid. After the transfer, TPP returns to its original state, ready to take on more pyruvate. Eventually the 2-carbon compound picked up by lipoic acid becomes acetyl CoA. Since acetyl CoA is essential in carbohydrate metabolism for operation of the Krebs cycle, the importance of the B vitamins in its formation becomes evident. Other points in metabolism which require TPP are shown in Figure 10-13.

Deficiency

As is the case in most vitamin deficiency diseases, scientists do not understand thoroughly why specific symptoms develop in thiamine deficiency. One of the early signs of deficiency is loss of appetite. As the deficiency becomes more

FIGURE 10-3. Simplified representation of a function of TPP in carbohydrate metabolism.

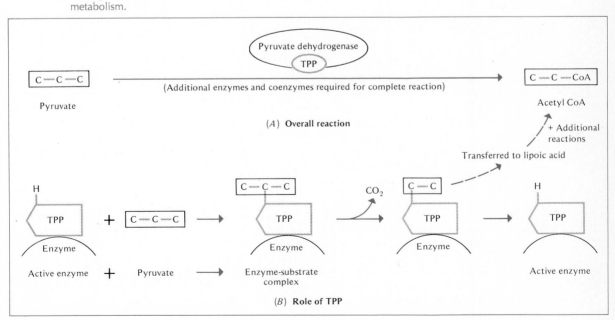

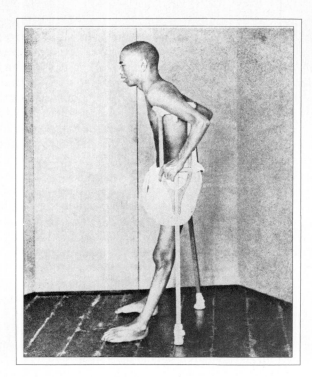

A patient with beriberi who is unable to walk without crutches. *(National Library of Medicine)*

severe, nausea, vomiting, and constipation develop. Loss of muscle tone in the intestinal walls accounts for the constipation. Nervous system disorders manifest themselves both physically and psychically. Physical signs include disappearance of knee and ankle reflexes, painful muscles, difficulty in walking, and, eventually, paralysis of leg muscles. Psychic disorders include irritability, depression, forgetfulness, thoughts of persecution, and fear of impending doom [2].

In severe deficiency the heart becomes enlarged. Edema may appear in the face, feet, and legs, a condition which has been called "wet beriberi." On the other hand, patients with "dry beriberi" (in which there is no edema) may suddenly develop edema [2].

In oriental countries where beriberi has been a public health problem,

A CLOSER LOOK

Many of the symptoms of vitamin deficiencies are nonspecific—they can result from diseases or disorders unrelated to vitamin deficiencies. A vitamin deficiency should be diagnosed only by a qualified physician who is skilled at nutritional assessment and diagnosis of disease. Self-proclaimed experts who hold mail-order degrees lack the qualifications needed. Unfortunately, our access to vitamin pills makes self-medication easy, but individuals should realize that such a practice can result in tragedy when symptoms are due to serious medical problems not involving vitamins.

infants subsisting only on the milk of thiamine-deficient mothers have developed beriberi. The infants usually are pale and ill-tempered, and may also have edema [3]. They may eventually become seriously ill, and can die of the deficiency.

Beriberi does not occur in countries such as India where rice is only lightly milled or parboiled—steamed under pressure to drive the nutrients from the bran and germ into the endosperm [3]. The enrichment of white rice with thiamine is an important public health measure to combat beriberi, but this technique has been successful only in countries where rice is centrally milled, enabling added thiamine to reach most segments of the population. Another obviously important preventive measure is to supplement the lactating mother's diet with thiamine sources. The incidence of beriberi decreases whenever improvement of economic conditions in a country results in consumption of a wider variety of foods, with a lower percentage of white rice in the diet [3].

In some areas of the orient, dietary practices such as chewing betel nuts or tea leaves (as stimulants) or consumption of raw fish may contribute to development of thiamine deficiency [4]. Raw fish contain an enzyme called *thiaminase* which destroys thiamine, but cooking the fish in activates the enzyme. Exactly how chewing tea or betel nuts contributes to thiamine deficiency is not understood, although the tannin content of these substances is thought to be involved [4].

In the United States and other developed western countries, thiamine deficiency is occasionally seen in some special conditions. Alcoholics may develop beriberi because alcohol decreases the absorption of thiamine [5] and the alcoholic liver may be unable to efficiently convert thiamine to its coenzyme form [6]. (See Box 13-3, Chapter 13.) Patients fed exclusively glucose by vein rapidly use up the thiamine in their tissues to aid in metabolizing glucose for energy. If thiamine is not provided in the glucose solution, thiamine deficiency rapidly develops. Patients suffering from feverish illnesses such as rheumatic fever and tuberculosis require a higher than normal intake of thiamine because the elevation of body temperature increases the rate of metabolism. An elevated rate of metabolism increases not only the kilocalorie need, but the need for all nutrients required for obtaining energy from food.

Food Sources

Thiamine tends to occur in the seeds of plants (grains, beans, and other seeds), but not in the leaves (Figure 10-4 and Appendix C). Pork muscle is unusually high in thiamine; liver is also a good source. Thiamine is one of the nutrients removed in the milling of flour and grains, but is added back when these products are enriched. Since not all states require that white flour used in baking be enriched, read labels on packages of white rice, bread, crackers, cookies, cakes, spaghetti, macaroni, cornmeal, and white flour to see if these products are enriched.

Thiamine in food is subject to losses due to its water solubility and its susceptibility to heat. High temperatures used to toast or puff ready-to-eat cereals destroy much of the thiamine. Manufacturers of many such products add thiamine after this procedure, however, a fact that should appear on the label. Roasting meat results in losses of 20 to 60 percent of the thiamine, the greater loss

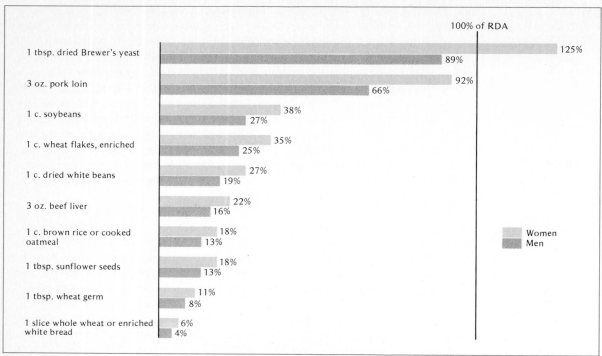

100% of RDA

Food	Women	Men
1 tbsp. dried Brewer's yeast	125%	89%
3 oz. pork loin	92%	66%
1 c. soybeans	38%	27%
1 c. wheat flakes, enriched	35%	25%
1 c. dried white beans	27%	19%
3 oz. beef liver	22%	16%
1 c. brown rice or cooked oatmeal	18%	13%
1 tbsp. sunflower seeds	18%	13%
1 tbsp. wheat germ	11%	8%
1 slice whole wheat or enriched white bread	6%	4%

FIGURE 10-4. Percentage of the thiamine RDA for the adult female (1.0 mg/day) and male (1.4 mg/day) furnished by selected foods. Values are for ready-to-eat foods. Dried brewer's yeast is shown for comparison purposes. (Source of values: Adams, C. F., *Nutritive Value of American Foods,* Agriculture Handbook No. 456, Washington, D.C.: U. S. Department of Agriculture, 1975.)

occurring with longer roasting. Practical suggestions for preventing excessive losses of thiamine and other nutrients in food preparation are discussed in Box 10-2.

Recommended Intakes

The thiamine RDA for adults has been set at 0.5 mg/1000 kcal (Appendix A), but higher intakes may be needed to saturate the tissues. Individuals consuming less than 2000 kcal/day should consume no less than 1 mg/day of thiamine [7].

Large oral doses appear not to be toxic, but there are no established benefits of large doses except in cases of thiamine deficiency.

RIBOFLAVIN

Riboflavin was isolated in pure form from milk in 1933. In their efforts to isolate the compound, scientists capitalized on the fact that riboflavin in solution is a yellow-green, fluorescent compound.

Functions

Riboflavin is more concentrated in the liver and kidneys than in other tissues, but all tissues contain some riboflavin. The tissues incorporate riboflavin into its

282

Saving Vitamins and Minerals in Foods

Water-soluble vitamins and minerals are subject to losses when foods are cooked in large amounts of water, if the water is then discarded. Some vitamins are also destroyed by heat, exposure to air, light, or alkaline medium. The following practical guidelines will aid in preserving vitamins and minerals in foods.

Harvesting and Storing

- Plan to harvest vegetables from a home garden immediately before they are to be cooked, frozen, or canned. Vitamin C and other vitamins are gradually lost from vegetables after harvesting, if stored improperly.
- Generally, fresh fruits and vegetables retain their vitamin content well when stored in wholesale warehouses under proper conditions of temperature and humidity. These foods should be kept cool in the store, too, and should be transported to the home refrigerator as quickly as possible.
- Purchase only the amounts of fresh vegetables that can be consumed within a short time (5 to 7 days). Fresh fruits retain a high percentage of their vitamin content over a period of weeks, however, if properly refrigerated.
- Prevent evaporation of water, and consequent wilting, by placing fresh vegetables and fruits in small covered containers or in plastic bags in the refrigerator. Vitamin C, for example, is rapidly lost as wilting occurs.

Preparation and Cooking

- Prepare vegetables just before they are to be consumed raw or cooked. Avoid soaking vegetables in water. When possible cook vegetables, such as potatoes, in their skins. Use a vegetable peeler to remove the thinnest possible peel when paring vegetables.

- Cook in as little water as possible; otherwise water-soluble vitamins and minerals dissolve in large amounts of cooking water. Bake, steam, or broil vegetables whenever possible. In boiling, add only small amounts of water and use a tight-fitting lid to diminish evaporation of water. Often, added water is unnecessary. (Contrary to popular belief, vitamins *do not* ''go off in the steam.'' They are *not* volatile.)
- Use the cooking water from freshly cooked or canned vegetables in soups or other dishes. Use meat or poultry drippings, after the fat is removed, in soups, gravies, or sauces.
- Cook vegetables as short a time as possible. Learn to prefer vegetables crisp in texture. Long cooking destroys more vitamin C, folacin, and vitamin B_6 than short cooking. Cooked green vegetables should still retain their bright green color. If they become olive-green, they are overcooked.
- Cook frozen vegetables in the frozen state. Use only a small amount of water and cook a short time. Cooking time is shortened by freezing.
- Avoid exposing cut vegetables to air for any period of time. Vitamin C is destroyed by exposure to oxygen, except when in an acid medium. Because of the acidity, little vitamin C is lost when orange juice is stored for several days in the refrigerator, if stored in a tightly covered glass container with a minimum of air space at the top.
- Avoid adding soda to preserve the green color of vegetables. Vitamin C and thiamine are more easily destroyed in an alkaline medium, and the texture quickly becomes mushy.
- Grating, chopping, and shredding vegetables increase the surface exposed to air, and the possibility of destruction of vitamin C and other vitamins. To diminish losses, use a sharp knife or grater to prevent macerating the tissues, which

releases enzymes that hasten destruction of vitamins. Shredded vegetables should be cooked quickly to a crisp stage, adding no water in the process. This procedure saves vitamins when compared with longer cooking in water.

- Cook rice in such a way that all the water is absorbed when the rice is done, preserving thiamine and other water-soluble vitamins.
- Serve vegetables, rice, and pasta immediately after cooking. Warming or keeping foods hot increases destruction of vitamin C, thiamine, folacin, and vitamin B_6.
- Direct contact of food with copper or iron during cooking hastens destruction of vitamin C. This is not to say that tomato sauce, for example, should *never* be prepared in an iron container, but some loss of vitamin C results from this practice.
- Protect milk, soups, and other liquids from long exposure to light since riboflavin and vitamin B_6, when in solution, are destroyed by light.

active forms, two coenzymes abbreviated FAD (*flavin adenine dinucleotide*) and FMN (*flavin mononucleotide*). A number of different enzymes in the body, called *flavoproteins* (Fp) require these coenzymes in the oxidation of pyruvate, fatty acids, and certain amino acids. They are also essential components of the electron transport system which produces large amounts of ATP (see Chapter 3). Riboflavin coenzymes function in oxidation-reduction reactions—in other words, they take up hydrogens from one compound and give them to another (Figure 10-5). They are therefore essential components of the complex system by which metabolism of carbohydrates, fats, and proteins takes place. An overall picture of some of the points in metabolism involving riboflavin coenzymes appears in Figure 10-13.

Deficiency

No deficiency disease ascribable to lack of riboflavin has occurred naturally in specific populations, as has happened for vitamin C and thiamine deficiency. Probably riboflavin deficiency has occurred along with other naturally occurring vitamin deficiencies, however, such as niacin deficiency, discussed later in this chapter.

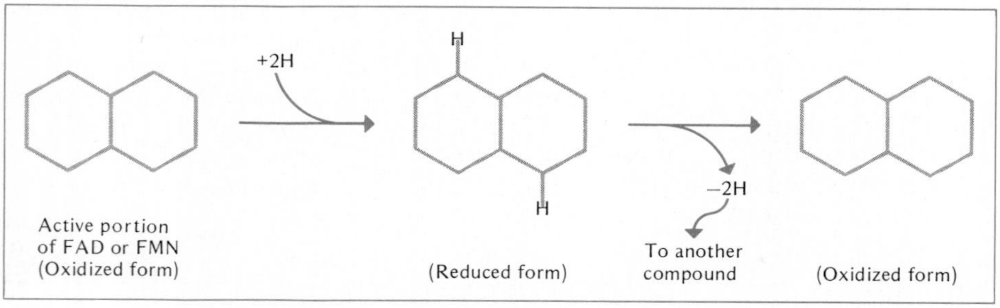

FIGURE 10-5. Mode of action of riboflavin coenzymes (simplified). These coenzymes take up hydrogens from a compound, oxidizing it, while becoming reduced themselves. They then give up hydrogens to a second compound, returning to their original oxidized form.

Active portion of FAD or FMN (Oxidized form)   +2H   (Reduced form)   −2H   To another compound   (Oxidized form)

Two groups of investigators [8,9] produced riboflavin deficiency in human volunteers, and found that their eyes became unusually sensitive to light (photophobia), tears formed easily, and sensations of burning and grittiness under the eyelids developed. In addition, subjects experienced soreness of the mouth. Lips became inflamed and fissures, sometimes encrusted with yellowish material, developed at the corners of the mouth; these changes are called *cheilosis*. The tongue may become inflamed and magenta red in color [10]. Whether or not riboflavin deficiency in humans eventually would become fatal is unknown.

Generally, signs of riboflavin deficiency do not appear until a person has been on a diet low in riboflavin for several months. Deficiency is more apt to occur during times when the dietary need is increased, such as in pregnancy, lactation, or rapid growth periods in children, or in feverish illnesses. Patients with chronic diarrhea may absorb insufficient riboflavin, and some patients with liver disease become unable to use the vitamin properly [2].

FIGURE 10-6. Percentage of the riboflavin RDA for the adult female (1.2 mg/day) and male (1.6 mg/day) furnished by selected foods. Values are for foods in the form usually eaten. (Source of values: Adams, C. F., *Nutritive Value of American Foods*, Agriculture Handbook No. 456, Washington, D.C.: U. S. Department of Agriculture, 1975.)

Food Sources

The best sources of riboflavin are shown in Figure 10-6. Grains (cereals) are not as good a source of riboflavin as they are of thiamine, but enrichment increases the amount in refined cereals and breads. Riboflavin is not destroyed by heat, but is destroyed by light when it is in solution. Milk stored in clear glass bottles and exposed to light loses more than 50 percent of its riboflavin in 2 h [2]. This is one reason that milk is frequently marketed in opaque cartons rather than in clear glass.

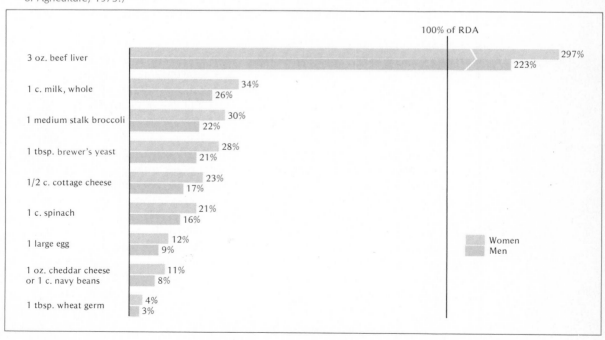

Although riboflavin is more widely distributed in foods than thiamine, avoiding milk and green vegetables will greatly decrease one's riboflavin intake. As mentioned in Chapter 6, total or strict vegetarians who consume no milk products need to include large intakes of legumes, green vegetables, grains, wheat germ, and seeds in their diets to obtain the RDA for riboflavin.

Recommended Intakes

The RDAs for riboflavin have been set at 0.6 mg/1000 kcal for people of all ages (Appendix A). For those with intakes of less than 2000 kcal/day, however, not less than 1.2 mg/day is recommended. The amount required to saturate the tissues appears to be between 0.5 and 0.75 mg/1000 kcal, since the urinary excretion of riboflavin increases greatly when the intake is increased to these levels or more. Large doses of riboflavin appear not to be toxic.

NIACIN

The discovery of the role played by niacin and tryptophan in the prevention and cure of pellagra constitutes one of the most interesting detective stories of the vitamin era. Pellagra has been associated with the eating of corn since 1730 when Casal first described this disease in Spain. Before 1900, explanations offered by investigators for the association of corn with pellagra were that the grain contained a toxin that produced the disease, or that corn failed to provide adequate protein, since vitamins were unknown [2].

In the first quarter of this century, pellagra occurred widely in the midwestern and southeastern United States, especially among people living in prisons, orphanages, and mental institutions. In fact, some mental institutions were populated chiefly by patients suffering from pellagra, as severe mental disorders are one manifestation of niacin deficiency [11]. Other symptoms include inflammation of the intestinal tract and dermatitis (skin inflammation).

In 1914, Joseph Goldberger, a physician with the U.S. Public Health Service, was assigned to determine the cause of pellagra. He first observed that inmates of many institutions contracted the disease, but that officials of the institutions, whose diets were more varied and of better quality than those of the inmates, never had pellagra. Furthermore, he noticed that pellagra began to appear in poor people at about the age of 6, yet never occurred among infants and children who drank milk. Goldberger began to suspect that the prevailing belief among physicians that pellagra was an infectious disease was incorrect, and that the real culprit was an inadequate diet.

In 1915, Goldberger placed 11 prisoners, who volunteered for the experiment, on the kind of diet he had observed to be consumed by poverty-stricken people who developed the disease. Foods allowed the prisoners were biscuits and cornbread (made with white flour and highly refined cornmeal), grits and rice (both highly refined), sweet potatoes, sugar, and coffee. Within a period of 6 months, 6 of the prisoners had developed clear-cut pellagra. Many physicans still were not convinced that pellagra was other than an infectious disease, however. Therefore, in 1916 Goldberger persuaded his wife and 14 of his colleagues to join him in trying to infect themselves with pellagra. They consumed pills made from the urine, feces, nasal secretions, and skin scrapings of pellagra patients. Solutions of these materials were also injected into their blood. Not one of the volunteers developed pellagra [2].

Although Goldberger was able to establish that the unknown substance that would prevent pellagra was in meat, milk, and yeast, and that the diet he used to produce pellagra in prisoners also produced a disease in dogs called *black tongue*, he died, in 1929, before he could isolate the active factor. His production of black tongue in dogs was a key experiment, however, because the solution to the mystery of pellagra came when scientists at the University of Wisconsin demonstrated that niacin, a substance they had just isolated from liver, cured black tongue in dogs [12,13]. Investigators immediately administered niacin to patients with pellagra, and found that it did indeed cure the disorder [2].

Some questions in the pellagra saga remained unanswered for a time, however. Scientists observed that corn contained more niacin than milk, but that milk was effective in curing or preventing pellagra. This mystery was solved when investigators learned that most of the niacin in corn occurs in a bound form called "niacytin." The niacin in corn is therefore unavailable to the body unless it is treated in an alkaline medium (limewater) as in Mexico and Central America where corn tortillas are a dietary staple, but where practically no pellagra has occurred.

A final bit of knowledge that fully solved the riddle of pellagra was the finding that the human body converts some tryptophan, an essential amino acid, to niacin. One reason that milk is effective in preventing or curing pellagra is that it is a good source of tryptophan (milk is rather low in niacin). Pellagra has been cured by administering large doses of tryptophan alone, without niacin [2].

Functions

Niacin is the term used to cover the two forms of this vitamin that are used by the human body, nicotinic acid and nicotinamide (or niacinamide). Both forms are absorbed easily from food by way of the portal vein, and are circulated throughout the body.

The coenzymes, abbreviated NAD (for *n*icotinamide *a*denine *d*inucleotide) and NADP (the P standing for *p*hosphate), are synthesized by body tissues if sufficient niacin and/or tryptophan are present in food. The coenzymes contain only nicotinamide and not nicotinic acid, but body tissues easily convert nicotinic acid to nicotinamide. Niacin coenzymes work in the body by accepting hydrogen atoms and electrons from specific compounds, then transferring these to other substances. In this process the oxidized forms of the coenzymes become reduced, and separate themselves from the enzymes and substrates. They then give up hydrogens and are oxidized again (Figure 10-7). Niacin coenzymes are essential in the electron transport system. Some of the points in metabolism that require nicotinamide coenzymes appear in Figure 10-13.

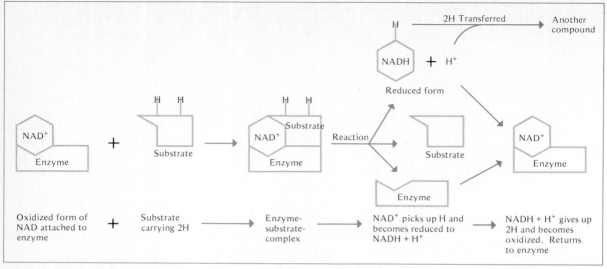

FIGURE 10-7. Mode of action of niacin coenzymes, simplified.

Metabolism

Excessive intakes of niacin are excreted in the urine as metabolites. During a deficiency of niacin and tryptophan, the urinary excretion of the metabolites of niacin decreases markedly.

Tissue cells convert some of the tryptophan in the cells to niacin, as mentioned earlier. Studies with human volunteers indicate that when 60 mg of tryptophan are consumed, enough is metabolized by the tryptophan-to-niacin pathway to produce 1 mg of niacin [7] (Figure 10-8). When large doses of

FIGURE 10-8.
Conversion of tryptophan to niacin. Tryptophan is involved in many metabolic pathways. Some of these are anabolic, leading to protein and serotonin synthesis, for example. The catabolism (breakdown) of tryptophan by one specific pathway produces niacin.

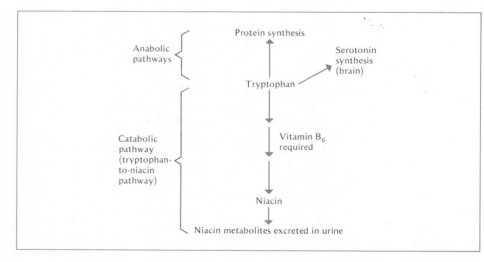

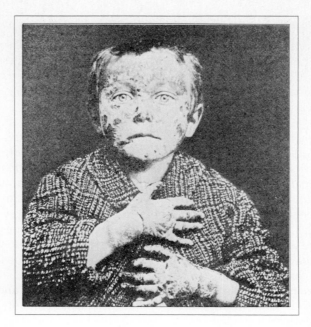

A child with pellagra, showing the typical dermatitis on parts of the body exposed to sun. *(National Library of Medicine)*

tryptophan are fed experimentally to normal subjects, excretion of niacin metabolites in the urine increases, indicating the metabolism of tryptophan by the tryptophan-to-niacin pathway. The coenzyme form of vitamin B_6 is needed for the conversion of tryptophan to niacin, another example of the interrelationships of vitamins in tissue metabolism.

Deficiency

Niacin deficiency results only when there is a low intake of both niacin and tryptophan. The earliest signs of developing pellagra include loss of appetite, weariness, feelings of weakness, heartburn, irritability, and depression. The classic deficiency signs then begin, and have been called "the three D's: dermatitis, diarrhea, and dementia." The dermatitis resembles sunburn in its early stages, and appears especially on parts of the body that are exposed to the sun: the face, neck, feet, arms, and hands. In well-developed pellagra, severe inflammation extends all along the intestinal tract, and diarrhea is common. Soreness of the mouth and esophagus prevents the patient from consuming much food, and rapid weight loss occurs [2].

The deficiency affects the nervous system, resulting in depression, fearfulness, disorientation, and finally delusions and hallucinations. Pellegra is fatal if allowed to progress. Probably, pellagra as it appeared in the United States and other countries was complicated by deficiencies of other B vitamins, including riboflavin, vitamin B_6, and pantothenic acid.

Food Sources

When considering niacin sources, foods that supply both tryptophan and niacin need to be taken into account. Tryptophan is present in largest amounts in meat, poultry, fish, eggs, cheese, legumes (dried beans), and seeds such as sunflower and sesame seeds. Good sources of niacin are meats, poultry, fish, whole grains, nuts, legumes, and dried yeast.

The 1980 RDAs for niacin are in terms of milligrams of niacin equivalents (NE). One NE is equal to either 1 mg of niacin or 60 mg of tryptophan. Most food composition tables report only the niacin in foods, however, and not the niacin equivalents. To estimate the niacin equivalents from tryptophan, one can assume that animal protein foods are about 1.4 percent tryptophan, while plant proteins are about 1.0 percent tryptophan [7]. Examples of the estimation of the niacin equivalents in food are given in Table 10-2. Figure 10-9 shows the percentage of the adult's RDA for niacin supplied by selected foods. Values for niacin itself in foods are in Appendix C. Since niacin and tryptophan are so widely available in present-day foods, only persons on highly restricted diets because of ignorance, poverty, or illness are apt to have a deficient intake.

Niacin is very stable in the presence of heat, light, and oxygen; cooking losses occur only when foods are cooked in large amounts of water, and the cooking water discarded.

FIGURE 10-9. Percentage of the niacin RDA for the adult female (13 mg NE) and male (18 mg NE) furnished by selected foods. Values are for foods in the form usually consumed. NE were calculated according to the method shown in Table 10-2.

Recommended Intakes

The RDA for adults and for children over 6 months old is 6.6 mg NE/1000 kcal (Appendix A). Not less than 13 mg NE is recommended for those whose

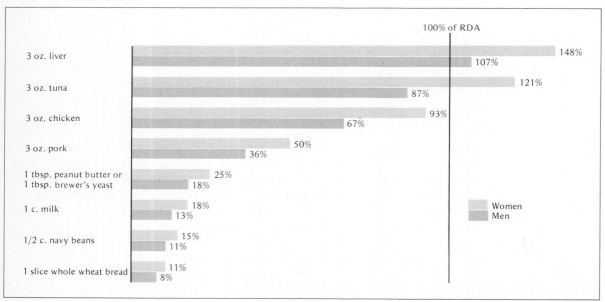

TABLE 10-2.   ESTIMATING THE MILLIGRAMS OF NIACIN EQUIVALENTS (NE) IN FOOD*

		COLUMN				
		I	II	III	IV	V
				NE FROM		TOTAL
	SERVING	PROTEIN,	TRYPTOPHAN,	TRYPTOPHAN,	NIACIN,	NE,
FOOD	SIZE	g	mg	mg	mg	mg
Hamburger, lean	3 oz	23	322	5.4	5.1	10.5
Chicken	3 oz	20	280	4.7	7.4	12.1
Milk (whole)	1 c	9	126	2.1	0.2	2.3
Peanut butter	1 tbsp	4	40	0.7	2.4	3.1
Whole wheat bread	1 slice	3	30	0.5	0.7	1.2

*Figures for protein in column I are from Appendix C. Tryptophan content (column II) is estimated by multiplying grams of protein by 1.4% (0.014) for foods of animal origin, and by 1% (0.01) for foods of plant origin. The resulting figure is in terms of grams and is multiplied by 1000 to obtain milligrams of tryptophan (1 g = 1000 mg). The milligrams of tryptophan are converted to niacin equivalents (NE) (column III) by dividing by 60. The amounts of niacin itself in foods (column IV) are from Appendix C. The total milligrams of NE in the food in column V are obtained by adding the values in columns III and IV.

kilocalorie intake is less than 2000 kcal/day. Average diets in the United States are thought to supply 16 to 34 mg NE/day.

Are Large Doses Harmful?

Drug doses of nicotinic acid, but not nicotinamide, have been used experimentally in human subjects to lower serum lipid levels [14]. Although these large doses appeared to protect to some extent against second heart attacks, serious side effects such as abnormal heart beat, gastrointestinal problems, and abnormal laboratory tests were of concern to the investigators. Large doses of nicotinic acid also cause flushing and consequent itching and discomfort of the face and neck, resulting from dilation of the blood vessels.

Claims have also been made that megadoses of niacin are effective in treating the mental disorder, schizophrenia. Carefully controlled studies have failed to support these claims, however [15]. The dangerous side effects of nicotinic acid should warn one against its indiscriminate use. Megadoses should be taken only under careful supervision by a competent physician.

VITAMIN B$_6$

Three forms of vitamin B$_6$ are active in the body: *pyridoxine*, *pyridoxal*, and *pyridoxamine*. Pyridoxine was isolated from food and synthesized in 1939.

The importance of vitamin B$_6$ in the diet was clearly demonstrated in the early 1950s when infants between the ages of 6 weeks and 6 months developed irritability and convulsions while consuming a well-known brand of infant formula which had undergone a processing change. Unknown to the manufacturer, the vitamin B$_6$ content of the formula was greatly reduced by the intensive heat

NUTRITION IN THE NEWS

NUTRITION

Dr. Jean Mayer and Jeanne Goldberg, R.D.,* *The Washington Post*, May 12, 1982

Q. Is it possible to get an allergic reaction from a vitamin? I read that niacin provides the same calming effect as a tranquilizer, so I bought a bottle of niacin pills. I took some, and about a half-hour later my face felt flushed and it turned red. Then my arms turned blotchy and began to itch. Far from calming me down, this reaction frightened me. Fortunately, the symptoms went away within a short period of time. I have not dared to take any of the pills again. What happened?

A. What you describe is not an allergic reaction to the vitamin but are the classic symp-toms of niacin toxicity. Fortunately, these symptoms are transient.

It is important to point out, however, that beyond the fact that these side effects are un-pleasant, there really is no justification for dos-ing yourself with niacin as a tranquilizer or for anything else, for that matter.

The fact is that mental symptoms respond to niacin only when they are caused by niacin deficiency in the first place. Thus, for individu-als eating virtually any sort of varied diet, this condition is extremely unlikely. . . .

ASK YOURSELF:
In what kinds of books, newspapers, or maga-zines are you apt to find unsubstantiated claims for a vitamin such as this one—that niacin is a tranquilizer? Why are individuals so willing to fall for such claims? What kinds of societal pressures cause some people to be willing to try out a vitamin as a tranquilizer or for some other special purpose? Where do you think the idea originated that a vitamin supplement may be used for a particular purpose (e.g., as a tranqui-lizer)?

*Dr. Mayer is a renowned nutritionist who is currently President of Tufts University, while Ms. Goldberg is a registered dietitian (R.D.). Their credentials are of the highest order, making their syndicated newspaper column a more reliable source of information than the questioner evidently used originally.

used in the new procedure. Pediatricians working with some of these infants realized that their symptoms were similar to those of vitamin B_6-deficient animals, and of an infant who had been intentionally placed on a vitamin B_6-deficient diet in an attempt to treat a brain disorder. An injection of pyridoxine stopped the convulsions within 4 to 5 min [16]. This story vividly dramatizes how vulnerable infants are to dietary deficiencies because their diet early in life is restricted to one source: either to a formula or to breast milk.

Functions

Each of the three forms of vitamin B_6 is easily absorbed in the upper part of the small intestine and reaches the liver by way of the portal vein. Enzymes in the tissues convert pyridoxine, pyridoxal, and pyridoxamine chiefly to the coenzyme pyridoxal phosphate (PLP), although pyridoxine phosphate is a coenzyme for some reactions. In metabolism PLP is needed as the coenzyme for more than 60

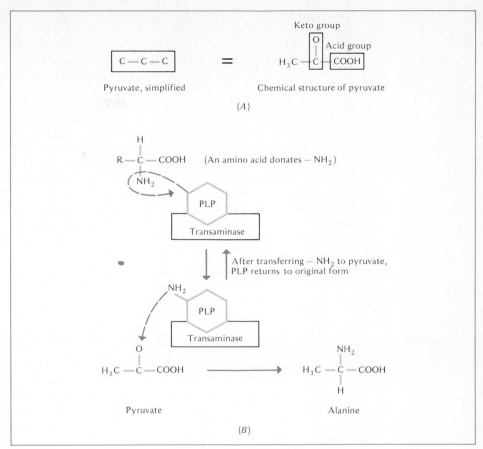

FIGURE 10-10.
Formation of alanine, a
nonessential amino acid,
from pyruvate. The
reaction requires a
specific transaminase
which requires PLP as a
coenzyme.

reactions involving amino acids [17]. It is required, for example, in the conversion of tryptophan to niacin, as already noted (Figure 10-8). One way that scientists determine vitamin B_6 deficiency is to test for urinary excretion products after giving a large oral dose of tryptophan. The large dose forces greater catabolism by the tryptophan-to-niacin pathway. If the individual is deficient in vitamin B_6, tests will show large amounts of abnormal compounds in the urine, but little of the normal metabolites of niacin.

Vitamin B_6 coenzymes are needed by enzymes called *transaminases* for the synthesis of nonessential amino acids. The transaminases, with the help of PLP, catalyze the transfer of the amino group (—NH_2) from an amino acid to a molecule such as pyruvate (a keto acid), forming a new, nonessential amino acid.

So far, we have represented pyruvate in a simplified way. By examining its complete chemical structure, however, you see that it has an acid group (—COOH), and that substituting an amino group (—NH_2) for the oxygen on the keto group ($>C = O$) produces alanine (Figure 10-10). PLP actually picks up and transfers the amino group.

Coenzymes of vitamin B_6 are also needed for the formation in the brain, from amino acids, of neurotransmitters (such as dopamine, tyramine, and serotonin) [17]. As noted in Chapter 9, neurotransmitters are required for normal brain function. PLP is also required for the synthesis of hemoglobin. Excessive amounts of vitamin B_6 in the body are excreted in the urine in the form of a metabolite.

Deficiency

Vitamin B_6 deficiency has never been reported in groups of adults consuming their usual diet, but has developed only in the unusual case of infants, discussed earlier. The development of convulsions in these infants signifies that the nervous system is adversely affected by deficiency. Adult volunteers in whom experimental deficiency was produced developed a greasy, scaly dermatitis around the nose and mouth, inflammation of the mouth accompanied by ulcers, and a rash on the forehead similar to acne. These subjects also were reported to suffer from depression, irritability, and a diminished sense of responsibility [17]. Anemia also has been reported in vitamin B_6-deficient patients.

Animal studies show that vitamin B_6 deficiency results in decreased immunity to infections, and studies in patients with severe kidney disease indicate that this also occurs in human subjects [18].

Circumstances in Which Deficiency May Occur

Use of Oral Contraceptives   Most women who take oral contraceptive drugs containing estrogen-progesterone excrete abnormal metabolites in the urine after taking a test dose of tryptophan. This same situation occurs in a person who is deficient in vitamin B_6, as noted earlier. Many years of research have been directed toward establishing whether or not oral contraceptive drugs induce a deficiency of vitamin B_6. Currently the judgment of researchers is that they do not, therefore the Food and Nutrition Board makes no additional recommendation for vitamin B_6 for women who take these drugs (see Chapter 14).

Doses of 25 to 50 mg of vitamin B_6 per day have been demonstrated to alleviate the following disorders in oral contraceptive users, however: (1) abnormal glucose tolerance, (2) elevated blood triglyceride levels, and (3) mental depression if accompanied by biochemical signs of vitamin B_6 deficiency (other than the abnormal urinary metabolites after a test dose of tryptophan) [19]. However, only 15 to 20 percent of oral contraceptive users exhibit biochemical signs of vitamin B_6 deficiency other than those after a tryptophan dose is given. Large doses of vitamin B_6 should be taken only under a competent physician's supervision for these specific disorders.

Other Circumstances   Recent studies indicate that as many as 50 percent of alcoholics may be deficient in vitamin B_6 because alcohol causes the breakdown of PLP and lowers the ability of body tissues to retain the vitamin [20]. Alcoholics may also have a low intake of vitamin B_6, especially during times when their alcohol intake is very high (see also Box 13-3, Chapter 13).

Several studies indicate that many elderly people may have borderline deficiency of vitamin B_6, but so far scientists are uncertain as to whether older people need more vitamin B_6 than younger ones [7].

Some drugs, such as *isoniazid*, used in treating tuberculosis, and *penicillamine*, used to treat rheumatoid arthritis and other diseases, increase the need for vitamin B_6 because they bind the vitamin and inactivate it [17]. Additional vitamin B_6 should be given to patients treated with these drugs.

Toxic effects of large doses of vitamin B_6 have rarely been observed in humans [21].

Food Sources

FIGURE 10-11.
Percentage of the vitamin B_6 RDA for the adult female (2.0 mg/day) and male (2.2 mg/day) furnished by selected foods. Most values are for raw (uncooked) foods. (Source of values: Orr, M. L., *Pantothenic Acid, Vitamin B_6 and Vitamin B_{12} in Foods*, Home Economics Research Report No. 36, Washington, D.C.: U. S. Dept. of Agriculture, 1969.)

Figure 10-11 indicates food sources of vitamin B_6. Other sources are indicated in Appendix D. Large amounts of the vitamin B_6 in whole grains are lost during the refining process when the bran and germ are removed. Parboiled rice retains large amounts of the vitamin B_6 present in brown rice because the steaming process drives vitamins from the bran into the grain before the bran is removed. "Instant" white rice, on the other hand, loses a considerable amount of vitamin B_6 during heat processing in addition to that lost during refining. Milk products and fruits, except for bananas, are only fair to poor sources of this vitamin. Vegetables can make a fairly good contribution to the vitamin B_6 in the diet, however, if sufficient amounts are consumed. Vitamin B_6 is destroyed by heat and by sunlight (when in solution). Canned foods tend to contain lower amounts than raw foods.

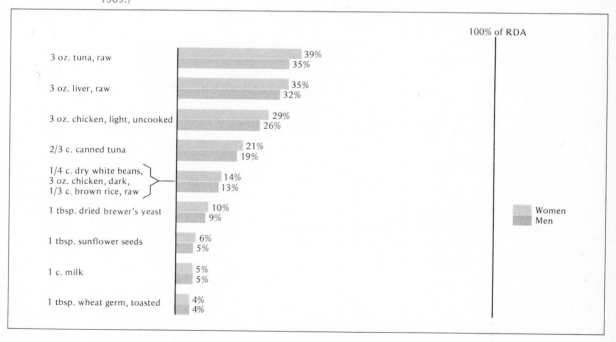

Recommended Intakes

The need for vitamin B_6 is known to be greater when the protein intake is high, since this vitamin is so intimately related to the metabolism of amino acids in the body. The RDA for adults, then, is based upon the assumption that 0.02 mg of vitamin B_6 per gram of protein in the diet is adequate. The average protein consumption for women in the United States is 100 g/day and for men, 110 g/day; therefore the RDA for adult women is set at 2.0 g/day and for men, 2.2 g/day (Appendix A).

PANTOTHENIC ACID

In 1933, Dr. R. J. Williams gave the name "pantothenic acid" to an unidentified substance that was necessary for yeast growth [22]. The name comes from the Greek word meaning "from everywhere," indicating its wide distribution in foods. By 1940, the chemical structure of pantothenic acid was determined and studies in the 1950s demonstrated that human beings require this nutrient in the diet [23].

Functions

Pantothenic acid performs a key role in metabolism as an essential part of two coenzymes: *coenzyme A (CoA)* and *acyl carrier protein (ACP)*. You are already familiar with an important function of coenzyme A, that is, its combination with acetate (a 2-carbon compound) to form acetyl coenzyme A (acetyl CoA) or "active acetate." Recall from Chapter 3 that acetyl CoA combines with a compound in the Krebs cycle to form the first intermediate in the oxidation of carbohydrates in that cycle (see Figure 3-18, Chapter 3).

Acetyl CoA also combines with choline to form *acetylcholine*, an important brain neurotransmitter. In addition, it detoxifies sulfa drugs by adding acetate to these compounds. Coenzyme A is also utilized in the catabolism of fatty acids in body tissue. Recall that when fatty acids are oxidized, they are broken down two carbons at a time in the form of acetyl CoA (Figure 4-17, Chapter 4). In addition, acetyl CoA is involved in the synthesis of ketones and cholesterol and is the basic building block for the synthesis of fatty acids (Figure 4-19, Chapter 4).

The second coenzyme form, acyl carrier protein (ACP), is involved in the synthesis of fatty acids, which occurs by the stepwise elongation of the carbon chain two carbons at a time. Active acetate (acetyl CoA) is the source of the 2-carbon building blocks, but the enzyme system responsible for the elongation process requires ACP. Clearly, pantothenic acid participates in fundamentally important anabolic and catabolic reactions throughout body tissues.

Deficiency

Pantothenic acid deficiency has never occurred spontaneously in any population group, although pellagra and perhaps other severe deficiencies as they have occurred in populations may have been complicated by a simultaneous but

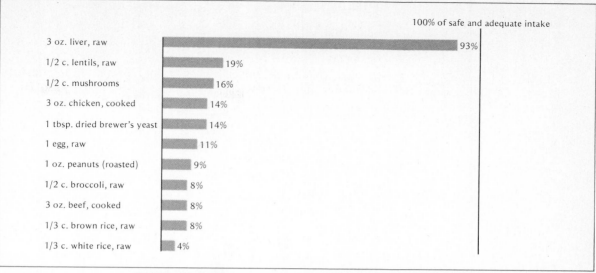

100% of safe and adequate intake

3 oz. liver, raw	93%
1/2 c. lentils, raw	19%
1/2 c. mushrooms	16%
3 oz. chicken, cooked	14%
1 tbsp. dried brewer's yeast	14%
1 egg, raw	11%
1 oz. peanuts (roasted)	9%
1/2 c. broccoli, raw	8%
3 oz. beef, cooked	8%
1/3 c. brown rice, raw	8%
1/3 c. white rice, raw	4%

FIGURE 10-12. Percentage of the adult estimated safe and adequate intake (7 mg/day) for pantothenic acid furnished by selected foods. Although a range of 4 to 7 mg/day is suggested, the authors chose the highest figure as a standard of comparison. [Sources of values: (1) Orr, M. L., *Pantothenic Acid, Vitamin B$_6$ and Vitamin B$_{12}$ in Foods*. Home Economics Research Report No. 36, Washington, D.C.: U. S. Dept of Agriculture, 1969. (2) Walsh, J. H., B. W. Wyse, and R. G. Hansen, "Pantothenic Acid Content of 75 Processed and Cooked Foods," Reprinted by permission from *Journal of the American Dietetic Association*, 78:140, 1981.]

undetected deficiency of pantothenic acid.

Human volunteers placed on a pantothenic acid–deficient diet for 10 weeks developed malaise, abdominal pains, vomiting, burning cramps, fatigue, and inability to sleep soundly [24]. Other investigators reported numbness and tingling of hands and feet, a sign of nervous system damage [23].

Deficiency in animals also produces poor growth, reproductive failure, dermatitis, and graying of dark hair. Gray hair produced by pantothenic acid deficiency in animals is ameliorated by feeding the vitamin. Pantothenic acid pills have been promoted as a "cure" for gray hair in human beings, but such attempts have proved to be ineffective. Only if a symptom is due to lack of a vitamin does dosing with the vitamin ameliorate the symptom.

Food Sources

Nearly all foods contain some pantothenic acid, but the richest sources are shown in Figure 10-12. Other sources appear in Appendix D. The refining of wheat flour and rice removes large proportions of this vitamin. Freezing and canning of foods also results in losses of pantothenic acid.

Recommended Intakes

Because data are insufficient on which to base an RDA for pantothenic acid, the Food and Nutrition Board has instead set estimated safe and adequate daily

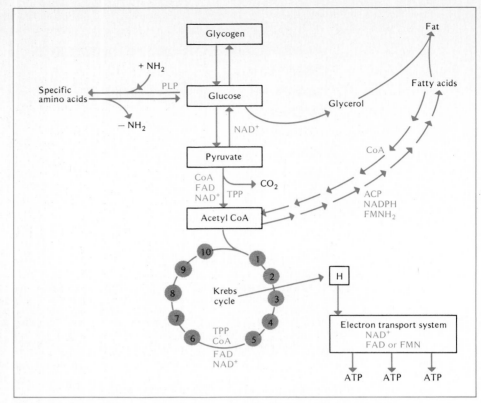

FIGURE 10-13. A
summation of some of
the points in metabolism
requiring B vitamins as
coenzymes. Some of the
metabolic pathways
involved in
carbohydrate, protein,
and fat metabolism are
indicated here.

dietary intakes of 4 to 7 mg/day for adults (Appendix A). Additional research on the need for this vitamin will make possible revisions of this estimate, and eventually an RDA will be developed.

The usual intake of pantothenic acid in the United States is thought to be about 7 mg/day [24], but some studies report lower intakes by low-income women [25] and by adolescent girls [26]. Large doses appear not to be harmful, except for some reports of diarrhea and water retention [27].

Figure 10-13 shows some of the important points in metabolism at which enzymes require pantothenic acid or other B vitamins as coenzymes.

FOLACIN

Folacin is the term used for a group of compounds required in the human diet for normal blood cell development, growth and reproduction, and important chemical reactions in the cells. Dr. Lucy Wills, working in India in the 1930s, reported that a specific kind of anemia existed there among pregnant women that could be cured by giving them a specially treated yeast [28]. Researchers found that monkeys fed the kind of diet the women normally consumed also developed anemia, and cured it by feeding a crude liver extract. Later research showed that the active substance present in the yeast and liver extract was folacin.

All the folacin compounds are related to *folic acid* in chemical structure and function. Folic acid was first obtained in pure form from 4 tons of spinach leaves, consequently investigators derived the name from the Latin word *folium* meaning leaf or foliage. Folic acid, the parent compound, is made up of three compounds linked together: (1) pteridine, a yellow pigment; (2) *para*-aminobenzoic acid (discussed in Box 9-1); and (3) glutamic acid, an amino acid. The technical name for folic acid is *pteroylglutamic acid* (PGA) (Figure 10-14). Folic acid is not present as such in foods nor is it active as such in the body because it must be changed in body tissues to coenzyme forms before it can be used.

Functions

Only 25 to 50 percent of the folacin in food appears to be absorbed [7]. Once folacin crosses the intestinal muscosal cell it is carried to the liver by way of the portal vein. Part of it accumulates in the liver while the remainder is distributed via the blood to all parts of the body. Body cells convert it to various coenzyme forms.

One of the most important functions of folacin coenzymes, along with those that contain vitamin B_{12}, is in the synthesis of DNA and RNA. DNA (*deoxyribonucleic acid*), as noted in Chapter 6, occurs in the nucleus of each cell, and contains the genetic information that directs the synthesis of all the cell's proteins. RNA (*ribonucleic acid*) works with DNA to synthesize cell proteins. Specifically, the folacin coenzymes function by transporting single-carbon groups from one compound to another during synthesis of DNA, RNA, or proteins. Examples of single carbon units are methyl groups ($-CH_3$) and hydroxymethyl groups ($-CH_2OH$). Folacin coenzymes participate in the synthesis of DNA and RNA by

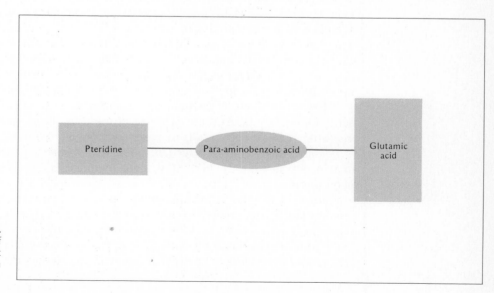

FIGURE 10-14.
Simplified structure of folic acid, the parent substance for folacin compounds.

FIGURE 10-15.
Participation of folacin
coenzymes in synthesis
of the purine nucleus.
Folacin coenzymes
transfer, from other
substances, the carbon
units at positions 2 and
8, completing the
synthesis of the purine
nucleus.

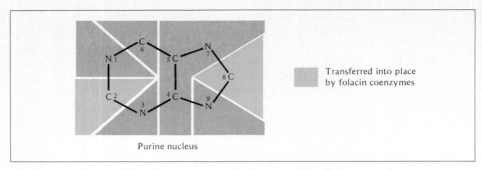

Transferred into place
by folacin coenzymes

Purine nucleus

providing single carbon units for the synthesis of purines which are essential components of DNA and RNA. In addition, purines are components of ATP and of the coenzymes FAD, NAD, and NADP. The role of folacin coenzymes in the body's synthesis of the purine nucleus, the foundation of the purines, is depicted in Figure 10-15.

Folacin coenzymes also participate in the synthesis of the nonessential amino acids glycine and serine, and in the catabolism of many amino acids in the body.

Excessive folacin is excreted from the body through the urine and bile. Much of that in bile is reabsorbed through the enterohepatic circulation (discussed in Chapter 4, Figure 4-14), a mechanism that apparently aids in maintaining the blood level of folacin [29].

Deficiency

Folacin deficiency strikes in particular those tissue cells having rapid turnover rates—those in which new cells fairly rapidly replace old ones. Blood and intestinal mucosal cells are therefore targets of this deficiency. *Macrocytic* (*macro* = large; *cytic* = pertains to cells) anemia is common in folacin deficiency. This anemia is identical with that of vitamin B_{12} deficiency and is characterized by the appearance of many unusually large red blood cells. These are immature cells called megaloblasts, and occur because folacin, by virtue of its involvement in DNA and RNA synthesis, is required for the normal maturation of these cells. White blood cells also show abnormalities resulting from maturational failure.

The anemia results eventually in symptoms of tiredness, weakness, headache, faintness, and extreme paleness of the skin. The effects of deficiency on intestinal mucosal cells results in a red, sore tongue, diarrhea, and weight loss. It is possible that nerve damage and mental disturbances may also develop in folacin deficiency [30]. Irritability, poor memory, hostility, and paranoia have been reported in deficiency [29].

Folacin deficiency occurs among pregnant women, particularly in the less-developed countries. The growing fetus requires a large amount of folacin for synthesis of new tissues, and the diet of many women may contain low amounts because prolonged cooking destroys much of the folacin in foods. In the United States, about 45 percent of pregnant women in low-income groups have been reported to have low amounts of folacin in their blood, possibly indicating beginning deficiency [31]. Concern about adequate folacin nutrition during pregnancy is based on studies in which folacin deficiency early in pregnancy in laboratory rats resulted in birth defects.

Additionally, observations in countries where a high percentage of pregnant women are folacin-deficient indicate that supplements increase the size of the placenta (through which the developing fetus receives nourishment), decrease the number of infants born prematurely, and increase the birth weights of infants [32]. Folic acid deficiency is not uncommon among children up to about age 2 in less-developed countries. Mild deficiency of folacin may also occur among elderly people in industrialized countries [31,32].

Oral contraceptive agents may induce folacin deficiency in some women [33]. A hypothesis recently offered is that extra folacin given to women who use oral contraceptives may reduce their chances of developing cancer of the cervix [34]. The hypothesis is that folacin deficiency induced by these drugs may result in changes in the cells of the cervix that can become cancerous. Further research should demonstrate whether or not this hypothesis is correct.

Food Sources

FIGURE 10-16.
Percentage of the folacin RDA for adults (400 µg/day) furnished by selected foods. (Source of values: Perloff, B. P., and R. Butrum, "Folacin in Selected Foods," Reprinted by permission from *Journal of the American Dietetic Association*, 70:161, 1977.)

Folacin occurs to some extent in nearly all foods in their natural state, but is highly susceptible to losses when foods, such as whole grains, are refined or when foods are canned or cooked for long periods of time. Folacin is not added back when refined grain products are enriched.

Figure 10-16 shows some food sources of folacin. Others appear in Appendix D. Eating a wide variety of minimally processed, traditional foods as opposed to highly processed foods enables one to obtain sufficient folacin. Routinely

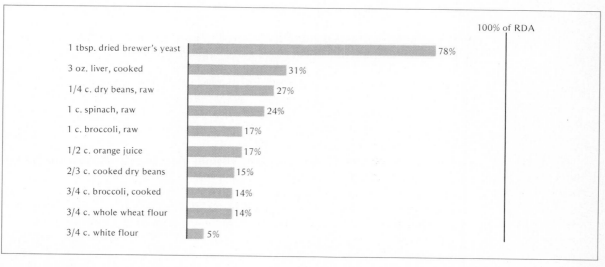

Food	% of RDA
1 tbsp. dried brewer's yeast	78%
3 oz. liver, cooked	31%
1/4 c. dry beans, raw	27%
1 c. spinach, raw	24%
1 c. broccoli, raw	17%
1/2 c. orange juice	17%
2/3 c. cooked dry beans	15%
3/4 c. broccoli, cooked	14%
3/4 c. whole wheat flour	14%
3/4 c. white flour	5%

100% of RDA

consuming some raw or lightly cooked green vegetables also contributes toward an adequate folacin intake.

Recommended Intakes

The RDAs for folacin assume that 100 to 200 μg are needed by the adult to maintain the body pool of this vitamin. The RDA therefore is set at 400 μg for the adult (Appendix A), taking into account that only 25 to 50 percent of dietary folacin may be absorbed.

Breast-fed babies from well-nourished mothers will receive sufficient folacin, but babies fed unsupplemented formulas from sterilized or powdered milk may need extra amounts. A recent study indicated that infants fed boiled pasteurized milk developed signs of folacin deficiency [35].

VITAMIN B_{12} (COBALAMIN)

Vitamin B_{12} was the last of the vitamins to be isolated, in 1948. This vitamin is unusual in that it contains a metal, cobalt, and is a very large molecule requiring a special mechanism for absorption.

The history of vitamin B_{12} can be traced back to a physician, Thomas Addison, working in London, who in 1849 described an anemia that occurred among middle-aged or elderly people resulting inevitably in death within a few years [36]. The name "Addisonian pernicious anemia" was given to the disease, the word pernicious meaning "tending towards death." A breakthrough occurred in 1926 when Minot and Murphy discovered that these patients survived if they were fed from ¼ to ½ lb of liver daily [37]. Soon after, W. B. Castle reported that pernicious anemia patients had a genetic defect of gastric secretion which resulted in failure to synthesize "intrinsic factor" required for absorption of an unknown "extrinsic factor" which was present in liver [38]. In 1948, pure vitamin B_{12} was isolated and found to be the "extrinsic factor." A single injection of as little as 3 to 6 μg of this compound resulted in production of normal red blood cells in pernicious anemia patients. Feeding large amounts of liver saved the lives of some pernicious anemia patients because small amounts diffuse into the intestinal mucosal cells without intrinsic factor when the intake is sufficiently large.

Functions

When a person swallows food containing vitamin B_{12}, stomach acid and enzymes free vitamin B_{12} from its linkages to food proteins. Then, intrinsic factor (IF), secreted by the normal stomach and required for vitamin B_{12} absorption, attaches itself to the free vitamin B_{12}, carrying it to the ileum. There, IF affixes itself to absorption sites, allowing vitamin B_{12} to be taken up by intestinal mucosal cells; IF is then released to the intestinal contents (Figure 10-17). Once vitamin B_{12} crosses the intestinal mucosal cell, it travels to the liver by way of portal blood. Normal individuals absorb between 30 to 70 percent of the vitamin B_{12} in food.

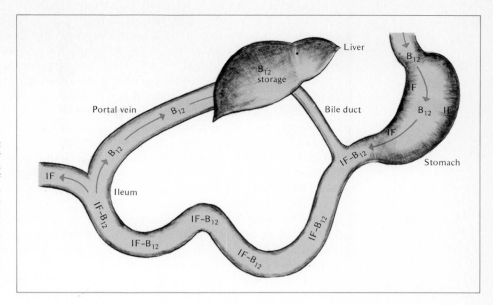

FIGURE 10-17. Intrinsic factor (IF), secreted by the normal stomach, is required for absorption of vitamin B_{12}. IF attaches itself to vitamin B_{12} in the stomach and travels with it to the ileum where it aids B_{12} in crossing into the intestinal mucosal cells. Vitamin B_{12} then is taken to the liver via the portal blood.

The liver serves as a storage site for vitamin B_{12}. Normally, a person stores enough vitamin B_{12} to prevent signs of deficiency for as long as 5 years after a defect in absorption begins. This is the only B vitamin stored in large amounts in body tissues.

When body cells need vitamin B_{12}, the liver releases some into the blood, and the cells then synthesize the B_{12} coenzymes, called *cobamides*. Cobamides perform several major functions in the body. First, they are required along with folacin coenzymes in the synthesis of DNA and RNA. These two vitamins are interrelated in such a way that a deficiency of vitamin B_{12} causes folacin to be "trapped" in the cells in a useless form. Normal DNA synthesis consequently cannot occur, and maturation of cells in the blood and gastrointestinal tract cannot proceed. Deficiency of either folacin or vitamin B_{12} results in the same macrocytic anemia because in either case the active form of folacin needed for maturation of blood cells is lacking. Second, vitamin B_{12} is required for synthesis of myelin, the fatty substance of nerve fibers. And third, vitamin B_{12} is involved in carbohydrate and fat metabolism. Little catabolism of vitamin B_{12} occurs in the body, and losses result only through excretion through the bile. Even then, the body conserves vitamin B_{12} by reabsorbing, via the enterohepatic circulation, most of that excreted in the bile [29].

Deficiency

As noted above, vitamin B_{12} deficiency results in macrocytic anemia, gastrointestinal symptoms, and dangerous nervous system damage. Failure of maturation of rapidly reproducing cells lining the gastrointestinal tract results in a sore, inflamed mouth and tongue. Loss of appetite, nausea, vomiting, and intestinal pain or discomfort commonly develop.

Damage to the nerves in vitamin B_{12} deficiency results in tingling and numbness of the hands and feet, unsteadiness on the feet, poor muscle coordination, forgetfulness, mental confusion and agitation, depression, and finally psychotic signs such as delusions, hallucinations, and paranoia.

Because of the seriousness of nervous system damage, accurate diagnosis of vitamin B_{12} deficiency must be made. If the diet contains large amounts of folacin, the anemia of vitamin B_{12} deficiency fails to develop because large amounts of folacin overcome the "trapping" problem mentioned earlier. As a consequence, the first symptoms of vitamin B_{12} deficiency are those signifying nervous system damage, which can be irreversible and fatal [32]. For this reason, the Food and Drug Administration specifies that vitamin pills sold without prescription cannot contain more than 0.1 mg (100 μg) of folacin per tablet, an amount too low to prevent the anemia of vitamin B_{12} deficiency.

Deficiency of vitamin B_{12} is rare. Addisonian pernicious anemia, as noted earlier, is due to a genetic defect that shows up in middle age or later, especially among people of northern European origin. Treatment involves routine injections of vitamin B_{12}, bypassing the intestinal tract.

Surgical removal of the stomach or ileum, or severe malabsorptive disorders such as sprue can also result in vitamin B_{12} deficiency. Vegetarians who consume only plant foods eventually develop low blood vitamin B_{12} levels, but rarely develop frank deficiency. Several cases of vitamin B_{12} deficiency have been reported, however, among infants fed entirely on breast milk from mothers who had long consumed strict vegetarian diets.

Food Sources

The original source of vitamin B_{12} is bacterial synthesis. Animal foods are all good sources because animals absorb this vitamin from bacterial synthesis in their intestinal tracts (see Appendix D). Until recently scientists believed that bacterial synthesis in human beings occurred only in the colon, preventing absorption of vitamin B_{12} from this source. Investigators have reported, however, that microorganisms in the ileum of human subjects synthesize significant amounts of vitamin B_{12} [39]. Presumably, if free IF happens to be present in the ileum, some of the vitamin from this source can be absorbed.

Scientists have been interested in why vegetarians who consume only plant, but no animal foods rarely develop full-blown cases of vitamin B_{12} deficiency. In addition to the possibility that they may obtain some of this vitamin from bacterial synthesis in their own digestive tracts, some may also be obtained from (1) microorganisms in the root nodules of certain legumes; (2) in some, but not all, seaweeds [40]; and (3) in some fermented soy products such as tempeh and natto [41]. Yeast ordinarily contains no vitamin B_{12}, but yeasts that have been grown on a medium to which vitamin B_{12} has been added provide this vitamin. Vegetarians living in countries where drinking water is contaminated with fecal matter may obtain some vitamin B_{12} from that source [29]. Vitamin B_{12} frequently is added to certain foods that strict vegetarians might use, such as soy milk and certain ready-to-eat breakfast cereals. The vitamin B_{12} commercially added to foods comes from bacterial synthesis and not from animal livers, therefore such foods are acceptable to many strict vegetarians.

Since vitamin B_{12} is needed for normal growth, protein synthesis, and health of the nervous system, it is important that strict vegetarians plan to obtain adequate amounts especially during pregnancy, lactation, infancy, and early childhood.

Vitamin B_{12} occurs in foods chiefly in coenzyme forms which are subject to losses by heat and light. "Flash" pasteurization of milk (exposure to heat only 2 to 3 seconds) destroys about 7 percent of the vitamin B_{12}, while boiling milk for 2 to 5 min results in about 30 percent loss [29].

Diets commonly followed in westernized countries contain generous amounts of vitamin B_{12}. Individuals consuming animal protein foods are apt to develop deficiency only if they are unable to absorb the vitamin.

Recommended Intakes

Vitamin B_{12} is the most potent of all the vitamins, for only a miniscule amount is needed daily. The RDA for adults is set at 3.0 μg per day, the lowest amount recommended by far for any vitamin (Appendix A). This amount appears to be adequate to maintain a sizable store of the vitamin in the body.

Infants obtain sufficient amounts from breast milk when their mothers receive the RDA of 4.0 μg/day. This amount seems also to be adequate for pregnant women.

Large doses of vitamin B_{12} have been taken by human subjects without obvious toxic effects [29]. However, the only known benefit of large doses is in the treatment of vitamin B_{12} deficiency.

BIOTIN

Biotin is a B vitamin that most people have heard little about, perhaps because deficiency has never developed naturally in any population group. This is probably because biotin is so widely distributed in foods, and because human beings apparently absorb some biotin that is synthesized by intestinal microorganisms.

Functions

Biotin is readily absorbed via the portal vein. It acts in the body as a coenzyme for certain enzymes that add carbon dioxide to carbon chains, elongating the chain. These reactions are important in carbohydrate and fat metabolism. Biotin coenzymes are also required for catabolism of some amino acids. Excess biotin is excreted in the urine.

Deficiency

Biotin deficiency was originally produced in animals by feeding very large amounts of raw egg white. Raw egg white contains a protein, *avidin*, which binds biotin, preventing its absorption. Investigators reported in 1942 that four human volunteers developed dry, scaly dermatitis, mild depression, muscle pains,

TABLE 10-3. AN OVERVIEW OF THE B VITAMINS

NAME	FOOD SOURCES	FUNCTIONS	DEFICIENCY SYMPTOMS	RDA FOR ADULTS (PER DAY)	ADVERSE EFFECTS (MEGADOSES)
Thiamine (vitamin B₁)	Pork, wheat germ, whole grains, dried beans, seeds, nuts, enriched flour and bread, brewer's yeast.	The coenzyme, TPP, is required by several enzymes for the oxidation of carbohydrates.	Loss of appetite; nausea; vomiting; constipation; loss of knee and ankle reflexes; depression; feeling of persecution; enlarged heart; edema. *Beriberi*	0.5 mg/1000 kcal (no less than 1.0 mg/day).	None reported.
Riboflavin	Liver, milk, dark green leafy vegetables, cheese, brewer's yeast.	The coenzymes FMN and FAD are required in oxidation of carbohydrates, fatty acids and amino acids. They are essential in the electron transport system.	Cheilosis (fissures at corners of mouth); sore, magenta-red tongue; photophobia; feeling of grittiness in eyes.	0.6 mg/1000 kcal (no less than 1.2 mg/day).	None reported.
Niacin (nicotinic acid, nicotinamide or niacinamide)	Niacin equivalents in liver, meats, poultry, fish, some nuts, whole and enriched grains and breads, dried beans.	The coenzymes NAD and NADP or their reduced forms are required for oxidation of carbohydrates, synthesis of fatty acids, and functioning of electron transport system.	Severe diarrhea; painfully sore mouth and GI tract; dark, peeling dermatitis; mental derangement. *Pellagra*	6.6 mg NE/1000 kcal (no less than 13 mg NE per day).	Nicotinic acid causes itching and flushing, abnormal heartbeat, gastrointestinal distress.
Vitamin B₆ (pyridoxal, pyridoxamine, or pyridoxine)	Liver, meats, poultry, fish, some nuts and seeds, whole grains, or beans, brewer's yeast.	B₆ coenzymes (one is PLP) required in amino acid metabolism. Required in conversion of tryptophan to niacin; in forming nonessential amino acids; forming neurotransmitters in brain from amino acids. Also involved in glycogen and fatty acid metabolism.	Convulsions in infants; greasy dermatitis; inflamed mouth with ulcers and rash on face in adults.	2.2 mg (males) 2.0 mg (females).	None reported.

NAME	FOOD SOURCES	FUNCTIONS	DEFICIENCY SYMPTOMS	RDA FOR ADULTS (PER DAY)	ADVERSE EFFECTS (MEGADOSES)
Pantothenic acid	Liver, peanuts, whole wheat, wheat germ and bran, eggs, chicken, broccoli, brewer's yeast.	Coenzyme A (CoA) required in oxidation of carbohydrates, fats, and proteins for energy: synthesis of acetylcholine, cholesterol, and ketones. Both ACP and CoA required in synthesis of fatty acids.	Fatigue; insomnia; abdominal pains; quarrelsomeness; numbness of hands and feet.	No RDA 4–7mgjudged safe and adequate.	One report of diarrhea and water retention.
Folacin (folic acid or folate)	Liver, dried beans, dark green leafy vegetables, orange juice, whole-grain breads and cereals, brewer's yeast.	Coenzymes required in transfer of single carbon units. Required in synthesis of DNA, RNA, and amino acids glycine and serine. Also required in catabolism of many amino acids.	Macrocytic anemia; red, sore tongue; diarrhea; weight loss; weakness; irritability; hostility; paranoia.	400 μg	Can obscure anemia due to vitamin B$_{12}$ deficiency.
Vitamin B$_{12}$ (cobalamin)	Animal foods: liver, meats, poultry, fish, eggs, milk.	Coenzymes (cobamides) required, along with folacin, in synthesis of DNA and RNA. Required for synthesis of myelin sheath of nerves, and for carbohydrate and fat metabolism.	Same macrocytic anemia as folacin deficiency; numbness of hands and feet; poor coordination; severe mental disorders. *Pernicious anemia*	3 μg	None reported.
Biotin	Liver, dried beans, nuts, whole grains, brewer's yeast, some fresh vegetables.	Coenzyme required by enzymes that elongate certain carbon chains in carbohydrate and fat metabolism.	Pallor; drowsiness; muscle pain; nausea; loss of appetite; scaly dermatitis.	No RDA. 100–200 μg/day judged safe and adequate.	None reported.

pallor, drowsiness, nausea, loss of appetite, and elevated blood cholesterol levels after consuming a low biotin diet in which raw egg white furnished 30 percent of the kilocalories. Urinary biotin excretion fell to very low levels. Injection of biotin cleared up all the symptoms within 3 to 5 days [42].

Food Sources

Biotin occurs widely in foods. Richest sources are dried brewer's yeast, liver, soybeans and egg yolks; nuts, oats, sardines, and mackerel contain moderate amounts. Removal of the bran and germ of grains in milling results in large losses of biotin.

Recommended Intakes

Since it appears that synthesis of biotin by intestinal bacteria makes a significant contribution to the body, it has been impossible to determine exactly how much dietary biotin is required. It is assumed, however, that some dietary biotin is needed. The Food and Nutrition Board has set estimated safe and adequate daily dietary intakes for adults of 100 to 200 µg/day (Appendix A). The American diet is thought to contain between 100 to 300 µg/day. The estimated adequate intake for infants is based on the average content of breast milk of 10 µg/1000 kcal. Most infant formulas contain 15 µg/1000 kcal [7].

CHOLINE AND INOSITOL

Two other substances, choline and inositol, require some comment, since extravagant claims are sometimes made about them. *Choline* is a fundamental part of the structure of the phospholipid, lecithin (Figure 4-10, Chapter 4). It also is incorporated into acetylcholine, an important neurotransmitter. Choline can be synthesized by some animals, yet some species require dietary choline because of inability to synthesize sufficient amounts. Scientists are uncertain as to whether or not this substance is a vitamin for human beings, since no clinical evidence of deficiency has ever been reported and no efforts have been made to produce a deficiency experimentally. Choline occurs widely in foods, however. Liver, egg yolks, whole grains, and muscle meats are excellent sources, while legumes contain moderate amounts [44].

Inositol is found in nearly all cells; in plants the most common form is phytic acid (phytate) in which inositol combines with phosphates. Inositol is widespread in foods and no cases of deficiency have been reported in human populations. Although animals are known to be able to synthesize inositol, experimental evidence is lacking to tell us whether or not human beings are dependent on the diet for inositol. The one kind of diet that might be low in choline or inositol consists of infant formulas made from nonmilk sources. To protect infants, the American Academy of Pediatrics recommends that choline and inositol be added to such formulas at levels equivalent to those in milk formulas [44].

SUMMARY

Table 10-3 contains an overview of the B vitamins.

1 The B vitamins function in body tissues as coenzymes that are essential for the activities of specific enzymes.

2 Deficiencies of B vitamins (and vitamin C) in body tissues can result from many causes other than poor dietary intake. Conditions which decrease absorption, diminish utilization, increase the rate of metabolism, or increase excretion may contribute toward a deficiency.

3 Steps should be taken to prevent losses or destruction of B vitamins in storage and preparation of foods. In addition to their water solubility, some B vitamins are subject to losses through exposure to heat or light.

4 Several of the B vitamins are interrelated in metabolism, so that a deficiency of one affects the ability of another to function properly.

5 Large doses of B vitamins appear not to be toxic except for nicotinic acid. Yet no benefit of large doses has been established, and megadosing is not recommended.

6 Except for vitamin B_{12}, the B vitamins are found in legumes, brewer's yeast, whole grains, seeds, and some nuts. In addition meats, poultry, and fish are sources of most of these vitamins, including vitamin B_{12}. Liver is a good source of most of them.

FOR DISCUSSION AND APPLICATION

1 Use the food record for Chapter 3 to calculate your daily intake of thiamine, riboflavin, niacin, vitamin B_6, pantothenic acid, folacin, and vitamin B_{12}. How do your intakes compare with the recommended intakes? What foods in your diet are rich sources of each of these vitamins? Do you need to improve your diet with respect to any of these vitamins?

2 Write a short article for your local newspaper's food section offering consumers suggestions for preserving vitamins and minerals during food preparation.

SUGGESTED READINGS

McGill, M., and O. F. Pye, "Vitamins," in *The No-Nonsense Guide to Food and Nutrition*, Maclean Hunter Learning Resources, Piscataway, N.J.: Century Publishers, 1981. A sound treatment of vitamins for the general reader by highly qualified nutritionists.

Nasset, E. S., "Utilization of Vitamins," in *Nutrition Handbook*, New York: Barnes and Noble Books, A Division of Harper & Row, 1982. A brief but interesting discussion of vitamins by a well-known nutrition researcher.

Johnson, G. T., and S. E. Goldfinger, eds., *The Harvard Medical School Health Letter Book*, New York: Warner Books, Inc., 1981. A recent synthesis of information originally published in *The Harvard Medical School Health Letter*. Many questions regarding vitamins are addressed.

11 THE FAT-SOLUBLE VITAMINS

Do large doses of vitamin E prevent aging or protect against heart disease? Are megadoses of vitamin A helpful in treating acne? Is it dangerous to swallow large doses of vitamins A, D, E, or K? This chapter attempts to answer these questions in addition to providing information about the important roles played by these vitamins in the body, the consequences of deficiency, and the foods that can supply the amounts needed.

The fat-soluble vitamins occur in the fatty portions of such foods as butter, cream, fish oils, vegetable oils, and meat fats. Since these vitamins are insoluble in water, they do not dissolve in cooking water, and are not excreted from the body in the urine. Because fat-soluble vitamins are stored in the body in considerable amounts, unlike water-soluble vitamins, deficiency signs do not begin to develop until body stores have been depleted. In well-nourished adults, then, several months to more than 2 years must elapse before deficiency develops after withdrawal of one of the fat-soluble vitamins from the diet.

310

VITAMIN A

Vitamin A, the first vitamin to be discovered, was identified as a result of experiments early in this century which sought to raise animals on purified diets containing polished rice, casein (a protein from milk), and minerals. The animals failed to grow normally unless a factor isolated from animal fats and fish oils was added to the diet [1]. As research continued, investigators realized that certain fats contained a substance required for normal growth. In 1920 this substance was given the name vitamin A [2].

Although vitamin A itself occurs only in foods of animal origin such as fatty fish, cream, butter, egg yolks, and liver, *carotenoids* present in green and yellow vegetables also have vitamin A activity. Carotenoids are substances in plants, some of which body cells convert to vitamin A. They are therefore *precursors* to vitamin A (a precursor is a substance which itself is nonfunctional as a nutrient but which body tissues directly convert to a nutrient). On food labels, the term *vitamin A* is used to include carotenoids as well as vitamin A itself. The terms *vitamin A activity* or *vitamin A value* refer to the combined contributions of vitamin A and carotenoids to the diet.

When discussing metabolism of vitamin A, nutritionists generally use chemical terms for the specific forms that occur. These include retinol, retinal, and retinoic acid. *Retinol* is vitamin A alcohol, the form present in animal foods. Body tissues convert retinol to the other forms.

Functions

Vitamin A performs several important functions in the body. It is required for vision in dim light, and for normal health of epithelial tissues which line the digestive tract, the respiratory tract, the genitourinary tract, the eyes, and the skin. This vitamin is also needed for normal bone growth and for maintenance of the structure of membranes.

Vision in Dim Light   Night blindness, or poor vision in dim light, was recognized many centuries ago. As early as 1500 B.C. Egyptian medical experts advocated consumption of ox liver for night blindness [3], but of course they had no knowledge of the active factor.

The way in which vitamin A enables us to see well in dim light is better understood than any other function of this vitamin. Light-sensitive cells lining the back of the eye make up the retina, which is the instrument of vision. These cells contain pigments which aid in vision. One of these pigments, called *rhodopsin* or visual purple, contains vitamin A in a form called *cis*-retinal, combined with a protein, *opsin* (Figure 11-1). Light splits *cis*-retinal from opsin, converting it to *trans*-retinal, an inactive form. In this process light energy is transformed into a nerve impulse which carries the visual image to the brain. Regeneration of rhodopsin is essential for the visual process to continue. Some of the split-off retinal drains away from the eye in the blood and must be replaced to permit vision in dim light. In the dark, the normal eye regenerates rhodopsin by converting *trans*- to *cis*-retinal, then combining it with opsin. Normally, this

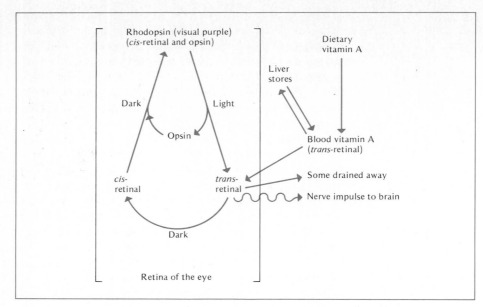

FIGURE 11-1.
Rhodopsin, containing
vitamin A as *cis*-retinal,
allows for vision in dim
light. Exposure to light
converts *cis*-retinal to
trans-retinal, which must
be converted again to
cis-retinal and combined
with opsin in the dark to
form rhodopsin before
night vision is possible.

regeneration occurs quickly so that, for example, one is able to see in a dark theater only 2 or 3 minutes after entering. In vitamin A deficiency, however, insufficient vitamin A reaches the eye by way of arterial blood to make up for losses, and *night blindness* (the inability to see in dim light) results.

Health of Epithelial Tissues   Epithelial cells are those that form the surface of the skin and the surface layer of mucous membranes. They therefore line the mouth, digestive tract, respiratory tract, genitourinary tract, the eyes, and the glands. Normally these lining tissues are moist, smooth, and slippery, like the inside of your cheeks, due to the secretion of mucus by epithelial cells. Mucus protects the lining from penetration by harmful substances such as bacteria and stomach acid. In addition, the epithelial cells lining the lungs and the reproductive tract have hairlike projections called *cilia* which use waving motions to move mucus along, ridding the area of any foreign substances adhering to the mucus. Vitamin A is needed to maintain the normal integrity of epithelial cells, including their ability to produce mucus.

Growth   Growth failure occurs in vitamin A-deficient animals and in infants and children. Although the exact reasons for growth failure are not completely understood, vitamin A deficiency appears to diminish the appetite, perhaps due to changes in the salivary glands and to keratinization of the taste buds [4]. In addition, vitamin A deficiency results in abnormal bone growth. In animals, deficiency results in paralysis due to crowding of the rapidly growing nervous tissue in a skull and vertebrae too small to accommodate it. Whether or not a similar problem occurs in vitamin A-deficient infants or children is yet to be determined.

Structure and Function of Membranes Recent evidence indicates that vitamin A probably plays an important role in regulating the structure and function of body membranes [5]. For example, the proper amount of vitamin A in the membranes of lysosomes in the cells ensures that the membranes remain intact. *Lysosomes* are structures containing hydrolytic or digestive enzymes that normally destroy worn-out parts of the cell or dead cells. In vitamin A deficiency, these digestive enzymes leak through the lysosomal membrane and presumably damage body cells.

Research continues in this important area, and others as well. Among these are vitamin A's function in reproduction, since it is known to be required for normal reproduction in animals, but its role, if any, in human reproduction is unknown. Vitamin A may also play important roles in the synthesis of certain hormones and proteins, and may have a significant influence on many enzymes. Clearly, vitamin A performs many important functions in the body.

Absorption and Metabolism

As noted earlier, the body may obtain vitamin A from certain animal foods or from carotenoids which the body converts to vitamin A. Among the carotenoids are alpha- (α), beta- (β), gamma- (γ), and delta- (δ) carotenes, but β-carotene is by far the most important precursor to vitamin A in foods. For absorption, both vitamin A and β-carotene require that fat and bile salts be present in the intestinal lumen. Bile salts render both vitamin A and carotenes more "mixable" with the watery medium of the intestinal lumen, thereby aiding absorption.

Only about one-third of the carotenoids in foods are absorbed, while vitamin A itself is almost completely absorbed. Once β-carotene crosses from the intestinal lumen into intestinal cells, about half of it normally is converted to vitamin A. For transport from mucosal cells to blood the remainder of the β-carotene and all the vitamin A are deposited in the chylomicrons (lipoproteins required for absorption of fat-soluble substances). (See Chapter 4.) The β-carotene and vitamin A therefore reach the liver by way of the lymph, the thoracic duct, and the bloodstream.

Vitamin A is stored in the liver. When needed in other parts of the body, the liver attaches vitamin A to two proteins, *retinol binding protein* (RBP), which is in turn attached to *pre-albumin*, both of which the liver synthesizes. If the liver is unable to synthesize these proteins, vitamin A cannot be removed from liver storage (Figure 11-2). In many cases of protein-calorie malnutrition, the low blood levels of vitamin A observed appear to be due to inability of the liver to synthesize RBP and pre-albumin [6].

Vitamin A as such is not lost from the body, but metabolites of vitamin A are excreted by way of the bile into the feces. Very small amounts of metabolites also appear in the urine.

Deficiency

Night blindness is one of the earliest signs that vitamin A deficiency is developing. Not everyone who develops night blindness is vitamin A-deficient, however,

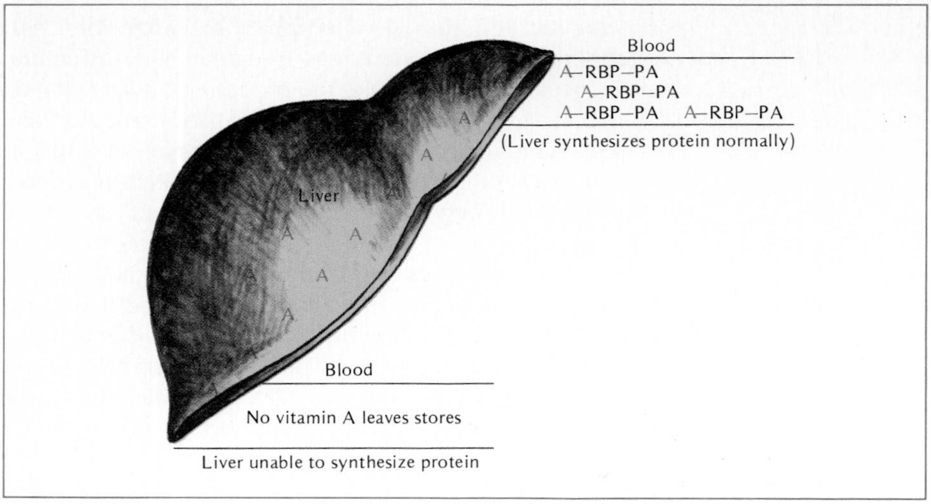

Blood

A—RBP—PA
A—RBP—PA
A—RBP—PA   A—RBP—PA

(Liver synthesizes protein normally)

Liver

Blood

No vitamin A leaves stores

Liver unable to synthesize protein

FIGURE 11-2. Removal of vitamin A from storage sites in the liver requires two specific transport proteins: retinol binding protein (RBP) and pre-albumin (PA), both of which the normal liver synthesizes.

since genetic defects can also produce this condition. As deficiency progresses, epithelial cells cease producing mucus, lose their cilia, and are converted to keratin, the hard, dry protein of hair and nails. Consequently, the protective effect of the normally smooth, slippery lining tissue is lost, and the deficient person becomes more prone to infections. Small, hard lumps of keratin plug the pores on the back of the arms, hands, or thighs once this stage of vitamin A deficiency is reached, taking on the appearance of "goose bumps."

The most serious result of vitamin A deficiency is a disease of the epithelial tissues of the eye, called *xerophthalmia*. This disease involves the epithelial cells of the *cornea*, the colored part of the eye, and of the *conjunctiva*, the membrane lining the eyelids and covering the whites of the eyes. As vitamin A deficiency progresses, first the conjunctiva, then the cornea become dry. Next, the cornea becomes cloudy. Sufficient amounts of vitamin A given at this stage completely reverse the disorder. Continued deficiency, however, results in ulceration and finally "melting" of the cornea into a gelatinous mass. The lens falls out of the eye, the fluid escapes, and the victim is now totally blind and in great danger of death unless vitamin A is supplied immediately. Xerophthalmia is, tragically, one of the major causes of blindness in infants and small children in underdeveloped countries.

In the fetus, vitamin A deficiency results in poorly developed tooth enamel, causing teeth to be more susceptible to decay in later life.

Deficiency may develop because of dietary lack of vitamin A (primary deficiency) or because other factors prevent the vitamin from reaching body cells (secondary deficiency). Deficiency does not occur until after liver stores have become exhausted, except in cases of secondary deficiency. This means that people who have unusually low blood levels of vitamin A are in danger of developing a deficiency.

Generally speaking, vitamin A deficiency is a disease of poverty. Dietary deficiency may occur because of scarcity of vitamin A sources in the food supply, or because of ignorance or lack of economic resources. In underdeveloped countries vitamin A may be very low in the diet of the landless poor, especially if rice or some other low-carotene cereal is the staple food. Frequently, green or yellow vegetables are unavailable, or by custom are not given to infants and small children.

Secondary deficiency of vitamin A may occur when lack of fat or protein in the diet or lack of bile secretion prevent adequate absorption of carotenes or vitamin A. Use of mineral oil as a laxative, if taken near mealtimes, prevents absorption of vitamin A and carotenes. Mineral oil is not a fat, but a hydrocarbon —hence it is not absorbed—but vitamin A and carotene dissolve in it. Prolonged diarrhea or serious malabsorptive diseases, such as celiac disease or sprue, prevent adequate absorption of this vitamin, and deficiency is possible.

Xerophthalmia with accompanying blindness is a public health problem among infants and small children in many Asian countries [7]. Since many children suffering from protein-calorie malnutrition also have low stores of vitamin A, proper treatment requires that sufficient kilocalories, protein, and vitamin A be supplied. If vitamin A is not given, the administration of protein alone allows the liver to synthesize RBP and pre-albumin, promoting removal of the remaining stores of vitamin A. As the stores vanish, vitamin A deficiency rapidly develops [5].

Although serious signs of vitamin A deficiency have not been observed in the United States and other affluent countries, individual cases of deficiency occa-

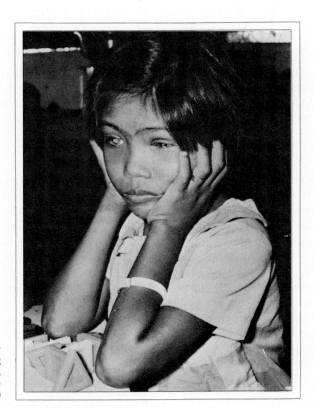

A Filipino girl blinded by xerophthalmia, resulting from vitamin A deficiency. *(WHO/Helen Keller International)*

TABLE 11-1. CALCULATION OF RETINOL EQUIVALENTS (RE) IN FOODS OR DIETS

1 RE = 1 μg retinol
    = 6 μg β-carotene
    = 12 μg other carotenoids
	1 RE = 3.33 IU vitamin activity from retinol
	    = 10 IU vitamin A activity from β-carotene

A. If retinol and β-carotene are given in μg, then: $\mu g \text{ retinol} + \dfrac{\mu g \ \beta\text{-carotene}}{6} = RE$

    Example: A diet contains 250 μg retinol and 2400 μg β-carotene. How many RE does it furnish?

$$250 + \frac{2400}{6} = 650 \ RE$$

B. If retinol and β-carotene are given in IU, then: $\dfrac{IU \text{ of retinol}}{3.33} + \dfrac{IU \text{ of } \beta\text{-carotene}}{10} = RE$

    Example: How many RE are furnished by a diet containing 999 IU of retinol and 4000 IU of β-carotene?

$$\frac{999}{3.33} + \frac{4000}{10} = 700 \ RE$$

C. If β-carotene and other carotenoids are given in μg, then:

$$\frac{\mu g \ \beta\text{-carotene}}{6} + \frac{\mu g \text{ other carotenoids}}{12} = RE$$

    Example: How many RE are in a serving of winter squash which contains 1800 μg of β-carotene and 288 μg of other carotenoids?

$$\frac{1800}{6} + \frac{288}{12} = 324 \ RE$$

Using the relationships shown, one can convert IU to RE, and μg of carotenoids to RE.

SOURCE: Food and Nutrition Board, *The Recommended Dietary Allowances*, 9th ed., National Academy of Sciences, Washington, D.C., 1980, p. 57.

sionally are seen by physicians in this country due to diets consisting chiefly of meat, potatoes, bread, cereals, and sweets for prolonged periods. However, most cases of vitamin A deficiency in affluent countries appear to be due to secondary causes such as illnesses and disease.

Recommended Intakes

Until recently the RDAs for vitamin A and values for vitamin A activity in foods were expressed in international units (IU). One IU is equivalent to 0.3 micrograms (μg) of retinol or 0.6 μg of β-carotene. But the IU system, which was based upon rat studies, fails to adequately take into account the lower absorbability of carotenoids compared with that of vitamin A itself. Therefore, the Food and Nutrition Board in 1974 adopted the retinol equivalent (RE) as the means of expressing the vitamin A value of foods. By definition, 1 RE is equal to 1 μg of retinol. Since only one-third of β-carotene in food is absorbed, and only half of that is converted in body tissues to retinol, 1 RE equals 6 μg β-carotene. This means that on a weight basis, retinol is six times as effective as is β-carotene. Other carotenoids are less well utilized than β-carotene, so that 1 RE is equal to 12 μg of carotenoids other than β-carotene. Practical uses of these relationships are shown in Table 11-1.

The RDA for adults is 800 μg RE for females and 1000 μg RE for males

(Appendix A). The larger body size of males accounts for their larger RDA. Although food composition tables generally still list the vitamin A value of foods in international units, newer tables list both μg RE and IU.

Food Sources

Figure 11-3 indicates good sources of vitamin A activity. Clearly, plant foods are the most important sources of vitamin A value in the diet, since liver is infrequently consumed.

Many foods supply little vitamin A value. Notice that in Table 11-2, a day's menu that meets the Basic Four Food Guide (but ignores the admonition to include a green or yellow vegetable) fails by far to reach the RDA for an adult woman. The addition of one carrot to this menu would add 7930 IU of vitamin A value. Dislike of vegetables may contribute to a low vitamin A diet. Many fast foods such as hamburgers, fried chicken, fried fish, and french fries are extremely low in vitamin A. Persons who routinely eat such foods should make a conscious effort to include good vitamin A sources in other meals.

Vitamin A itself is stable to heat and does not dissolve in cooking water, but can be destroyed by exposure to air. Cooking or canning reduces the vitamin A activity of the carotenes by about 15 to 35 percent, however, because these

FIGURE 11-3. Percentage of the RDA for vitamin A for the adult female (800 RE) and male (1000 RE) furnished by selected foods. Values obtained from Appendix C (in IU) were converted to RE according to methods shown in Table 11-1. For this purpose, all the carotenoids in plant foods were assumed to be present as β-carotene.

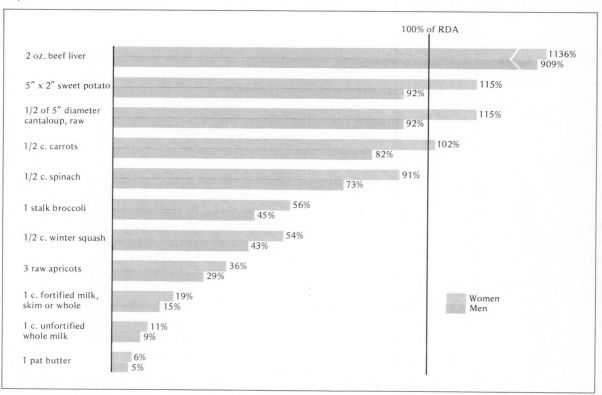

100% of RDA

Food	Women	Men
2 oz. beef liver	1136%	909%
5" x 2" sweet potato	115%	92%
1/2 of 5" diameter cantaloup, raw	115%	92%
1/2 c. carrots	102%	82%
1/2 c. spinach	91%	73%
1 stalk broccoli	56%	45%
1/2 c. winter squash	54%	43%
3 raw apricots	36%	29%
1 c. fortified milk, skim or whole	19%	15%
1 c. unfortified whole milk	11%	9%
1 pat butter	6%	5%

TABLE 11-2.   ONE DAY'S MENU PLANNED ACCORDING TO THE BASIC FOUR, BUT INCLUDING NO DARK GREEN OR YELLOW VEGETABLE

	VITAMIN A VALUE IU
Breakfast	
½ grapefruit (white)	10
1 shredded wheat biscuit	0
1 c whole milk (no vitamin A added)	310
1 slice toast	0
1 tsp jelly	0
1 pat butter	150
1 c coffee	0
Lunch	
1 c onion soup (dehydrated mix)	30
2 slices rye bread	0
2 oz tuna	46
1 tbsp mayonnaise	40
½ stalk celery	55
1 brownie (from mix)	20
1 glass iced tea	0
Dinner	
½ chicken breast	70
½ c mashed potatoes (milk added)	25
½ c yellow (wax) beans	145
Wedge of iceberg lettuce	450
Italian dressing	0
1 piece apple pie (⅕ of 9″ pie)	40
1 c yogurt (made with nonfat milk)	20
Total	1411 IU
RDA, adult women	4000 IU

SOURCE OF VALUES: Appendix C.

processes cause the molecules to undergo a change in arrangement of atoms [8]. Drying vegetables or fruit by exposing them to air results in large losses of vitamin A activity. Rancid fats destroy both vitamin A and carotenes, but storing fats or fatty foods at proper refrigeration temperatures delays development of rancidity, as does freezing or addition of antioxidants during processing.

Toxicity

Excessive intakes of vitamin A, but not carotenoids, can be toxic or poisonous. Toxicity may occur in a short time (acute toxicity) or only after a long period of high intake (chronic toxicity). The toxic condition that results is called *hypervitaminosis A*. Toxicity rarely occurs from eating foods, but generally results from taking supplements (pills). Symptoms of *acute* toxicity include violent headache, nausea, vomiting, sluggishness, dizziness, and peeling of the skin. In infants, bulging of the fontanel (the soft spot on the top of the head where bones have not yet fused) and drowsiness develop.

In infants and children, chronic toxicity usually has developed when caretakers have given larger doses of vitamin A supplements than the physician recommended. Infants develop toxicity after taking 14,000 to 20,000 IU per day over several weeks [9] (the RDA in infancy is equivalent to 1400 to 2000 IU). In adults, chronic toxicity has developed among health enthusiasts who mistakenly believed that large doses would be beneficial, or among those who had previously received large doses for skin disorders but who continued the dosage without a physician's guidance. (The use of large doses of vitamin A to treat acne is discussed in Box 11-1.)

Symptoms of *chronic* toxicity include dryness, itching, and peeling of the skin, loss of hair, bone and joint pain, headache, enlargement of the liver, loss of appetite, great fatigue and weakness, cessation of menstruation in women, and increased cerebrospinal fluid pressure.

Because of the danger of toxicity, the Food and Nutrition Board recommends that only under a physician's supervision should infants and children receive as much as 10,000 IU (3000 RE) per day of vitamin A. The Board also notes that for adults an intake of more than 25,000 IU (7500 RE) per day "is not prudent [18]." Intakes of 25,000 IU occasionally from liver or a combination of foods is of no concern, but *daily* intakes of this amount are not recommended even from foods. Infants and young children should not be fed liver daily, for example, since such a diet presents a danger of chronic toxicity. Often such a practice means one is not consuming a wide variety of foods, but is instead including only a select few in the diet.

The carotenes, unlike vitamin A, are not toxic. In large amounts, carotenes will turn the skin yellow as is sometimes observed in small children who go on carrot-eating binges. No harm is known to result, and cessation of the practice quickly alleviates the condition.

Vitamin A Derivatives as Anticancer Agents

Currently, synthetic derivatives of vitamin A called *retinoids* are under investigation for the prevention of certain epithelial tissue cancers. So far, research indicates that retinoids, to be effective, must be administered at an early stage during which the affected cells are gradually developing into cancer cells [19].

Interest in retinoids as anticancer agents came about from the observation that in vitamin A deficiency epithelial cells structurally resemble cells in the early stages of cancer development. One might expect, then, to find a greater incidence of cancers of epithelial tissues among animals or human beings deficient in vitamin A. This has been demonstrated in rats [20,21], and epidemiological studies suggest that this may also be the case in human subjects. Norwegian cigarette smokers whose diets were low in sources of vitamin A had a greater occurrence of lung cancer than smokers whose diets included greater amounts of vitamin A food sources [22]. Another study reported that patients with lung cancer had lower blood levels of vitamin A than patients with other lung diseases [23]. While these studies do not *prove* that low intakes of foods

11-1 Is Vitamin A the Answer to Acne?

BOX

Acne, a common skin disorder among adolescents, is dreaded because of concern about physical attractiveness and because in severe forms it can be disfiguring. Acne is thought to result from increased androgen (sex hormone) production at puberty which, in sensitive persons, brings about overproduction of sebum, a greasy material secreted by the sebaceous glands which causes unsightly pimples. Sensitivity to androgens is thought to be hereditary, since acne tends to run in families [10].

Recently, various forms of vitamin A have been used to treat acne. One group of investigators reported effectively treating over 300 patients with severe inflammatory acne (not mild acne) with oral doses of 300,000 to 500,000 IU of retinol (vitamin A alcohol) daily for 4 to 5 months [11]. Adverse effects included dryness and peeling of the skin, minor nosebleeds, dryness of the nasal mucosa, and headaches, but were not considered serious enough to merit cessation of treatment. Since individuals vary widely in their susceptibility to toxicity, such large doses should never be taken except under close supervision by a knowledgeable physician. Treatment with very large oral doses of retinol is not recommended for longer than 5 or 6 months [11] and unfortunately is not a cure, as the acne tends to recur after treatment is stopped. Other forms of vitamin A may prove useful, however. Peck and coworkers treated 14 patients suffering from severe scarring acne with very large doses of 13-*cis*-retinoic acid, a different form of vitamin A than occurs naturally. After 4 months of treatment, 13 of the 14 showed complete healing, while the 14th showed 75 percent improvement. Acne had not recurred in these patients 20 months after the treatment ended [12]. Other investigators have confirmed the effectiveness of 13-*cis*-retinoic acid [13]. Further work must be done to assure that 13-*cis*-retinoic acid causes no damage to the body, but it appears to be a promising experimental drug for acne treatment.

Creams or lotions containing retinoic acid, called tretinoin, have also demonstrated their effectiveness in treating acne. Applications of tretinoin to the skin can cause redness and peeling and should be used only under a physician's guidance [10]. Frequently, tretinoin is used in combination with orally administered antibiotics, since a study of 238 patients in Denmark demonstrated the effectiveness of this combined treatment [14,15].

An interrelationship of zinc with vitamin A may play a role in acne. Patients with severe acne had lower blood levels of vitamin A, retinol binding protein (RBP), and zinc than a group of controls [16]. Since zinc is believed to be required for secretion of RBP by the liver, and RBP carries vitamin A into the blood from liver stores, zinc deficiency might explain the low serum levels of vitamin A and RBP in these patients with severe acne. Although not all studies indicate that supplemental zinc improves acne, others demonstrate a beneficial effect in some patients [17]. Further work should clarify the relationship of zinc and vitamin A in acne. Obviously, vitamin A is not *the* answer to acne.

Exactly how various forms of vitamin A aid in the treatment of acne is not fully understood, just as the precise way in which vitamin A maintains the health of epithelial tissues remains to be determined. Therapy for acne today is far more effective than it was 20 years ago, however, and doubtless will continue to improve as research continues. However, it should be stressed again that attempts at self-medication with vitamin A are fraught with danger and should be avoided.

furnishing vitamin A play a causative role in cancers of epithelial tissues, they indicate that this is a promising area for future research.

VITAMIN D

Rickets, a disease in which the developing bones in infants and children become bent and misshapen, has been known since antiquity. Around the 1820s cod-liver oil was a popular folk remedy for rickets and by the end of the nineteenth century we knew that sunshine would cure rickets. The reasons for the effectiveness of either cod-liver oil or sunshine remained a mystery, however, until 1922 when

E. V. McCollum demonstrated that cod-liver oil exposed to oxygen to destroy the vitamin A still cured rickets in animals. Later the curative factor in cod-liver oil was called vitamin D.

Vitamin D can be formed from precursors. One of these precursors, *7-dehydrocholesterol*, exists in human and animal skin and is converted to vitamin D_3 (*cholecalciferol*) when exposed to ultraviolet rays from the sun or sunlamps. Vitamin D_3 occurs naturally in fish-liver oils. *Ergosterol* is a precursor occurring in some strains of yeasts and molds which, upon exposure in the laboratory to ultraviolet light, is converted to vitamin D_2 (*ergocalciferol*). Vitamin D_2 is the most important synthetic form used commercially. Humans use vitamin D_2 and D_3 with equal facility.

Functions

Vitamin D is essential for normal *mineralization* (calcification) of bones. Bone mineralization occurs when calcium and phosphorus crystals are deposited in the soft collagen matrix which forms the foundation of bones. Without proper calcification, bones bend and become misshapen. Before we discuss how vitamin D participates in bone mineralization, let's look at how this vitamin is absorbed and metabolized in body tissues.

The absorption of vitamin D from food requires the presence of fat and bile salts in the intestinal tract. The absorbed vitamin D is deposited in chylomicrons in the intestinal mucosal cells, and reaches the blood by way of the lymphatic route. Vitamin D synthesized in the skin from exposure to ultraviolet light also enters circulating blood. Most of the vitamin D absorbed from food or synthesized in the skin is taken up by the liver [24].

Any vitamin D lost from the body is excreted chiefly through the bile in chemical forms not yet identified. Very little is lost through the urine.

Vitamin D itself is not active in the body, as recent research has shown [24]. Vitamin D_2 and D_3 are changed to their active forms by a two-step process, beginning in the liver and concluding in the kidney. In the liver an —OH (hydroxyl) group is placed on position no. 25 of vitamin D, forming 25-hydroxyvitamin D (25(OH)vit D). This compound is sent to the kidney by way of the blood where a second —OH group is added to position no. 1, forming the active form, 1,25-dihydroxyvitamin D (1,25(OH)$_2$vit D) (Figure 11-4).

While the exact mechanism by which active vitamin D promotes bone mineralization has yet to be identified, it is known that the fluid bathing the bones must contain very high concentrations of calcium for calcification to occur. Active vitamin D brings about such high concentrations at the specific sites in the bone where mineralization is needed in at least three ways: (1) by increasing the absorption of calcium in the intestines; (2) by moving calcium from already calcified bone to the fluids bathing the bone; and (3) by increasing the reabsorption into the blood of calcium by the kidneys, preventing its loss in the urine (Figure 11-4).

Active vitamin D is believed to aid in the absorption of calcium in the intestines by stimulating the synthesis of a calcium transport protein by intestinal mucosal cells. Apparently this protein carries calcium across the intestinal

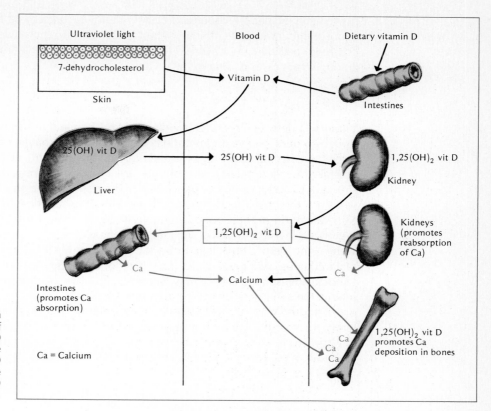

FIGURE 11-4. Formation and functions of 1,25-dihydroxyvitamin D (1,25(OH)$_2$vit D), the active form of vitamin D in metabolism. The action of 1,25(OH)$_2$vit D is shown in color.

mucosal cell membrane from the intestinal lumen to the interior of the mucosal cell [24].

The way in which the body regulates movement of calcium in and out of bones and body fluids is discussed in Chapter 12. At this point, we need only emphasize that while vitamin D plays a role in regulating calcium in fluids bathing bone, in the end its major function is to promote bone calcification.

Thinking over all we have just said about vitamin D, it becomes apparent that by accepted definitions vitamin D can be classified both as a vitamin and as a hormone. A *hormone*, you will recall from the Introduction to this book, is a substance produced by specialized cells in the body and sent by way of the blood to its target tissues. According to this definition, 1,25(OH)$_2$vit D is a hormone that is formed in the kidneys and sent by way of the blood to its target tissues, the intestines, bones, and kidneys. Precursors of this hormone are 7-dehydrocholesterol and vitamins D$_2$ and D$_3$ obtained from food.

A *vitamin*, on the other hand, is necessary for specific functions in body tissues, but must be provided in the diet. Clearly, those who are exposed sufficiently to sunlight do not require vitamin D in food—technically it is not a vitamin for them. On the other hand, those who lack sufficient exposure to sun are dependent upon dietary vitamin D—for them it is a vitamin. A large percentage of people require dietary vitamin D because climatic conditions, atmospheric pollutants, living indoors, and covering the body with clothing combine to drastically diminish their exposure to sunlight. Vitamin D is unique among vitamins in its duality as a vitamin and hormone.

Deficiency

Vitamin D deficiency results in *rickets* in children and in *osteomalacia* in adults. Both disorders involve abnormalities of the bones. We have noted that the mature bone consists basically of a foundation of the protein, collagen, into which crystals of calcium and phosphorus are embedded, imparting hardness and strength. Collagen is limber like the tip of the nose and the ears. Infants' bones are soft since they consist chiefly of collagen and little calcification has yet occurred. Mineralization of their bones gradually increases after birth so that, by the time they have learned to walk, sufficient calcification has occurred to support their weight and permit their legs to be straight. If insufficient calcification has taken place, the legs will bend under the weight of the body, resulting in bowed legs or "knock knees." The chest may become shrunken or deformed, and in young infants the skull may become enlarged.

Children with rickets frequently have enlarged joints at the wrist or knees, or knots in the ribs, giving the appearance of a string of beads, called "rachitic (referring to rickets) rosary." These signs all result from overgrowth or overaccumulation of collagen. In normal growth, bones of the arms, legs, and ribs increase

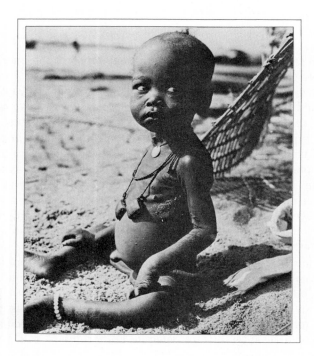

A child with rickets. Notice the protruding abdomen, curvature of the lower legs, and enlarged wrist. *(The Bettmann Archive, Inc.)*

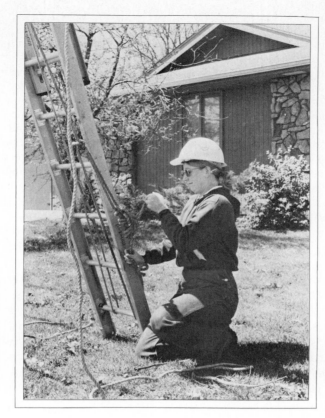

Adults who routinely
work in the sun
synthesize nearly all the
vitamin D they need,
even though during part
of the year only their
faces and hands are
exposed. *(J.R.
Holland/Stock, Boston,
Inc.)*

in length by the laying down of new collagen near the ends of the bones, followed by calcification of the collagen. When vitamin D is lacking, the laying down of collagen continues, but calcification fails to occur, resulting in enlargements in the wrists, knees, and ribs. Administration of sufficient vitamin D brings about orderly calcification of the bone and disappearance of excessive collagen.

For unknown reasons, muscles become weakened in rickets, producing a markedly protruding abdomen. Delayed tooth eruption occurs, and tooth enamel of permanent teeth is sometimes absent and often thin and pitted [25]. Although vitamin D cures rickets, damage may be severe enough that misshapen bones persist into adulthood, resulting in bowed legs or deformities of the chest or spine.

Osteomalacia results from the development of vitamin D deficiency in adulthood. Even in adulthood, calcium and phosphorus are withdrawn from the bones daily and must be replaced to maintain their strength. Since calcification requires vitamin D, deficiency in adults can result in soft, deformed bones. The disease causes deformities of the pelvis and the shafts of the leg bones [25]. Osteomalacia is uncommon in the United States but still occurs in northern China, Japan, and northern India. It occurs in women who subsist on diets low in vitamin D and calcium and who have lost much body calcium through many pregnancies and lactations. Furthermore, they are little exposed to sunlight [25].

Recently a resurgence of rickets has been reported in the United States and in Scotland [26]. Most cases reported have been among dark-skinned people following strict vegetarian diets and, in many cases, also avoiding exposure to the sun. (Dark skin apparently prevents much ultraviolet light from reaching the deep layers of the skin.) Because plant foods contain no vitamin D, a pregnant woman consuming only plant foods is likely to have a baby with low stores of vitamin D. If she nurses her infant, little vitamin D will be in her milk and early development of rickets is likely. Teenagers following strict vegetarian diets may also develop vitamin D deficiency, since the adolescent growth spurt increases their requirements for this vitamin. Persons following strict vegetarian diets should make certain they consume foods fortified with an adequate amount of vitamin D, such as soymilk. Other alternatives might be vitamin D supplements or ample exposure of the skin to sunlight.

Recommended Intakes

The 1980 RDAs list the allowances for vitamin D in micrograms (μg) rather than in international units (IU), as was done in previous RDAs. This was done in accordance with the recommendations of the Expert Committee of the Food and Agriculture Organization (FAO)/World Health Organization (WHO) of the United Nations [18]. One IU of vitamin D is defined as the activity in 0.025 μg of cholecalciferol (vitamin D_3). The RDAs for vitamin D (Appendix A) are 5 μg (200 IU) per day in adults and double this amount during pregnancy, lactation, and other periods of growth.

Food Sources

Few foods contain vitamin D naturally. For both animals and humans, exposure of the skin to sunlight converting 7-dehydrocholesterol to vitamin D, has always been an important source of this vitamin. Foods that in their natural state contain vitamin D include egg yolks, liver, butter, and fatty fish, but the amount in these foods depends upon the amount in the animal's diet and upon the extent of exposure to sunlight. The most important source of this vitamin in the current American diet is probably milk fortified with vitamin D. All evaporated milk and most fluid milk in the United States is fortified with 400 IU per quart. Vitamin D is also added to many ready-to-eat breakfast cereals and margarines.

Although for many years we believed that human milk supplies too little vitamin D to meet the needs of infants, rickets is relatively uncommon among breast-fed infants of well-nourished mothers. A more detailed discussion of this topic is in Chapter 15.

Toxicity

Vitamin D, like vitamin A, is toxic in large amounts because the body's metabolic machinery is unable to handle excessive amounts. Doses of 3000 to 4000 IU (75 to 100 μg) have been reported to delay growth in infants [27,28]. Larger doses

(10,000 IU or 250 μg in infants, and 75,000 IU or 1875 μg in adults) cause high concentrations of calcium in the blood, eventually resulting in calcification of soft tissues such as kidneys and blood vessels. Death or irreversible damage can occur as a consequence. Among the symptoms of vitamin D toxicity are loss of appetite, nausea and vomiting, excessive urination, excessive thirst, lack of muscle tone which may lead to constipation, itchiness of the skin, slow heart beat, and disorders of the heart rhythm.

Generally, the intake of vitamin D should not exceed the RDA. Care should be taken to avoid overdosing infants by giving only amounts of "baby vitamins" prescribed. Routinely feeding several infant foods, each of which has vitamin D added, also should be avoided. Smaller amounts are toxic for infants than for adults because of the smaller body size.

VITAMIN E

Vitamin E cures sterility! Sexual impotence prevented with vitamin E! Vitamin E prevents heart attacks! Vitamin E cures muscular dystrophy! Vitamin E keeps you young! Vitamin E erases scars! All these emphatic claims have been made for vitamin E, but is this vitamin truly such a panacea? In this section we will examine the functions of vitamin E, paying particular attention to the popular claims noted above.

The technical name for the most active form of vitamin E is alpha-tocopherol. Seven other tocopherols also occur in nature, but alpha-tocopherol is more than twice as active as beta-tocopherol, the next most active form.

Functions

A long-standing controversy about whether vitamin E acts in the body only as a biological antioxidant or whether it also acts as a component of an enzyme system has yet to be resolved. It may be that this vitamin acts in both ways, but at present the hypothesis that vitamin E acts as an antioxidant is well established, while its function as a component of an enzyme system has yet to be convincingly demonstrated.

According to the antioxidant theory, vitamin E collects in the cell membranes and in membranes of other cellular components. There it comes in contact with phospholipids and cholesterol, major structural components of membranes. Each of these contains polyunsaturated fatty acids, and vitamin E protects these easily oxidized compounds against destruction by free radicals. *Free radicals* are compounds having unpaired electrons and as such are highly reactive and capable of heavily damaging the cell. Polyunsaturated fatty acids themselves give rise to free radicals when they begin to undergo oxidation. The presence of sufficient vitamin E in membranes inactivates free radicals, thereby protecting polyunsaturated fats from deterioration and preventing cell damage (Figure 11-5). The mineral selenium, as a part of an enzyme, acts synergistically with vitamin E in protecting polyunsaturated fatty acids in cell membranes from oxidative destruction—yet another example of important nutrient interactions (Chapter 13).

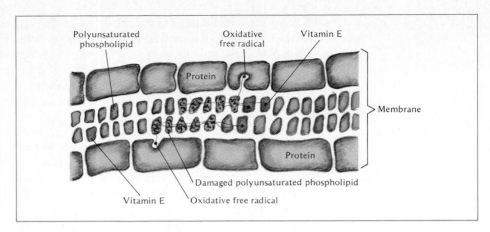

Polyunsaturated
phospholipid

Oxidative
free radical

Vitamin E

Protein

Membrane

Protein

Damaged polyunsaturated phospholipid

Vitamin E

Oxidative free radical

FIGURE 11-5. Vitamin E protects membranes in cells from damage by free radicals. In the absence of vitamin E, free radicals damage polyunsaturated fats and proteins (including enzymes), destroying membranes and therefore destroying cell functions.

Membrane damage by free radicals in the absence of vitamin E results in accumulation in the tissues of fluorescent pigments called *ceroid pigments* or lipofuscin. These are regarded as evidence that oxidative destruction of membranes has occurred. They are sometimes called aging pigments since they tend to occur in aged animals, including humans. (See Box 11-2 for a fuller discussion of the possible relationship between vitamin E and aging.)

Vitamin E absorption depends upon normal secretions of pancreatic lipase and bile salts into the duodenum. Once inside the intestinal mucosal cells, vitamin E is deposited in chylomicrons and absorbed by way of the lymphatic system.

Only about 20 to 40 percent of dietary vitamin E is absorbed [29]. After absorption, vitamin E travels in the blood from one tissue to another attached chiefly to the low-density lipoproteins (LDL). It is stored in adipose tissue, muscles, and liver. It also occurs in high concentrations in the adrenal and pituitary glands, and in testes and blood platelets [29].

Although vitamin E is not excreted in the urine, consumption of large doses results in biochemical modification of the vitamin and these products may be excreted in the urine [29].

Deficiency

In animals, a great many disorders are attributable to vitamin E deficiency, a fact that may be partly responsible for the extravagant claims made for this vitamin. Reproductive failure occurs in both male and female rats. In the chick, hemorrhaging in the brain and underneath the skin of the breast and abdomen occurs as does damage to the nervous system. Several species of animals develop "nutritional muscular dystrophy," a disorder different from human muscular dystrophy, an inherited disease.

In the 1950s adult men were fed a diet low in vitamin E (3 mg of alpha-tocopherol a day) for over 6 years [30]. The only effect noted was that erythrocytes (red blood cells) survived a somewhat shorter time than normal. Red blood cells normally survive about 120 days; as old cells are destroyed new ones must replace them. The shorter survival time meant new cells were needed to replace old ones within a shorter time span. No anemia developed, but supplementation with vitamin E resulted in a small but significant increase in synthesis of new red blood cells [30]. Apparently, body stores of vitamin E in normal adults are large enough so that many years are required to exhaust them.

Vitamin E deficiency has never been reported to occur in any human population group subsisting on its usual diet [30]. In diseased states in which children or adults absorb fats poorly, however, signs of deficiency have been reported. For example, children with cystic fibrosis (who absorb little fat) frequently have erythrocytes that survive a shorter time than normal [29], and a small number of these patients have also developed various skeletal muscle abnormalities. Many of these children excrete unusually high amounts of creatine in the urine, an indicator of muscle wastage [30]. Giving them a water-soluble form of vitamin E (a form available to physicians) clears up all these deficiency signs.

Premature infants may be prone to develop vitamin E deficiency [31]. These infants are born with low levels of vitamin E in their bodies, and tend to absorb it inefficiently. Injection of a water-soluble form prevents deficiency from developing [29].

Although many studies have reported no ill effects when 200 to 1000 IU of vitamin E have been consumed daily by adults for several weeks to years, a few cases of abdominal discomfort, fatigue, and skin rash have been reported [29].

Recommended Intakes

The most recent RDA uses milligrams of alpha-tocopherol equivalents (mg αTE) as the unit for expressing recommended amounts of vitamin E, whereas in previous years the international unit (IU) was used. The activity of 1 milligram (mg) of naturally occurring alpha-tocopherol is equivalent to 1.49 IU. Most food composition tables still use international units, although newer tables use milligrams.

The adult RDA is 8 mg αTE (12 IU) for females and 10 mg αTE (15 IU) for males (Appendix A). The need for vitamin E is related to the polyunsaturated fat content of cellular and subcellular membranes (membranes surrounding lysosomes, mitochondria, and other cellular components. See Figure 0-1, Introduction). The RDAs assume an average intake of polyunsaturated fat (about 5 to 7 percent of total kilocalories). Higher intakes of vitamin E are recommended for individuals whose polyunsaturated fat intake is higher than average. Since the major food source of polyunsaturated fatty acids are oils and margarines which are also excellent sources of vitamin E, it is assumed that individuals consuming large amounts of these fats also consume adequate vitamin E. Those who have become accustomed to a high polyunsaturated fat intake and suddenly change to a low intake may develop a deficiency eventually because they no longer have a sufficiently high vitamin E intake to protect their polyunsaturated fat stores [29]. Vitamin E is lost from body stores more rapidly than polyunsaturated fat; therefore in such cases vitamin E intakes equal to the previous level should be continued for some time.

Food Sources

Figure 11-6 indicates that animal foods, except for fish-liver oils, are generally low in vitamin E. Plants, on the other hand, can synthesize vitamin E and frequently contribute large amounts to the diet.

Considerable losses of vitamin E may occur in cooking, processing, and storage of foods. Vitamin E is lost from some foods during freezer storage, and canning results in significant losses. One study reported that canned entrees contained only one-third to one-half as much vitamin E as the same entree prepared at home [32]. Refining whole wheat results in significant losses and bleaching white flour results in further losses. Potato chips stored at room temperature for 2 weeks lost about half their vitamin E content during that time [33]. Losses of vitamin E from tightly closed bottles of oil are usually minimal but increase during exposure to air and heat.

FIGURE 11-6. Percentage of the vitamin E RDA for adult women (8 mg αTE) and adult men (10 mg αTE) supplied by selected foods. Values are for total vitamin E, including α-, β-, τ-, and δ-tocopherols. (Source of values: McLaughlin, P. J., and J. L. Weihrauch, "Vitamin E Content of Food," Reprinted by permission from *Journal of the American Dietetic Association*, 75:647, 1979.)

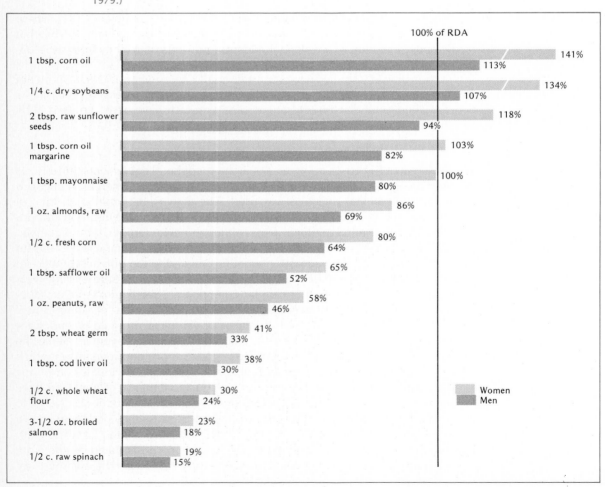

Is there any basis for popular claims that large doses of vitamin E are beneficial? Is it the "miracle vitamin?" These questions are addressed in Box 11-2.

VITAMIN K

Intestinal bacteria are capable of synthesizing many vitamins, but in human beings this phenomenon occurs chiefly in the colon, which means that the newly synthesized vitamins are excreted in the feces rather than absorbed. Vitamin K is an exception to this rule. Apparently bacteria higher in the intestinal tract, probably in the ileum, synthesize vitamin K which the normal person absorbs; consequently, healthy individuals are not dependent on dietary vitamin K alone.

Function

The liver synthesizes several different proteins necessary for blood clotting. Vitamin K is required for the synthesis of four of these proteins, including prothrombin [45]. If insufficient vitamin K is present in the liver the clotting factors are not formed, and hemorrhaging or bleeding results.

The absorption of vitamin K, whether from food or from bacterial synthesis, requires the presence of bile salts and normal secretions of pancreatic juice. Vitamin K, like other fat-soluble vitamins, is deposited in the chylomicrons by the intestinal mucosal cells and absorbed by way of the lymphatic system. Large amounts are then stored in the liver, but skin and muscle also contain fairly large amounts. Any vitamin K leaving the body appears chiefly in the feces by way of bile.

Deficiency

Vitamin K deficiency is unusual, and does not develop among normal people living under normal conditions. Newborn infants, however, may become deficient because they are born without bacteria in their intestinal tracts, and very little, if any, vitamin K crosses from mother's blood to baby's blood during pregnancy. The low level of clotting factors in the infant's blood during the first week of life may result in bleeding, a disorder called *hemorrhagic disease of the newborn*. To prevent the disease, the American Academy of Pediatrics recommends that an injection of vitamin K be given to all infants at birth. After about a week, the bacterial flora develop sufficiently for vitamin K synthesis to begin, but infant formulas and mother's milk also supply some vitamin K.

Adults tend to develop vitamin K deficiency only if (1) there is very poor absorption of fat for a prolonged period; (2) the bacterial flora are destroyed by long-term intakes of antibiotics; (3) liver disease prevents synthesis of the clotting factors, even if vitamin K is present; or (4) a vitamin K antagonist, such as dicumarol, is used. Dicumarol may be prescribed to prevent blood clots, as in heart patients, and accomplishes this by preventing vitamin K from forming clotting factors. Too much dicumarol can result in hemorrhaging, making it

Is Vitamin E a Cure-all?

Despite the fact that healthy individuals consuming their usual diet are not deficient in vitamin E, popular publications claim that large doses of this vitamin will prevent or cure a wide variety of disorders. Is there any truth in such claims?

In cases of real deficiency, as in premature infants or when there is prolonged malabsorption of fats, vitamin E deficiency can be cured by giving the vitamin. In addition, certain other disorders appear to respond to vitamin E therapy. Older people with intermittent claudication, a disorder in which blood circulation in the lower legs is so poor that walking becomes impossible because of cramplike pain and muscle weakness, have been successfully treated with large daily doses of vitamin E for 3 months or longer [34,35].

Premature infants are subject to eye damage because their immature eye retinas are exposed to much higher concentrations of oxygen in their incubators than they received in the uterus. Whether or not vitamin E guards against oxidative damage to the retinas is a matter of controversy [36,37], but vitamin E appears to lessen oxidative damage in the lungs of small premature infants treated in an atmosphere high in oxygen [38,39].

For a number of years, doctors at the Shute Clinic in Canada have claimed that large doses of vitamin E prevent and cure heart disease, including *angina pectoris*, a disorder in which chest pains occur due to inadequate blood and oxygen supply to the heart muscle. Physicians at the Shute Clinic have never performed studies using placebos, however, because they were certain that vitamin E was beneficial. A well-controlled study, using the dosage and duration of vitamin E supplementation recommended by the Shute Clinic, showed no alleviation of angina pain when patients received vitamin E compared with those receiving a well-disguised placebo [40]. Earlier studies also failed to support the contention that vitamin E is effective in

treating heart disease [41]. In light of its effectiveness in intermittent claudication, however, it is clear that further research on its usefulness in circulatory disorders is justified.

Claims that vitamin E is effective in improving sexual performance or in preventing sterility or impotence in the male are not supported by scientific studies [42]. Much of the hope in this area was based on the fact that vitamin E was discovered because of reproductive failure in experimental rats, but these animals were severely deficient in the vitamin, while human beings are not deficient.

Although studies show that vitamin E protects the lungs of animals against damage from air pollutants such as ozone and nitrogen dioxide, further research must be done before we know whether these results apply to human beings [43].

Because ceroid pigments accumulate as tissues age, it is tempting to think that vitamin E might prevent not only the accumulation of these pigments but also the aging process. In mice, however, although vitamin E prevented accumulation of ceroid pigments, it did not prolong the lives of the animals [44]. The aging process is very complex, and it is highly unlikely that swallowing a vitamin will prevent it.

The claim that vitamin E rubbed on scars causes them to disappear is also unsubstantiated by scientific studies. This claim has come from personal testimonials and is an excellent example of why controlled placebo studies are needed to establish the efficacy of a vitamin in treating a disorder. The suggestion that vitamin E will clear up a scar can easily cause one to believe, upon daily examining of the scar, that it is gradually disappearing. But one has no basis for comparison without a placebo, large numbers of subjects, and an unbiased examiner of scars.

Clearly, then, there are some legitimate medical uses for vitamin E, but claims that it cures or prevents heart disease, muscular dystrophy, sterility, or aging appear to be without foundation. As for all nutrients, one needs to be skeptical of claims made for vitamin E until convincing evidence is available, while nonetheless remaining open-minded about possible beneficial effects.

necessary to balance the amount of dicumarol and vitamin K so as to prevent both clotting and hemorrhaging [45].

Generally, deficiency does not occur in adults unless both intestinal synthesis and dietary intake are curtailed simultaneously. In deficiency, the "prothrombin time," or the time required for the blood to clot, is prolonged.

Recommended Intakes

No RDA has been set for vitamin K because the fact that normal individuals absorb some from bacterial synthesis makes determination of the dietary need difficult. The Food and Nutrition Board suggests an estimated safe and adequate daily intake of 70 to 140 μg for adults (Appendix A). The lower level of the range given for each age group in Appendix A assumes that only one-half the need is supplied by the diet, while the upper extreme of the range assumes that the entire amount needed is supplied by diet. The total amount of vitamin K needed, from both intestinal synthesis and from diet, is estimated to be 2 μg per kilogram of body weight. The estimated safe and adequate intake (Appendix A) can easily be obtained from food since the usual American diet is calculated to furnish 300 to 500 μg/day.

Food Sources

The vitamin K content of foods is shown in Figure 11-7. The best sources are green vegetables and liver. Fruits are low in this vitamin. Meats and milk contain intermediate amounts.

An overview of the fat-soluble vitamins appears in Table 11-3.

FIGURE 11-7. Percentage of the safe and adequate intake of vitamin K suggested for adults (140 μg) furnished by selected foods. Although a range of 70 to 140 μg/day is suggested, 140 μg is used as the standard of comparison here. (Source of values: Olson, R. E., "Vitamin K," in Goodhart, R. S., and M. E. Shils, (eds.), *Modern Nutrition in Health and Disease*, 6th ed., Philadelphia: Lea & Febiger, 1980, p. 172.)

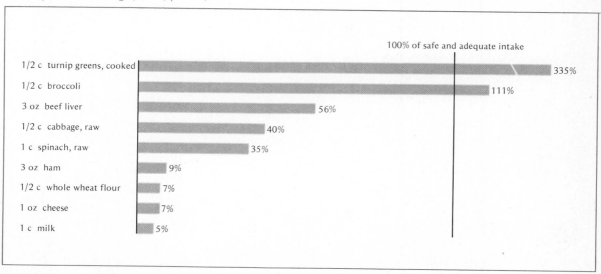

100% of safe and adequate intake

Food	Percentage
1/2 c turnip greens, cooked	335%
1/2 c broccoli	111%
3 oz beef liver	56%
1/2 c cabbage, raw	40%
1 c spinach, raw	35%
3 oz ham	9%
1/2 c whole wheat flour	7%
1 oz cheese	7%
1 c milk	5%

TABLE 11-3. AN OVERVIEW OF THE FAT-SOLUBLE VITAMINS

NAME	FOOD SOURCES	FUNCTIONS	DEFICIENCY SYMPTOMS	RDA FOR ADULTS (PER DAY)	ADVERSE EFFECTS (MEGADOSES)
Vitamin A (retinol)	Liver, whole or fortified milk, cheese, butter, margarine. Carotenoids: orange-colored vegetables and fruits; deep green vegetables.	Maintains integrity of epithelial tissues; required for night vision; growth; regulates structure and functions of cellular and subcellular membranes.	Night blindness; epithelial cells become dry and keratinized; conjunctiva and cornea become dry. *Xerophthalmia*.	800 μg (females) 1000 μg (males).	Itching, peeling skin; bone and joint pain; liver enlargement; weakness; headache.
Vitamin D (cholecalciferol (D$_3$), ergocalciferol (D$_2$)	Fortified milk, liver, fatty fish, butter, egg yolks.	Promotes mineralization of bones by promoting absorption of calcium in the intestines; moves calcium from bones to fluid bathing bones; increases reabsorption of calcium by kidneys.	Misshapen bones, enlarged wrists and knees, potbelly in children, deformed bones in adults. *Rickets* in children *Osteomalacia* in adults.	5 μg	Calcification of kidneys and blood vessels; excessive thirst and urination; slow heart beat.
Vitamin E (α-tocopherol)	Vegetable oils, dried beans, sunflower seeds, nuts, wheat germ, whole wheat, dark green leafy vegetables.	Protects membranes from oxidative breakdown by inactivating free radicals.	Deficiency unlikely to occur.	8 mg αTE for females 10 mg αTE for males.	A few cases of fatigue, skin rash, and abdominal discomfort reported.
Vitamin K	Green leafy vegetables, liver. Some absorbed from intestinal synthesis.	Required by liver for synthesis of blood-clotting factors.	Hemorrhaging; prolonged blood-clotting time.	No RDA. Estimated safe and adequate intake 70 to 140 μg.	None reported for naturally occurring vitamin K.

SUMMARY

1 Fat-soluble vitamins require bile for absorption. In the intestinal mucosal cells they are deposited in chylomicrons and absorbed by way of the lymphatic route.

2 Fat-soluble vitamins can be stored in the body in significant amounts, prolonging the time required for deficiency to develop. Vitamins A, D, and K are stored primarily in the liver while vitamin E is stored in adipose tissue, liver, and muscle.

3 Body stores generally must be exhausted before deficiency signs begin, except when some defect prevents mobilization of stores.

4 Circumstances that prevent fat absorption are apt to induce deficiencies of fat-soluble vitamins, given sufficient time.

5 Vitamins A and D are toxic at high levels of intake.

6 Some forms of vitamin A are under study for prevention or treatment of acne and some forms of cancer.

Vitamin E may be useful for some medical disorders, but is not the panacea it is popularly claimed to be.

7 Precursors to both vitamins A and D exist in foods, and in the case of vitamin D also in the skin.

8 Liver and green leafy vegetables are good sources of all the fat-soluble vitamins, except that green leafy vegetables are poor sources of vitamin D.

FOR DISCUSSION AND APPLICATION

1 Use the food record from Chapter 3 to calculate your daily intake of vitamin A. How does your intake compare with the recommended intake? What foods in your diet are rich sources? Do you need to modify or improve your diet with respect to vitamin A?

2 From your diet record, list foods that were good sources of vitamins D and E. Do you need to be concerned about your vitamin K intake? Explain.

3 Which of the fat-soluble vitamins is most apt to be low in the diet of a strict vegetarian? Visit a store which serves many strict vegetarians. Which products available there supply this vitamin? How much would a strict vegetarian need to consume to obtain the adult RDA for this vitamin? The RDA for children?

12 WATER AND THE MAJOR MINERALS

Manuel is a college senior who plans to train for marathon running. He has questions about his need for water and salt. Should he take salt tablets? Can he rely on thirst as a guide to his needs for water?

Megan's father has high blood pressure. His doctor says the entire family should consume a low-sodium diet. Because Megan has read conflicting reports in newspapers about low-sodium diets, she asks: "Should I go on a low-sodium diet? What are the arguments for and against low-sodium diets as preventive measures for high blood pressure?"

Erin heard on television that blood calcium should be maintained at a certain level for normal nerve transmission to occur. She wonders: "Does this mean that nerve function is normal only if you consume lots of calcium every day?"

This chapter addresses these questions, among others. In previous chapters, we discussed carbohydrates, fats, proteins, and vitamins—compounds made up almost entirely of four elements: carbon, hydrogen, oxygen, and—for protein and

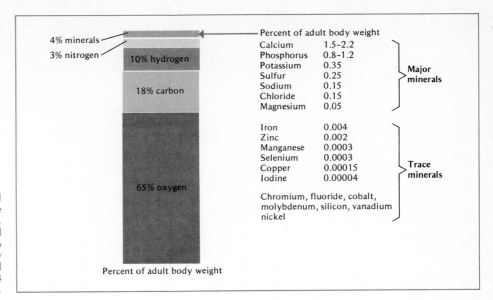

FIGURE 12-1. Elemental
composition of the
human body. Oxygen,
carbon, hydrogen, and
nitrogen constitute 96
percent of the body
weight, while mineral
elements make up only 4
percent.

some vitamins—nitrogen. These elements constitute the major portion of the body weight while the remaining elements—called *mineral elements* or simply *minerals*—make up a very small percentage of body weight (Figure 12-1). (Recall from the Introduction to this book that an *element* is any one of the 103 or so pure chemical substances which combine to make up chemical compounds. Elements cannot be broken down chemically.)

Minerals differ from vitamins in many ways, although both classes of nutrients are required in the diet in relatively small amounts. Minerals are inorganic substances (they contain no carbon) while vitamins are organic (or carbon-containing) molecules. Furthermore, minerals cannot be synthesized by any form of life, whereas many bacteria, plants, and other organisms synthesize some of the vitamins. Vitamins are destroyed by a variety of treatments, but minerals are indestructible by ordinary chemical methods. In fact, if you burn a food completely so that only the ash is left, you still have not lost the minerals—they *are* the ash. The ultimate sources of minerals are the earth's soils and sea water, although humans obtain them through eating plants that have grown on soils or in the sea, or animals that have consumed plants, or through purified sources such as salt (sodium chloride).

The *major minerals* or *macronutrient elements* are those required in the diet in amounts greater than 100 mg/day and present in the body in amounts greater than 0.005 percent of body weight. *Trace elements* (minerals) or *micronutrient elements* are those required in the diet and occurring in the body in smaller amounts (Figure 12-1). This chapter discusses the major minerals while Chapter 13 considers the trace elements.

Minerals are water-soluble and capable of forming ions when placed in water. As noted in Chapter 9, an ion is an atom or group of atoms that carries an electrical charge. A substance that dissociates into ions when placed in solution is an *electrolyte*. The major minerals form electrolytes in water and as such play extremely important roles in regulating the distribution of water in the body, in maintaining the slight alkalinity of the blood, and in maintaining the contractility of muscles and normal nerve impulse transmission. Because of the fundamental relationship of the major minerals with body water, this chapter discusses in turn water; the electrolytes sodium, potassium, and chlorine; and finally calcium, phosphorus, and magnesium. Although these last three minerals play important roles as electrolytes, they also participate in the building of bones and teeth. Sulfur is not discussed in this chapter because it is used in the body chiefly as a constituent of the sulfur-containing amino acids methionine, cysteine, and cystine.

WATER

Functions

We take water very much for granted, even though it is probably the most important constituent of the body, except for oxygen. Water is the compound occurring in largest amounts in the body. All metabolic processes and all exchanges among body tissues take place in a medium of water. It is the solvent for many substances in the body and diffuses freely through membranes. It participates in delivering nutrients to cells and in removing wastes and toxic substances from them. It serves as a lubricant in the form of fluids bathing the joints, and in saliva and mucus secreted by the respiratory, gastrointestinal, and genitourinary tracts. Within cells, not only is water a reactant in many chemical reactions, but it is also an integral part of the cell structure. Cellular activities as we know them could not take place without water.

Water performs additional crucial functions. It is essential for maintaining body temperature, for example. As body heat becomes excessive, water from sweat glands accumulates on the skin surface where it can evaporate. Water evaporation rids the body of large amounts of heat, since about 600 kcal are needed to evaporate 1 g of water. "Insensible skin losses" of water occur constantly as a means of cooling the body. Individuals are unaware of these losses since they do not involve sweat losses.

Distribution

As noted above, water is the largest component of the body, making up about 73 percent of the lean body mass (fat-free body weight). Because body fat holds little water (only 0.2 lb of water per pound of fat), a fat person has a lower percentage of body weight as water than a slim individual (1 lb of protein holds about 4 lb of water). Researchers use their knowledge of water distribution in lean and fat tissue as one means of roughly estimating body fatness [1]. How this is done is beyond the scope of this book, but we would expect to find a lower percentage of body water in the average adult female than in the male because females have more body fat. In fact this is the case, for the average adult female's body is about 49 percent water while the male's is 54 percent [2].

Body water occurs within the cells and outside the cells. That within the cells is called *intracellular fluid (ICF)*, while that outside the cells is called *extracellular fluid (ECF)*. Extracellular fluid includes the water in the fluid component of blood (the plasma), between the cells (interstitial fluid), and the water in tendons, skin, connective tissue, and the skeleton. In the adult, about two-thirds of all body water is found within the cells, while about one-third is located outside the cells.

Most people are unaware that one source of body water results from catabolism of carbohydrates, protein, and fat for energy. Complete oxidation produces 1.07 g of water from 1 g of fat, 0.41 g of water from 1 g of protein, and 0.60 g of water from 1 g of carbohydrates. Generally, metabolic water makes up 13 to 15 percent of the body's water.

Water Balance

Maintaining the amount and distribution of water in the body is critical for health and well-being, and several mechanisms operate together to make this possible. As Table 12-1 indicates, normally the amount excreted or lost from the body is balanced by intake from food and drink. How does your body know how much to take in or to excrete? For one thing, when it needs water, you feel thirsty and are prompted to drink. A thirst center in the brain is triggered when the blood flowing through the thirst center becomes too concentrated in dissolved substances. Other important mechanisms involve hormonal actions. *Antidiuretic hormone* (ADH), secreted by the pituitary in the brain when the blood becomes too concentrated, circulates to its target organ, the kidneys. Normally, the kidneys filter water from the blood into the kidney tubules, eventually excreting much of it as urine. ADH causes the kidney tubules to move needed water back into the blood, a process called the *reabsorption* of water. A second hormone, *aldosterone*, causes the kidneys to reabsorb sodium from the kidney tubules when blood

TABLE 12-1. BALANCE OF BODY WATER IN AN ADULT WHEN NO SWEAT LOSSES OCCUR

LOSSES		mL
Exhaled air		250–600
Insensible skin losses*		300–550
Urine		670–1750
Feces		80–200
	Totals	1300–3100
SOURCES OF WATER		
Beverages		500–1500
Foods		600–1200
Metabolic water†		200–400
	Totals	1300–3100

*Evaporated water from the skin's surface.

†Water formed in body tissues when energy nutrients are oxidized.

salts become low; water is reabsorbed with it because in solution sodium ions always hold "shells" of water around them. This is a second mechanism, then, for maintaining normal blood volume.

Urine volume may become very low if the body needs to retain water in the blood. A minimal volume of urine is required, however, to excrete excessive sodium, potassium, and urea (derived from protein catabolism). The need for water for excretion of these substances is greatest when the diet is high in protein, salt (sodium chloride), and potassium.

The need for water increases dramatically when there are large sweat losses. People living in a hot, dry climate may experience water losses through sweat and expired air that are twice as high as those of people living in a cool climate. Athletes or persons performing hard physical labor in hot environments may lose ten times as much water as they would have in a cool environment [3].

A healthy adult can live only a few days without water to drink. Water losses of only 1 percent of body weight trigger the thirst mechanism. By the time losses amount to 5 percent, an individual experiences great fatigue, apathy, and loss of desire to work or exercise. He or she is unable to work or exercise when losses reach 8 to 10 percent of body weight, and death occurs when 20 percent is lost.

Infants and children need proportionately larger water intakes than adults to maintain water balance. This is because (1) their body surface area per kilogram of body weight is greater, resulting in proportionately greater evaporative losses; (2) their basal metabolic rate per kilogram of body weight is higher, requiring increased utilization of water; and (3) their physical activity is often greater, resulting in greater sweat losses. Adults under comfortable environmental conditions need 1 mL of water per kilocalorie expended, while infants should have 1.5 mL/kcal [4]. This amounts to about 6 cups of fluid per day for an adult requiring 1500 kcal or for an infant requiring 1000 kcal daily. The need for water increases when there are abnormal losses, as in prolonged vomiting or diarrhea.

ELECTROLYTES

We noted earlier that electrolytes are those substances that dissociate into ions when placed in water. Some ions, called *cations*, have positive charges while others, called *anions*, have negative charges. These charges are due either to gain of electrons, in the case of anions, or their loss in the case of cations (Figure 12-2, see also Figure 9-2, Chapter 9 and Figure 3-2, Chapter 3). Common table salt (sodium chloride) in crystalline form is made up of positive sodium ions alternating with negatively charged chloride ions in a three-dimensional repeating pattern (Figure 12-3). The bonds holding the ions together, called *ionic* or *electrovalent* bonds, exist because of the mutual attraction between positive and negative charges. When sodium chloride crystals dissolve in water the ions dissociate and move around freely in the water. Cations in body fluids, other than sodium, include potassium, calcium, and magnesium. Important anions include chloride, phosphate, bicarbonate, and ions of protein. Sulfate ions also occur in small amounts.

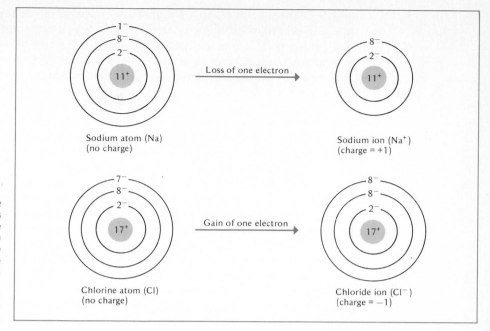

FIGURE 12-2. The sodium atom becomes an ion having one positive charge (Na⁺) when it loses one electron, while the chlorine atom, upon gaining an electron, becomes the chloride ion (Cl⁻), having one negative charge.

Functions

Distribution of Body Fluids   Normally, the concentration of water and electrolytes within and outside the cells remains constant. As a result, the cells neither swell from too much water retention, nor shrivel from loss of water. Electrolytes—particularly sodium and potassium—are effective in maintaining normal water distribution through their participation in *osmosis*. To demonstrate the process of

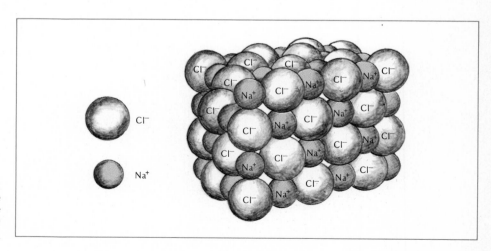

FIGURE 12-3. The structure of crystalline sodium chloride (NaCl) or table salt.

osmosis, suppose we place a concentrated solution of sodium chloride on one side of a semipermeable membrane and a dilute solution on the other (Figure 12-4). Suppose, too, that this membrane allows water to pass through freely but is impermeable to sodium or chloride, hence the term, *semipermeable*. Under these circumstances water diffuses into the more concentrated salt solution—that is, the movement is to dilute the concentration of salt. *Osmosis*, therefore, is the process of net movement of water across a membrane due to differences in concentration of *solute* or dissolved substances—in this case, sodium chloride—on the two sides of the membrane. Electrolytes very effectively control the movement of water from one body compartment to another through osmosis.

Cell membranes are more complex than the semipermeable membrane just described—some sodium and potassium ions can cross them, for example. Body cells therefore use some special mechanisms for distributing electrolytes between the extracellular (ECF) and intracellular (ICF) fluids. Normally the blood plasma (the liquid portion of blood) and the fluids bathing the cells (the ECF) contain sodium (Na^+) as the chief cation and chloride (Cl^-) as the chief anion. The fluids inside the cells (ICF) contain potassium (K^+) as the chief cation, along with some sodium and magnesium (Mg^{2+}). The chief anions in the cells are phosphate (HPO_4^{-2}) and ionized protein (Figure 12-5).

A "pump" mechanism is thought to be responsible for keeping sodium out of the cell, while keeping potassium inside. The "pump" consists of an enzyme system which uses the energy from adenosine triphosphate (ATP) to move sodium ions from an area of low concentration (within the cell) to one of high concentration (outside the cell). For each sodium ion pumped out, a potassium ion is pumped in. Since sodium ions are surrounded by water (hydrated), the pump mechanism constantly removes water from the cells with sodium, controlling the cell size. If the pump mechanism fails, the cells swell, even to the point of bursting.

Electrolytes are not alone in their ability to regulate shifts of fluid from one

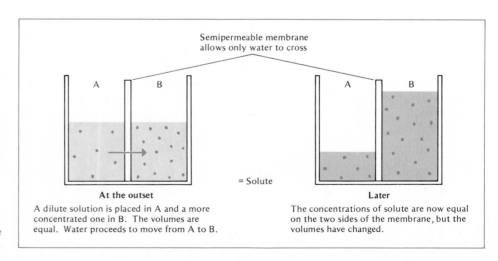

Semipermeable membrane
allows only water to cross

A   B

A   B

= Solute

At the outset

A dilute solution is placed in A and a more concentrated one in B. The volumes are equal. Water proceeds to move from A to B.

Later

The concentrations of solute are now equal on the two sides of the membrane, but the volumes have changed.

FIGURE 12-4. The process of osmosis.

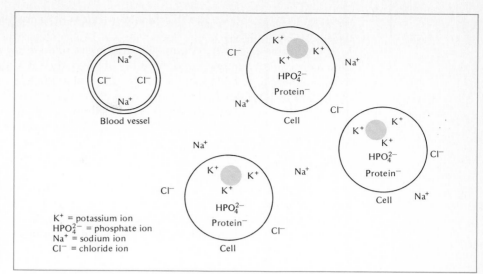

FIGURE 12-5. Potassium
is the chief cation in
intracellular fluid (ICF),
while sodium is found in
extracellular fluid (ECF).
Anions are chiefly
phosphate and protein
ions in ICF and chloride
in ECF.

compartment to another. Protein within cells and in the blood plasma exerts an osmotic effect, accounting for some movement of fluids. Plasma proteins enable fluid to remain in the blood vessels despite the force of the blood pressure, which otherwise would push it out (see Chapter 6). The kidneys also play a vital role in regulating the amount of water in extracellular fluid by excreting or reabsorbing water and sodium as needed. In addition, the gastrointestinal tract plays a major role in maintaining water balance. Digestive secretions amount to approximately 8000 mL/day in the adult, and contain water and electrolytes obtained from blood plasma. Normally, both water and electrolytes are reabsorbed into the blood in the colon after digestion is completed.

Acid-Base Balance   Electrolytes also play a role in regulating the acid-base balance of the body. *Acid-base balance* refers to maintenance of the normal hydrogen ion concentration in body fluids. Whether or not body fluids are acidic or alkaline (basic) depends upon their concentration of hydrogen ions (H^+). If the concentration of hydrogen ions increases, the fluid becomes more acidic; if the concentration decreases, the fluid becomes more alkaline. The degree of acidity or alkalinity is frequently designated by a system called *pH*, in which values below 7.0 indicate acidity, 7.0 indicates neutrality, and values above 7.0 indicate alkalinity. Normally the blood is slightly alkaline, maintaining a pH range between 7.35 and 7.45. Very slight deviations above or below the normal blood pH indicate acid-base imbalance, and death may result if the deviation is too great. Consequently, the body has elaborate mechanisms for maintaining normal blood pH.

Some electrolytes, particularly sodium and phosphates, aid in regulating acid-base balance as essential components of buffers. *Buffers* are substances which prevent a change in pH by either removing or releasing hydrogen ions as required. The exact way in which electrolytes function in buffer systems is beyond the scope of this book, but this function represents another significant role of minerals in the body.

In addition to buffer systems, the respiratory and kidney systems function in intricate ways to maintain the normal pH of the body fluids and cells. Conditions that are essential to life—such as maintenance of acid-base balance—are always controlled by complex mechanisms. They are never left to chance controls, such as diet. Some self-styled "nutritionists" recommend that one carefully choose foods so as to balance acid- and base-forming foods, in an attempt to control blood or tissue pH. While it is true that some foods are acid-forming, and others base-forming, the normal individual easily controls acid-base balance regardless of the diet consumed.

Electrolytes are required for additional essential functions. Both muscle and nerve cells must be bathed in electrolyte-containing tissue fluids for nerve impulse transmission and muscle contractility to occur in a normal way. Sodium, potassium, calcium, and magnesium all contribute to these vital functions.

SODIUM

One should not confuse *sodium* and *salt*. Sodium refers to the *element* (abbreviated Na), while salt refers to the compound, sodium chloride (NaCl). To convert milligrams of sodium to salt, divide sodium (in milligrams) by 0.40. To convert milligrams of salt to sodium, multiply salt (in milligrams) by 0.40.

Sodium (or salt) has been much in the news because of its possible relationship to hypertension (high blood pressure), a risk factor for coronary heart disease and stroke (see Chapter 5) and a contributor to heart and kidney failure. Of even greater interest is the fact that experts disagree on whether or not everyone should be advised to cut back on salt. Furthermore, other electrolytes—including potassium and calcium—may be related to hypertension along with sodium. What is the source of conflict among investigators about advice the public should receive regarding sodium? How are other electrolytes implicated in hypertension? This section focuses on these questions, examining some of the problems inherent in finding answers to nutrition problems in human populations. Before we discuss the relationships of sodium and potassium to hypertension, we shall look briefly at their functions, metabolism, recommended intakes, and food sources.

Functions

As noted earlier, sodium is the chief cation of extracellular fluid, regulating the volume of fluid in this component. Sodium plays a vital role in acid-base balance; it is chiefly responsible for the alkalinity of gastrointestinal secretions, for example. It is essential for normal nerve impulse transmission and muscle contractility and, through the sodium pump mechanism, participates in maintaining electrolyte and water balance between extracellular and intracellular fluid.

Water and Sodium Needs of Athletes

Water is essential for the chemical reactions that occur in muscle cells during exercise. As soon as exercise begins, water is transferred into muscle cells from the extracellular fluid to expedite energy production. Extracellular fluid losses are immediately replaced with fluid from the blood, lowering the blood volume. The lower blood volume results in decreased urine production, a mechanism that helps to conserve body water as sweat losses and heavy breathing increase water losses [3].

A progressive decline in blood volume does not occur as exercise continues, however, because that would jeopardize the functions of body organs. Eventually, continued exercise without water replacement results in dehydration of muscle cells (loss of intracellular water), producing a significant decline in athletic performance [3]. Although athletes should routinely consume sufficient water to replace losses incurred during a workout or competition, they unfortunately cannot rely upon thirst to indicate how much water is needed. They should therefore weigh themselves before and after an exercise period to determine their water loss, and drink sufficient amounts to replace it. If they drink insufficient amounts and continue to work out daily, then the extent of their dehydration intensifies and can become serious within 2 to 3 days [3].

Sweat losses result not only in water loss but also in sodium (salt or sodium chloride) loss. Should athletes immediately replace salt losses along with water losses? The answer is no—not unless water loss (body weight loss) is greater than 6 to 7 lb due to practice or competition [4]. Otherwise, plain water should be taken to replace losses. The reason for caution in consuming salt is that it increases the fluid in the extracellular fluid at the expense of that inside the cells. This dehydrates muscle cells and cuts down on performance [3]. It is important to realize that sweat contains lower concentrations of salt than does extracellular fluid; therefore, sweat losses should never be replaced with fluids containing higher salt concentrations than sweat.

When body water loss is great enough to merit salt replacement, the athlete may simply salt food heavily at mealtimes or may consume limited amounts of fluids containing low amounts of salt (⅓ tsp per quart of water) [3]. Although highly advertised beverages of known salt concentrations are available to athletes, these are expensive and are not superior to properly made salt-water solutions. Athletes should never use these beverages to replace all water losses because too much salt would be ingested by doing so [3]. Salt tablets should never be used, for these increase the danger of consuming too much salt.

Maintaining an adequate state of hydration is essential for preventing heat stroke. An athlete's muscles produce a large amount of heat, which normally is removed from the body as sweat evaporates from the skin surface. If environmental temperature and humidity are high, or too much clothing prevents evaporation, or if *too little body water is present to allow adequate sweating*, body temperature begins to rise until the athlete collapses of heat stroke. Severe brain damage, kidney failure, and death may result [3].

Although we have focused here on athletes, the principles discussed apply also to individuals who make their living by heavy physical labor.

Metabolism

Sodium is readily and completely absorbed from foods. About half the body's sodium is in extracellular fluid, 10 percent or less is in intracellular fluid, and the remaining 40 percent is in bones. The kidneys, through the action of the hormone aldosterone, are responsible for regulating the amount of body sodium. They excrete practically no sodium when the sodium intake is extremely low, but excrete large percentages of high intakes. Measuring the sodium excretion in a 24-hour collection of urine is a good way to estimate the level of intake in a normal individual. Significant sodium losses may occur in sweat, particularly in unusually hot weather. Methods of replacing losses for the athlete are discussed in Box 12-1.

Recommended Intakes

Sodium needs depend upon growth rate and losses through the feces and skin. Infants, children, and pregnant women are expected to be in slightly positive sodium balance because they retain sodium in the extracellular fluid of newly forming tissues. Normal, nonpregnant adults, on the other hand, should be in sodium balance or equilibrium.

The amount of sodium required for growth and to replace unavoidable losses is low—in the range of 100 to 200 mg of sodium per day (250 to 500 mg of salt per day or 0.03 to 0.08 tsp). The Food and Nutrition Board has set 1100 to 3300 mg of *sodium* (roughly 3 to 8 g or ½ to 1½ tsp of *salt*) as the safe and adequate intake for adults and reinforced this recommendation in their publication *Toward Healthful Diets* [5]. (Remember that this amount refers to all dietary sources of sodium, and not just to salt.) The rationale is that many Americans consume excessively high amounts of sodium (ten or more times than needed) and that this practice may be harmful to the estimated 10 to 20 percent of Americans who are at risk for developing hypertension. There is no evidence that reducing the salt intake to the Board's lowest recommended amount would be harmful for normal adults. Many people in nonindustrialized parts of the world have lived for generations on salt intakes of less than 2.5 g/day with no known detrimental effects [6]. Indeed, many experts argue that low intakes of sodium might be beneficial, as noted below in the section on hypertension.

Food Sources

If one wishes to consume a fairly low sodium intake (between 1 to 3 g/day), one cannot assume that simply cutting out salt at the table or in cooking will do the job. Today's food supply includes many processed foods which are often very high in sodium. As little as 10 percent of the sodium in the diet of Americans may be added by the individual at home [7]. Table 12-2 shows that reliance on highly processed foods can lead to a high sodium intake, and gives alternative choices that decrease the intake to within the range recommended for adults.

Among food processing practices that account for high sodium levels are curing meats with sodium nitrates and nitrites, sorting peas and lima beans in

TABLE 12-2. SODIUM CONTENT OF ONE DAY'S MENU BASED ON HIGHLY PROCESSED VS. HOME-PREPARED FOODS

HIGHLY PROCESSED FOODS	mg Na	ALTERNATIVE FOODS	mg Na
Breakfast			
Wheaties, 1 c	355	Regular oats, cooked, ¾ c	1
		¹⁄₁₆ tsp salt	121
Milk, whole, 1 c	122	Milk, whole, 1 c	122
Dehydrated orange drink, 1 c	35	Frozen orange juice, diluted, 1 c	6
Cocoa mix, water added, 1 c	232	Coffee, 1 c	2
Coffee whitener, 1 tbsp	12	Milk, 1 tbsp	8
Lunch			
Dehydrated chicken noodle soup, 1 c	1284	Homemade chicken noodle soup, 1 c	400*
Grilled cheese and meat sandwich—2 slices pumpernickle bread	364	2 slices whole-wheat bread	264
1 oz American processed cheese	406	1 oz natural cheddar cheese	176
1 oz ham	371	1 oz lean beef	18
Dill pickle, 1	928	Celery stalk, 1	25
Instant chocolate pudding, ½ c	470	Homemade chocolate pudding, ½ c	73
Low-calorie soda, 8 oz	21	Iced tea, 8 oz	1
Snack			
Potato chips, 20 chips	400	Unsalted peanuts, ½ c	4
Beer, 1	25	Beer, 1	25
Dinner			
Frozen turkey pot pie	1018	Homemade turkey pot pie	400*
Frozen green beans with almonds, 3 oz	335	Plain frozen green beans	3
Frozen carrots in butter sauce, 3.3 oz	350	Frozen carrots, plain, 3.3 oz	43
Lettuce, 1 c	4	Lettuce, 1 c	4
Bottled French dressing, 1 tbsp	214	Homemade French dressing, 1 tbsp	92
Devil's food cake (from mix), ¹⁄₁₂ of cake	402	Devil's food cake, homemade, ¹⁄₁₂ of cake	235
Total mg Na (rounded)	7350	Total mg Na (rounded)	2025
g NaCl	18.4	g NaCl	5.0†

*Estimated by authors

†To reach the lower range suggested by the Food and Nutrition Board of 1100 mg of Na (2.75 g of salt) could be done by substituting plain fruits for the desserts, substituting ½ roasted chicken breast for turkey pot pie and omitting the soup at lunch.

SOURCE: Home and Garden Bulletin No. 233, *The Sodium Content of Your Food,* U.S. Department of Agriculture, Washington, D.C., 1980.

brine (highly concentrated salt solution) before freezing, buffering some canned and bottled fruit drinks with sodium citrate, and use in foods of certain chemical additives such as monosodium glutamate (MSG) (a flavor enhancer), sodium saccharin (a sweetener), sodium phosphates (emulsifiers, stabilizers, buffers), sodium caseinate (a thickener and binder), and sodium benzoate (a preservative). Many condiments and seasoning agents are also high in sodium, including soy sauce, worcestershire sauce, miso (a fermented soybean product used in oriental cooking), catsup, and garlic, onion, and celery salts. Baking powder and baking soda are both high in sodium. Antacids and many other drugs also contain sodium. Some wines are also sources of sodium, as are many bottled mineral waters.

The sodium content of drinking water varies from one location to another. In the United States, county or city departments of public health can supply information on the amount of sodium in local water supplies. Water softeners increase the amount of sodium in water.

Naturally good sources of sodium are milk, cheese, shellfish, meats, poultry, fish, and eggs. Most unprocessed fruits, vegetables, and cereals are low in sodium (Appendix D).

Consumers often want to know how much sodium is present in a food, but manufacturers are not currently required to place such information on the label. The Food and Drug Administration has proposed that sodium labeling be required whenever a manufacturer uses nutrition labeling (see Chapter 17), but only about 40 percent of all foods have nutrition labels. They propose further that manufacturers not required to use nutrition labeling could volunteer to put only sodium content on labels if they desired. At this writing, these proposals have not yet become regulations. Currently, food labels indicate that salt or sodium is present, but not how much. Health professionals have recently suggested that the food industry decrease the amount of salt in cereals, breads, and canned foods [8].

POTASSIUM

Potassium, as mentioned earlier, is found inside while sodium occurs outside body cells, for as sodium is pumped out, potassium is pumped in. These two electrolytes also may be interrelated in hypertension, a subject to which we will turn shortly. But first let's gain some perspective on potassium.

Functions

Potassium, as the chief cation in intracellular fluid, plays a major role in maintaining fluid balance in this component. In addition it is needed for some enzymatic reactions in cells. For example, both protein and glycogen synthesis require potassium. When either glycogen or protein is catabolized, potassium is released. Even though potassium is found in small concentrations in extracellular fluids, it is essential there for nerve and muscle activity, particularly in the heart muscle. Because potassium is present almost entirely inside cells in lean tissues, the measurement of body potassium is sometimes used as a way of estimating the relative amounts of lean and fat tissue in the body (see Chapter 8).

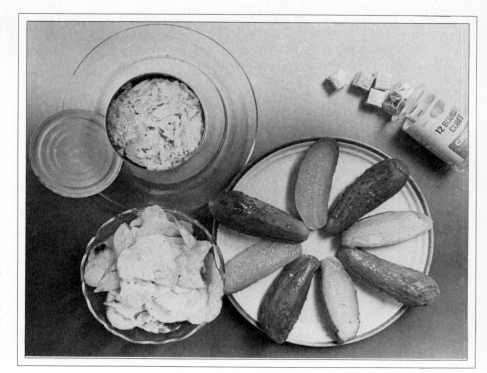

Many processed foods including canned tuna, potato chips, pickles, and bouillon cubes are high in sodium. Rinsing products such as tuna in water removes much of the sodium.
(Randy Matusow)

Metabolism

Potassium is well-absorbed. About 97 percent of that in the body is located inside cells making up lean tissues. Some potassium is secreted into digestive juices but this is reabsorbed in the colon; therefore excessive potassium intakes are excreted in the urine. The kidneys fail to conserve potassium as efficiently as they conserve sodium. Even when tissue levels are low and none is in the diet, the kidneys continue to excrete potassium.

Deficiency

When potassium deficiency results from dietary lack, an aberration affecting food intake is usually responsible such as alcoholism, severe illness producing loss of appetite, or anorexia nervosa. Although potassium deficiency is uncommon, most cases seen in the United States are due to excessive losses of body potassium, occurring, for example, when excessive body protein is catabolized—as in starvation, serious burns, or chronic fevers. Chronic diarrhea or vomiting may prevent adequate absorption to replace losses. Prolonged use of those kinds of *diuretics* (drugs that promote urinary water and sodium excretion) that induce potassium excretion are widely believed to induce deficiency, but this has been questioned [9].

Symptoms of potassium deficiency include marked weakness, lethargy, modification of the heart rhythm, and eventually muscle paralysis. Death from paralysis of the heart muscle or those muscles affecting respiration may result.

Recommended Intakes and Food Sources

No RDA is set for potassium, but safe and adequate intakes of 1875 to 5625 mg daily are designated for the adult (Appendix A). The usual adult diet in the United States is estimated to contain amounts very close to this amount. Fruits, vegetables, and whole grains are excellent sources, while fresh meats, poultry, and fish are good sources. (See Appendix C for details on potassium sources.)

Large doses of potassium are toxic if they raise blood potassium levels beyond a certain level, and eventually cause cardiac arrest. This can happen when kidney disorders prevent patients from excreting potassium normally. One investigation reported high blood potassium levels in patients who were consuming the salt substitute potassium chloride [10]. Some experts believe that the common practice of prescribing potassium supplements for hypertensive patients taking diuretics may result in potassium toxicity [9].

Hypertension, Sodium, and Potassium: A Look at the Research

Some experts in hypertension are now questioning whether the general public is apt to benefit by lowering salt intakes as advised by the Food and Nutrition Board, the American Medical Association, the American Heart Association, *Dietary Goals for the United States*, and *Dietary Guidelines for Americans* [11]. The crux of the disagreement lies in whether or not (1) high-sodium diets *cause* hypertension, and (2) whether moderate restriction of sodium, as suggested by the Food and Nutrition Board, is apt to prevent hypertension in the general population.

The basic causes of hypertension are poorly understood. Epidemiological studies show that people living in remote, nonindustrial areas who consume very low amounts of sodium have practically no hypertension, and their blood pressure does not rise with age as is usual in the United States. They are not all genetically protected against high blood pressure, for as they migrate to more industrialized areas and adopt the diet there, a certain percentage develops hypertension, and higher blood pressure with age [6]. Yet these data do not *prove* that sodium *causes* high blood pressure, for other factors may be operating. In primitive societies, people tend to lose weight with age, while the opposite generally occurs in industrialized countries. Obesity is known to be associated with high blood pressure. Other factors that must be considered are that people in primitive societies generally are more physically active, are subjected to different kinds of stresses, and consume more potassium than those in highly developed countries. Researchers who have worked in primitive groups say their data show that low sodium is much more strongly implicated in low blood pressure than leanness or absence of stress in these societies, however [6].

Investigators are pursuing the possibility that high potassium intakes may protect against hypertension. Diets in industrialized societies tend to be high in sodium and low in potassium largely because during canning, freezing, and other food processing methods, sodium is added while potassium is lost [12]. Some studies in human populations indicate that high blood pressure is associated with low intakes and thus low excretions of potassium [13,14,15]. Further studies are needed to (1) determine whether potassium can lower high blood pressure levels and (2) delineate the relative importance of high sodium or low potassium intakes in causing hypertension.

Sodium excess may increase blood pressure by expanding the extracellular fluid, promoting the constriction of blood vessels, or inducing hormonal changes. On the other hand, potassium may dilate blood vessels and may also increase urinary sodium excretion [16].

Some authorities believe that whether or not dietary sodium causes hypertension by middle age depends upon one's genetic susceptibility. Susceptible individuals are said to be able to avoid developing hypertension by a lifetime low sodium intake of less than 1380 mg, equivalent to about 3.5 g or ⅔ tsp of salt daily [6]. Many also believe that it is normal to react to a high salt intake by developing hypertension with age; the few who do not are genetically resistant [17]. Although there is no sure way to determine one's genetic susceptibility, authorities say individuals at high risk are those who (1) have a family history of hypertension; (2) have high blood pressure readings in early life; (3) have a more rapid resting heart rate than expected, taking into account their physical condition; and/or (4) are more than 15 percent over ideal body weight [6].

Scientists need to learn a great deal more about the relationships not only of sodium and potassium but also of calcium, magnesium, and dietary fiber to hypertension. In the meantime, should the general public be advised to lower their sodium intakes to amounts suggested by the Food and Nutrition Board and other groups? Of should we wait until research gives us more insights into the relationship?

Some have argued that since grain foods, flesh foods, and milk products furnish most of the sodium in the American diet, eliminating these in an effort to cut down on sodium would result in deficiency of important nutrients such as B vitamins, iron, and calcium. But there is a serious flaw in this argument. These foods are high in sodium *only* if highly processed; minimally processed grains,

A CLOSER LOOK

Young children from families with hypertension have higher blood pressures than those from families with no hypertension. Many experts believe that high-sodium diets early in life may induce hypertension later among those who are genetically predisposed [17]. In 1970, a subcommittee of the Food and Nutrition Board suggested that the amount of salt added to infant foods should be reduced, even though it was not possible to *prove* that high salt intakes in infancy will result in hypertension in adulthood [18]. The food industry since that time has removed salt from most infant foods, for it is clear that infants consume salt-free foods just as readily as they consume salted ones. Parents should not add salt to baby foods made at home, and should allow infants and small children to have salty foods only in small amounts at infrequent intervals.

meats, poultry, and fish are quite low in sodium (see Appendix D). In the milk group, processed cheeses and some natural cheeses are high in sodium, but fluid milk and certain cheeses are moderately low sources. A nutritionally adequate diet can be achieved easily while adhering to the intake suggested by the Food and Nutrition Board.

Those who argue for cutting down on salt make the point that since it is impossible to identify the 20 percent of the population prone to hypertension, the only way to protect them is for everyone to cut back. Those on the opposite side argue that we lack evidence that this will do any good.

The issues are similar to those discussed in Chapter 5 in relationship to dietary fat and cholesterol. Some experts prefer to wait until they understand thoroughly all the relationships of diet to hypertension before advising changes in diet for the general population. Others believe we already have enough information to tell us that high sodium intakes are dangerous. They believe that moderate restriction can do no harm and might be beneficial. You can decide which of these views to accept in choosing your diet.

If you decide to decrease dietary sodium and increase potassium, we suggest that you stay within the amounts suggested by the Food and Nutrition Board. It is sensible to rely on *food* for potassium and not pills; taking potassium tablets without a competent physician's supervision can be dangerous [9]. Consult a physician before using a potassium substitute for common salt, since these should be avoided if certain medical disorders are present. To change the American diet to one lower in sodium and higher in potassium would mean reducing the use of highly processed convenience foods, fast foods, salty snacks, and condiments, while increasing minimally processed fruits, vegetables, and cereals. Meats, poultry, and fish used would be fresh, not processed.

CHLORIDE

Chlorine is a toxic gas used to disinfect drinking water. It occurs in the body as the chloride ion and is an essential element that is frequently forgotten or ignored in nutrition. This mineral is a constitutent of hydrochloric acid (HCl) secreted by the stomach mucosa, which, among other functions, prevents bacterial growth in that organ. Chloride ions, like sodium ions, are present chiefly in extracellular fluids, and are important for normal nerve impulse transmission and maintenance of the body's acid-base balance.

Chloride occurs in the diet chiefly as sodium chloride, and its metabolism in the body is closely associated with that of sodium. If salt intake is high, large amounts of both sodium and chloride are excreted in the urine. In prolonged sweating and severe diarrhea, both sodium and chloride are lost. In cases of prolonged vomiting, however, more chloride than sodium is lost from the body.

In 1979, the removal of salt from specific soy-based infant formulas (because of concern for the sodium content) produced chloride deficiency in infants consuming nothing but the formula [19]. Approximately 1 percent of the infants fed this formula became ill enough to require hospitalization. Among the symptoms were failure to gain weight as expected, retardation in growth of the head, poor appetite, alkalosis (the blood became more alkaline than normal), and in some, behavioral and learning problems developed [20]. The alkalosis, growth retardation, and poor appetite were cleared up by administering chloride. The National Institutes of Health has launched a 5-year study to determine whether or not infants who developed this disorder have suffered any permanent damage in growth or development [21].

When changes are made in infant formulas, manufacturers now are required to conduct tests before putting the new formula on the market. The unfortunate occurrence of chloride deficiency dramatizes the vulnerability of infants to nutritional problems because of their dependence typically on only one food source. This event also illustrates the importance of the interrelationships of nutrients and the consequent dangers of considering individual nutrients in isolation.

No RDA has been set for chloride but the estimated safe and adequate intake for adults is 1700 to 5100 mg/day. The dietary source is almost exclusively from sodium chloride.

Thus far we have considered those mineral elements that function chiefly in distributing water throughout body tissues. Let's turn now to the elements that form structural components of the body.

CALCIUM

As children you probably learned that calcium helps to build strong bones and teeth, but calcium plays fundamentally important roles in body fluids as well.

Functions

Since we have just discussed the functions of other minerals in body fluids, let us see how calcium functions in these fluids before proceeding to its structural functions.

Calcium in Body Fluids   Although 99 percent of body calcium occurs in the skeleton, the remaining 1 percent in body fluids is vital for several purposes. It is required for normal blood coagulation, transmission of nerve impulses, muscle contractility, activation of certain enzyme reactions and hormonal secretions, the integrity of intracellular cement substances, and cell membrane functions. To perform these functions, the body uses a complex mechanism to maintain the calcium concentration of blood and other fluids at normal levels. This mechanism involves the action of three hormones: 1,25-dihydroxyvitamin D ($1,25(OH)_2vitD_3$) (Chapter 11), parathyroid hormone (PTH), and calcitonin.

When the blood calcium concentration begins to fall below normal, *parathyroid hormone* (PTH) is released from the parathyroid glands, located in the neck immediately behind the thyroid gland. This hormone raises the blood calcium level by stimulating synthesis in the kidneys of $1,25(OH)_2vitD_3$, which then stimulates intestinal calcium absorption. In addition, PTH works with $1,25(OH)_2vitD_3$ to (1) bring about reabsorption of calcium into the blood from the

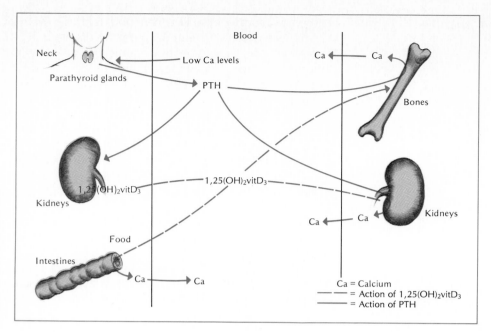

FIGURE 12-6.
Parathyroid hormone
(PTH) stimulates synthesis
of 1,25(OH)$_2$vitD$_3$ by the
kidneys. This hormone
works with PTH to
release calcium (Ca) from
bones and to stimulate
reabsorption of Ca by the
kidneys. 1,25(OH)$_2$vitD$_3$
also stimulates absorption
of Ca by the intestines.

kidney tubules and (2) move calcium from bones into the blood. As the blood calcium rises, PTH secretion is suppressed, in turn suppressing 1,25(OH)$_2$vitD$_3$ secretion [22]. Figure 12-6 illustrates these interactions.

If blood calcium levels rise above normal, *calcitonin* is released by the thyroid gland. It stops the removal of calcium from the bone and may also increase excretion of calcium by the kidneys, restoring calcium to normal [22]. Figure 12-7 illustrates the action of calcitonin.

Calcium in Bones Bones support and give shape to the body, protect some vital organs, such as the brain, and serve as points of attachment for muscles. They consist of a foundation of cartilage into which crystals of calcium phosphate are embedded, hardening the bone. Magnesium, sodium, and carbonate ions are also deposited in the calcium phosphate crystalline structure.

The ends of the long bones of the body are capable of storing calcium phosphate crystals on their inner surfaces. These storage sites are called the *trabeculae* of the bones. Calcium stored in the trabeculae is more readily available to the blood than calcium in other parts of the bones. The extent of development of trabeculae depends upon the adequacy of calcium intake—the higher the intake, the more extensive the trabeculae.

For years, scientists assumed that calcium was deposited in bone permanently, but are now aware that bone is in a dynamic state. Some calcium phosphate crystals are constantly deposited, forming new bone, while at the same time others are torn down. As the crystals are torn down, calcium and phosphorus are taken up by the blood in a process called *resorption*. The extent of deposition and resorption of bone minerals is called the turnover rate. The younger the person, the more rapid the turnover of skeletal calcium. In the first year of life, 100 percent of the bone calcium appears to turn over, while in older children yearly turnover amounts to about 10 percent, and in adults it is between 2 and 4 percent [23].

Between 40 and 50 years of age, bone resorption begins to occur to a greater extent than bone deposition, resulting in a gradual loss of bone mass. This loss begins earlier in females than in males, and shorter persons of both sexes lose bone mass more rapidly than taller ones. In many women, the loss increases after menopause. Since young whites have less skeletal mass than young blacks, and young males within a given race have greater skeletal mass than females, the person most apt to have the greatest loss of bone mass is the small, white, postmenopausal female [23]. *Osteoporosis* is the name given to the disease in which there is excessive loss of bone mass. The relationship of a lifetime of low calcium intake to development of osteoporosis in old age needs to be clarified by further research, and is discussed in Chapter 16.

Calcium and phosphorus crystals also are deposited in the teeth, accounting for their hardness. There is very little turnover of calcium and phosphorus in the teeth, however. Once decay has caused disappearance of calcium and phosphorus crystals from the teeth, the body cannot repair the damage.

Absorption and Metabolism

Calcium is absorbed chiefly from the upper small intestines by a process requiring the active form of vitamin D. Absorption increases when the blood calcium level falls below a certain level, demonstrating that the rate of absorption is geared to need. In infancy and childhood, when active skeletal growth is occurring, as much as 75 percent of dietary calcium is absorbed. Adults, on the other hand, absorb 20 to 30 percent of the intake, excreting the remainder in the feces [24].

Several dietary factors influence calcium absorption. The presence of vitamin

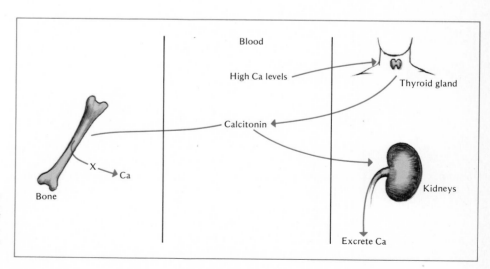

FIGURE 12-7. Calcitonin lowers blood calcium to normal by shutting off removal of Ca from bone and by stimulating the kidneys to excrete Ca.

D, lactose, and the amino acids lysine and arginine at the absorption site increase absorption. On the other hand, foods high in oxalates (spinach, kale, cocoa) and phytates (bran or whole wheat) may combine with calcium to form insoluble complexes that cannot be absorbed. Dietary fiber may also bind calcium, thereby decreasing its absorption. These negative factors do not apparently have adverse practical consequences, however, if calcium intake is sufficienctly high [24].

After absorption via the portal vein, calcium enters the circulating blood and rapidly exchanges with bone calcium. Small amounts are lost from the body in urine and sweat and through secretions into the intestinal tract. Most of the calcium in feces consists of unabsorbed food calcium.

Calcium metabolism is frequently studied by using the calcium balance technique in which the intake and excretion are measured and the difference between them noted. The technique is similar to that of nitrogen balance studies discussed in Chapter 6. Growth periods (infancy, childhood, and pregnancy) call for positive calcium balance, while normal adults should be in calcium balance or equilibrium. Negative calcium balance is generally viewed as an undesirable condition, since excessive bone calcium is lost. Negative calcium balance has been observed when the body is immobilized (in a cast, or during enforced bed rest), during periods of intense emotional stress or physical injury, during an adjustment period after the intake of calcium is changed from a high to low level, and when dietary protein is increased while dietary calcium and phosphorus levels remain unchanged [25].

Deficiency

Calcium deficiency in animals results in poor growth, small adult size, and fragile and deformed bones. Small body size for age in children and short stature in adulthood in many parts of the world may be related to routine low calcium intakes. Although people adapt to low calcium intakes, one means of adaptation is slower growth and smaller size for age.

While rickets more commonly is due to vitamin D deficiency, inadequate calcium intake can result in failure of bone mineralization and full-blown rickets, as described in Chapter 11. Adult rickets, or *osteomalacia*, similarly is more often due to vitamin D than calcium deficiency, but may be exacerbated by low calcium intakes.

Recommended Intakes

Dietary surveys indicate that adults in western countries ordinarily vary widely in the amount of calcium consumed: from 400 to 1300 mg/day. The Food and Agriculture Organization/World Health Organization of the United Nations set an adult allowance of 400 to 500 mg/day, noting that there is no evidence of calcium deficiency in countries where this amount is customarily consumed, and no evidence that larger intakes are beneficial [26]. For a number of years, however, the adult RDA in the United States has been set at 800 mg/day (Appendix A), based on calcium balance studies, and, more recently, on the knowledge that the

NUTRITION IN THE NEWS

LOW CALCIUM TIED TO HIGH BLOOD PRESSURE

The New York Times, July 13, 1982

Too little calcium in the diet may be a hitherto unrecognized factor contributing to high blood pressure, according to a study done at the Oregon Health Sciences University in Portland.

The study, based on a survey of the dietary habits of a group of 90 adults, found the 46 persons who had high blood pressure had consumed significantly less calcium than the 44 with normal blood pressure. . . .

Dr. David A. McCarron, associate professor of medicine at the university, and chief author of the report, said he considered the calcium findings to be much more striking than earlier evidence linking salt to high blood pressure. It is widely believed that excess salt in the diet contributes to high blood pressure, but Dr. McCarron said it has been impossible to prove this on the basis of American dietary habits. . . .

The report noted that the trend in the United States in recent years has been toward reduced consumption of dairy products as Americans have lowered their intake of fats, cholesterol and salt, hoping to cut the risk of heart disease and perhaps cancer. However, the new study suggests that, for some people at least, the resulting loss of calcium may increase the risk of high blood pressure.

ASK YOURSELF:

Is hypertension present in more than 50 percent of the adult population, as the sample used in this study would suggest? Is it likely that one study of 90 adults represents all those adults with and without hypertension in the United States? How would you choose subjects representative of these two groups? What other nutrients besides calcium would have to be ruled out before one could conclude that calcium was the important factor? How do you suppose the investigators found out how much calcium their subjects consumed? By questionnaire? By interview? By observing what they ate? Did investigators try to find out how much calcium their subjects *currently* consume, as opposed to their consumption in infancy and childhood? How can you reach the adult RDA for calcium while consuming the fat and cholesterol intake recommended by the *Dietary Goals for the United States*? Must you cut out dairy products to do so?

---

high consumption of protein and phosphorus in the United States may increase the need for calcium. The Board observes that persons consuming less protein and phosphorus than is typical in this country will remain in calcium equilibrium on calcium intakes lower than the RDA [3].

It is important to realize that in short-term experiments, individuals accustomed to intakes of 800 mg/day will require this intake to maintain calcium equilibrium. Over a period of time, however, most people appear to be able to adapt to (achieve calcium equilibrium on) lower intakes, even as low as 200 mg/day. Such very low intakes are not recommended, however, because an individual's actual need may be higher.

During growth periods calcium needs are increased, as indicated by the RDA during pregnancy, childhood, and adolescence. Although the RDA for ages 1 to 10 years is the same as for adults, 800 mg/day represents a higher intake per unit of weight in children than in adults. During the very rapid growth periods of puberty and pregnancy, the RDA for calcium is at its highest. Lactation is also a time of greater dietary calcium need for milk production and protection of the mother's calcium reserves.

The calcium needs of the elderly appear to be at least as great as those of young adults, and in people who adjust poorly to low intakes the need may be greater.

Food Sources

Milk and milk products contribute more calcium to the American diet than other food groups. Appendix C indicates that a person who consumed no milk or milk products would need to include routinely in the diet: green, leafy vegetables such as turnip and collard greens (not spinach, because oxalate makes the calcium unabsorbable), canned salmon or sardines, sesame seeds, soybeans, soybean curd (tofu), and blackstrap molasses. Persons unable to consume milk or milk products who choose to use calcium supplements should choose the soluble salts calcium gluconate or lactate.

PHOSPHORUS

Functions

Phosphorus, in conjunction with calcium, is essential for bone mineralization, but performs many other functions independently of calcium. Although 85 percent of the body's phosphorus exists in bones, that in fluids and soft tissues performs crucial roles in the body. Phosphorus is an essential component of ATP and other high-energy compounds required for muscle contractions and many anabolic reactions in metabolism. The tissues use phosphorus to produce the active coenzyme forms of thiamine, riboflavin, niacin, vitamin B_6, and pantothenic acid. Many metabolites in metabolic pathways are activated by attaching phosphate groups. For example, glucose cannot be oxidized in metabolism until a phosphate group is attached. In addition, this mineral is an integral part of DNA and RNA, without which cellular reproduction and protein synthesis could not occur. In the form of phospholipids, phosphorus is an important component of cell membranes and of the lipoproteins required to transport blood lipids. It also aids in maintaining normal blood pH by acting as a part of inorganic phosphate buffers.

Absorption and Metabolism

About 70 percent of dietary phosphorus in the usual adult diet is absorbed, in contrast to absorption of only 30 percent of dietary calcium. Some forms of phosphorus, such as phytates of whole-grain cereals and seeds, are not well absorbed, but this poses no practical problems since generous amounts are absorbed from other sources. Although phytates prevent absorption of some calcium, zinc, and iron by forming insoluble complexes, this is of practical significance only if diets are low in these minerals and unusually high in phytates.

The kidneys regulate the level of phosphorus in the blood by either excreting excessive amounts or preventing urinary phosphorus excretion when blood levels become low. The active form of vitamin D and parathyroid hormone aid the kidneys in performing this function.

Deficiency

Phosphorus deficiency does not exist among people consuming their usual diets unless antacids are used in large amounts over long periods. Antacids prevent phosphorus absorption and can eventually lower blood phosphate levels. Deficiency symptoms include weakness, loss of appetite, and skeletal aches. This disorder appears to be rare, however [23].

Recommended Intakes

The RDA for phosphorus from age 1 year through adulthood is the same as that for calcium; the ratio of calcium to phosphorus (Ca:P) is therefore 1:1 (Appendix A). For infants, however, the Ca:P ratio is set at 1.5:1. The recommendation for infancy is in part due to the fact that human milk has a high Ca:P ratio of 2:1. (Most of the RDAs in infancy are based on the nutrient composition of breast milk.) Undiluted cow's milk, having a lower ratio of 1.2:1, is unsuitable for newborn infants because of its high phosphorus content (see Chapter 15).

The daily intake of phosphorus in the United States is much higher than the RDA, averaging 1500 to 1600 mg [27]. Milk, cheese, meat, fish, poultry, legumes, and grains contribute major amounts of phosphorus to the American diet (Appendix C) but soft drinks containing phosphoric acid and other foods containing phosphate additives may contribute a significant amount also.

The Ca:P ratio of the current United States diet is about 1:1.6 [27]. Whether or not this ratio is undesirably high in phosphorus is unknown at present. In lower animals, a Ca:P ratio of 2:1 appears to be optimal, resulting in minimal loss of calcium from the bones and maximal calcium absorption. Although human beings appear to be able to adjust to Ca:P ratios varying between 2:1 and 1:2, a recent authoritative review suggested that the ideal ratio is 1:1 [28]. Future research should clarify the significance of the Ca:P ratio in human nutrition.

MAGNESIUM

Functions

Magnesium performs many essential functions in the body as an activator of enzymes, particularly those which use ATP for energy. It is also required in the synthesis of DNA and RNA, and performs other roles in protein synthesis. In addition, this mineral is essential for normal nerve conductivity and normal muscle functioning. It also is deposited in the crystalline structure of bones.

Absorption and Metabolism

About 30 to 40 percent of magnesium in the usual adult diet is absorbed, but absorption is dependent on how much is consumed. About 75 percent of a very low intake is absorbed, while only about 25 percent of a very high intake is absorbed [29]. The amount absorbed may be diminished by a high calcium intake, especially if the magnesium intake is low, apparently because the two minerals compete for the same transport mechanism. Absorption of magnesium also may be lessened somewhat by the presence of phytates or oxalates in the intestinal tract.

About 55 percent of the magnesium in the adult body exists in the bones, while 27 percent is in the muscles [29]. Small amounts are found in body fluids, including the blood. Magnesium ions are also present in small but significant amounts in intracellular fluid.

Blood levels of magnesium are controlled chiefly by the kidneys. As blood levels decrease, the kidneys reabsorb more magnesium; high blood levels, on the other hand, result in increased urinary excretion of magnesium.

Deficiency

Magnesium deficiency has never been documented in normal population groups consuming their usual diets, but is occasionally seen in unusual circumstances. Alcoholics sometimes develop the deficiency because alcohol promotes urinary excretion of magnesium. Infants who develop kwashiorkor (protein-calorie malnutrition) often have magnesium deficiency. Severe malabsorptive disorders, long-term use of those diuretics which promote urinary losses of magnesium, and kidney diseases, in which the ability to reabsorb magnesium is diminished, all may result in a deficiency. Patients requiring prolonged intravenous feeding have also developed magnesium deficiency.

Symptoms of deficiency include loss of appetite, nausea and vomiting, muscle tremors and weariness, poor coordination, and, in infants, convulsions [29].

Recommended Intakes and Food Sources

The RDA for magnesium is set at 300 mg/day for the adult female and 350 mg/day for the adult male (Appendix A). The American diet appears to contain about 120 mg/1000 kcal, an apparently adequate amount.

Magnesium occurs in highest amounts in nuts, seeds, dried beans, green vegetables (the green pigment, chlorophyll, contains magnesium) and in whole grains (Appendix D). The refining of wheat flour results in large losses of magnesium, since most of this mineral occurs in the bran and germ. Some hard waters contain a considerable amount of magnesium, while soft waters are always low in magnesium.

In recent years some health-conscious people have taken dolomite pills which are promoted in health food stores as a source of magnesium and calcium. A physician recently reported that chemical analysis of these pills found that they contained toxic metals, including arsenic, lead, cadmium, mercury, and aluminum [30]. This report draws attention to possible dangers associated with consuming preparations of unknown composition.

TABLE 12-3. AN OVERVIEW OF THE MAJOR MINERALS

MINERAL	FUNCTIONS	DEFICIENCY SYMPTOMS	FOOD SOURCES	TOXICITY	ADULT RDA PER DAY
Sodium	Fluid balance, acid-base balance, nerve and muscle function.	Rare. Excessive sweat losses cause nausea, giddiness, muscle cramps, fatigue.	Common salt (NaCl); occurs naturally in milk products and meats, poultry, fish, eggs. Highly processed foods often high.	Suspected of leading to hypertension.	No RDA. Estimated safe intake: 1100–3300 mg.
Potassium	Fluid balance, acid-base balance, nerve and muscle function, required for enzyme reactions.	Weakness, lethargy, change in heart rhythm, muscle paralysis, can be fatal.	Fruits, vegetables, whole grains, fresh meats, poultry, fish.	Occurs from supplements only.	No RDA. Estimated safe intake: 1875–5625 mg.
Chloride	Fluid balance, acid-base balance, component of stomach acid.	Growth failure, slow growth of head, poor appetite, more alkaline blood, behavioral and learning problems.	Sodium chloride (common salt).	Unlikely from diet.	No RDA. Estimated safe intake: 1700–5100 mg.
Calcium	Structural component of bones, blood coagulation, nerve and muscle function, required for enzyme reactions and cell membrane functions.	May rarely be involved in producing rickets and osteomalacia. Possibly involved in osteoporosis.	Dairy products, green leafy vegetables, legumes, almonds, soybeans, tofu.	Unlikely.	800 mg.
Phosphorus	Structural component of bones, component of ATP, DNA, RNA, B vitamin coenzymes, phospholipids, lipoproteins, buffers.	Rare.	Milk, cheese, meats, poultry, legumes, cereals.	Large intakes may lower calcium absorption.	800 mg.
Magnesium	Enzyme activator, required for synthesis of DNA, RNA, protein synthesis, nerve and muscle functions, bone structure.	Poor appetite, nausea, muscle tremors, poor coordination, weariness, convulsions.	Nuts, seeds, legumes, green vegetables, whole grains.	Unlikely.	300 mg—females; 350 mg—males.

SUMMARY

An overview of the major minerals is given in Table 12-3.

1 The electrolytes sodium, potassium, and chloride play important roles in distributing water between intracellular and extracellular fluid compartments. These electrolytes, in conjunction with calcium and magnesium, are also required for regulating nerve response and muscle contractility.

2 Potassium occurs chiefly in intracellular fluid while sodium and chloride occur in extracellular fluid. The sodium-potassium pump maintains this differential.

3 Most authorities agree that, in an attempt to prevent hypertension, it is prudent to avoid high sodium intakes, and consume more potassium than sodium. The estimated safe and adequate suggestions of the Food and Nutrition Board reflect this viewpoint.

4 The majority of body calcium is deposited in bones, but the small amount in body fluids performs essential regulatory functions.

5 Normal adults are in calcium equilibrium, excreting the same amount of calcium that they consume. During growth, calcium is retained in the body and the individual is in positive balance, excreting less than is consumed.

6 Phosphorus is needed for calcification of bones and for many important compounds required for energy metabolism, protein synthesis, cellular reproduction, and for metabolism of carbohydrates and transport of lipids.

7 Magnesium, in addition to its functions in nerve conductivity and muscle contractility, is an activator of many enzymes, and is essential for RNA, DNA, and protein synthesis.

FOR DISCUSSION AND APPLICATION

1 From your food record (Chapter 3) calculate your average daily intake of calcium and phosphorus.
   a. What was the ratio of calcium to phosphorus?
   b. How close was your calcium intake to the RDA? Your phosphorus intake?
   c. If one's calcium intake is low while phosphorus intake is high, what possible difficulty might develop? Explain.
   d. If your calcium intake was low, is there any reason to increase your intake? Explain. What foods could you add to your diet as calcium sources?

2 Suppose that at a party you consumed a large amount of potato chips, pretzels, salted nuts, and olives. What would happen regarding your desire for water? Why? Mentally trace the passage of the excess sodium ions into your blood and out of your body. What would happen to the volume of ECF for a short time? Why? What mechanisms would prevent any permanent change in the fluid balance in your body?

3 Suppose a physician had prescribed a 1000-mg sodium diet for your mother because of high blood pressure. Plan 1 day's menu that would supply all the nutrients needed, but would furnish 1000 mg of sodium or less.

SUGGESTED READINGS

Lecos, C., "Potassium: Keeping a Delicate Balance", *FDA Consumer*, February 1983, pp. 21–23. An article discussing the FDA's regulations regarding potassium chloride as a salt substitute.

Miller, R. W., "*How to Ignore Salt and Still Please the Palate,*" *FDA Consumer*, April 1982, pp. 19–22. An article listing of a great many sources of information on how to cook with little, if any, added salt.

Johnson, G. T., and S. E. Goldfinger, eds., *The Harvard Medical School Health Letter Book*, New York: Warner Books Inc., 1981. Many questions about minerals are addressed in this synthesis of information originally published in *The Harvard Medical School Health Letter*.

13

TRACE ELEMENTS (MINERALS)

Loretta is taking her first course in nutrition, but she already knows that she wants to become a nutrition educator. During Nutrition Month, sponsored by the American Dietetics Association, the local dietetics group planned "Ask the Dietitian" booths at local supermarkets. Loretta knew one of the participating dietitians who invited Loretta to help her hand out information packets. Loretta jumped at the chance because this gave her the opportunity to learn what questions people were concerned about and how the dietitian answered them. Loretta was particularly intrigued by the questions on trace elements. They included: (1) "A new clinic opened in my neighborhood that does hair analysis. That's a good way to find out if you are deficient in vitamins or minerals, isn't it?" (2) "I'm diabetic. Should I start taking brewer's yeast to get chromium?" (3) "Does fluoridated water cause cancer?'' (4) ''Should I take superoxide dismutase for my arthritis, as promoted by health food stores? What *is* this substance, anyway?'' This chapter answers these and other questions about trace minerals.

But first, are these elements found in tissues only in trace amounts, as the name implies? Early investigators reported that certain minerals occurred in animal tissues only in trace amounts because analytical methods at that time were too insensitive to determine exact concentrations. Today, new technology allows us to determine exceedingly small concentrations of these elements, yet we persist in calling them trace elements even though some are in tissues in markedly greater amounts than others (see Figure 12-1).

All those trace elements listed in Figure 12-1 are considered dietary essentials, but nonessential elements, such as lead, aluminum, cadmium, and mercury, also may be found in body tissues. Technical difficulties and ethical problems preclude inducing trace mineral deficiencies in humans to pinpoint those that are essential. Consequently, a trace mineral is considered essential if (1) it is present in the tissues of all animal species, and (2) its dietary withdrawal produces the same biochemical and functional abnormalities in each species, which are reversed by feeding the mineral [1]. Proving a trace mineral's essentiality in several lower animals is therefore sufficient to gain its classification as essential in human diets.

Trace elements—essential and nonessential alike—share a characteristic not shown by any other class of nutrients; they are all toxic if consumed in large enough amounts for long enough time periods. They differ in how wide the margin is between amounts that are biologically active and those that are toxic—some have quite small margins.

In this chapter we focus on those trace elements about which most is known. These include iron, zinc, iodine, chromium, fluorine, copper, and selenium. For each of these, we consider not only its functions, metabolism, deficiency signs, and recommended intakes, but also questions of current concern surrounding it. Furthermore, some of the interrelationships of trace elements with one another or with other nutrients are examined, particularly those having practical applications.

IRON

Functions

The overriding function of iron in the body is to enable tissues to utilize oxygen and get rid of waste carbon dioxide. You are probably already familiar with *hemoglobin*, the iron-containing substance in red blood cells that combines with oxygen in the lungs, releases it in the tissues, picks up carbon dioxide there and returns it to the lungs. Iron in hemoglobin exists in an organic complex called *heme*. Heme is an essential component not only of hemoglobin but also of myoglobin, a similar compound that stores oxygen in muscles until needed there for energy metabolism [2]. Furthermore, enzymes (called cytochromes) in the electron transport system also contain heme; without it they are unable to participate in the oxidation of carbohydrates, lipids, and protein for energy. Other enzymes involved in oxygen utilization also are heme-containing.

Absorption

Our understanding of iron absorption surged ahead in recent years when researchers found that some forms of iron in foods are much better absorbed than others. Heme iron found in meats, poultry, and fish (as hemoglobin and myoglobin) is better absorbed than nonheme, or inorganic, forms found in both plant and animal foods. Heme iron is absorbed directly as the heme complex, and its iron is then released in the intestinal mucosal cells [2].

Most of the iron in food is in the form of nonheme iron. This form must be soluble and in ionic form to be absorbed. Stomach acid solubilizes both ferrous (Fe^{2+}) and ferric (Fe^{3+}) iron, but generally ferrous iron is better absorbed than ferric iron. Many food components form soluble chelates with ferrous or ferric iron, aiding in absorption. The most important of these is vitamin C (see Chapter 9). An undefined "meat factor" present in meat, poultry, and fish also enhances absorption of nonheme iron [3]. Acid foods solubilize some of the iron in iron cooking utensils, making it available for absorption.

Among substances that inhibit absorption of nonheme iron are tannic acids of tea, phosvitin of eggs, EDTA (a food additive), phytates from whole grains, antacid drugs, and salts of calcium and phosphorus such as those that may be added to certain highly processed foods [4]. Practical considerations regarding these substances in diets are discussed later under food sources.

An individual's nutritional status affects iron absorption, for iron-deficient individuals absorb a higher percentage of their dietary intake than do those who are well-nourished. Women during their reproductive years have lower iron stores than men, and are therefore more apt to become deficient. Exactly how the body regulates absorption relative to its need for iron is not understood, but the mechanism cannot protect against deficiency if too little available iron is in the diet.

One group of investigators arrived at a practical way to estimate how much iron is absorbed from a given meal [3]. Although details of their method are beyond the scope of this book, their estimate assumes that no nonheme iron is absorbed unless some heme-containing food (meat, poultry, or fish) or vitamin C is consumed with it. Table 13-1 indicates that the percentage of nonheme iron absorbed is always less than that of heme iron. Furthermore, heme iron absorption is the same regardless of meal composition, while absorption of nonheme iron is dependent upon presence in the meal of vitamin C or heme-containing foods. The percentage of iron absorbed from either heme or nonheme iron is greatly influenced by the extent of body iron stores. Men, having markedly larger stores of iron than women, absorb lower percentages of both nonheme and heme iron than do women.

Metabolism

Upon crossing the intestinal mucosal cells from the intestinal lumen, iron reaches the liver by way of the portal vein. The liver puts iron into the circulating blood

TABLE 13-1. FACTORS FOR ESTIMATING PERCENT ABSORPTION OF DIETARY IRON, TAKING INTO ACCOUNT MEAL COMPOSITION AND BODY IRON STORES

TYPE OF MEAL	PERCENTAGE ABSORPTION OF IRON IN A MEAL							
	DIETARY NONHEME IRON				DIETARY HEME IRON			
	STORES* 0 mg	STORES* 250 mg	STORES* 500 mg	STORES* 1000 mg	STORES* 0 mg	STORES* 250 mg	STORES* 500 mg	STORES* 1000 mg
Low availability meal < 1 oz meat, poultry, fish or < 25 mg vitamin C	5	4	3	2	35	28	23	15
Medium availability meal 1–3 oz meat, poultry, fish or 25–75 mg vitamin c	10	7	5	3	35	28	23	15
High availability meal > 3 oz meat, poultry, fish or > 75 mg vitamin C or 1–3 oz meat, fish, poultry plus 25–75 mg vitamin C	20	12	8	4	35	28	23	15

*Iron stores in women and men may range from 0 to 1000 mg. There is a progressive decrease in percentage of iron absorbed as the stores increase from 0 to 1000 mg.

SOURCE: Modified from Monsen, E. R., L. Hallberg, M. Layrisse, D. M. Hegsted, J. D. Cook, and W. Mertz. "Estimation of Available Dietary Iron," *American Journal of Clinical Nutrition*, 31:134, 1978.

attached to a protein, *transferrin*. This form of iron is called *serum iron*, since it is in the liquid portion of the blood (the serum) and not yet incorporated into hemoglobin. The bone marrow then picks up iron as needed from the blood serum and uses it to synthesize hemoglobin, which it incorporates into newly formed red blood cells. The new red blood cells, having their full component of hemoglobin, enter the circulating blood, transporting oxygen from the lungs to body cells and removing carbon dioxide from cells for expiration by the lungs. Red blood cells exist for about 120 days in the adult. When the body destroys old red blood cells, it conserves the iron by storing it in the liver and bone marrow or by reusing it immediately for synthesis of new red blood cells (Figure 13-1). Storage forms of iron are called *ferritin* and *hemosiderin*.

Small amounts of iron are lost from the body daily through bile, urine, sweat, and loss of intestinal mucosal cells. In male adults, this loss amounts generally to about 1 mg/day, while in females, menstrual losses bring the total average daily iron loss to 1.5 mg or more.

Deficiency

Iron deficiency is unique in that it is found in both highly industrialized and developing countries. Although the body conserves iron by keeping its excretion

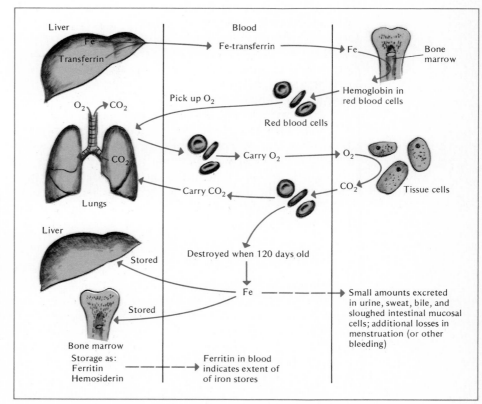

FIGURE 13-1. Schematic summary of iron metabolism. Iron (Fe), transported in the blood attached to transferrin, is used to synthesize hemoglobin, placed in red blood cells. These carry oxygen (O_2) to cells and carbon dioxide (CO_2) from cells to the lungs. Red blood cells are destroyed after approximately 120 days, but their Fe is stored for later use. Only small amounts of Fe are lost daily.

low, the lack of absorbable dietary iron makes iron deficiency the world's most common nutrient deficiency [5]. In addition, iron losses from the body through bleeding due to menstruation, intestinal parasites, or various gastrointestinal diseases contribute to the occurrence of iron-deficiency anemia. Groups that are most prone to develop this anemia include (1) infants, because their body stores of iron at birth are sufficient to last at best only 6 months, while their major food source of human or animal milk is low in iron; (2) children and adolescents during periods of rapid growth, due to needs for synthesis of new tissues and to keep blood hemoglobin concentrations constant as body fluids expand; (3) women during their reproductive years because of menstrual losses of iron and their generally low iron stores; and (4) women during pregnancy because of needs for expansion of maternal blood volume, the requirement of the fetus and placenta for iron, and loss of blood during childbirth.

In fully developed (severe) iron-deficiency anemia, the red blood cells are decreased in number, unusually pale in color (hypochromic), and small in size (microcytic). As the anemia develops, the concentration of serum iron and the percentage bound to transferrin decreases. Hemoglobin concentrations and the hematocrit (volume of red blood cells) also fall below normal.

However, iron-deficiency anemia does not develop until all the storage iron has been used up. Physicians use, as an indicator of low iron stores, a decreased level of ferritin in the blood, since normally a certain level of blood ferritin is maintained. Iron deficiency is defined as diminution or disappearance of body iron stores, even if anemia has not yet appeared [6]. Arresting iron deficiency at an early stage, before there are changes in the red blood cells, prevents development of symptoms and makes treatment less difficult for the patient. In assessing nutritional status regarding iron, individuals are considered to be well-nourished if their hematocrit and blood levels of ferritin, hemoglobin, serum iron, and percentage of serum iron bound to transferrin are all normal.

The most common symptoms or complaints in moderate to severe iron-deficiency anemia include great fatigue, paleness of mucous membranes (lining the eyelids, for example), shortness of breath on physical exertion, and consciousness of a rapid or fluttering heartbeat. Patients often also complain of having cold hands and feet. Although iron-deficiency anemia rarely is a direct cause of death, the disorder is a serious public health problem because it contributes to poor work performance and ill health in many people throughout the world [5].

Recommended Intakes

The iron needed in the diet is that amount that will allow absorption of sufficient amounts to replace daily losses and maintain iron stores. Women in their reproductive years lose more body iron but consume less iron than men. It is not surprising to find, therefore, that women in their reproductive years generally have iron stores amounting to 300 mg or less, while men are more apt to have stores of about 1000 mg. Women would be better able to avoid iron-deficiency anemia if their iron stores were larger than this.

Since men, on the average, lose about 1 mg of iron per day, the RDA sets the allowance for men at 10 mg/day, assuming that 10 percent of total dietary iron will be abosrbed. For adolescent girls and women in their reproductive years and for male adolescents, the allowance is set at 18 mg. This means that 1.8 mg/day needs to be absorbed to replace losses and for adolescents to use for growth (Appendix A). As noted earlier, the amount and form of iron in each meal as well as the amount of vitamin C per meal needs to be taken into account in estimating whether sufficient iron is absorbed to meet the RDA.

Food Sources

Appendix C lists sources of iron in foods. Although these are not divided into heme and nonheme sources, you can estimate these by assuming that iron in meats, poultry, and fish is 40 percent heme iron [3]. The remainder is considered to be nonheme iron, as is iron in plants and in all animal foods other than meat, poultry, and fish. Legumes, dried fruits, and leafy green vegetables contribute the largest amounts of nonheme iron in plant foods. Although eggs contain iron, phosvitin in eggs inhibits iron absorption, not only from eggs but from other foods consumed with them [3].

In planning diets for women of childbearing years and young children, consideration should be given to factors apt to enhance or inhibit iron absorption. Including a source of vitamin C and/or a source of heme iron in each meal increases the availability of iron. This does *not* mean that one should go overboard, consuming huge amounts of meat, poultry, or fish or taking vitamin C tablets. It means instead distributing good food sources of vitamin C and/or heme-containing foods throughout the day's meals and snacks within the context of a varied, moderate diet. Vegetarians, because they do not include heme iron in their diets, should consume a source of vitamin C in each meal for better iron absorption. Enhancing factors can quadruple the amount of iron absorbed from a meal of otherwise low iron availability [7].

One should remember that vitamin C is easily destroyed by heat. One study showed that iron absorption was diminished by 33 to 35 percent by keeping meals warm for 4 hours as might be done in a cafeteria line. Iron availability was completely restored by adding vitamin C to these meals [8].

Among factors that may inhibit iron absorption is tannic acid, found in tea and in many plants. Consuming tea with meals may decrease iron absorption by half, but this can be overcome if sufficient vitamin C is present in the meal or snack [7]. Foods containing large amounts of EDTA, a food additive, may inhibit absorption of nonheme iron by forming an insoluble iron chelate (check the label for presence of EDTA and consult the manufacturer to find out amounts used) [7].

Manufacturers add iron to many foods, including enriched breads and cereals, fortified breakfast cereals, and infant cereals and formulas. Many of the iron compounds used in fortification are poorly absorbed, however [7].

Toxicity

Toxicity from iron is most common in industrialized countries when small children accidentally consume large amounts of vitamin or mineral supplements containing iron [9]. Prolonged consumption of iron supplements by adults not in need of extra iron can also result in iron overload, for this practice overcomes the mechanism that normally balances absorption with need [5].

A small number of individuals have a genetic defect resulting in failure to block iron absorption. These individuals slowly accumulate larger and larger stores of iron throughout life. Eventually, scarring of the liver develops (cirrhosis), dark pigmentation of the skin occurs, diabetes develops because pancreatic cells that produce insulin are destroyed, and finally heart failure may develop. This disorder has been named *hemochromatosis*.

Alcoholics who consume large amounts of wine daily are susceptible to iron overload because alcohol increases absorption of iron and some wines contain a significant amount of iron. Iron overload in the Bantus of Africa results from habitual consumption of alcoholic beverages prepared in iron pots [5].

ZINC

Interest in zinc as an important nutrient in human nutrition escalated in recent years as borderline deficiency was reported among some children in the United States.

Functions

Zinc functions chiefly as an essential *cofactor* (an activator of enzymes) or structural component for over 70 enzymes in body cells. Enzymes requiring zinc are involved in alcohol, carbohydrate, and protein metabolism, in bone calcification, in protein digestion, in the synthesis of DNA, RNA, and proteins, and in ridding the blood of carbon dioxide. Zinc is essential for growth and reproduction in animals. It aids wound healing and is believed to be required for mobilizing vitamin A from storage sites in the liver. Little wonder, then, that most systems of the body are affected by changes in zinc metabolism.

Absorption and Metabolism

Scientists believe that normal zinc absorption is facilitated by a substance thought to be secreted by the pancreas, classed as a zinc-binding ligand. The nature of the substance and how it aids in zinc absorption are presently unknown [10]. So far, the only food proved to enhance zinc absorption is breast milk, which contains a zinc-binding ligand. Several dietary substances inhibit zinc absorption, however. These include dietary fiber and phytates from whole grains and legumes and inorganic (nonheme) iron [10]. Thus, zinc and iron are involved in an important interaction.

As zinc enters the intestinal mucosal cells, some is absorbed by way of the portal blood while another portion is trapped in mucosal cells bound to protein. When mucosal cells are sloughed off into the intestinal lumen, this zinc goes with them. That zinc reaching the liver, if not needed in that organ's tissues, is distributed to all body tissues. Relatively large amounts of the body's zinc is deposited in bones and teeth, but this does not appear to interchange very rapidly with that of soft tissue and body fluids. About one-fifth of the body's zinc occurs in the skin. Zinc is secreted daily into the small intestines in pancreatic juices and other intestinal secretions. A large percentage of this zinc is reabsorbed to be used over and over in the body [10]. Little zinc is normally excreted in the urine.

Deficiency

Human zinc deficiency was first observed in villages of the Middle East where *unusually* high intakes of phytates and dietary fiber were thought to play a major role in decreasing absorption of zinc [11]. Since that time marginal zinc deficiency has been observed among infants and children in the United States from both middle [12] and lower-income [13] families.

Symptoms of zinc deficiency depend upon duration and severity of the deficiency, as well as on age. In infants and small children, growth retardation and loss of appetite (anorexia) are common signs [12]. Loss of taste acuity is also common at all ages. In adolescents, delayed sexual maturation and stunted growth have been reported [11]. Scaliness of the skin may develop, as well as delayed wound healing, mental depression, lethargy, loss of hair, diarrhea, and increased susceptibility to infections [14]. Zinc deficiency is associated with deficiencies in immune systems observed in protein-calorie malnutrition [15].

In early pregnancy in animals and perhaps also in humans zinc deficiency results in birth defects [14]. Zinc added to commercial formulas fed to a group of infants resulted in increased growth of male, but not female, infants indicating that the original formula had been inadequate in zinc for male infants [16]. As a result of this study, most manufacturers now add zinc to infant formulas.

Food Sources

Zinc appears to be much better absorbed from animal than from plant foods. Animal sources of zinc include oysters and other seafoods, liver, meats, and eggs. Although whole grains supply a significant amount of zinc (Appendix D), their content of phytates and dietary fiber can adversely affect absorption of zinc. However, recent studies of women who had consumed lacto-ovo-vegetarian diets high in phytates and dietary fiber for some time indicated that their zinc nutritional status was normal [17,18]. Further studies of this nature are needed to give us perspective on the influence of current dietary practices on zinc nutritional status.

The zinc currently available in the United States diet is 12.5 mg/day, the same as in 1909, but sources have changed over that 70-year period (Figure 13-2). Today we obtain more zinc from meats, poultry, fish, and dairy products and less from grain products than in 1909–1913. This change probably has resulted in greater absorbability of dietary zinc.

Recommended Intakes

The Food and Nutrition Board set 15 mg/day of zinc as the RDA for adults, assuming that about 40 percent of dietary zinc is absorbed (Appendix A). The RDA assumes that animal products, with their higher zinc availability, are

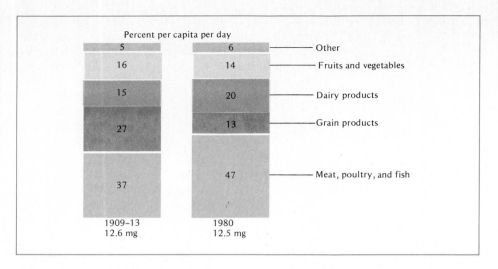

FIGURE 13-2. Zinc contributed to the food supply by major food groups. Although the amount of zinc in today's food supply is the same as in 1909–1913, a higher proportion today comes from meats and dairy products, and a lower proportion from grains. (Source: 1981 Handbook of Agricultural Charts, Agriculture Handbook No. 592, Washington, D.C.: U. S. Dept. of Agriculture, 1981.)

Percent per capita per day

5	6	Other
16	14	Fruits and vegetables
15	20	Dairy products
27	13	Grain products
37	47	Meat, poultry, and fish

1909–13
12.6 mg

1980
12.5 mg

included in the diet. Individuals who restrict their intakes exclusively to plant foods may need larger intakes [19].

IODINE

Simple goiter, or enlargement of the thyroid gland, has afflicted groups of people since antiquity. The ancient Egyptians, Chinese, and the Incas of South America all treated this disorder with seaweed and burnt sponge, not knowing that the active substance was iodine. Despite early recognition that goiter could be successfully treated, it was not until 1917–1918 that scientific studies established that iodine supplements could prevent simple goiter [22].

A CLOSER LOOK

It may be tempting to think that you should take zinc supplements if your diet is high in dietary fiber and low in animal zinc sources. Although the margin between adequacy and toxicity is wider for zinc than for some other trace elements, large intakes produce nausea and vomiting. More subtle effects may occur with lower doses. For example, daily intakes of a little less than 500 mg/day decreased blood concentrations of high-density lipoprotein (HDL), the form of lipoprotein thought to be protective against heart disease [20] (see Chapter 5). Excessive zinc intakes also tend to precipitate marginal copper deficiency [21]. Researchers are becoming more aware of the importance of the interactions of nutrients with one another, and therefore believe it unwise to assume that supplements of a given nutrient have no effect on others. It seems preferable to depend upon a diet composed of a variety of minimally processed foods rather than on supplements to supply zinc and other minerals.

A SIGNIFICANT PROPORTION OF THE AMERICAN POPULATION MAY NOT CONSUME ENOUGH ZINC

Jane E. Brody, *The New York Times*, July 28, 1982

. . . Concern has focused on the fact that a significant proportion of the American population, including those in middle-income and upper-income families, may not be consuming enough zinc. And the mineral is now known to play many vital roles in health, including protection against infection and possibly cancer.

A survey of apparently normal children from well-to-do families in Denver revealed that a sizable proportion had marginal zinc deficiencies and experienced such symptoms as taste insensitivity, poor appetite and retarded growth. For many other children, zinc intake is only barely adequate.

A similar situation exists among adults, especially among adolescent girls and adult women. Nutritional surveys of adults indicate that the intake of zinc generally falls below the Recommended Dietary Allowance (R.D.A.) for all age and sex categories, with the average intake being only 46 to 63 percent of the R.D.A.

The problem is more extensive in low-income families, where eating habits tend to be erratic and menus often depend heavily on packaged foods, which lose much of their natural zinc in processing.

People who consume a diet rich in whole grains and low in animal foods may also develop a marginal zinc deficiency because animal foods are the best sources of zinc, and substances in some plant foods can interfere with zinc absorption. . . .

An accurate assessment of zinc deficiency is tricky. In some disorders, zinc may be redistributed to other tissues, creating an apparent shortage in the tissue analyzed, even though the total body supply may be adequate.

Hair analysis is unreliable. . . . Blood tests are more dependable but must be carefully done. . . .

When zinc deficiency is suspected, the most reliable way to confirm it may be to monitor the response to a zinc supplement; if symptoms of zinc deficiency disappear, then the usual supply of the nutrient can be assumed to be inadequate. . . .

ASK YOURSELF:
If individuals consume on the average only 46 to 63 percent of the RDA for zinc, is this convincing evidence that they are deficient in zinc? Why or why not? Since food available in the United States supplies only 12.5 mg/day of zinc, is it possible that the RDA for zinc is unrealistically high? Why or why not? What methods of zinc assessment are discussed in this article?

Function

The only known role played by iodine is in the formation of the thyroid hormones, *thyroxine* (T_4) and *triiodothyronine* (T_3). These hormones are formed in the thyroid gland from the amino acid tyrosine and iodine. Their most important function is to regulate the rate of metabolism in body tissues (see Chapter 7). This fundamental role explains their essentiality for normal growth and development in infancy and childhood.

Hypothyroidism, in which low amounts of thyroid hormones are secreted, results in an unusually low basal metabolic rate, sluggish mental and physical activity, and a tendency to gain weight. People with *hyperthyroidism*, on the

373

other hand, have high basal metabolic rates, tend to be thin and nervous, and frequently have rapid heartbeat and protruding eyes.

Absorption and Metabolism

Iodine in food is rapidly and completely absorbed in the upper small intestines. A high percentage of the total iodine in the body is concentrated in the thyroid gland, where it is used to synthesize thyroid hormones. The remainder circulates in the blood and other extracellular fluids. Iodine is excreted from the body by the kidneys. Losses in the urine continue when the dietary intake is low, since the kidneys are unable to completely conserve iodine.

Deficiency

Simple goiter is a classic sign of iodine deficiency, and continues to be a problem in many parts of the world. A dietary deficiency leads to simple enlargement of the thyroid gland, apparently because cells in the thyroid gland enlarge and/or multiply in an effort to synthesize sufficient thyroid hormones when dietary iodine supply falls below a critical level. In simple goiter, the enlargement suceeds in producing normal blood levels of thyroid hormones, and the person's basal metabolic rate remains normal.

Lack of dietary iodine is not the only factor that can produce simple goiter.

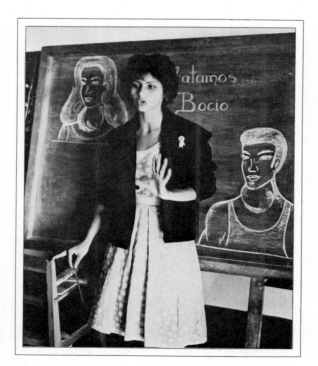

A teacher in a rural school in the Asunción region of Paraguay, where goiter is still common, explains how iodized salt will prevent the disorder. *(WHO photo by Paul Almasy)*

Certain drugs, such as sulfonamides, lithium, and even *excessive* iodine (discussed later) may inhibit the secretion of or interfere with the tissue metabolism of thyroid hormones. In addition, *goitrogens*, substances occurring in food or water, may prevent proper synthesis or activity of thyroid hormones. Goiter probably rarely develops from goitrogens alone, but they may contribute to goiter development [23]. Goitrogens have been found in such foods as turnips and rutabagas and, in some parts of the world, in drinking water.

Simple goiter is common in mountainous parts of the world and areas surrounding freshwater lakes, such as the Great Lakes, because soils in such areas are very low in iodine. Not everyone living in these regions develops goiter, leading authorities to postulate that the disorder develops chiefly in individuals who may have genetic defects in enzymes involved in the synthesis of thyroid hormones. Another possibility is that some individuals are exposed to more goitrogens than others [23]. Dietary iodine is successful in reducing the size of the thyroid gland to normal only if the goiter is small and relatively newly developed.

A particulary severe manifestation of iodine deficiency is *cretinism*, which occurs in infants whose mothers have markedly low secretions of thyroid hormones during pregnancy. Such infants are born with little or no functioning thyroid tissue, and are doomed to stunted bodies and mental retardation unless they are effectively treated with thyroid hormones at birth and for the remainder of their lives. Cretinism occurs chiefly in isolated mountanious regions of the world where soil iodine is extremely low.

Food Sources

The ultimate source of iodine is the sea; therefore, seafoods and certain seaweeds are excellent sources, as are foods grown on soils that were at one time covered by the sea. Recently, the Food and Drug Administration noted, however, that a sample United States diet not only contained a high amount of iodine (4½ times the RDA), but that the chief source of this mineral was dairy products (Figure 13-3). This was an unexpected finding [24].

Iodine gets into milk through the use of iodine-containing chemicals used to clean and disinfect equipment. In addition, iodine is frequently added to the feed of dairy cows to prevent goiter, but some farmers have fed their cattle many times more than the amount needed [24].

The amount of iodine found in grain and cereal products and in sugar and adjuncts (jams, jellies, puddings, candy bars) was also unexpected (Figure 13-3). Iodine-containing chemicals used to clean processing equipment account for some of this, but other practices also make a contribution. Dough conditioners that contain iodine have been used in some forms of bread-making. Iodine makes up about 50 percent of red dye no. 3, the common red coloring dye used in candies, maraschino cherries, breakfast cereals, and vitamin pill coverings. The extent to which the human body absorbs iodine from red dye no. 3 is unknown, however.

Food additives, such as carrageenan, which are derived from algae also are very high in iodine. Fast foods such as hamburgers, french fries, milk shakes, and

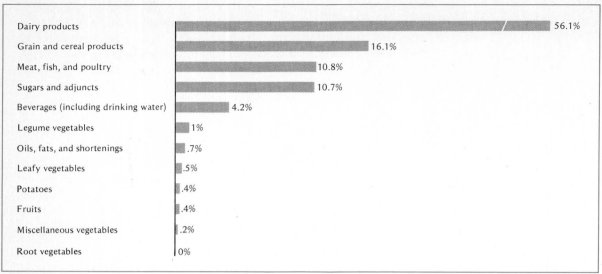

Dairy products	56.1%
Grain and cereal products	16.1%
Meat, fish, and poultry	10.8%
Sugars and adjuncts	10.7%
Beverages (including drinking water)	4.2%
Legume vegetables	1%
Oils, fats, and shortenings	.7%
Leafy vegetables	.5%
Potatoes	.4%
Fruits	.4%
Miscellaneous vegetables	.2%
Root vegetables	0%

FIGURE 13-3. Sources of iodine in adult diet furnishing 2850 kcal daily according to 1978 Total Diet Study by the Food and Drug Administration. (Source: Adapted from Taylor, F., "Iodine," *FDA Consumer*, Washington, D.C., April 1981.)

frozen fried chicken dinners have also been shown to contain large amounts of iodine [24].

The American Medical Association reported that intakes of 2000 μg/day by adults and 1000 μg/day by children, amounts consumed by many Americans, do not appear to be harmful based on present evidence [24]. Large intakes are known to induce goiter, however. Intakes of 10,000 to 200,000 μg/day produced goiter in 6 to 12 percent of Japanese fishermen consuming large amounts of seaweed [25].

The FDA has urged industry and dairy officials to use iodine-containing chemicals and feeds sparingly. Persons who prepare their own food at home using minimally processed ingredients stand to have lower iodine intakes than those using highly processed foods. Even then, milk from dairies might still contribute large amounts of iodine to the diet.

Recommended Intakes

The RDA for ages 11 through adulthood is 150 μg/day (Appendix A). In setting this recommendation, the Food and Nutrition Board assumed that 50 to 75 μg/day will prevent goiter in adults. This amount was increased to 150 μg to allow for individual differences in need and for any goitrogens that might be in the diet [19]. In pregnancy and lactation, the recommendation is increased enough to provide for the needs of the developing fetus and to allow for iodine secretion into milk (Appendix A).

Although experts recently declared that the present intake of iodine in the United States is both adequate and safe [26], the Food and Nutrition Board states that "any additional increases should be viewed with concern" [19]. As a result of these increases in availability of iodine in the food supply, nutritionists no longer encourage the public to use iodized salt.

CHROMIUM

Chromium is a mineral of particular interest, not only because deficiencies may exist among children suffering from protein-calorie malnutrition in some less-developed countries, but also because deficiencies may occur to some extent in the United States and other affluent countries [14].

Function

The most important presently known role of chromium is to potentiate insulin action. Without chromium, insulin is unable to perform its function, resulting in impaired glucose tolerance (see Chapter 4).

Absorption and Metabolism

The physiologically active form of chromium in the body appears to be an organic form in which chromium is complexed with nicotinic acid and amino acids [27]. This form is called *glucose tolerance factor* (GTF). Animals, including human beings, may require some GTF in the diet since their ability to synthesize it from inorganic chromium may be limited.

While less than 1 percent of inorganic chromium may be absorbed, at least 10 percent of GTF appears to be absorbed [14]. Both forms reach the liver by way of the portal blood. Much of it remains in the liver to be released into the blood whenever elevated blood glucose levels trigger insulin release. Once insulin action is completed, this chromium is believed to be excreted in the urine.

Although urinary chromium excretion after an oral glucose dose once was assumed to indicate that an individual had some tissue chromium stores [27], more recent investigation reported that this method fails to indicate chromium nutritional status [28]. The only reliable method for assessing chromium nutritional status appears to be to determine whether or not supplementation with chromium improves glucose tolerance [28].

Deficiency

Chromium deficiency has been found in certain countries (Jordan, Turkey, and Nigeria) in infants having protein-calorie malnutrition [29]. Impaired glucose tolerance occurred in these infants, which was normalized by giving inorganic chromium. Impaired glucose tolerance observed in some (but not all) American diabetics and elderly people responded to chromium treatment [30]. While it appears that some diabetics and some elderly individuals in the United States may be chromium-deficient, we cannot say that all diabetes is *caused* by chromium deficiency. Individuals who are diabetic, like the one mentioned at the beginning of this chapter, need to understand that only if one is actually deficient in chromium is administration of chromium (in brewer's yeast) apt to improve glucose tolerance. A competent physician should supervise any supplementation in diabetic individuals.

Tissue levels of chromium decline with age in the United States, and are lower among United States adults than among those of the Far East, Africa, and

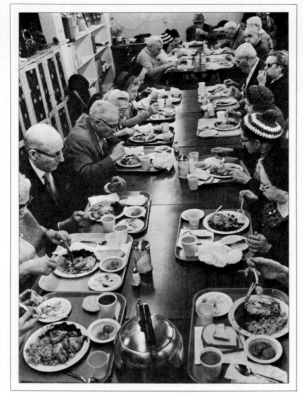

Scientists are interested in finding out whether or not chromium deficiency is more common among the elderly in the United States than in less developed countries. (© *Barbara Pfeffer/Photo Researchers, Inc.*)

the Middle East [31]. This may indicate that many people in the United States become chromium-deficient, especially in later life.

Several studies have indicated that inorganic chromium fed to adults is poorly absorbed, and therefore less effective than feeding GTF. A major drawback to research efforts, however, is that pure GTF has been technically impossible to obtain. Further progress in determining the extent to which chromium deficiency actually exists awaits improvement in techniques for determination of chromium in biological materials [27].

Food Sources

People who consume diets containing large amounts of highly refined grain products and sugars may have low chromium intakes [32]. Bran and germ from whole grains, and raw sugar cane contain chromium, whereas refining these foods removes high percentages of the element. Since chromium must be mobilized from body tissues to permit the insulin action required to metabolize carbohydrates, consumption of refined carbohydrates results in excretion of chromium from the body without replacing the losses.

The best sources of GTF include brewer's yeast and liver [30]. Beef, poultry, whole-grain cereals, bran and germ of wheat, and cheese are also good sources of available chromium [33]. Refined white flour, rice, sugar, butter, and margarine are all poor sources. Cooking acidic foods in stainless steel containers may make some of the chromium in the steel available to the body [30].

Recommended Intakes

The exact amount of chromium needed in the diet is unknown because the availability of this element from foods depends upon its chemical form. The Food and Nutrition Board has tentatively set safe and adequate amounts at between 50 to 200 μg/day for adults (Appendix A). The typical American diet is thought to supply between 50 and 100 μg/day, although some diets are known to supply very low amounts.

FLUORIDE

The importance of fluoride, the ionized form of fluorine, has long been recognized for its role in preventing tooth decay (dental caries).

Function

Carefully executed studies in many parts of the world have clearly established that adding fluoride to drinking water at the level of one part of the element per million parts of water reduces the occurrence of dental decay by 50 percent or more in children who consume the water from early infancy. Fluoride guards against dental caries by causing the tooth enamel to become more resistant to acids. Greatest protection occurs if adequate fluoride is ingested from infancy, before the teeth erupt. One author estimated that fluoridation of the water supply in a specific American city would result in a savings of $7 million a year in dental bills [34].

Fluoride has an unusual affinity for bones and teeth. As fluoride intake increases, the amount deposited in bones and teeth increases in the growing animal, but the rate of increase diminishes as the animal reaches maturity. Nonetheless, amounts of bone fluoride increase with age. Fluoride becomes a part of the crystalline structure of bones—that part made up chiefly of calcium and phosphate crystals, called *hydroxyapatite*. Studies show that fluoride increases the crystal size and is associated with the formation of more nearly perfect crystals [35].

Fluoride may be important in the maintenance of normal bone, since investigators have reported a higher incidence of osteoporosis—a bone disease seen in aging—in individuals who lived in areas with little natural fluoride in drinking water compared with those having high fluoride levels (4 mg/L) in water [36]. Fluoride is currently under study as a possible means of treating osteoporosis (Chapter 16).

Absorption and Metabolism

Fluoride in foods and water is easily absorbed by way of the portal system, and becomes concentrated in bones and teeth, but all tissues contain some fluoride. Excessive intakes are excreted by way of the urine.

Sources

In 1975 the United States Public Health Service estimated that about one-half the total United States population lived in areas where the water supply was fluoridated [37]. Other sources, such as unprocessed and processed foods, fluorides applied to the tooth surface by dentists, and fluoridated toothpastes, contribute significantly to the total daily intake [38]. The amount of fluoride in minimally processed foods depends upon the amount in the soil, water, and air for plant foods; or the amount in feed and water for animal foods. Most foods contain less than one part per million, but seafoods (if bones are consumed) and tea contain large amounts.

Processed foods containing or made from bones, such as gelatin, mechanically deboned meat (meat containing small amounts of bone), and bone meal (as sold in health food stores) are high in fluoride. Use of fluoridated water in processing foods—such as fluid infant formulas, baby foods, and other processed foods requiring water—significantly increases their fluoride content [38].

Recommended Intakes

No formal RDA has been set for fluoride, but the safe and adequate intake for adults is 1.5 to 4.0 mg/day (Appendix A). A total intake of at least 1.5 mg/day is necessary to prevent tooth decay [39].

Fluoride intakes of young male adults in the United States were estimated to vary between 0.9 mg/day in a city in which water was not fluoridated to 1.7 mg/day where water was fluoridated [40]. Although the fluoride intake in some parts of the United States may be too low to protect against dental caries, there is evidence that dental caries is declining in the nation as a whole. The decline is credited to increased intakes of fluoride by routes already discussed [38].

Toxicity

No harm has been demonstrated from daily consumption of fluoride at the level recommended for prevention of tooth decay—that is, one part per million. In parts of the United States where fluoride occurs naturally in water at higher levels—two to four parts per million—mottled tooth enamel developed in children who consumed the water from birth. In this disorder, the tooth enamel loses its luster, becoming chalky in appearance; the chalky areas then become stained and turn brown. Although unsightly, mottled teeth have been found to be highly resistant to decay [35].

Claims made in recent years that fluoridated water increases the death rate from cancer have been shown to be erroneous [42]. Use of inappropriate statistical methods and failure to examine all the available data were the chief errors made by those who made these claims. Studies in many parts of the world indicate that water fluoridation does not increase the chances of dying from cancer [42].

Intakes of fluoride between 20 to 80 mg/day over a period of years results in crippling deformities of the skeleton [39], and amounts as high as 150 mg/day produced loss of appetite, stomach pains, and damage to the retina and optic nerve [41]. These amounts are unlikely to be obtained from the diet, but fluoride tablets should never be taken without competent medical supervision.

COPPER

Functions

Copper is an integral part of many enzymes in the body. One of these is essential for the normal production of hemoglobin in the body, explaining the iron-deficiency anemia commonly observed in copper deficiency. Another is located in the electron transport system; consequently copper is essential for ATP production. Copper also is needed for normal development of connective tissue proteins in the arteries and bones.

Absorption and Metabolism

Copper is absorbed chiefly from the stomach or duodenum [43]. About 30 percent of dietary copper is absorbed by adults. Its absorption is inhibited by phytates, and in experimental animals the presence of vitamin C in the intestines decreases copper absorption. Other trace elements such as zinc, cadmium, and molybdenum also decrease the absorption of copper.

Copper may become somewhat more concentrated in the liver, brain, heart, and kidneys, but is present in all tissues [44]. In the blood plasma, copper is attached to a transport protein, *ceruloplasmin*. In red blood cells, it is associated with the enzyme superoxide dismutase. Ceruloplasmin performs enzymatic functions—for example, it oxidizes ferrous to ferric iron, an important reaction in formation of transferrin, the iron transport protein. This is another example of the interaction of minerals.

Deficiency

Copper deficiency has never occurred among normal people on their usual diets, but has been reported in very small premature infants fed formulas low in copper [43]. Premature infants are born with lower stores of copper than full-term infants, and cow's milk is low in copper. Anemia and skeletal changes have been reported in premature infants [45] and in infants suffering from severe protein-calorie malnutrition who were rehabilitated on milk diets low in copper [46]. These symptoms were cured by giving copper.

A CLOSER LOOK

Recently, superoxide dismutase has been advertised in health food stores to prevent aging and cancer and to treat arthritis, radiation therapy side effects, and muscular dystrophy. Superoxide dismutase, a copper- and zinc-containing enzyme, is produced in the fluid portion of cells. It is a scavenger of a free radical called the superoxide ion—oxygen which has picked up an extra electron (O_2^-). The superoxide ion is generated in cells during oxidation of carbohydrates, protein, or fat for energy. Free radicals can be very damaging to cells, as previously discussed (see Chapter 11).

Health food stores are promoting tablets purportedly containing superoxide dismutase. Is it sensible to believe that these tablets might be useful to the body as free radical scavengers? Are enzymes absorbed *as such* by the body? Can this product reach your cells to do any scavenging?

Enzymes are proteins. Any enzymes in the intestinal lumen eventually are destroyed there for they are digested like any other protein. The only form of superoxide dismutase that can protect body cells from free radicals is that *synthesized in your own cells*. Taking pills won't help that process.

Although a product such as this one may be promoted using much scientific terminology that you may not understand, you need not be confused by it. Always stop to think whether you have fundamental information that places the whole sales pitch into proper perspective.

Food Sources

Foods highest in copper include oysters, liver, dried yeast, and lobster (Appendix D). Good sources are crabmeat, fresh vegetables and fruits, nuts, seeds, and legumes. Foods very low in copper are refined sugars, cereals, and milk (except hunan milk, which is relatively high, particularly at the beginning of lactation). Highly refined diets of low kilocalorie levels may be low in copper.

Recommended Intakes

The estimated safe and adequate intake proposed by the Food and Nutrition Board is 2 to 3 mg/day for the adult (Appendix A). Investigators recently noted, however, that "the majority of diets in the United States analyzed since 1966 contain less copper than 1.3 mg" per day [47].

The Food and Nutrition Board assumes that occasional intakes of up to 10 mg/day are safe, but amounts greater than this can be toxic [19].

SELENIUM

Selenium is a component of an enxyme, glutathione peroxidase, that defends cell membranes and such vital molecules as DNA against oxidative damage. Vitamin E plays a similar role in the body, and animal experiments have shown that the presence of selenium in the diet can decrease the amount of vitamin E needed under certain circumstances [48]. Selenium is known to maintain the integrity of muscle and red blood cells, and of keratins (the tough proteins of hair and nails). In addition, it is essential for sperm motility, immune mechanisms, and pancreatic function [49]. Animal studies triggered interest in selenium as a cancer inhibitor. Although research in mice indicates that selenium inhibits early tissue changes that otherwise develop into cancer, there is no indication yet that this has any application to humans [50].

Absorption, Metabolism, and Deficiency

Selenium is well absorbed from food, and becomes most highly concentrated in the liver, kidneys, heart, and spleen. The urine is the chief excretory route, although some is lost through sweat and the intestines.

In animals, selenium deficiency produces poor growth and a wide variety of disorders, depending upon the species studied. Children with kwashiorkor often have low body stores of selenium [51], but no clear-cut deficiency disease exists even in populations living in regions where the soil is low in selenium.

Food Sources

The dietary intake of population groups depends upon the amount of selenium in the soils on which foods are grown, and on the types of food chosen. The richest sources of selenium in the American diet are organ meats, seafoods, and muscle meats. Grains are excellent sources if grown on high-selenium soils. Eggs and dairy products vary in selenium content depending upon the animal's diet. Fruits and vegetables tend to be low in this nutrient.

Recommended Intakes

The Food and Nutrition Board suggests as safe and adequate amounts between 0.05 and 0.2 mg/day (50 to 200 μg/day) for the adult (Appendix A).

Although the dietary intake of New Zealanders is three to four times lower than that in the United States due to low levels of selenium in the soil, there is no indication that the lower intake in that country is determental to health [52]. Soils in some regions of the United States are low in selenium, but since a high percentage of foods locally consumed are grown in distant regions, it is unlikely that selenium deficiency would develop because of low selenium in local soils. There is no evidence at present that the U.S. diet is either too high or too low in selenium [53].

Supplementation of diets with selenium without competent medical guidance is foolhardy since the margin between adequate and toxic amounts is rather small. The Food and Nutrition Board notes that "a maximal intake of 200 μg/day for adults . . . should not be exceeded habitually if the risk of long-term chronic overexposure is to be avoided" [19]. Symptoms of toxicity (called selenosis) include loss of hair, fatigue, irritability, odor of garlic on the breath, and brittle nails [53].

As noted at the beginning of this chapter, one often hears that hair analysis is a good way to determine whether or not one is well-nourished regarding minerals, as well as vitamins. Is this a legitimate way of assessing nutritional status regarding these nutrients? Box 13-1 addresses this question.

MANGANESE

Manganese is known to be an essential nutrient for many species of animals, and is assumed to be essential for humans. The element is required by several enzymes involved in energy and protein metabolism. In animals, manganese is essential for lipid metabolism, reproduction, bone growth and development, and the utilization of glucose.

The body absorbs only a low percentage of dietary manganese. It becomes widely distributed in body tissues, and is excreted largely through the bile and pancreatic juices.

The Food and Nutrition Board considers a range of 2.5 to 5 mg/day to be safe and adequate for adults and adolescents (Appendix A). The usual adult dietary content appears to vary from 2 to 9 mg/day. Manganese deficiency has never been reported in human populations.

Richest food sources are whole grains and nuts, while vegetables and fruits furnish moderate quantities. Meats, milk, and seafoods are poor sources.

MOLYBDENUM

Molybdenum is required for the function of several important enzymes, including those having to do with uric acid production. The human diet appears to supply the amounts needed, however, since a deficiency has never been reported in any human population.

The estimated safe and adequate intake for adults is 0.15 to 0.5 mg/day (Appendix A). Toxicity of molybdenum is a problem in animal nutrition because high intakes result in losses of copper from the body. In addition, a gout-like disorder due to accumulation of uric acid in the blood has been reported in an area of Russia where the molybdenum intake is high [19].

Good food sources of molybdenum include organ meats, legumes, and whole-grain cereals.

OTHER TRACE ELEMENTS

The remaining trace elements thought to be essential in human diets include cobalt, silicon, vanadium, nickel, tin, and arsenic. Cobalt is used in the human body only in the form of vitamin B_{12} which the body cannot synthesize. Therefore, the essential nutrient for human beings is actually vitamin B_{12} and not cobalt. The remaining essential elements have been demonstrated to be essential in animals and are assumed to be essential in human beings. All these appear to be present in adequate amounts in the diet.

Although some trace elements now classified as nonessential may be found

Hair Analysis as an Assessment Tool

Commercial laboratories devoted to multi-element hair analysis have sprung up around the country. Some health food stores, beauty salons, and self-styled "nutritionists" may pressure clients into providing a sample of hair for analysis. For a sizable fee, the client receives from the laboratory a computer printout showing the sample's concentration of a long list of minerals and a "normal range" for each. Some laboratories provide a computerized dietary analysis in addition. The results usually lead to the client's being advised to purchase mineral and/or vitamin supplements [54].

Is hair analysis, under these conditions, a legitimate method of assessing an individual's nutritional status regarding vitamins and minerals?

The answer is clear: No! Hair contains no vitamins, so vitamin supplements are pointless. As far as minerals are concerned, "normal ranges" are fictitious, for these are as yet unknown. The difficulties in interpreting the meaning of the amount of minerals found in hair are enormous. Even after standard washing procedures,

minerals remaining in hair may have come from the environment rather than from the body. Bleaching, dyeing, and permanent waving either elevate or diminish the concentration of specific minerals in hair. Some shampoos contain trace elements which will contaminate those elements in hair that originated from the body. Hair color, coarseness or fineness, location on the scalp, sex, age, and season all may affect mineral concentration in hair [54].

Competent researchers find hair analysis of some use in studying mineral nutrition in a specific population. Qualified nutritionists never use this technique when assessing the nutritional status of individuals, however, because the method is not yet well enough developed to provide any definitive information [54].

Since hair analysis by commercial laboratories almost invariably leads to recommendations for mineral supplementation, remember that many interrelationships exist among minerals. Taking large amounts of one may adversely affect utilization of another.

to be essential as research progresses, current concern about nonessential trace elements focuses on their possible toxicity. For example, lead toxicity may occur among children who chew on toys or other surfaces covered with paints containing lead. Lead can also enter the body from consumption of plants grown in areas where the air is polluted with lead from automobile exhausts or industrial wastes.

Toxic levels of mercury, lead, or cadmium sometimes enter the food supply through discharges of industrial waste into the environment. Consumers need to take an active role in working with organizations and agencies in efforts to keep toxic substances at low levels in the food supply.

Now that we have completed our discussion of the vitamins and minerals, we can examine the effects of heavy alcohol consumption on vitamin and mineral nutrition (Box 13-2).

TABLE 13-2. AN OVERVIEW OF THE TRACE MINERALS

MINERAL	FUNCTION	DEFICIENCY SYMPTOMS	FOOD SOURCES	TOXICITY	ADULT RDA PER DAY
Iron	As component of heme, enables tissues to utilize oxygen and eliminate carbon dioxide. Components of enzymes required in oxygen utilization.	Anemia—hypochromic, microcytic. Fatigue, paleness, shortness of breath on exertion.	Meats, poultry, fish, legumes, dried fruit, leafy green vegetables.	Individuals with genetic defect develop hemochromatosis.	10 mg for men and postmenopausal women. 18 mg for women in reproductive years.
Zinc	Required by enzymes in alcohol, protein and carbohydrate metabolism and in synthesis of DNA and RNA. Needed for growth and reproduction in animals and in wound healing.	Growth retardation, anorexia, loss of taste acuity, delayed sexual maturation, scaly skin, mental depression, deficiencies in immune systems.	Oysters, liver, meats, eggs, dairy products, whole grains, legumes.	Low. Supplements can result in toxicity.	15 mg
Iodine	Used to form thyroid hormones, thyroxine and triiodothyronine, which are essential in regulating rate of tissue metabolism.	Simple goiter, cretinism in severe deficiency during fetal life.	Dairy foods, grains, cereals, and other processed foods from iodine cleaning agents. Seafoods.	Very high intakes may induce goiter.	150 μg
Chromium	Potentiates insulin action, thus aiding in glucose metabolism.	Abnormal glucose tolerance.	Brewer's yeast, liver, beef, poultry, whole grains, cheese.	Unlikely from diet.	Safe and adequate intake: 50–200 μg

MINERAL	FUNCTION	DEFICIENCY SYMPTOMS	FOOD SOURCES	TOXICITY	ADULT RDA PER DAY
Fluoride	Prevents tooth decay.	Tooth decay.	Fluoridated water, tea, some processed foods if made with fluoridated water.	Mottled enamel. Very high intakes can deform bones and damage optic nerve and retinas.	Safe and adequate intake: 1.5–4.0 mg
Copper	Required by many enzymes including those in heme synthesis, and connective tissue formation.	Anemia, skeletal changes.	Oysters, liver, dried yeast, fresh vegetables, fruits, nuts, seeds, legumes.	Amounts over 10 mg/day can be toxic.	Safe and adequate intake: 2–3 mg
Selenium	Component of enzyme that protects membranes and compounds against oxidative destruction.	None known in humans except low blood levels.	Organ meats, seafoods, muscle meats, grains grown in high-selenium soils.	Amounts greater than 200 μg may produce chronic toxicity. Loss of hair, fatigue, odor of garlic on breath.	Safe and adequate intake: 50–200 μg
Manga-nese	Required by enzymes involved in energy and protein metabolism.	Rare.	Whole grains, nuts.	Unlikely from diet.	Safe and adequate intake: 2.5–5 mg
Molybde-num	Required by enzymes involved in uric acid metabolism and other functions.	Rare.	Organ meats, legumes, whole grains.	Unlikely from diet.	Safe and adequate intake: 0.15–0.5 mg

13-2 Alcohol: Its Effects on Vitamin and Mineral Nutrition

BOX

Alcohol consumption adversely affects vitamin and mineral nutritional status. Studies are lacking on the influence of *moderate* drinking on nutritional status, but heavy drinkers are clearly in danger or developing nutritional problems regarding vitamins and minerals. Although the majority of studies have been done on diagnosed alcoholics, one should keep in mind that a great many heavy drinkers, including many who view themselves as moderate or social drinkers, are in fact undiagnosed alcoholics. Furthermore, many "moderate" drinkers sometimes engage in weekend periods of heavy drinking.

While poor nutritional status may result from multiple causes, including inadequate diet during bouts of heavy drinking, we focus our attention here on the effects of *alcohol itself* on absorption, metabolism, and excretion of vitamins and minerals. The overall health risks of heavy alcohol consumption are summarized in Chapter 3.

Water-Soluble Vitamins Alcohol damages the intestinal absorptive surface and diminishes the absorption of thiamine, folacin [55], and vitamin B_{12} [56]. In addition, the body's ability to form the active coenzyme forms of thiamine and vitamin B_6 becomes impaired [55,57]. Ability to utilize folacin is also diminished [55]. Alcohol damages the precursor blood cells in the bone marrow, increasing the need for folacin, vitamin B_6, and vitamin B_{12}, all of which are required in the maturation of red and white blood cells [57]. Anemias characteristic of folacin and vitamin B_6 deficiencies are common in alcoholics [57]. Disorders of the nervous system observed in alcoholics most commonly involve thiamine deficiency, but may also involve vitamin B_6 and niacin deficiencies. Such deficiencies may result in part from the toxic effects of alcohol or its metabolites on nervous tissue [57].

Fat-Soluble Vitamins Alcohol may damage the intestinal mucosa sufficiently to prevent efficient fat absorption, resulting in poor absorption of fat-soluble vitamins [56]. In addition, liver disorders, common in heavy drinkers, may reduce vitamin A storage in that organ [56]. Night blindness may develop because the enzyme required in the eye to convert retinol to retinal, needed to form rhodopsin (see Chapter 11), is alcohol dehydrogenase (see Chapter 3). Blood alcohol competes with retinol for use of this enzyme in the eye. Furthermore, alcohol dehydrogenase requires zinc as a cofactor, and alcoholics sometimes are deficient in zinc [56]. Liver damage due to alcohol may also prevent utilization of vitamin K for formation of blood-clotting factors [56].

Osteomalacia and other skeletal problems are frequently seen in heavy drinkers. Although poor dietary intake or poor absorption may be underlying causes, the damaged liver may be unable to accomplish the first step in the activation of vitamin D—the formation of 25-OH-vitD [56] (see Chapter 11).

Minerals Heavy drinkers may suffer from low blood potassium levels due to losses through the kidneys, or through vomiting or diarrhea. If severe enough, abnormalities in the heart rhythm result [56]. Liver disease in heavy drinkers often results in edema due to retention of sodium and water [56].

When the intestinal absorptive surface is damaged sufficiently to prevent fat absorption, calcium absorption is impaired because dietary calcium combines with the unabsorbed fats to form insoluble calcium complexes. This may contribute to the bone disorders observed in some heavy drinkers [56]. Magnesium and zinc excretion are increased during periods of drinking; if intakes are also low, deficiencies are apt to develop [57].

Iron overload is a more frequent problem among heavy drinkers than iron deficiency. Stimulation of stomach acid secretion by alcohol increases the conversion of ferric to ferrous iron, increasing iron absorption. Furthermore, the fact that many red wines supply iron, coupled with the propensity for certain pancreatic and liver disorders to increase iron absorption explain iron storage disorders seen in many alcohol abusers [56].

Our present knowledge of the extent to which the toxic effects of alcohol can jeopardize one's vitamin and mineral nutritional status underscores the need for moderate alcohol consumption. Generally, one to two drinks a day is considered to be a moderate intake, except that two drinks might be excessive for individuals of small body size.

SUMMARY

Table 13-2 presents an overview of the trace minerals.

1 Iron is required for hemoglobin formation and hence for supplying cells with oxygen. Iron in plant foods is best absorbed if consumed with either a source of vitamin C or with meats, poultry, or fish.

2 Severe zinc deficiency has been reported in Middle Eastern villages, while marginal deficiency has been observed in some infants and children in the United States. Zinc from animal sources is better absorbed than that from plant sources.

3 Iodine deficiency results in simple goiter. The current dietary intake appears to be relatively high due to use of iodine-containing cleaning compounds and additives in food processing.

4 Chromium appears to be active in the body as glucose tolerance factor (GTF), which potentiates the action of insulin. The extent of chromium deficiency in human beings cannot be determined until techniques for determining chromium in biological materials are improved.

5 Fluoride has proved extremely beneficial in preventing dental caries. Whether or not it may also be useful in preventing or treating osteoporosis is under investigation.

6 Copper is essential for synthesis of hemoglobin; in a deficiency, iron-deficiency anemia develops.

7 Selenium plays a role in defending cell membranes and certain vital compounds such as DNA against oxidative destruction.

8 Despite frequent claims to the contrary, hair analysis alone is a poor way of assessing one's nutritional status regarding minerals.

9 Trace elements are all toxic if consumed in large enough amounts. For many trace elements, however, one is unlikely to obtain toxic amounts from foods.

FOR DISCUSSION AND APPLICATION

1 Calculate from your food record your average daily intake of iron.
   a. What percentage of the RDA did your intake represent?
   b. Suppose an individual's intake amounted to only 50 percent of the RDA. Does this fact alone mean that the person is *deficient* in iron? Explain. How can you find out whether or not you are iron-deficient—or are getting close to becoming iron-deficient?

2 How many students in your nutrition class have consumed fluoridated water since early infancy? What percentage do not know? What percentage have not done so because of having lived in several localities? Has anyone lived in a community in which there was organized opposition to water fluoridation? Find out what the arguments are for and against fluoridation. Which do you think are the stronger arguments? Why?

3 Suppose the latest craze to sweep the campus was trace element supplementation. What arguments would you make for or against supplementing the diet with one or all of the following: selenium, zinc, copper, chromium, manganese, and molybdenum.

4 What would you say to a fellow student who told

you he was planning to spend $500 to find out what his dietary mineral deficiencies were by having a sample of his hair analyzed?

SUGGESTED READINGS

Henderson, D., "Cookware as a Source of Additives," *FDA Consumer*, March 1982, pp. 11–13, A discussion of the possible contamination of foods with copper, lead, or other trace elements when utensils made of unlined copper or improperly formulated ceramic materials are use. Whether or not health problems are apt to develop from routine use of aluminum utensils is also discussed.

Corwin, E., "On Getting the Lead Out of Food," *FDA Consumer*, March 1982, pp. 19–21. What the FDA and the canning industry are doing to cut down on the amount of lead consumers ingest from canned foods.

PART IV

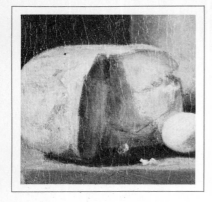

PART IV

NUTRITION
THROUGHOUT
THE LIFE CYCLE

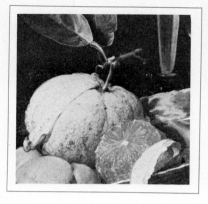

Up to this point we have focused our attention on individual nutrients as they relate to the needs of normal adults from youth through middle life. If we stopped here, however, our study of nutrition would be incomplete. The nurrient needs and how they can be supplied differ in young and middle adulthood from those required by the developing embryo, fetus, infant, child, and adolescent, on the one hand, and by the aging adult, on the other.

Women pregnant for the first time seem suddenly to brim over with questions about diet and nutrition, as you may have noticed when a close relative or friend became pregnant. Some of these questions include: "Does it matter what I eat?" "Is it all right if I continue with cocktails before dinner?" "Does it matter how much I gain during pregnancy?" "What is this I hear about toxemia of pregnancy? And of diabetes in pregnancy?" "Are there any practical guidelines for diet during pregnancy and lactation?" Chapter 14 supplies answers to these and other questions.

Once the baby arrives, parents are faced with new problems of nurturing the infant to foster normal growth and development. Chapter 15 discusses nutritional considerations from infancy through adolescence. Topics examined include breast feeding, preparing infant foods at home, monitoring growth patterns of infants and children, building good food habits in children, diet and hyperactivity, food allergies, and complexion problems in adolescence.

Many Americans remain vigorous into old age. Chapter 16 looks at theories of aging, factors that influence nutritional needs of the elderly, and some special considerations, such as drug–nutrient interactions, since many elderly people receive drugs for various aliments. Lastly, planning adequate diets for older adults is discussed.

These chapters should reinforce the conviction that good nutritional practices throughout life are essential components of one's personal plan for health care.

14 PREGNANCY AND LACTATION

Pregnancy is a time when most women become interested in instruction in nutrition because they want healthy babies. The nutritional status of the mother both before conception and during pregnancy is one of several factors that affect the health of the mother and infant. This chapter describes how the unborn child is nourished, changes that occur in the mother's body during the 40 weeks of normal pregnancy, nutrient requirements during pregnancy, and how nutrition is related to the birth weight of the infant and to certain complications of pregnancy. The importance of nutrition for the lactating mother is emphasized and practical dietary guidelines for pregnancy and lactation are discussed.

THE BABY BEFORE BIRTH

Nourishment

The mother's body normally provides means of nurturing the baby-to-be from the moment of conception, when a sperm penetrates an ovum or egg. Conception usually occurs high up in one of the two fallopian tubes that lead from the ovaries

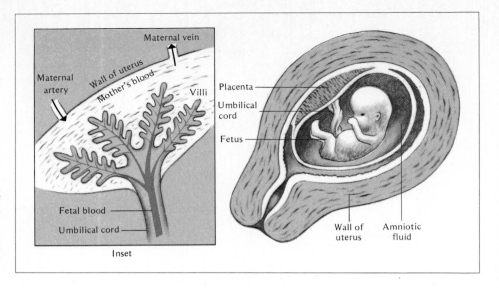

FIGURE 14-1. The uterus at about 10 weeks of pregnancy, showing the fetus in the amniotic sac, and the umbilical cord, placenta, and uterine wall. The inset shows the placenta in greater detail.

to the uterus. Cell division begins immediately upon fertilization. The fertilized ovum travels down the fallopian tube to the uterus over a period of about 4 days. During this time, the ovum obtains from secretions of glands that line the fallopian tubes nutrients needed to support its rapid proliferation of new cells.

Upon conception, the mother's body secretes a hormone, human chorionic gonadotropin (HCG), that prevents shedding of the lining of the uterus, as would occur had she not conceived. Consequently, she will miss her next menstrual period. The fertilized ovum, on about the sixth or seventh day after conception, embeds itself in the swollen lining of the uterus. The process of becoming embedded in the lining of the uterus is called *implantation*. Immediately upon implantation, the rapidly dividing *embryo* (the term applied to the unborn baby during the first 8 weeks of pregnancy) taps into the mother's blood, which is enriched by nutrients held in the swollen uterine lining. The lining furnishes glycogen from which glucose is obtained, protein from which amino acids are obtained, lipids supplying fatty acids, and vitamins, minerals, and water.

The *platenta* begins to form at 9 to 10 days after conception, and becomes capable of supplying the baby-to-be with nourishment after about 10 weeks of gestation (pregnancy). The placenta is attached to the uterine wall and consists of spongy tissue contaiing mother's blood in its spaces. The embryo is connected to the placenta by the umbilical cord, which contains fetal arteries and veins. Fingerlike projections, called villi, carrying fetal blood protrude into the pools of maternal blood in the spaces of the placenta (Figure 14-1). Fetal blood is separated from maternal blood by a thin membrane—normally the two blood sources do not intermingle. Up to about 10 weeks, the embryo obtains nutrients by diffusion from maternal blood, but the placenta has been developing all this time. By the tenth or eleventh week, the placenta takes over the task of nurturing the fetus (Figure 14-1).

After 8 weeks of gestation, the baby-to-be is no longer an embryo, but a *fetus*. During the last weeks of normal pregnancy, after the placenta takes over nurturing the fetus, vitally needed oxygen and nutrients cross from the maternal to fetal blood in the placenta. At the same time, carbon dioxide and other waste products cross from fetal to maternal blood in the placenta and are excreted through the mother's lungs and kidneys. The placenta also synthesizes several hormones that are essential for maintenance of the pregnancy. The placenta must grow normally throughout pregnancy to foster normal growth and development of the fetus.

Differentiation

The ovum at the time of fertilization is about the size of a period on this paper. As soon as the fertilized ovum is implanted in the uterine wall, *differentiation* begins—that is, organs and tissues begin to develop. The fetus is 1 to 1½ in long by the end of the eighth week, and all the basic organ systems and supporting structures such as bone, skin, and muscles have begun to form. Although the fetus could not survive if delivered at this time, the foundations for all body structures have been laid by this early date.

Since all the organs and bodily structures are established during the first 8 weeks, this is the period during which birth defects can occur. Many women do not realize they are pregnant during these early weeks. Obviously, then, it is important that they have good dietary habits *before conception* to increase the likelihood of having healthy babies. Women of childbearing age also should avoid drugs, chemical pollutants, and alcohol that might result in birth defects. Long-established good dietary and health practices will not *guarantee* a normal pregnancy, however, since the process is exceedingly complex, and many factors must operate simultaneously to produce a healthy baby.

Growth

The fetus grows very rapidly during the fourth month, increasing in length from 3 to 4 in to about 8 or 10 in. At the twentieth week or halfway point of the pregnancy, the fetus is about 12 in long (from head to toes) and weighs about 1 lb. The brain and lungs are still too immature to permit survival if the fetus were born at this time. Growth is rapid during the last 3 months. The average gain in weight of the fetus as pregnancy progresses is as follows:

BY END OF	AVERAGE WEIGHT OF FETUS IN POUNDS
Sixth month	2
Seventh month	3½
Eighth month	5
Ninth month (birth)	7½

Fat accumulates underneath the fetal skin during the last 2 months of pregnancy. A baby born prematurely at 7 months, for example, has little body fat, but has developed sufficiently to have a fair chance of surviving if given specialized care. The longer a fetus is carried in the mother's body—up to 40 to 42 weeks—the better its survival chances, in normal circumstances.

It is reasonable to expect that the chances of having a well-nourished fetus are greater if the mother is well nourished at the time of conception, and continues to be well nourished throughout her pregnancy.

CHANGES IN THE MATERNAL BODY

A great many changes, most of them dictated by hormonal secretions, occur in a woman's body as a result of pregnancy. After the first 2 to 3 months, the woman becomes conscious of weight gain. Figure 14-2 indicates that less than half the average weight gain of 24 lb over the course of pregnancy is due to the weight of tissues related to the fetus. More than half the weight gain is due to increases in maternal tissues, including the uterus, mammary glands, blood and other tissue fluids, and maternal stores. Maternal stores consist chiefly of fat, but include some protein.

Changes in the activity of the nervous system, thought to be due to hormonal secretions, often produce morning nausea and vomiting during the first 2 or 3 months. In the last 3 months mothers often notice fatigue and decreased physical coordination. Hormonal secretions also result in relaxation of the smooth muscles of the uterus and gastrointestinal tract. Apparently this change allows the uterus to expand more easily as the pregnancy progresses, but it also results in diminished stimulus in the rectal area. Constipation is therefore a common complaint of pregnancy. In addition, the sphincter muscle between the esophagus and

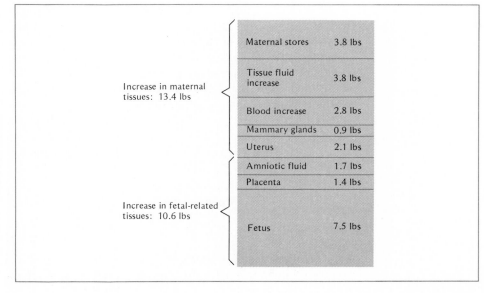

FIGURE 14-2.
Distribution of weight gain among body components during normal pregnancy (40 weeks). Average expected weight gain is 24 lb. (Source of values: Hytten, F. E., and S. Leitch, *The Physiology of Human Pregnancy*, Oxford: Blackwell Scientific Publications, Ltd., 1971, p. 332.)

Maternal stores	3.8 lbs
Tissue fluid increase	3.8 lbs
Blood increase	2.8 lbs
Mammary glands	0.9 lbs
Uterus	2.1 lbs
Amniotic fluid	1.7 lbs
Placenta	1.4 lbs
Fetus	7.5 lbs

Increase in maternal tissues: 13.4 lbs

Increase in fetal-related tissues: 10.6 lbs

stomach relaxes more easily, resulting in a burning sensation called heartburn whenever the acid stomach juice is regurgitated into the esophagus.

Blood volume normally increases by about 50 percent by the end of the first 6 months of pregnancy. Both the blood plasma (the liquid portion of the blood) and the total weight of red blood cells increase, but the plasma increase is proportionately greater than the red cell mass increase. The total ability of the blood to carry oxygen increases as a result of the increase in red cell mass.

By the time a woman is in her thirtieth week of pregnancy, the amount of blood her heart pumps per minute increases by about 30 percent, compared with her pre-pregnancy rate, and her blood vessels dilate. These changes help nurture the fetus by increasing the blood supply from the mother. The mother also gradually increases the volume of air she moves with each inspiration and expiration, enabling her to effectively remove fetal carbon dioxide from her blood. Her kidneys also change in ways that allow them to efficiently excrete waste products put into maternal blood by the fetus.

Many of the changes that occur in the mother's body as a result of pregnancy may affect food intake or may be partially alleviated by certain dietary practices. These are discussed under the section on dietary guidelines.

NUTRITIONAL NEEDS DURING PREGNANCY

Because the mother's body must synthesize rather large amounts of new tissues during pregnancy, the need for energy (kilocalories) and nutrients increases markedly. The extent of the increased need varies with specific nutrients. The Recommended Dietary Allowances for adolescent and adult women during pregnancy and lactation are compared with those of the nonpregnant state in Table 14-1.

Both the fetus and placenta must take from the mother's blood those nutrients that cannot be synthesized in the amounts needed. These include glucose, the chief nutrient the fetus uses for energy, the essential amino acids, the essential fatty acid (linoleic acid), and all the vitamins, minerals, and water required by the human being. The placenta stores some nutrients for fetal use, including glycogen, many water-soluble vitamins, and iron.

The placenta passes some nutrients on to the fetus against a concentration gradient. For example, the levels of amino acids, water-soluble vitamins, and calcium in fetal blood near the time of delivery are higher than in maternal blood. The fat-soluble vitamins tend to be lower in fetal than in maternal blood, however. Perhaps this mechanism protects the fetus, since in general those nutrients that are high in fetal blood tend to be those the mother cannot store (except for calcium). On the other hand, the nutrients that are low in fetal blood tend to be those, such as vitamins A and D, that can be toxic in large amounts.

Energy

The pregnant woman's energy needs generally increase by approximately 15 percent when compared with her nonpregnant needs, but there is little increased

TABLE 14-1. RECOMMENDED DIETARY ALLOWANCES (RDA) FOR NONPREGNANT AND PREGNANT OR LACTATING ADULTS AND ADOLESCENTS

NUTRIENT	NONPREGNANT ADULT (23–40 years), 55 kg (120 lb), 163 cm (64 in)	NONPREGNANT ADOLESCENT (11–14 years), 46 kg (101 lb), 157 cm (62 in)	NONPREGNANT ADOLESCENT (15–18 years), 55 kg (120 lb, 163 cm (64 in)	INCREASE DURING PREGNANCY OVER NONPREG-NANT	INCREASE DURING LACTATION OVER NONPREG-NANT
Calories	2000	2200	2100	+ 300.0	+ 500.0
Protein (g)	44.0	46.0	46.0	+ 30.0	+ 20.0
Vitamin A (μg RE)*	800.0	800.0	800.0	+ 200.0	+ 400.0
Vitamin D (μg)	5.0	10.0	10.0	+ 5.0	+ 5.0
Vitamin E (mg αTE)†	8.0	8.0	8.0	+ 2.0	+ 3.0
Vitamin C (mg)	6.0	50.0	60.0	+ 20.0	+ 40.0
Thiamine (mg)	1.0	1.1	1.1	+ 0.4	+ 0.5
Riboflavin (mg)	1.2	1.3	1.3	+ 0.3	+ 0.5
Niacin (mg NE)‡	13.0	15.0	14.0	+ 2.0	+ 5.0
Vitamin B$_6$ (mg)	2.0	1.8	2.0	+ 0.6	+ 0.5
Folacin (μg)	400.0	400.0	400.0	+ 400.0	+ 100.0
Vitamin B$_{12}$ (μg)	3.0	3.0	3.0	+ 1.0	+ 1.0
Calcium (mg)	800.0	1200.0	1200.0	+ 400.0	+ 400.0
Phosphorus (mg)	800.0	1200.0	1200.0	+ 400.0	+ 400.0
Magnesium (mg)	300.0	300.0	300.0	+ 150.0	+ 150.0
Iron (mg)	18.0	18.0	18.0	+30–60.0	+30–60.0
Zinc (mg)	15.0	15.0	15.0	+ 5.0	+ 10.0
Iodine (μg)	150.0	150.0	150.0	+ 25.0	+ 50.0

*μg RE = μg retinol equivalents.
†mg αTE = mg Alpha tocopherol equivalents.
‡mg NE = mg niacin equivalents.
SOURCE: Food and Nutrition Board, Recommended Dietary Allowances, 9th ed., National Academy of Sciences, Washington, D.C., 1980.

need during the first 2 months. Toward the end of the third month, however, the mother's energy needs increase markedly and remain rather constant thereafter until the baby is born [1]. Physicians divide the 9 months of pregnancy into 3 month segments called *trimesters*. The mother needs extra kilocalories during the second trimester chiefly to support growth of the uterus, mammary glands, and expansion of blood volume. During the last trimester, she uses extra kilocalories chiefly for the growth of the placenta and fetus [2].

A pregnant woman requires sufficient kilocalories to support desirable weight gain. Because the RDAs for kilocalories are set for the *average* person, the figures given in Table 14-1 for energy may be inappropriate for a given individual pregnant woman. Most authorities consider an average gain of 24 to 28 lb (11 to 12 kg) to give the best results from the point of view of the health of the infant [2]. Furthermore, weight gain should occur at a specific rate. Only 1 to 3 lb should be gained in the first trimester, followed by a steady gain of about 0.8 to 0.9 lb (0.35 to 0.40 kg) per week thereafter until delivery (Figure 14-3). For optimal care, a pregnant woman's weight gain should be routinely plotted on the grid shown in Figure 14-3 to compare with gain that is considered normal. Preferably, she should plot her own gain so that she is fully aware of her progress. Some women

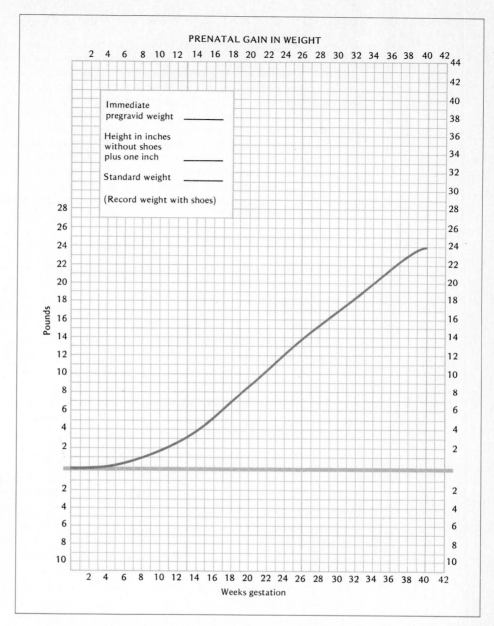

PRENATAL GAIN IN WEIGHT

Immediate
pregravid weight _____

Height in inches
without shoes
plus one inch _____

Standard weight _____

(Record weight with shoes)

Pounds

Weeks gestation

FIGURE 14-3. Pattern of
normal weight gain
during pregnancy.
(Source: Committee on
Maternal Nutrition, Food
and Nutrition Board,
National Research
Council, Maternal
Nutrition and the Course
of Pregnancy.
Washington, D.C., 1970,
p. 175.)

become less physically active toward the end of pregnancy, which may result in
their needing fewer kilocalories than if they had continued to be active.

Protein

Because both maternal and fetal tissues must synthesize large amounts of protein
during pregnancy, a generous daily allowance of 30 g plus 0.8 g/kg pregnant

A CLOSER LOOK

Pregnant adolescents who have yet to attain adult size should gain on the average 24 lb plus the amount they would have gained had they not been pregnant. Women who are underweight by 10 percent or more at conception should gain more weight during pregnancy than the average woman. Women with twins are also expected to gain more weight than the average.

Overweight women should never lose weight during pregnancy, but instead should gain 20 to 24 lb. Either failure to gain weight or actual weight loss may damage the fetal brain due to the state of ketosis (see Chapter 4) that develops under these circumstances in the maternal body. Since ketosis develops with unusual ease in pregnancy, merely skipping breakfast in the morning after an overnight fast can induce it. The pregnant woman can detect ketosis by testing her urine for ketones. Women needing to lose weight should do so *between* and not *during* pregnancies.

body weight has been set [2]. For the adult woman referred to in Table 14-1, the allowance during pregnancy is 44 g + 30 g = 74 g/day. This is not an unusually large intake, since many Americans routinely consume more than 100 g per day. Pregnant adolescents should receive 0.9 g/kg for ages 15 to 18, or 1.0 g/kg for ages 11 to 14, plus an additional 30 g.

Allowances set for protein assume that the kilocalorie intake will be sufficient to maintain desirable weight gain during pregnancy. As noted in Chapter 6, insufficient caloric intake causes the body to use dietary protein for energy, preventing its use for synthesizing new protein tissues.

The pregnant woman may obtain protein from plant or animal foods, or from a combination of these. Vegetarians should follow the guidelines in Chapter 6 for complementing protein foods.

Nutrients Needed for Blood Formation

Pregnancy results in stress on the blood-forming system due to the need to increase maternal blood volume and the demands of both the placenta and fetus for blood-forming nutrients. The two nutrients involved in blood formation that may be low in the diet during pregnancy are iron and folacin.

Iron   The RDA for iron (Table 14-1) assumes that the needs are too great during pregnancy to be met by dietary intake, and supplements of 30 to 60 mg of ferrous iron daily are recommended. Most women enter pregnancy with relatively low stores of iron in their bodies (300 mg or less), while the extra iron need imposed by pregnancy amounts to 500 mg for maternal blood expansion plus an additional 300 mg for the fetus and placenta. The usual American diet can be expected to supply only enough iron to allow absorption of 1 to 2 mg/day, while the pregnant woman needs to absorb 3 mg/day. To prevent the pregnant woman from exhausting her iron stores, and to prevent iron-deficiency anemia during pregnancy, the Food and Nutrition Board recommends iron supplementation in the form of ferrous sulfate, fumarate, or gluconate for all pregnant women.

Some investigators disagree that *all* pregnant women should be given iron supplements, regardless of their iron nutritional status. These scientists argue that supplementation should be given only after iron-deficiency anemia has been diagnosed. Iron supplements often cause constipation and abdominal discomfort, and have been shown to result in unusually enlarged red blood cells in some normal pregnant woman [3]. The RDA of 30 to 60 mg of supplemental iron is designed to *prevent* anemia. Once iron-deficiency anemia actually develops, doses higher than 30 to 60 mg are required to alleviate it.

Iron-deficiency anemia in pregnancy is diagnosed by a hemoglobin concentration of 10 g/100 mL of blood or less, a hematocrit of 30 percent or less, and serum iron levels below 50 to 60 μg/100 mL. In addition, microscopic examination of the blood reveals unusually small (microcytic) and pale-colored (hypochromic) red blood cells. A pregnant woman who has anemia must pump more blood to nourish the fetus, resulting in greater stress on her heart. She also resists infections less well than a nonanemic woman, and is prone to greater danger if hemorrhaging develops. The fetus tends to obtain whatever iron it needs, and if born at term is unlikely to be iron-deficient. However, studies of women who, during pregnancy, had moderate to severe iron-deficiency indicated there were higher occurrences than among normal women of low birth weight babies, babies who were born dead, or who died soon after birth [4].

It is important to realize that *high* hemoglobin and hematocrit values are not beneficial, and may be associated with impaired ability to expand blood volume [5].

Folacin Folacin requirements are elevated during pregnancy, not only for synthesis of maternal and fetal blood cells, but also to supply the rather large amounts needed to synthesize new tissues in the placenta and fetus. The RDA during pregnancy is double that of the nonpregnant state (Table 14-1). Since folacin is easily destroyed in cooking and storage, many women may subsist on relatively low intakes of this vitamin. Low blood levels of folacin were noted in 64 percent of a group of low-income pregnant women in New York, and 16 percent had low levels in red blood cells, taken to indicate that their tissue levels were also low [6]. Generally, only a small number of pregnant women in the United States show the macrocytic anemia of folacin deficiency, however. Whether or not low serum folacin levels are a reason for concern in pregnancy is unknown at present, since there is some evidence that the action of hormones secreted in pregnancy may lower blood folacin levels. Nevertheless, folacin deficiency occurs more commonly in pregnant women than in any other group. The Food and Nutrition Board therefore recommends that supplements be given to pregnant women to ensure they obtain the 800 μg/day recommended [2]. If the dietary intake is good, a supplement of only 200 to 400 μg/day may be prescribed.

Nutrients Needed for Bone Formation

The needs for calcium, phosphorus, and vitamin D increase in pregnancy because of bone formation in the fetus. The normal fetus accumulates approximately 30 g (30,000 mg) of calcium in its bones by the end of normal gestation. Calcification of fetal bones begins in the last trimester of pregnancy, but it is recommended that calcium intake be increased from the onset of pregnancy. The extra allowance is set at +400 mg/day for a total of 1200 mg for adult and 1600 mg for adolescent pregnancy (Table 14-1).

The allowance for phosphorus is the same as for calcium, since these two minerals are deposited together in bones. In addition, a calcium-to-phosphorus ratio of 1:1 is thought to be optimal during adolescence and adulthood. Vitamin D is needed for absorption of calcium and deposition of calcium and phosphorus in bones; therefore the RDA for vitamin D is increased during pregnancy by 5 μg/day (Table 14-1).

Some pregnant women experience painful spasms of the muscles in the calf of the leg, thought to be caused by decreasing blood calcium levels resulting from rising blood phosphorus levels. In the past, this condition has sometimes been treated by removing milk from the diet because of its high phosphorus content [7]. Other studies have failed to support the usefulness of removing or decreasing milk consumption, however [8]. More recently, the suggestion has been made that foods high in phosphate additives but low in calcium, such as soft drinks, snack items, and many processed foods such as processed cheese, be restricted, and that aluminum hydroxide gels, which prevent absorption of phosphorus, be given. Because milk is such a highly nutritious food, it seems unreasonable to restrict milk consumption in pregnant women unless absolutely necessary.

Other Minerals

Zinc has special significance in pregnancy because it is involved in DNA synthesis, and because, in experimental animals, zinc deficiency in early pregnancy results in fetal malformations. The recommendation of 20 mg during pregnancy takes into account that zinc may be poorly absorbed from some types of diets, and provides a large margin of safety [2]. It is doubtful, however, that most pregnant women consume this amount, since recent studies indicate that diets consumed by educated middle-class nonpregnant adults that were adequate in kilocalories and protein contained, on the average, only 8.6 mg of zinc [9]. Studies are needed to establish whether or not the zinc RDA for pregnancy is unrealistically high.

Iodine needs increase during pregnancy because the maternal rate of metabolism increases as pregnancy progresses, and because the fetus also requires iodine. Iodine deficiency in a mother who has goiter can produce cretinism in the infant, as described in Chapter 13. The usual American diet is likely to supply all the iodine needed without using iodized salt, however (see Chapter 13).

Sodium is required for normal growth of the fetus and normal expansion of maternal blood and tissue fluids. About 18,000 mg of sodium must be retained in the mother's body to achieve this increase in body fluids. Normal pregnant women should consume at least 2 to 3 g (2000 to 3000 mg) of sodium per day, which is equivalent to 5 to 7.5 g of salt. This level of intake is advisable even for women who before pregnancy became accustomed to lower intakes. Generally, the American diet tends to be considerably higher in sodium than this, so there is no difficulty in obtaining this amount.

Vitamins

Table 14-1 indicates that recommendations for all vitamins increase in pregnancy. In experimental animals, deficiency early in pregnancy of vitamins A, D, or E, and of riboflavin, folacin, or vitamin B_{12}, have resulted in birth defects. Whether or not human diets are ever as deficient as those used in these studies is unknown, so the extent to which deficiencies of any of these vitamins cause birth defects in humans is uncertain.

Excessive intakes of certain vitamins may also result in malformed young. Recently a case was reported of a mother who consumed 150,000 IU of vitamin A daily early in her pregnancy. Her baby was born with several serious defects of the nervous system [10]. Although cause and effect is not certain in this case, it is possible that the excessive vitamin A caused the defects.

Excessive intakes of some of the water-soluble vitamins by the mother during pregnancy may have detrimental effects on the fetus. One investigator reported scurvy in two infants whose mothers had consumed large amounts of vitamin C during pregnancy [11]. Presumably the infants became conditioned to a large intake during fetal life, but developed deficiency on the much lower intake after birth, an amount that would be adequate for normal infants. Although many questions can be raised about the thoroughness of this study, nevertheless it seems sensible to avoid unusually high intakes of any nutrient during pregnancy.

The need for vitamin B_6 in pregnancy merits some special discussion. Much research in recent years has attempted to solve a mystery concerning vitamin B_6 needs in pregnancy. The problem is that in apparently normal pregnant women certain biochemical changes in vitamin B_6 metabolism occur that in nonpregnant persons indicate deficiency. Is it possible that the human race has survived in spite of vitamin B_6 deficiency during pregnancy? At present, many authorities tend to believe that this is not the case, since routine B_6 supplementation during pregnancy fails to improve the health of mothers and babies, as should occur if the women had been B_6-deficient before supplementation [12]. It may be that the immense hormonal changes that occur in the maternal body during pregnancy are responsible for modifications observed in vitamin B_6 metabolism, modifications that perhaps are normal in pregnancy.

Some attention to vitamin B_6 intake may be appropriate for women who, prior to conception, have used oral contraceptive agents (OCA) for periods longer than 30 months. These women may have lower-than-normal amounts of vitamin B_6 in their bodies and may therefore require higher amounts in their diets during pregnancy than women who have never used OCA [13].

At present the RDA for vitamin B_6 in pregnancy is only 0.6 mg greater than in the nonpregnant state. Many pregnant women may consume low amounts of vitamin B_6 since the best sources are whole grains, wheat germ and bran, nuts, seeds, legumes, and some meats and fish.

Obviously, pregnant women need to avoid excessive intakes of vitamins, but should consume sufficient amounts for normal growth and development of maternal and fetal tissue. The RDAs for vitamins during pregnancy constitute a logical guideline to follow. Some physicians automatically prescribe prenatal vitamins without inquiring into the mother's dietary habits. If a vitamin prepara-

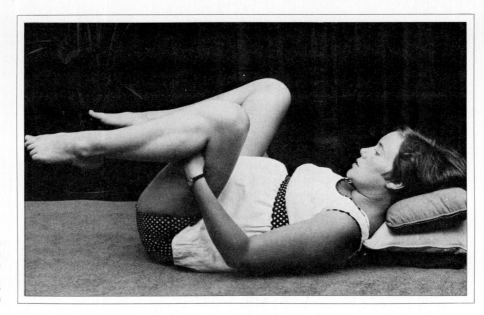

Exercise is just as
important for the
pregnant as for the
nonpregnant woman.
*(Erika Stone
Peter Arnold, Inc.)*

tion is used by the normal pregnant woman, the amounts per tablet should not exceed the RDAs. Normal pregnant women who conscientiously consume adequate diets need not take prenatal vitamins.

NUTRITION AND COMPLICATIONS OF PREGNANCY

Several conditions of pregnancy appear to be related to nutrition, but in most cases it is impossible to point to nutritional status as the only causative factor. Genetic factors, infections, exposure to drugs or other chemical hazards, and economic and social conditions are often intertwined with nutritional factors, making it very difficult to designate nutrition as the culprit.

Low Birth Weight

Birth weight is one of the most important indicators of whether or not a new-born baby can be expected to grow and develop normally, without complications. Unusually small babies are at much higher risk than normal-weight babies for early death or complications such as mental retardation, visual and hearing problems, and behavioral and learning problems. The medical profession in this country designates a low birth weight (LBW) infant as one who weighs 2500 g (5½ lb) or less at birth. These babies are divided into two groups:

1. Premature (or preterm) infants: those born before the 37th week of gestation
2. Small-for-date or small-for-gestational-age infants: those born at 40 weeks of gestation who weigh less than 2500 g or those born earlier than 40 weeks who weigh less than appropriate for age

Premature infants may be the proper weight for their gestational age or they may be growth-retarded. Small-for-date babies are all growth-retarded, however. Growth retardation may be the result of poor dietary habits, or conditions in the mother or placenta that prevent sufficient nutrients from reaching the fetus, resulting in malnourishment of the fetus. Based on studies in animals, Rosso postulates that the fetus suffers growth retardation whenever the placenta fails to grow normally, or when blood flow through the placenta is reduced [14]. Maternal malnutrition contributes to both of these conditions, not only by supplying an inadequate quantity of nutrients, but also by preventing the normal expansion of the blood volume. As a consequence, the normal increase in cardiac output fails to occur. The fetus, as a result, is deprived of sufficient nutrients to allow normal growth (Figure 14-4). Every effort should be made to prevent fetal growth retardation because of the increased danger for the infant of illness, disability, or early death. Special facilities required for mentally retarded children or those with behavioral or learning problems are very costly to society and parents, in terms of both money and emotional trauma.

It is clear from statistics kept by public health agencies that the chances of having an infant of low birth weight are greatest if the mother:

1. Fails to gain the recommended amount of weight during pregnancy
2. Was markedly underweight at conception and fails to gain as recommended during pregnancy
3. Smokes cigarettes or drinks alcohol during pregnancy
4. Has her first baby before age 17 or after age 35
5. Has a history of previous fetal or infant death
6. Is from a low socioeconomic group, which usually means a low level of education, poor medical care, and poor nutrition throughout the mother's life

FIGURE 14-4. Postulated mechanisms of placental and fetal growth retardation caused by maternal malnutrition. (Source: Rosso, P., "Nutrition and Maternal-Fetal Exchange," *American Journal of Clinical Nutrition*, 34:744, 1981.)

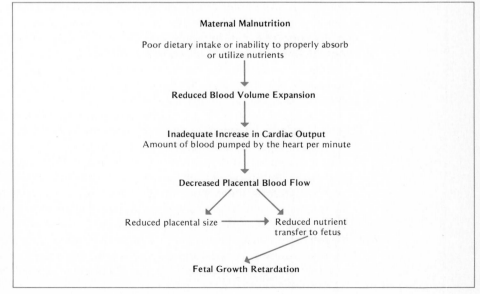

Women who are genetically small are apt to produce small babies (although not necessarily under 5½ lb at birth), while taller, heavier women tend to produce larger babies. A recent study indicated that maternal genetic factors are responsible for 25 percent of the variance in birth weight, while the father's genetic contribution accounts for only 1 to 2 percent of the variance in birth weight [15].

Two of the most important factors related to the birth weight of an infant are the height and weight of the mother at conception, and the amount of weight the mother gains during pregnancy. A singular responsibility of health professionals working with pregnant women is to convince them of the importance of gaining the recommended amount of weight at the proper rate in order to increase their chances of having a normal-weight baby. In the face of the societal norm for slenderness in women, this is sometimes a difficult task. Adolescent pregnant girls offer a special challenge since they are often rebellious about conforming to adult suggestions concerning food, and may lack the maturity and realism needed to accept responsibility for properly nurturing the baby.

Preeclampsia–Eclampsia (Toxemia of Pregnancy)

This disorder occurs only in pregnancy—a sure way to cause all symptoms to disappear is to terminate the pregnancy. The old term "toxemia of pregnancy" is misleading in that no toxin exists in the blood as the word "toxemia" implies. The disease, which occurs in the last 20 weeks of pregnancy, is divided into two stages. The first, *preeclampsia*, is characterized by sudden high blood pressure, protein in the urine, and edema or excessive fluid accumulation in the tissues. More specifically, the blood pressure is considered high if the systolic pressure (upper reading) increases over the individual's normal reading by 20 to 30 mmHg, and/or if the diastolic pressure (lower reading) increases by 10 to 15 mmHg.

Edema of the lower legs is a normal occurrence during the later stages of pregnancy, and diminishes when the woman lies down for a period of time. The edema of preeclampsia, on the other hand, is over many parts of the body and occurs suddenly, causing rapid weight gain. Because rapid weight gain is one warning of edema—and consequently of preeclampsia—a good health care plan in pregnancy provides for routine checking of weight gain during the last half of pregnancy. Symptoms of the second stage of the disease, called *eclampsia*, consist of convulsions and coma. Death can result.

Preeclampsia and eclampsia occur most frequently in first pregnancies, in teenage pregnant women, in women having multiple fetuses, in diabetic women, in women who already have high blood pressure or kidney disease when pregnancy begins, and in women from lower socioeconomic groups. Although the cause of this disorder is unknown, the most widely accepted theory is that, for unknown reasons, there is poor blood flow through the wall of the uterus and the placental-fetal unit. The insufficiency of blood alters the mechanisms controlling sodium and water balance, and edema results. At the same time, substances are released that cause constriction of blood vessels in the uterus, placenta, and kidneys, resulting in hypertension and leaking of protein into the urine.

Because preeclampsia occurs more frequently in women in low rather than high socioeconomic groups, the possibility that poor nutrition may be involved in the onset of the disorder has long been postulated. Various studies have suggested that low intakes of kilocalories, protein, vitamin B$_6$, vitamin C, or calcium, or high intakes of sodium may play a role in development of the disease. To date, however, none of these has been established to be the cause.

Experts point out that advising normal pregnant women to *restrict* sodium intake and use diuretics (to cause water excretion) in an effort to *prevent* preeclampsia is completely outdated and probably dangerous. Sodium is necessary for normal expansion of body fluids in pregnancy, as noted earlier. Hormonal changes in the mother's body during pregnancy result in greater excretion of sodium through the kidneys than occurs in nonpregnant women. This situation triggers a second hormonal system (the renin-angiotensin-aldosterone system) which results in significant reabsorption of sodium by the kidneys, allowing fluid volume expansion to occur normally. *Restricting dietary sodium may so tax this hormonal system that it fails,* resulting in low blood sodium levels and inability to expand fluid volume.

Good medical care throughout pregnancy, including an adequate diet as described below, significantly decreases the number of cases of preeclampsia. This is not to say that the disorder never occurs among women receiving excellent medical care who are conscientious about diet, but the number of such cases is relatively small.

Gestational Diabetes

Diabetes which develops during pregnancy, but subsides at termination of pregnancy, is called *gestational diabetes*. About 20 to 30 percent of these women become diabetic sometime after pregnancy, however. In pregnancy, intricate hormonal changes occur, some of which antagonize the action of the insulin. The normal pregnant woman overcomes this antagonism simply by secreting more insulin, but a woman who is genetically prone to develop diabetes may be unable to secrete sufficient insulin. She then will show abnormal glucose tolerance and has gestational diabetes.

Glucose tolerance is determined by observing the individual's blood glucose level while fasting and at intervals after taking an oral dose of glucose. Diabetic individuals tend to show unusually high levels for several hours after the glucose dose, while levels in normal individuals peak within 1 hour and return to fasting levels at 2 hours. Testing for gestational diabetes should take place early in pregnancy and again at about 26 weeks when hormones antagonistic to insulin are at high levels in the body.

Among normal pregnant women, a certain percentage excrete glucose in the urine (which also occurs in untreated diabetes). Since untreated diabetes in pregnancy constitutes a danger to both the mother and fetus, every effort should be made to diagnose gestational diabetes. Women at risk for gestational diabetes include those who (1) excrete glucose in the urine; (2) have a history of diabetes in the family; (3) have had a baby weighing 9 lb or more at birth; (4) have had previous stillbirths, spontaneous abortions, or infants with birth defects; or (5) are excessively obese.

If the abnormal glucose tolerance is mild, the woman with gestational diabetes will require no extra insulin. Depending upon the characteristics of her particular case, she may be treated, however, in the same way as women who are known to have diabetes when they become pregnant. Such methods of treatment are beyond the scope of this book, but the important point is that gestational diabetes should be detected and effectively monitored and treated.

Fetal Alcohol Syndrome

Fetal alcohol syndrome (FAS) is the name given to a pattern of birth defects in infants of mothers with chronic severe alcoholism. These infants are at high risk for early death, and survivors have a high incidence of mental retardation. They tend to be retarded also in height, weight, and head size; and fail to experience catch-up growth in later years. Eye and heart defects occur frequently, as do abnormalities of facial development. These children also may be more prone to infection than normal children [16].

The critical time for fetal birth defects to develop is during the first few weeks of pregnancy—a period during which many women are unaware they are pregnant. The chances of abnormalities developing in the infant appear to be small if the average daily intake is less than 1 oz of absolute alcohol, but increase as the intake increases [17]. Heavy alcohol consumption during pregnancy greatly increases the risk of low infant birth weight. One study compared the birth weights of infants of three groups of mothers: those who had never consumed alcohol, those who drank heavily before but not during pregnancy and those who drank heavily both before and during pregnancy. Birth weight was significantly lower in those who drank heavily throughout pregnancy. Infants of those women who drank heavily before but not during pregnancy weighed significantly less than those of women who never drank alcohol [18]. The safest strategy is to avoid alcohol prior to starting and during pregnancy.

Whether or not the damage observed in FAS is due to alcohol itself or a nutrient deficiency brought about by displacement of food with alcohol is uncertain. In animals, the severity of defects increases with increasing maternal blood alcohol levels [19]. However, maternal malnutrition could have been one factor influencing the lower birth weight in women who had been heavy drinkers before pregnancy but abstained during pregnancy, as mentioned earlier [18]. Further research should clarify this question.

DIETARY GUIDELINES

For Dietary Cravings and Aversions

Everyone is familiar with stories of the long-suffering husband who must go out in the middle of the night to find some ridiculous combination of foods—such as pickles and ice cream—to satisfy a sudden craving his pregnant wife has developed. Cravings are not universally experienced by pregnant women, but are frequently reported. A recent study pointed out that pregnant women crave only

NUTRITION IN THE NEWS

ALCOHOL IN PREGNANCY FOUND TO CUT OFF OXYGEN TO FETUS

C. Russell, *The Washington Post,* Nov. 5, 1982

Government scientists are reporting today that moderate to heavy alcohol consumption during pregnancy can cut off oxygen temporarily to the developing fetus, possibly leading to brain damage.

Although the study was conducted on monkeys, "We suspect that moderate or heavy drinking by pregnant women may have a similar effect on human fetuses," said Dr. Anil B. Mukherjee of the National Institute of Child Health and Human Development. . . .

The scientists conducted their research on monkeys far along in their pregnancies. They were given alcohol until it reached a level in their blood equivalent to that found in humans after a woman had consumed three to five drinks.

Mukherjee and Dr. Gary D. Hodgen, . . . recommend that women "consider total abstinence" from alcohol throughout pregnancy. . . .

In the new study, the federal researchers looked at the effects of alcohol in the mother's bloodstream on the function of the umbilical cord, which connects the placenta and the fetus. It delivers oxygen and nutrients from the mother and carries away waste products.

They found, to their surprise, that soon after the five pregnant monkeys in the experiment received injections of an alcohol solution, all of the blood vessels in their umbilical cords collapsed.

The doctors said that the "striking interrup-

tion" in blood flow had a "markedly adverse" effect on the fetuses, who all developed severe oxygen deficiency and dangerously abnormal blood acidity.

This gradually improved as the umbilical cord function returned. But severe fetal oxygen deprivation "may lead to irreversible brain damage," concluded the National Institutes of Health scientists. They noted that a single brief deprivation "may or may not have discernible consequences."

Adverse effects were not observed in the mothers or in the fetuses of monkeys who received a nonhazardous sugar or salt solution or no injection at all. . . .

They found about one-third of the maternal alcohol level in the fetuses, but the alcohol and its byproducts persisted far longer in the developing babies.

"These monkeys are the closest thing you can come to humans. But this kind of experiment could not be done in humans," said Mukherjee. To answer the unsolved questions, he hopes to follow up with experiments involving lower amounts of alcohol that would be orally ingested. . . .

While much of the concern has been directed at the early stages of pregnancy, when the major organs are developing, the new study suggests that the fetus remains at risk even during late pregnancy.

ASK YOURSELF:

Why might researchers decide to inject alcohol into the test animals rather than have them drink it? Why are scientists more apt to think that results found in monkeys are more applicable to human beings than those found in rats or other animals? Is it legitimate to conclude that a woman who has had one bout of heavy drinking during her pregnancy has damaged her baby? What advice would you give a woman who worries that such an incident has damaged her baby?

those foods or substances they are already familiar with. The most commonly reported foods craved were fruit, milk or other dairy products, and sweet foods [20].

Pica   *Pica* is a craving, sometimes developing during pregnancy, for non-food items such as raw starch, dirt, clay, plaster, air-freshener blocks, ground-up bricks, or blocks of magnesia. A special form of pica is the compulsive consumption of ice or refrigerator frost. Generally, pica occurs in certain cultural groups—in other words, the pregnant woman rarely craves one of these substances unless she has observed the practice in someone else.

Pica has been reported to occur in 25 percent of pregnant women diagnosed as having iron-deficiency anemia [21]. For some time, the assumption was that the practice of pica prevented absorption of iron and therefore resulted in anemia. Craving for these substances has been shown to disappear with iron therapy, however [22]. Furthermore, compulsive ice-eating, which probably has no influence on the absorption of iron, has been reported to disappear with iron therapy [23]. It may be, then, that iron deficiency affects the appetite centers in the brain in some fashion, or causes deficiency of enzymes in the lining of the mouth, bringing about these unusual cravings [23]. The craved substances do not provide the body with iron, however, and do not solve the problem. On the contrary, they can displace needed food from the diet, and compromise the mother's nutritional condition. All pregnant women with iron deficiency should be questioned to determine whether or not they practice pica. At the same time, women known to practice pica should be examined for iron-deficiency anemia.

There is no evidence for the common superstition that cravings for "pickles and ice cream"'' and other such combinations must be indulged, else the fetus will be damaged. If the pregnancy is progressing normally with no signs of iron-deficiency anemia, no significance should be attached to desires for specific foods.

Aversions   It is not uncommon for pregnant women to experience aversions to coffee, meats, fried foods, and foods flavored with oregano [20]. The cause is unknown, but so many hormonal changes occur during pregnancy that it is not surprising that the senses of taste and smell and other mechanisms affecting the desire for food are affected. Fortunately, a nutritionally adequate diet can be planned by omitting all these foods, if necessary.

For Discomforts

Nausea and Vomiting of Early Pregnancy   Hormonal changes in the mother's body probably are the chief cause of nausea and vomiting—or "morning sickness"—common to early pregnancy. Usually, this disorder is mild and does not last long. Consuming some kind of dry food, such as crackers, dry cereal, or melba toast before getting out of bed in the morning helps many women. Eating small, more frequent meals, and confining liquid intake to between-meal periods is also effective. If severe and prolonged vomiting occurs, medical treatment is required.

Constipation and Hemorrhoids   Constipation, as noted earlier, is related to the relaxation of the muscles of the gastrointestinal tract during pregnancy. Hemorrhoids, or enlarged veins in the anus, also may cause discomfort, especially in the latter part of pregnancy when the fetus is growing rapidly, resulting in pressure in the lower back area. Alleviating or preventing constipation can help to prevent discomfort from hemorrhoids. Routine consumption of whole-grain breads and cereals, bran, fresh fruits, and dried prunes and figs together with plenty of fluids should aid in preventing constipation. Laxatives should be used only in unusual conditions, and always under a physician's guidance.

Heartburn   Regurgitation of acid stomach contents into the lower esophagus results in the burning sensation called heartburn. This disorder tends to become more bothersome as the fetus enlarges in the latter part of pregnancy. Dividing the food into several small meals and avoiding specific foods—often highly seasoned ones—if found to cause heartburn, can help diminish discomfort. Eating slowly and under relaxed circumstances can also help.

Dietary Planning

The kind of diet advocated by nutritionists for pregnant and lactating women is like that for nonpregnant women in that it provides sufficient but not excessive kilocalories, includes a wide variety of foods, and avoids excessively high intakes of any one food component.

The kilocalorie intake during pregnancy should allow for the amount and rate of weight gain discussed earlier. Nutritionists tend to calculate the kilocalorie need for an individual pregnant woman by allowing 40 kcal/kg of pregnant weight (18 kcal/lb). Kilocalorie intakes of less than 36 kcal/kg (16 kcal/lb) in pregnancy have been shown to prevent utilization of protein for protein synthesis, and should be avoided [24]. Furthermore, sufficient carbohydrate should be consumed to prevent ketosis; therefore, a minimum of 5 g of carbohydrate/100 kcal of the diet is recommended. Most diets will contain more carbohydrate than this, however, and a great deal more if one is choosing a wide variety of foods. The major portion of the carbohydrate should come from starchy foods rather than from those high in sugar.

A food guide for diet during pregnancy and lactation designed to meet the Recommended Dietary Allowances appears in Table 14-2. The following features of this guide should be noted.

1. For economic reasons, the serving size for animal protein foods is small: 2 oz.
2. Two servings of protein foods of plant origin are recommended daily, one of which should be legumes. One cup of legumes contains more vitamin B$_6$, folacin, iron, magnesium, and zinc than is found in a 2-oz serving of animal protein or in ½ c of nuts. If economy is no barrier, and an individual is reluctant to consume plant protein foods, two 3-oz servings of red meat may be consumed and only one serving of plant protein food.
3. Whole-grain breads and cereals should be chosen over white or enriched white. Whole-grain products, in addition to their dietary fiber, supply more

TABLE 14-2. **FOOD GUIDE FOR PREGNANCY AND LACTATION**

| FOOD GROUPS | SERVING SIZE | NO. OF SERVINGS PER DAY | |
		PREGNANCY	LACTATION
Protein Foods			
Animal	Meats, poultry, fish, 2 oz Eggs, 1	2	2
Plant	Legumes, 1 c cooked Nut butters, ¼ c Nuts, ½ c	1	1
	Seeds, ½ c Tofu (soybean curd), 1c	1	1
Milk, cheese, etc.	Milk, 1 c; cheddar cheese, 1½ oz; cottage cheese, 1⅓ c; yogurt, 1 c; tofu (soybean curd) 1 c	4	5
Breads and cereals (whole-grain preferable)	Bread, 1 slice or piece; rice, ½ c; pasta (spaghetti, etc., ½ c); cooked cereal, ½ c; Ready-to-eat cereal, ¾ c; wheat germ, 1 tbsp; crackers, 4	4	4
Vitamin C-rich fruits and vegetables	4 oz orange juice; 12 oz tomato juice; ½ grapefruit or cantaloupe; ¾ c strawberries; ¾ c cooked greens; ½ raw green pepper; 1 stalk broccoli	1	1
Dark green vegetables	1 c raw or ¾ c cooked: broccoli, spinach, collards, turnip or mustard greens, kale, dark green lettuce such as romaine	1	1
Other fruits and vegetables (including yellow ones high in vitamin A)	½ c carrots, yams, squash, eggplant, corn, cucumber, zucchini, etc. 1 piece fresh fruit or ½ c frozen or canned	1	1
Fats and oils	1 tbsp oil (not palm or coconut oil), margarine, mayonnaise, or salad dressing	2	2

SOURCE: *Nutrition During Pregnancy and Lactation,* Maternal and Child Health Branch, California Department of Health, 1977.

zinc, magnesium, vitamin B_6, pantothenic acid, and folacin than enriched white breads and cereals.

4. Two tablespoons of fats and oils are recommended each day to supply linoleic acid and vitamin E.
5. Dark green vegetables, in addition to supplying vitamin A, are good sources of vitamin B_6, iron, and magnesium, and, if leafy, also supply vitamin E, vitamin C, folacin, and riboflavin.

The foods listed in this food guide do not supply sufficient kilocalories for the weight gain recommended in pregnancy. Additional foods may be chosen from some of the same groups, preferably vegetables, fruits, or bread and cereals. Generally, most foods in the diet should be high-nutrient-density foods—high in nutrients relative to the number of kilocalories in the food.

Women who are strict (total) vegetarians should consult a knowledgeable dietitian or nutritionist to be certain their diet meets the RDA for all nutrients with emphasis on calcium, riboflavin, vitamin B_{12}, and vitamin D. In addition, a source of vitamin C should be consumed in each meal to increase the absorption of iron from plant foods.

Instruction in sound dietary practices should be a routine part of medical care during pregnancy. Too frequently, attention is paid only to the weight gain during pregnancy, and not to other aspects of nutrition. The food record is a good tool to use in helping the mother evaluate her diet. When using this tool, the health professional instructs the mother in details of how to record her food and beverage intake for a 1-week period. The professional then helps the mother analyze her food record, pointing out the strengths and weaknesses of her present diet. Together they agree upon what foods or groups of foods need to be added, deleted, or modified in amounts. Since the mother's dietary habits frequently serve as a model for other family members, any improvement in her diet is apt to have a positive influence over that of others.

NUTRITIONAL NEEDS DURING LACTATION

During lactation, the diet should furnish energy and nutrients needed for the production of milk, but also should protect the mother's body reserve of nutrients.

Energy

Energy needs during lactation depend on the amount of milk produced, which varies as lactation progresses and differs from woman to woman. The production of 1 L of human milk requires about 900 kcal. During the first 3 months of lactation, body fat stored during pregnancy can be counted on to supply some of the energy needed for milk production. If body fat provides about one-third of the kilocalories needed for milk production, an extra 500 kcal/day will be required in the diet during the first 3 months of lactation. This is the basis on which the RDA for energy is calculated for the lactating woman. Lactation appears to be nature's

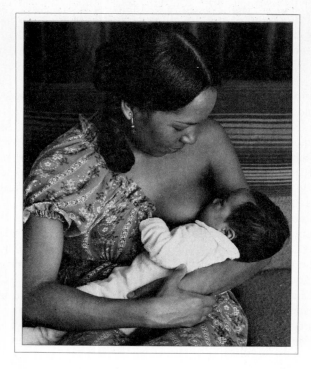

Consuming a nutritious diet during lactation prevents depletion of the mother's body stores and maintains the quantity and quality of milk her infant needs. *(Erika Stone/Peter Arnold, Inc.)*

way of using up body fat stores that accumulate during pregnancy. Many lactating women observe that, for the first time in their lives, they can eat all they want without fear of gaining weight, while others find they still need to be careful about quantities of food eaten to prevent undesirable weight gain.

The lactating mother should be content to lose body fat accumulated during pregnancy gradually because moderate to severe kilocalorie restriction can diminish the amount of milk produced. For many women who continue lactation beyond 3 months, the kilocalorie intake will need to be increased to prevent weight from falling below desirable levels.

Protein and Other Nutrients

The protein RDA is somewhat lower during lactation than in pregnancy—that is, 20 g of protein in addition to the nonpregnant allowance of 0.8 g/kg body weight. Table 14-1 indicates that the RDAs for many vitamins and for zinc and iodine are somewhat higher during lactation than during pregnancy.

The amounts of many, but not all, water-soluble vitamins in human milk are directly related to the levels in the mother's blood. For example, cases of deficiency of thiamine, vitamin B_6, and vitamin B_{12} have all been reported in breast-fed infants of mothers poorly nourished in these nutrients. Vitamin C levels in milk also depend to some extent upon the mother's intake. On the other hand, folacin levels in milk remain at normal levels for a long time after the maternal blood levels fall to deficient levels [25].

The influence of the mother's diet on the levels of fat-soluble vitamins and minerals in her milk is uncertain at present. Maternal iron supplementation does not increase the iron level of milk, however.

Severe malnutrition of mothers in less-developed countries is known to result in diminished volume of milk. Frequently, in this country, on the other hand, well-nourished mothers report inability to produce enough milk to support their infants. The reason for this is lack of knowledge of the nursing process and lack of psychological support from physicians, nurses, other health professionals, and family members. Before the advent of infant formulas, practically all babies were breast-fed. Women learned how to nurse from their mothers and other female relatives and friends. Furthermore, physicians and other health professionals knew how to help them with any problems encountered.

When bottle-feeding became the norm, medical and nursing students were taught how to bottle-feed, and breast-feeding skills were no longer passed along from one generation of women to the next. If a normal woman wholeheartedly desires to nurse her infant, she will be able to do so if she obtains competent help from a person who is knowledgeable about the process, and if those family members closest to her support her psychologically.

Women who use oral contraceptive agents (OCA) made up of combinations of estrogen and progesterone are apt to suffer diminished milk supply, adversely affecting infant growth [26]. An alternative is to use agents containing only progesterone, or those with progesterone and low amounts of estrogen. Many physicians advise forms of contraception other than OCA during lactation.

The lactating mother may find that some foods she eats disturb the baby. These foods differ from individual to individual, so trial and error must be used to discern them. Caffeine passes into the milk, so a baby may become overstimulated if the mother consumes as much as six to eight caffeine-containing beverages daily [27]. Alcohol also passes into breast milk; the nursing mother should therefore consume only moderate amounts, if she consumes any.

DIETARY PLANNING FOR LACTATION

Studies in countries where some lactating women have obvious malnutrition show that generally the maternal body is damaged more by poor diet than is the nursing infant [28]. Lactating women need to realize that many nutrients will be mobilized from maternal tissues as lactation progresses if their diets fail to supply them.

Physicians, dietitians, and nutritionists frequently place little emphasis on diet during lactation, but the need for kilocalories and many nutrients is greater during lactation than during pregnancy. The food guide for lactating women in Table 14-2 is similar to that in pregnancy except that a larger milk intake is recommended. The total kilocalorie intake should be adjusted to maintain normal body weight.

Continued iron supplementation for the first 2 or 3 months of lactation is recommended to replenish iron stores lost during pregnancy. If a lactating woman is unable to consume milk because of allergy or lactose intolerance, she should be guided to choose adequate alternative sources of calcium to protect her bones from calcium depletion. She should also be certain her vitamin D intake or exposure to sunlight is adequate to permit normal absorption of calcium.

Lactating women who adhere to a nutritious diet for themselves generally find other family members following their example. As indicated in the following chapter, a cardinal rule in teaching a child good food habits is to "set a good example."

SUMMARY

1 A mother's nutritional status before conception is an important factor in influencing nourishment of the baby-to-be. Proper growth of the placenta is vital for proper growth and development of the fetus.

2 A normal phenomenon in pregnancy is expansion of maternal blood and tissue fluids. Sodium restriction during pregnancy may prevent this process from occurring.

3 Normal weight gain during pregnancy amounts to 24 to 28 lb and should occur at the rate of 1 to 3 lb during the first 3 months, and 0.8 to 0.9 lb per week thereafter.

4 The nutrient requirements during normal pregnancy can be obtained from food except for iron and folacin. Supplements of both these nutrients are recommended.

5 Low birth weight (LBW) babies are at increased risk for early death, mental retardation, visual and hearing problems, and behavioral or learning problems. Inadequate maternal weight gain during pregnancy increases one's chances of having a LBW infant.

6 Food guides suggested for pregnancy and lactation emphasize inclusion of a wide variety of foods of high nutrient density.

7 Fat stored during pregnancy may be oxidized during lactation to supply some of the energy needed for milk production.

8 The need for kilocalories and many nutrients is greater during lactation than during pregnancy. Just as much emphasis should be placed on the importance of a nutritious diet during lactation as during pregnancy.

FOR DISCUSSION AND APPLICATION

1 Collect popular publications written for pregnant and lactating women, such as baby magazines or women's magazines. Is the nutrition information in these publications accurate? What type of dietary recommendations are made? Are the suggestions helpful to pregnant women or new mothers? Do you notice any misinformation?

2 Jennifer is a 21-year-old woman in her third month of pregnancy. For the past 2 years she has followed a lacto-ovo-vegetarian diet. She includes generous amounts of eggs, dairy products, beans, whole-grain products, fresh fruit, and vegetables. Can you recommend this type of diet for her? Is she likely to be deficient in any nutrients?

3 Once Jennifer has delivered her baby, she plans to breast-feed. Is her lacto-ovo-vegetarian diet acceptable during lactation?

4 Roberta is a 24-year-old college graduate, pregnant with her second child. She is 5'4" and weighs 110 lb. She is in her second month of pregnancy. Roberta is very weight-conscious and prides herself on the fact that she gained only 15 lb during her first pregnancy. She plans to curtail her food intake during this one, too, to again limit total weight gain to 15 lb. What suggestions can you make for Roberta? Do you think her strategy may be harmful? Who is most likely to be at risk, Roberta or her baby?

5 Survey the class or a group of your friends to determine attitudes toward breast-feeding. Are they positive or negative? What factors may influence attitudes toward nursing?

SUGGESTED READINGS

Reaching Out to the Pregnant Teenager. This is a nutrition education resource developed by the Department of Health and Human Services, the Department of Agriculture, and the March of Dimes Birth Defects Foundation. It stresses the importance of catering to the special needs and lifestyles of the pregnant adolescent. It may be obtained from Nutrition and Technical Services Division, Food and Nutrition Service, USDA, Alexandria, Va, 22302.

Pregnancy and Nutrition. Society of Nutrition Education. This is a bibliography of over 100 books, papers, audiovisual materials, and references useful in learning about pregnancy or counseling the pregnant mother.

Breast Feeding. Bureau of Community Health Services, Health Services Administration, 5600 Fishers Lane, Rockville, Md, 20857, No. (HSA) 79-5109; 1979. A single copy is free. This pamphlet provides suggestions on preparing for breast-feeding before the birth, how to begin nursing, and how to eat during the nursing period.

Hess, Mary Abbott, and Anne Elise Hunt; *Pickles and Ice Cream.* New York: McGraw-Hill Book Co., 1982. Written for the general reader, this book discusses nutrition in pregnancy and lactation, covering many of the questions often asked.

INFANCY, CHILDHOOD, AND ADOLESCENCE

Infants, children, and adolescents have special nutrient needs. These phases of the life cycle are times of rapid growth and physical development, and nutrient requirements parallel these changes. Children's food habits and their nutritional status will have a great impact on their adult eating behavior and nutritional status. It is therefore important to help children and adolescents develop sound food habits. This chapter will consider the nutrient needs during normal physical growth from infancy through childhood and adolescence. Psychosocial factors influencing eating behavior and practical aspects of feeding children will be discussed. The possible relationship between diet and hyperactivity in children will also be examined.

PHYSICAL GROWTH AND DEVELOPMENT IN INFANCY

Human beings reach physical maturity as a result of a remarkably complex process requiring almost 20 years to complete. During this period, individuals develop from only two germ cells and become adults composed of more than 100,000 billion cells.

Infancy constitutes the age period from birth to 1 year of age. Although the fetal period is the time of greatest growth rate for humans, there is also a dramatic growth rate during early infancy. In fact, after birth, the periods of maximal growth are those occurring during the first year of life and during the adolescent years. The infant typically doubles his or her birth weight in 4 to 6 months and triples it by the age of 1 year. If a 21-year-old, 110-lb female grew at this rate, she would weigh 330 lb by the age of 22. A baby gains an average of 15 lb during the first year, but the rate of gain declines to about 5 lb per year by the age of 5 [1].

Figure 15-1 illustrates the rate of normal physical growth of girls from birth to 3 years and is the chart that physicians use to assess their growth rates. Percentile charts for boys are similar to this one. These percentile charts are marked from the 5th to the 95th percentile. The 95th percentile means that out of 100 girls of a given age, 95 would be at or below that height (length) or weight.

In using these charts, an infant's length and weight would be recorded at intervals of every 1 to 2 months in infancy and every 6 months thereafter. The length measurement would be plotted on the length (upper) chart, and weight on the lower chart for the appropriate age. An infant or child growing normally would tend to stay fairly near the same percentile as she gets older. In other words, if she began at about the 50th percentile she would be expected, normally, to continue close to that percentile.

During the first year of life, many other physical changes occur in addition to weight gain. Length increases by about 50 percent and blood volume triples. The percentage of body weight due to water decreases from about 75 percent at birth to about 55 to 60 percent at age 1. Lean body mass increases, body fat accumulates, bones and teeth grow and become more calcified. The brain and nervous system grow rapidly; internal organs such as the gastrointestinal tract, kidney, and liver become more mature and efficient in their ability to digest, absorb, and metabolize food.

All infants grow and develop in a generally predictable manner, but often at different rates. Growth normally occurs in spurts rather than at a steady pace, and

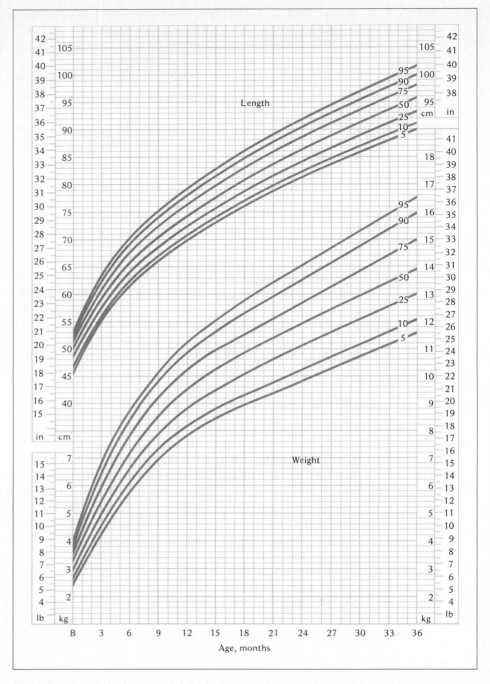

FIGURE 15-1. Girls (birth to 36 months): Physical growth, National Center for Health Statistics (NCHS) percentiles. (Source: Adapted from Hamill, P. V. V., T. A. Drizd, C. L. Johnson, R. B. Reed, A. F. Roche, and W. M. Moore, "Physical Growth: National Center for Health Statistics Percentiles," *American Journal of Clinical Nutrition,* 32:607, 1979. © 1980 Ross Laboratories.)

occurs in two general ways: *hyperplasia*, an increase in the number of cells, and *hypertrophy*, an increase in the size of cells.

The concept of a critical growth period is important in development. *Critical growth periods* are times when a given event will have its greatest impact on development. There is a critical period of growth for each organ system, during which rapid cell division takes place. Nutritional deprivation during critical periods may cause irreversible damaging effects on a given organ. Examples of the harmful consequences of malnutrition during critical growth periods are the smaller head circumference or the shorter height of individuals who suffered from malnutrition during infancy. Overnutrition during infancy may promote the onset of obesity (Chapter 8).

NUTRIENT REQUIREMENTS

Kilocalories

An infant's energy needs are much higher per unit of body weight than for the older child or adult because of the more rapid rate of growth. As one's growth rate decreases with age, so do kilocalorie needs per unit of weight. From birth to 6 months, infants require an average of 115 kilocalories per kilogram of body weight. From 6 to 12 months, the recommendation is 105 kilocalories per kilogram of body weight or 1000 kcal/day by the time the infant weighs around 22 lb (10 kg). In comparison, average adult kilocalorie recommendations are usually over 2000 kcal/day. The recommended average energy intake for a 70-kg male aged 23 to 60 years old is 2700 kcal, which is less than 40 kcal per kilogram of body weight.

Protein

Sufficient dietary protein is necessary for synthesis of body proteins during the normally rapid growth rate of infancy. Protein needs during the first year are higher per unit of body weight than at any other time in life. The same nine essential amino acids required by the adult are needed by the infant. Protein recommendations are also determined on the basis of body weight:

- From birth to 6 months, the protein recommendation is 2.2 g per kilogram of body weight.
- From 6 to 12 months, it is 2.0 g per kilogram of body weight.

If kilocalorie needs are not met, protein may be used for energy. At low levels of kilocalorie intake, when protein is used to supply energy, protein is not available to supply the essential amino acids, and deficiency may develop. An insufficient amount of protein can lead to growth retardation. Too much protein, however, can be hazardous for the infant. The infant's kidneys and renal system are not mature enough to handle an excessive amount of the residues of protein metabolism such as urea, phosphorus, and potassium. Excess protein intake increases the need for water; if sufficient water is not consumed, the infant may become dehydrated. Thus, feeding too much protein can be almost as harmful as a protein deficiency.

Fats and Other Lipids

While there is no set recommendation for fat during the early months of life, fat is an important source of kilocalories for infants. Moreover, it is a carrier of fat-soluble vitamins and also a source of linoleic acid, a deficiency of which may result in skin rash and retarded growth. Because of the possible relationship between dietary fat and coronary heart disease, there is considerable controversy over recommended fat and cholesterol intakes for infants. Most infant formulas have only 15 to 20 percent as much cholesterol as human or whole cow's milk, and comparable total fat content. The source of fat in most infant formulas is corn or soy oils rather than butterfat; thus, the ratio of polyunsaturated to saturated fatty acids is higher than that in either human or cow's milk.

Surveys have indicated that about 80 percent of American infants are given infant formula during their first 3 months of life; an estimated 40 percent continue with formula until the age of 6 months [2]. Thus, a majority of U.S. infants consume diets relatively low in cholesterol and high in polyunsaturated fat. This changes around 6 months of age when whole, 2 percent, or skim milk is frequently introduced.

The research to date remains inconclusive as to whether or not relatively low intakes of cholesterol and saturated fat during early infancy are advantageous. Based on limited data, one hypothesis suggests that body systems which break down cholesterol need a type of early "priming" exposure to relatively high cholesterol levels [2]. However, other investigators have reported that infants whose cholesterol intakes were low during early infancy had lower serum cholesterol levels at the age of 8 or 9 than did other children who had higher cholesterol intakes [2]. Whether or not this lower serum cholesterol level at age 8 or 9 is advantageous, however, is uncertain.

Some parents give their infants nonfat (skim) milk in an effort to reduce saturated fat or kilocalories. This practice has been questioned since nonfat milk may lead to insufficient kilocalorie intake or a deficiency of linoleic acid, the essential fatty acid. In addition, nonfat milk may provide excessive intakes of protein and minerals, resulting in difficulty in excreting minerals or urea. Thus, using skim milk as the major milk is not recommended until a child is at least 2 years old.

Carbohydrates

While there is no Recommended Dietary Allowance for carbohydrates, this nutrient is important as a source of energy for infants. Newborns are able to digest lactose, the primary form of carbohydrate in milk, but cannot digest more complex carbohydrates efficiently until the age of 2 to 3 months. Therefore, starches are not well digested by very young infants.

Water

Water is crucial to the infant's health. Infants lose proportionately more water through evaporation than do older children or adults. Their renal systems are also immature; therefore, relatively more water is needed to process and excrete their waste products. Because the relative water needs of infants are higher than those of the adult, infants are more prone to suffer from dehydration. If they are fed cow's milk, which has more protein, and hence results in greater residues from protein digestion than human milk, additional water should be offered. During periods of high fevers or with symptoms such as vomiting or diarrhea, additional water should also be given and medical attention should be sought.

Minerals and Vitamins

Requirements for minerals and vitamins for infants up to the age of 6 months are usually estimated on the basis of the average amounts consumed by healthy infants who are breast-fed by healthy, well-nourished mothers. The basis for this is the assumption that human milk contains nutrients in a well-balanced combination suitable for growing, active infants. Nutrient requirements for infants aged 6 months to 1 year are determined on the basis of consumption of infant formula and gradually increased quantities of solid foods [3].

The optimal ratio of *calcium* to *phosphorus* for infants is similar to that found in human milk (2.4:1) rather than that found in undiluted cow's milk (1.2:1). Calcium and phosphorus are both needed for hardening of the bones. Too much phosphorus may result in too high an excretion load for the kidneys and, in rare cases, in a disorder called tetany, characterized by muscle twitchings, cramps, and convulsions. Newborn infants should never be fed *undiluted* cow's milk because of its high phosphorus content. By the age of 6 months, however, most infants can consume undiluted cow's milk without problems if less than 1 qt per day is consumed.

Iron is the mineral most often deficient in the infant's diet, and iron-deficiency anemia is the most common nutritional problem in infants 6 months to 2 years old. The full-term infant is born with a store of iron, although this is usually depleted by the age of 6 months. Premature infants generally have lower iron stores. Both human and cow's milk are poor sources of iron. However, iron in human milk is more efficiently absorbed than that in cow's milk, and normal infants fed only breast milk during the first 3 or 4 months of life are unlikely to develop iron-deficiency anemia. They should receive an iron supplement at the age of 4 or 5 months, however, because their iron stores need to be replenished by that time. It is important to note here that too much iron could lead to iron toxicity. The sample menu in Table 15-1 illustrates how easy it is for a child to receive too much iron. Since iron is added to infant cereals and formulas, the total amount of iron in an infant's diet should be monitored so it does not greatly exceed the recommended level of 10 mg/day for the infant under 6 months old and 15 mg/day for the infant aged 6 months to 1 year.

Fluorine is another mineral for which supplements are commonly prescribed. Breast milk and cow's milk are low in fluorine so physicians may advise

TABLE 15-1. A HIGH-IRON MENU FOR AN 8–12-MONTH-OLD INFANT

	IRON CONTENT
Breakfast	
4 oz apple juice	—
3½ oz infant cereal with milk	10 mg*
Lunch	
3½ oz strained egg yolks	2.7 mg
3½ oz strained vegetables	0.6 mg
3½ oz strained fruit	0.4 mg
Milk	
Dinner	
3½ oz strained liver	5.0 mg
3½ oz strained vegetables	0.6 mg
3½ oz strained fruit	0.4 mg
Milk	
Before Bed	
3½ oz infant cereal with milk	10 mg
Daily total	29.7 mg

*Approximate iron content.

The high-iron menu in this table demonstrates how easy it is for the infant to consume an excessive amount of iron.

fluorine supplements to guard against tooth decay. Infants consuming formula may not require supplementation if the water supply is fluoridated. Recommendations for the level of supplementation vary according to the amount of fluorine in the water supply.

Of the fat-soluble vitamins in human milk, *vitamin D* is of greatest concern from a practical standpoint. Although rickets is uncommon among breast-fed babies of well-nourished white mothers in sunny parts of the country, authorities recommend supplements of 400 IU (10μg) of vitamin D daily for breast-fed babies under the following circumstances: (1) if the mother has had a poor intake of vitamin D, as might be the case for a strict vegetarian or a woman who is rarely exposed to sunlight; (2) if the infant is rarely exposed to sunlight because of climate, environmental pollution, or style of clothing worn; and (3) if the infant has dark enough skin to prevent efficient conversion of 7-dehydrocholesterol in the skin to vitamin D when exposed to the sun [4,5].

Exactly how much vitamin D is in breast milk is unclear at present, but there appears to be little of the active forms in the fat portion of milk [6], and little vitamin D sulfate in the watery portion [7,8]. Nevertheless, light-skinned, well-nourished mothers living in sunny areas probably do not need to give their breast-fed babies vitamin D supplements [5].

Infants fed formulas or cow's milk fortified with vitamin D require no additional supplementation. Excessive intakes of vitamin D can be toxic to infants.

Human milk is rich in *vitamin E*. Colostrum, the first milk produced by the lactating mother, is very high in vitamin E. As noted previously, the requirements for vitamin E vary depending on the level of polyunsaturated fatty acids in the diet. Infant formulas high in polyunsaturated fatty acids usually also have higher levels of vitamin E.

Newborn babies are apt to have low levels of *vitamin K* in their blood because intestinal bacteria which normally synthesize vitamin K do not become established until infants begin to consume milk. Human milk is relatively low in vitamin K, while cow's milk contains larger amounts. Most infants are given a vitamin K supplement at birth to avoid problems in blood clotting.

Most commercially available infant formulas have *ascorbic acid* added to them; if not, a source of ascorbic acid must be provided either as "baby drops" or as a vitamin C-rich food. Some infants are allergic to substances in orange juice, so it should be fed cautiously.

Other vitamins and minerals are commonly supplied in adequate amounts by both human and cow's milk. Thus, additional supplementation with these nutrients is not generally considered necessary. The Recommended Dietary Allowances for minerals and vitamins in infancy are given in Appendix A.

EATING HABITS

Comparing Human, Cow's, and Formula Milk

Milk is the primary source of nutrients during infancy. The newborn infant is usually fed either human milk, or a commercially prepared infant formula. Because undiluted cow's milk is inappropriate for newborn infants, most formula milks are modified to result in a composition closer to that of human milk than is undiluted cow's milk.

Is it more desirable to breast-feed a baby, or to offer the infant formula? Let's take a look at the composition of the various milks, and also at some of the advantages and disadvantages of breast-feeding. Table 15-2 summarizes some of the major characteristics of these different milks, while Table 15-3 gives the nutrient composition of human, cow's, and formula milk. In interpreting these tables, it should *not* be assumed that *more* is *better*. Undiluted cow's milk is designed to nurture an animal that is born at a more advanced stage of maturity and that grows more rapidly than does the human infant.

To Breast-Feed or Bottle-Feed

Nutritionists generally agree that breast-feeding, in most cases, is the best method of infant feeding [9,10]. During the first 4 to 6 months of life, mother's milk supplies all the nutrients the normal baby needs for growth and development. After this early period, breast milk must be supplemented with other foods, but it can still serve as an important source of essential nutrients. Some facts about breast-feeding are presented in Box 15-1.

We have been aware of the differences between human and cow's milk for years. In fact, this knowledge has helped producers to make commercial formulas that approximate human milk in many respects. But current research continues to

TABLE 15-2. COMPARISON OF HUMAN, COW'S, AND FORMULA MILK

	HUMAN MILK	UNDILUTED COW'S MILK	INFANT FORMULAS
Protein	Relatively low. Curds formed in the stomach are easily digestible.	More protein than human milk. High in casein, which forms tough, hard-to-digest curds. Heat treatment, as in evaporated milk, results in softer, easier-to-digest curds.	Protein content slightly higher than human milk. Protein forms a more easily digested curd than does undiluted cow's milk.
Lipids	Rich in cholesterol. High in linoleic acid especially if diet is high in linoleic acid. Saturated fat is somewhat lower than in cow's milk.	Low in linoleic acid. Less cholesterol than human milk, but more than infant formulas. Relatively high in saturated fat.	Usually high in polyunsaturated fat (linoleic acid) and low in cholesterol and saturated fat.
Carbohydrate	High in lactose, which may aid in absorption of calcium, magnesium, and iron.	Lower in lactose than human milk.	About same amount of carbohydrate as in human milk, but frequently is a mixture of glucose and dextrins rather than lactose.
Vitamins	Richer in vitamin E than cow's milk. Adequate in ascorbic acid and vitamin A to meet infant's needs. Vitamin D content may be insufficient to meet RDA. Vitamin B content adequate if mother's diet is adequate.	Pasteurization results in low ascorbic acid content. Higher in vitamin K, and most B vitamins than human milk.	Vitamins fortified to meet the RDAs.
Minerals	Ratio of calcium to phosphorus is 2.4:1. Calcium better absorbed than in cow's milk. Iron is in a more available form than in cow's milk. Poor source of fluorine.	Four times the calcium and six times the phosphorus of human milk, but low in iron. Poor source of fluorine.	Special "humanized" formulas have sodium and potassium levels similar to those in human milk, but nearly all formulas have calcium and phosphorus levels considerably higher than in human milk.
Immune factors	Such factors as immunoglobulins (secretory IgA, for example), lactoferrin, and living leukocytes provide immunologic protection against gastrointestinal and respiratory infections.	None	None

Human milk is generally lower in protein, calcium, and phosphorus, but higher in linoleic acid, lactose, vitamin E, and cholesterol than cow's milk. Formulas are designed to more closely resemble human milk than does undiluted cow's milk, but no formula exactly simulates human milk. Human milk is unique in its ability to protect the infant against certain infections.

TABLE 15-3. COMPOSITION OF MATURE HUMAN MILK, COW'S MILK, AND COMMERCIALLY PREPARED MILK-BASED FORMULAS

COMPOSITION	HUMAN MILK	UNDILUTED COW'S MILK	ENFAMIL (MEAD) SIMILAC (ROSS)
Water (mL/100 mL)	87.1	87.2	—
Energy (kcal/100 mL)	75	66	—
Protein (g/100 mL)	1.1	3.5	1.5–1.6
P/S ratio	0.4–0.8	0.4	2.0–4.5
Fat (g/100 mL)	4.5	3.7	3.6–3.7
Carbohydrate (g/100 mL)	6.8	4.9	7.0–7.2
Cholesterol (mg/8 fl oz)	35–52	22–32	5–10
MINERALS (PER LITER)			
Calcium (mg)	340	1170	550–600
Phosphorus (mg)	140	920	440–455
Sodium (meq)	7	22	11–17
Potassium (meq)	13	35	16–28
Chloride (meq)	11	29	12–24
Magnesium (mg)	40	120	40–48
Sulfur (mg)	140	300	130–160
Copper (mg)	0.4	0.3	0.4–0.6
Zinc (mg)	3–5	3–5	2.0–4.2
Iodine (μg)	30	47	40–69
Iron (mg)	0.5	0.5	Trace–1.5
VITAMINS (PER LITER)			
Vitamin A (IU)	1898	1025	1700–2500
Thiamine (μg)	160	440	400–650
Riboflavin (μg)	360	1750	600–1000
Niacin (mg)	1470	940	7–8.5
Pyridoxine	100	640	320–400
Pantothenate (mg)	1.84	3.46	2.1–3.2
Folacin (μg)	52	55	50–100
B_{12} (μg)	0.3	4	1.5–2.0
C (mg)	43	11	55
D (IU)	22	14	400–423
E (IU)	1.8	0.4	8.5–12.7

A comparison of the nutrient content of human, cow's, and formula milk illustrates important differences as well as similarities among the milks.

SOURCE: Fomon, S., *Infant Nutrition,* Philadelphia: W. B. Saunders Co., 1974, pp. 362, 363, 379.

uncover the unique properties of mother's milk. It is made up of more than 100 constituents which are present in very different proportions than in milk produced by other mammals. In general, the nutrient composition of the milk of each species is best suited to the growth and development needs of the offspring of that species.

Breast milk is valuable for its anti-infective properties which offer protection against gastrointestinal and respiratory disorders common in babies [11]. In addition, many allergists contend that bottle-fed babies develop more allergies than breast-fed babies.

Breast-Feeding Facts

- A healthy and well-nourished mother will produce milk that is qualitatively good. In general, a very poorly nourished mother produces a reduced quantity of milk.
- Milk production is greatly influenced by the mother's emotions. Most women who are confident of their ability to successfully breast-feed their infants are able to do so.
- The size of a woman's breasts is not related to the quantity or quality of milk produced.
- As the baby nurses and empties the breast, additional milk production is stimulated. A breast that is only partly emptied will produce less milk at a later feeding; a breast totally emptied will tend to produce more milk. Thus, there is a relationship between the appetite and needs of the infant and the quantity of milk available to satisfy the infant.
- The nursing time needed to satisfy the infant is very short. Approximately half the milk available is received by the baby during the first few minutes of nursing. The breast is emptied in about 6 to 12 minutes. Some babies nurse for 15 to 20 minutes, however. This may indicate that there is not enough milk to satisfy and that the baby is still hungry; or it may mean that the infant desires the closeness and warm feeling derived from nursing.

Nursing at the breast makes possible an emotional sense of security, warmth, and well-being for both mother and child. If the mother has a positive attitude toward breast-feeding, the nursing experience can offer a way of continuing the intimate physiological relationship between infant and mother that began before birth. In addition to the psychological benefits, there are other advantages for the mother who nurses her baby. An early benefit is the stimulation of uterine contractions after birth that help to reduce blood loss. In addition, these contractions help the uterus regain its normal size earlier than might otherwise occur.

Rarely are infants unable to tolerate their mother's milk. Health professionals interested in promoting breast-feeding are concerned that certain drugs, pesticides, and herbicides can be transmitted to the infant through mother's milk. For example, DDT has been found to be present in some human milk samples at higher levels than the government allows to be present in cow's milk [12]. The only solution to this problem appears to be to work toward lowering such contaminants in the environment.

Usually mothers can continue to nurse their babies even during maternal illnesses. But some diseases such as *staphylococcal* and *streptococcal* infections may be transmissible through mother's milk. Mothers with these illnesses are usually advised not to nurse until they have recovered. Mothers with tuberculosis or cancer of the breast also should not nurse their infants.

Despite the advantages of breast-feeding, it is not necessarily appropriate for all. Breast-feeding can be very demanding for the mother. Some mothers may find that breast-feeding takes too much time away from other responsibilities. Others are psychologically unprepared for breast-feeding, while still others encounter strong resistance to breast-feeding from their spouses or other family members.

Numerous infants thrive on infant formulas. The psychological closeness of being held, caressed, touched, and loved can occur with bottle-feeding. Bottle-feeding allows the father or other family members to take an active part in feeding the baby, something which can't be done with breast-feeding. When the family can afford the formula, where facilities ensure sanitary preparation and feeding conditions, and when the mother prefers not to nurse the baby, bottle-feeding is a satisfactory alternative. In such cases, the mother should be provided support in her decision, and she can generally be assured that her baby will thrive and prosper on an appropriate infant formula.

Introducing Solid Foods

The ability to eat different types of foods depends upon the maturation of infants' central nervous systems, which control motor skills affecting the way in which babies suck, chew, and swallow food. At birth, the "rooting reflex," in which touching the skin near the mouth causes an infant to turn the head toward the stimulus, trying to find the nipple, and the sucking reflex, in which placing a nipple in the mouth causes involuntary sucking movements, enable a newborn to take in liquid nourishment. Milk is sucked from a nipple by an action in which the tongue moves up and down and strokes the liquid from the nipple, pulling it to the back of the mouth. Newborn infants also have a protrusion reflex. If a solid food is placed in the mouth, an infant involuntarily pushes it out with the tongue. By 3 to 4 months of age, this reflex begins to disappear and the infant learns to move food with the tongue from the front to the back of the mouth. Therefore, to attempt to feed the baby solid food before the body has matured sufficiently to handle it is frustrating for both caretaker and baby, and may prompt the beginning of problems centering around food.

A Closer Look

Putting a small child to bed with a bottle of milk or other sweet liquid can result in "nursing bottle syndrome," a disorder affecting the teeth. As the child falls asleep sucking on the bottle, the sweet liquid pools around the upper teeth because saliva that normally would wash it away is no longer secreted during sleep. Any liquid containing sugar, such as sugared water, baby formula, sodas, fruit juice, or even plain milk provides the sugar on which oral bacteria grow to produce acid. The result can be complete destruction of the upper primary or "baby" teeth. The upper teeth are most affected because the tongue protects the lower teeth. Loss of the upper primary teeth means that the child will be handicapped in learning not only eating styles but also speaking skills. To avoid this syndrome, the infant or small child should be given formula or milk only while awake and should never be put to bed with a bottle. Fruit juice is best given to a baby by cup; sodas and other drinks high in sugar should never be given to infants.

STUDY ON INFANT FORMULA USE

The New York Times, Oct. 27, 1981

Despite the natural childbirth and nursing movement that has led many women back to breast-feeding, 68 percent of the mothers who gave birth in all types of hospitals in New York City last year planned to use infant formula, according to a study by the New York City Department of Health.

In municipal hospitals, where most maternity patients are lower-income women, the figure was 82 percent. . . .

A Vast Sampling The study involved 22,211 mothers at private and city hospitals from January to March 1979 and 7,447 in November 1980. And in 1979, the Health Department's Bureau of Nutrition surveyed 1,300 low-income mothers at city child health stations and found that 94 percent of them were using infant formula. This indicated that even some of the mothers who originally planned to breast-feed their babies used formula instead, according to Health Department officials. . . .

City maternal health professionals . . . argue that most low-income women use infant formula because . . . a city hospital policy of giving mothers free samples of infant formula on discharge "implies that the hospital endorses the product". . . .

Under a contract the Health and Hospitals Corporation signed in 1974 with Ross Laboratories, the makers of the infant formula Similac, city hospitals buy the formula for general use in the maternity departments. The contract also guarantees that every new mother will leave a municipal hospital with a free one-day supply of Similac.

Josephine Williams, spokesman for the Health and Hospitals Corporation, disagreed that the free-sample policy influenced a mother's decision to use formula. "Nobody is forcing a mother to take the infant formula home," she said. . . .

A Ross Laboratories representative, Thomas Craig, defended the gift packages by noting that despite free samples, breast-feeding in the nation is "increasing significantly among all socioeconomic groups."

Bronx Municipal Hospital discontinued the distribution of the free gift packages a year ago at the urging of Dr. Katherine Lobach, director of the Comprehensive Family Care Center at the Albert Einstein College of Medicine, who is affiliated with the Bronx hospital.

Free samples, she said, are "free advertising for the infant formula companies and the companies know it." Dr. Lobach said a recent marketing study conducted by one company showed that the formula fed in hospitals and brought home was what the mothers would use for the next six to 12 months. . . .

Other doctors believe that the dispute over free samples overlooks another factor: many low-income women must return to work soon after giving birth, which makes formula the simplest feeding method.

Dr. Pakter and other advocates of breast-feeding counter that working women can remove enough milk with a breast pump—which they say is cheap, sanitary and simple to use—and store it for feedings during the day. . . .

Another major stumbling block to getting lower income women to breast-feed, Dr. Pakter . . . said, is not that they work, but that they do not hear about other options—such as the breast pump—or learn how to breast-feed properly, because they receive insufficient counseling in the prenatal care centers for low-income mothers.

"Breast-feeding is a learned response," said Elaine Kaplan, the mid-wife for Metropolitan Hospital. She said that if women are not taught how to breast-feed, they inevitably run into complications and turn to formula.

ASK YOURSELF:
How were the data gathered in this study? What are the arguments for and against giving mothers infant formula packets when they leave the hospital with their new infants? What aspects of breast-feeding does a mother need to learn? Why might a woman in a lower-income group be less inclined to breast-feed than one in a higher-income group?

Table 15-4 summarizes developmental milestones from birth to 18 months of age and the relationship between some of these milestones and eating behavior.

As we have noted, the majority of infants in this country receive either breast milk or infant formula as their main source of kilocalories during the first 3 months. The importance of formula and milk as kilocalorie sources declines by the age of 6 months and declines even further by the age of 1 year. Almost half of U.S. infants receive either whole or low-fat cow's milk by the age of 6 months and almost all take one or more of these forms of milk by the age of 1 year. Commercial baby foods are popular during the period from 4 to 9 months of age. By the age of 1 year, most infants are eating primarily table food. Figure 15-2 illustrates the sources of kilocalories in the typical infant diet at different ages.

Weaning refers to the period when the infant changes from the breast or bottle to other food sources. Weaning usually occurs gradually and depends upon

TABLE 15-4. DEVELOPMENTAL MILESTONES—BIRTH TO 18 MONTHS

APPROXIMATE AGE*	ACTIVITIES
1 to 2 weeks	Lifts head from prone position. Clenches fists when awake. Responds to loud noise. Rooting reflex causes head to turn in direction of stimulus. Sucking reflex enables baby to suck from breast or bottle. Needs holding, warmth, and sucking. Has poor motor control of head, neck, and trunk. Demonstrates protrusion reflex, making it difficult to eat solid foods.
1 month	Watches objects in direct line of vision. Looks at mother's face, listens attentively to music. Begins to put thumb or fingers in mouth.
2 months	Holds objects in hand but doesn't look at them. Follows moving objects with eyes. Smiles and coos.
3 months	Relaxes hands when awake. Sucks fingers. Recognizes breast or bottle as source of food and may help to hold bottle. Begins to transfer food from front to back of mouth with tongue. Bites and drools. Rooting reflex diminishes.
4 months	Grabs objects. Holds head erect. May begin to roll over from stomach to back. Laughs out loud. Notices hands. Tongue begins to move back and forth rather than up and down, and protrusion reflex disappears. This facilitates spoon feeding.
5 months	Begins to get teeth. Is now able to swallow small lumps of food and bite destructively. Able to sit up, reach for objects, and put them in mouth. Recognizes familiar persons.
6 to 8 months	Plays with rattle. Able to roll over from stomach to back and from back to stomach. Smiles at self in mirror. Begins uttering syllables such as da-da. May begin to drink from a cup. Begins chewing movements, demonstrating a readiness for foods requiring chewing such as crackers or teething biscuits.
9 to 10 months	Creeps, crawls. May get in sitting position without help. Tries to stand without support. Holds bottle. Picks up finger foods and feeds self. Waves bye-bye. Understands "no."
1 year	Toddles, walks unsteadily. Holds cup to drink by self. Is now able to eat many foods from table with family.
18 months	Walks with ease. Climbs stairs. Begins saying words. Uses spoon to eat. Drinks liquids well from a cup.

*As noted, the ages listed are approximate ones and should not be interpreted as the "right" age for an infant to achieve the corresponding milestones. There is a wide range of normal and acceptable individual differences among infants which should be kept in mind when reading this table.

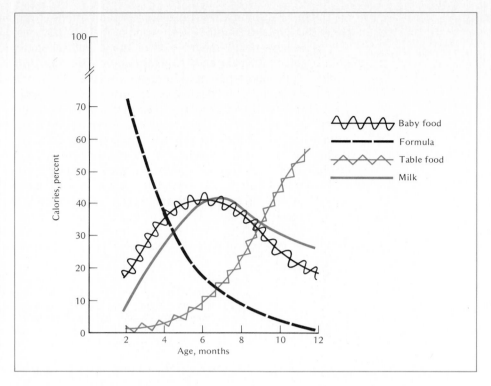

FIGURE 15-2. Sources of kilocalories in the infant diet at various ages. During the first few months of life most infants receive either milk or formula. From about 4 months to 1 year, baby foods become increasingly important food sources. (Source: Winick, M. (ed.), *Year One: Nutrition, Growth and Health,* New York: Medcom for Ross Laboratories, Columbus, Ohio, 1975.)

the growth and developmental rate of the infant. Some infants appear to need the extra kilocalories they get from solid foods earlier than others, but most are at least 4 months old before this stage is reached. After the initial introduction of solid foods, several months generally elapse before the weaning process is completed.

A century ago children did not eat vegetables and potatoes until the age of 3. In contrast to this view, a pediatric text in the early 1960s recommended feeding infants cereal the consistency of putty at 2 or 3 days of age, strained vegetables at 10 days, strained meat at 14 days and combinations of meat and vegetables at 17 days [13]. Most authorities now believe that there is no benefit to early feeding and suggest that feeding solid foods should be delayed until the age of 4 to 6 months. The Nutrition Committee of the American Academy of Pediatrics recommends that solid food be delayed until the baby weighs 6 to 7 kg (13 to 15 lb) and that it not be given before 3 months of age [14].

Why are parents often eager to feed solid foods to their infants early in life? Some consider this step a milestone in their infant's development, while others believe that their babies are not satisfied with milk or formula alone, or that solid food will help their infants sleep through the night. Most babies, however, begin to sleep through the night around the age of 9 weeks, whether or not solid foods have been introduced [15].

When solids are introduced, a few commonsense guidelines should be considered:

1. Offer only a small portion (a teaspoonful or two) of a new food at first. Every new food is a new adventure for a baby, as well as an experiment for the person feeding the child. A new food may upset the child—it is better to start slowly rather than risk an adverse reaction from too large a first feeding.
2. Allow 5 days between adding two new and different foods to a baby's diet. This will simplify the identification of a food that upsets the baby. If an infant develops diarrhea or becomes irritable after a new food has been introduced, don't offer the food again for several days to determine if the food was responsible for the upset.
3. Don't offer a new food to the baby if she is ill, or even if she has a cold.
4. If the baby resists a food, don't force, or bribe, but wait a period of time and then reintroduce the food. Mealtime should be a pleasurable experience. As the infant grows, likes and dislikes will change.

A suggested schedule for introducing solid foods is as follows:

FOOD	AGE
Dry cereal	4–5 months
Strained vegetables	5–6 months
Strained fruit	6–7 months
Teething foods	6–8 months
Strained meat	7–8 months
Strained or mashed egg yolk	8 months

Because cereals are very easy to digest, they are usually chosen as baby's first solid food. Cereals are good sources of the B vitamins and iron, and are highly nutritious and inexpensive. One serving of iron-fortified cereal (1/2 oz or approximately 5 level tbsp) contains 45 percent of the infant's RDA for iron, and 60 kilocalories. Rice cereal is not likely to result in food allergies, so it is usually the first cereal given the infant. Next to be offered are oat and barley cereals; later wheat, mixed cereals, corn, and high-protein cereals may be given. Other high-carbohydrate foods such as rice and breads may be offered, but they should not replace other nutritious foods.

After cereal, fruits and vegetables are usually the next foods offered to the infant. These foods contribute dietary fiber, carbohydrate, vitamins A and C, B vitamins, and a small amount of iron to the baby's diet. A very common complaint of parents is that their child dislikes vegetables. Perhaps if we followed Dr. Spock's advice, "Eat your applesauce or I won't allow you to have your carrots," the baby would want the vegetables. The first vegetables usually offered are strained squash and carrots. Later, string beans and peas, then other vegetables such as spinach, beets, and mixed vegetables can be tried. First fruits to be offered are applesauce, ripe bananas, and strained pears. Next are peaches, apricots, and pineapple. Some nutritionists suggest introducing vegetables before fruits because all babies like sweet foods, (and thus do not need to "learn" to like fruits) and may reject vegetables if first accustomed to fruits.

Meat and egg yolks, usually the last groups of new foods offered to the infant, are a significant source of animal protein, fat, vitamins, and iron. Strained beef, lamb, and chicken are usually the first meats offered. Later liver, turkey, and veal, then pork and fish are offered. Egg whites are usually not given until the infant is about 1 year old, since many infants are allergic to egg whites. Dairy products such as cottage cheese, yogurt, and mild cheeses (Swiss, American, cheddar) can serve as supplements or substitutes for some of the milk.

In recent years, as a result of greater consumer interest in and awareness of the importance of good nutrition, there have been changes in the composition of commercially prepared baby food [16]. In 1969 the Food and Nutrition Board of the NAS–NRC suggested that only minimal levels of salt be added to baby foods (added salt should not exceed 0.25 percent or 100 mg of sodium per 100 g of food) [17]. In response to this recommendation, manufacturers of baby food significantly reduced the sodium content of their products. Manufacturers decided about the same time to stop adding monosodium glutamate (MSG) to baby foods, further reducing the sodium content of infant foods. Levels of added sugar to baby fruits and desserts have also been reduced.

Alternatives to Commercial Baby Foods: Home Preparation

Some 150 million American children have eaten commercial baby foods since their introduction about 45 years ago. They provide kilocalories, protein, vitamins, and minerals for rapidly growing babies when breast milk or infant formula no longer meets total nutrient needs. However, many parents believe they can make more nutritious and less expensive baby food at home.

FIGURE 15-3. Changes in body proportions during growth, keeping height constant. This figure illustrates the fact that human development proceeds from the head to the foot, with the head developing first. (Source: Adapted from Scammon, R. E., and L. A. Calkins, *The Development and Growth of the External Dimensions of the Human Body in the Fetal Period,* Copyright 1929 by the University of Minnesota, University of Minnesota Press, Minneapolis, in Beal, Virginia, *Nutrition in the Life Span,* New York: John Wiley & Sons, 1980, p. 15.)

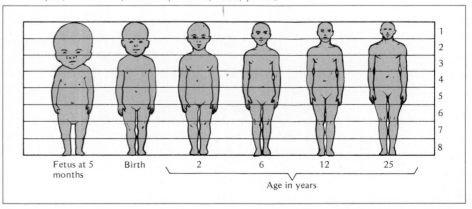

Fetus at 5 months   Birth   2   6   12   25

Age in years

Homemade baby foods, compared with commercial ones, tend to be slightly higher in kilocalories because water is usually added to commercial products [16]. Modified food starches such as corn or tapioca starch are sometimes used to improve the consistency and stability of commercial foods. These starches add carbohydrates to the food, but no other significant nutrients. Commercial baby foods are often more expensive than homemade foods. However, some mothers are willing to pay for the convenience.

If baby foods are prepared at home, parents should avoid adding sugar, fat, salt, or spices, and should follow good sanitary practices. Fresh ripe fruits such as bananas and cooked vegetables may be mashed or cut in fine pieces. Since it is difficult to cut meats finely enough for the infant to easily manage, parents have found it helpful to use a blender, grinder, or food processor to puree meats and other foods. Small hand grinders are available relatively inexpensively (under $10), and can be used at the table to grind foods for the infant. Pureed food may be frozen in ice cube trays, then stored in a freezer bag until ready to be used, one cube at a time. Babies need pureed food only until they are able to chew efficiently—usually between 9 and 12 months of age.

PHYSICAL GROWTH AND DEVELOPMENT IN EARLY CHILDHOOD

In contrast to the rapid growth that takes place during the first year of life, growth after infancy through childhood progresses much more slowly. By 1 year, the "average" boy has reached a height of 30 in and a weight of 22 lb. By 2, he is about 35 in tall and will have achieved about half his adult height. By 3, he is approximately 38 in tall. After the third birthday, his growth rate will level off; he will grow about 2½ in taller each year. Girls follow similar growth trends, and are, on the average, slightly smaller than boys [18]. During the preschool years, boys and girls develop at a similar rate, but girls tend to have more fatty tissue while boys have more muscle.

Body proportions of children also change as they grow. Development proceeds from the head to the foot. Thus, an infant's head, brain, eyes, and ears develop earlier than the lower body and are larger, relative to the lower body, than is true at the age of 5 or 10. The brain of a 1-year-old child, for example, has reached 70 percent of its adult weight, while the rest of the body is far behind. Coinciding with this, young children learn to use the upper body before they gain use of the lower body. Infants can do many things with their hands while having little control over their legs. Young children sit before they stand, and can control eye movements before they can control the lower body. Changes in body proportions during growth are illustrated in Figure 15-3.

NUTRIENT REQUIREMENTS

As with infants, physical changes and development affect nutrient needs of children. As their rate of growth slows, so kilocalorie needs per unit of body weight tend to decrease. However, *total* kilocalorie, protein, and many vitamin and mineral needs increase.

There are fewer studies on the nutritional requirements of young children than of any other age group. Because preschoolers do not routinely attend baby clinics or visit physicians' offices unless they are sick, there were few places researchers could go to study groups of such children. This situation has changed now, with the initiation of the Head Start Program and the Special Supplemental Food Program for Women, Infants and Children (WIC Program), described later in this chapter. In 1968 national nutrition surveys were undertaken, also providing data on the nutritional status of children over the age of 1 year [1].

Kilocalories

Since total kilocalorie needs of young children are not extremely high, care must be taken to see that they don't consume too many low-nutrient-density foods (those high in kilocalories but low in essential nutrients). As the growth rate slows in early childhood, appetites diminish. Parents should be aware that it is normal for a 2-year-old to eat less ravenously than during infancy, and should not be overly concerned about the small quantity of food their child will be willing to eat, as long as they are certain that she is not ill.

TABLE 15-5. COMPARISON OF CHARACTERISTICS INDICATIVE OF ADEQUATE AND LESS THAN ADEQUATE NUTRITION

ADEQUATE (GOOD)	LESS THAN ADEQUATE (POOR)
General appearance of vitality, well-being, and alertness.	Strained expression; dull and listless; apathetic.
Bright, clear eyes; smiling, happy expression; no dark circles under eyes.	Sad-looking; dark circles under eyes; little smiling; prone to tears.
Recovers quickly from fatigue; endurance during activity.	Chronic fatigue; tires easily; takes excessive time to bounce back from physical activity; lack of endurance.
Full of energy; vigorous.	Lack of energy; weakness.
Smooth, glossy hair.	Dry, brittle, easily "pluckable" hair.
Good appetite; curious and eager to try new foods.	Poor appetite; unwilling to try new foods; may have many food dislikes.
Good posture; stands erect; well-developed muscles.	Poor posture; slumping; muscles weak and underdeveloped.
Skin is firm, resilient, and "feels alive"; subcutaneous fat layers.	Skin is dry; has little or no tone; little or no subcutaneous fat.
Interested in environment; curious; responsive.	Irritable, nervous, slow to react; indifferent, passive, unresponsive; unable to cope with stimuli.
Good growth, adequate weight and height for age.	Stunted growth; thin, small for age; overweight for height.
Attentive, eager to learn and experiment.	Shortened attention span; reduced capacity to concentrate.

While it is not easy to evaluate marginal inadequate nutrition, some of the characteristics listed here may be helpful.

SOURCE: Alford, B., and M. Boyle, *Nutrition During the Life Cycle*, Englewood Cliffs, N.J.: Prentice-Hall, Inc., 1982, p. 56.

How can we tell if a child is well nourished? Certain characteristics of appearance and behavior suggestive of adequate nutrition or of nutrition problems are summarized in Table 15-5.

Protein

Because of rapid growth, protein needs during early childhood are relatively high in proportion to body weight. Nonetheless, most people have exaggerated ideas of the importance of protein in the diet, as we saw in Chapter 6. Most American children obtain sufficient protein in their diets. Protein needs can be met if a child consumes two glasses of milk and a serving of meat or meat alternate each day.

Carbohydrates and Fat

No allowances have been set for either carbohydrates or fat. However, children should be discouraged from eating foods high in sugar and fat because these tend to be low in nutrient density. It is important that young children receive adequate intakes of the essential fatty acid, linoleic acid. Three percent of total kilocalories as linoleic acid is considered adequate [3].

Minerals and Vitamins

Iron is the nutrient most often low in the diets of young children, as it is in infant diets. Meeting the RDA for iron—15 mg—is difficult unless a child routinely consumes fortified or enriched foods such as grain and cereal products or liver. One cause of iron deficiency in young children may be an overconsumption of milk, which is low in iron, along with a relatively low intake of iron-rich foods. Calcium, phosphorus, magnesium, and riboflavin needs can be met by consuming daily two glasses of milk and a serving of meat or meat alternate. The vitamins most often low in the diets of young children are vitamin A and ascorbic acid. A rich source of each of these foods should be served daily. The Recommended Dietary Allowances for children ages 1 through 6 are presented in Appendix A.

PSYCHOSOCIAL CHARACTERISTICS AND FOOD HABITS

The young child develops not only physically, but also socially and psychologically. Developmental levels attained by children affect their food preferences, their appetites, and hence, the types of foods offered to them.

Considerable literature exists on feeding infants but surprisingly little data exist regarding foods consumed by toddlers. Parents' major concerns about food habits of young children include concerns about food choices and dawdling over food. Table 15-6 summarizes problems parents often encounter with their children at mealtimes and offers suggestions for dealing with these difficulties.

Young children sometimes have "roller coaster" appetites. Their desire for food changes greatly from day to day as well as from month to month. Some days they may have voracious appetites, while on other days, nothing catches their

TABLE 15-6.   DEALING WITH FOOD PROBLEMS

THE PROBLEM	AS THE CHILD SEES IT	AS THE PARENTS SEE IT	WHAT TO DO ABOUT IT
Introducing new foods	Here's something new. He's curious but probably distrustful of the unknown.	They want the child to learn as early as possible to eat and enjoy a variety of foods.	Introduce only one new food at a time. Offer a very small amount at first, at beginning of the meal. When appropriate, mix with milk or cereal or another food the child likes. Be aware that many small children reject mixtures, however. Allow plenty of time for the child to look at and examine the food. Don't try to introduce a new food when a child doesn't feel well or is cross and irritable. If the food is turned down, don't make a fuss. Offer again a few days later.
Food dislikes	She's asserting her independence by rejecting something unappealing. Or she may dislike the taste.	They want their child to overcome the dislike if possible.	Refrain from making an issue of the situation as this is likely to make the child more determined to refuse. Try combining the food with other favorites. Offer small servings. Prepare in a different way. A fruit or vegetable might be served raw. Milk might be incorporated into cooked dishes. Set a good example. (Of course, children, as well as adults, are entitled to a few dislikes.)
Refusal to eat	He may be asserting his independence or may actually not feel like eating. He may just have no appetite for some reason.	They feel the child needs the food and must in some way be made to eat.	If this happens occasionally and the child appears to be healthy, simply remove the food and let him wait until the next meal. No bribes or punishment. A skipped meal will not damage a healthy child. If the child is ill, consult a doctor. Few healthy children starve themselves unless food becomes a weapon against parents.

TABLE 15-6.   DEALING WITH FOOD PROBLEMS *(Continued)*

THE PROBLEM	AS THE CHILD SEES IT	AS THE PARENTS SEE IT	WHAT TO DO ABOUT IT
Dawdling or playing with food	She may not be hungry or she may be trying to attract attention.	They probably become irritable and feel that they must "take over" and make her hurry and eat.	Allow a reasonable amount of time. Offer help if it's needed. Explain to the child that you will remove the food when she is finished. Refrain from making a scene. This may be what the child is looking forward to. Once the food is removed, there's no more until the next meal. A child who has just been playing actively may be too tired to eat. Allowing her to eat sooner, or planning a quiet, relaxing time before eating may help.
Wants to feed himself or herself	Eating is a way to be independent. He's eager to do things for himself, pour his own milk, serve himself, and so forth.	Feeding himself often leads to a mess—spilled milk, food in hair, food on the floor. It seems much easier to feed the child.	The wise parent will promote the desire for independence. By offering as many choices as possible among desirable foods, the parent can help a child learn to make decisions and become independent. Children like finger foods such as raw vegetables and strips of fruit, meat in bite-size pieces, sandwiches in quarters. Thinking ahead, serving food in ways to reduce spillage, such as offering soup in a cup, rather than in a bowl with a spoon, can help to solve problem.

Adapted from C. G. Hussy and N. Kanoff. "Toddler and Preschool Nutrition." In *Maternal and Child Nutrition: Assessment and Counseling*, J. S. Slattery, G. A. Pearson, and C. T. Toue, eds. New York: Appleton-Century-Crofts, 1979, pp 11-12, as adapted from *Tots at the Table: A Food Guide for Use by Parents With Children from 1 to 5 Years*. National Livestock and Meat Board, 407 South Dearborn Street, Chicago, Illinois.

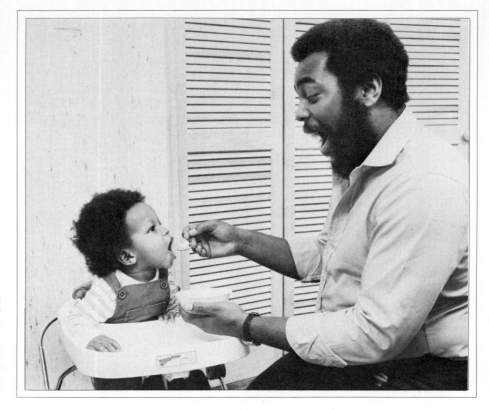

Parents influence the food habits of their children, not only through their own food choices but also through their attitudes toward child feeding. *(© Michal Heron 1980/Woodfin Camp & Assoc.)*

interest. Often these shifts parallel shifts in their rate of physical growth. Parents face the challenge of understanding their children's responses to food, including disinterest, while at the same time encouraging the development of sound food habits. Young children often go on food jags in which they will only eat certain foods for a period of time. For example, the child may want nothing but peanut butter and jelly sandwiches for lunch for weeks. This may be an attempt to establish a degree of independence or to attract attention.

In the 1920s, Dr. Clara Davis [19] studied the food habits of infants and young children who were allowed to choose their own foods. At each meal over a study period ranging from ½ to 4½ years the children were offered at each meal a tray of food containing 11 to 14 different foods. They were allower to eat as much as they wanted of any of the foods offered, but only highly nutritious foods such as meat, fish, cereal, milk, eggs, fruits, and vegetables were offered. Frequently, the children chose only a few specific foods for several days, then suddenly switched to a small number of different foods. The research showed that young children allowed to select their own diets tend to go on food "jags," eating large quantities of some foods for some time, but that preferences for foods changed. Because no sugar or other foods of low nutrient density were offered, this study *does not* support the conclusion that small children will eat what they need over a period of time or that they can select whatever foods their bodies need. Investigators could not ethically offer them foods having little nutritive value.

What advice can you offer a parent if the child refuses all but one or two foods? First, parents shouldn't panic. Rarely will the problem last for long. Offer the child a well-balanced diet, including foods that interest the child, such as finger foods or foods that are colorful or taste good to the child. Parents shouldn't make a big fuss if their child refuses these foods. Understanding that such jags are a normal part of the child development process, and that soon the child will outgrow this phase and accept a wider variety of foods is important. Often it is possible to slip in a food unnoticed by the child. For example, if a child will not accept milk but seems addicted to peanut butter, dried milk can be mixed with the peanut butter until the child again accepts milk as a beverage.

What types of foods do children prefer? Because they have acute senses of taste and smell, they usually prefer mildly seasoned foods. Thus, foods with a sharp taste, such as overcooked broccoli, acid fruits, and sharp cheeses should be introduced very gradually. Textures of foods must also be considered. Children often dislike foods that are lumpy, mushy, slimy, or stringy, and enjoy crunchy, chewy, crackly, and smooth foods.

Young children love to touch and feel their food. Not only food but anything that comes into contact with the fingers is likely to reach the toddler's mouth. This can include dirt, sand, toys, tools, and so forth. Offering the toddler finger foods such as a graham cracker, a piece of apple, a carrot stick, or a piece of mild cheese to experiment with can stimulate interest in foods. By the time the child is 18 months old or so, he or she can grasp a spoon and eat with it. Allowing the

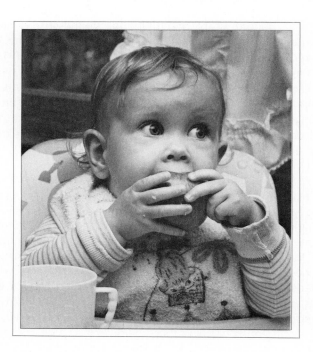

By the end of the first year, the child enjoys eating many foods without help. *(Erika Stone/Peter Arnold, Inc.)*

child freedom in feeding himself will probably promote an enjoyable eating experience as well as independent behavior.

Frequently, small children need to eat five or six small meals rather than three larger ones because of their limited stomach capacities. Snacks can help to provide needed nutrition. It is important to plan snacks carefully, offering foods such as cheese, fruit, and vegetables, rather than sweet or salty snacks.

Children love to experiment. Often they will imitate what they see parents, siblings, or the nursery school teacher do. Thus, it is extremely important to set a good example. The early years of childhood should set the stage for the development of sound food habits to carry on into the middle and later years of childhood.

PHYSICAL GROWTH AND DEVELOPMENT IN THE MIDDLE YEARS OF CHILDHOOD

The period from ages 6 to 12 is characterized by a slowing down of physical development. The school-aged child has reached a growth plateau between the early infancy growth spurt and the one that signals puberty. During this 6-year period, the child's weight doubles from an average of 40 to 80 lb. The average 6-year-old is about 3½ ft tall; the average 12-year-old is 5 ft tall. The average 6-to-12-year-old has a good appetite, and may eat rapidly and with gusto.

NUTRIENT REQUIREMENTS

During the middle years of childhood, youngsters engage in considerable physical activity and have high energy requirements. The RDA for energy for children 7 to 10 averages 2400 kcal, with a range of 1650 to 3300 kcal, depending upon physical activity and growth rate.

The RDA for protein for both sexes ages 7 to 10 years is 34 g (Appendix A). Although there is no official RDA for carbohydrate or fat, care should be taken to include generous amounts of complex carbohydrates with minimal amounts of refined carbohydrates. Thirty percent of total kilocalories from fat is a prudent level to aim for in dietary planning.

PSYCHOSOCIAL CHARACTERISTICS AND FOOD HABITS

During the middle years of childhood, the child's world greatly expands beyond the home. In early childhood, the family can rather easily control food patterns, but as the child starts school, teachers and friends exert increasingly strong influences on important aspects of the child's life, including food habits. Peer acceptance becomes very important and the child has a great need to feel she belongs and is accepted by classmates and friends. She learns that some foods are accepted by the group, and by adopting these foods she will feel more accepted herself. Some foods, such as those belonging to a certain culture, for example,

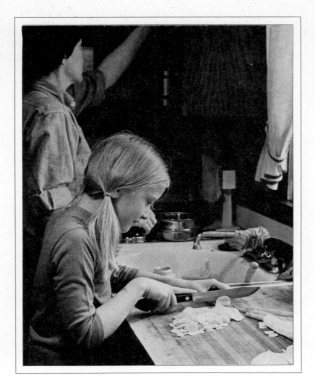

Children generally enjoy helping prepare meals and are more likely to try a new dish if they helped prepare it. *(© Ron Engh/Photo Researchers, Inc.)*

may be scorned by the group out of ignorance and, as a result, the child may refuse to accept these previously liked foods at home.

School-aged children typically eat four or five times a day, eating lunch, and possibly breakfast at school. They often snack after school, preferring to prepare these snacks themselves. The school-aged child often accepts an increasing number of foods, but may still reject many vegetables and foods such as casseroles and liver.

Why do some children like all kinds of food while others are picky eaters? Many factors influence a child's food preferences. Parents' knowledge of good nutrition, as well as their own food preferences greatly affect the child's knowledge of food, dietary habits, and consequently food preferences [20]. Methods of food preparation also affect children's food preferences. As previously mentioned, children tend to prefer simply prepared foods and may be more likely to eat vegetables if they are not mixed in casseroles or prepared with rich cream sauces.

Television advertising exerts an important influence on children's food preferences. Most television advertising aimed at children is for food. Cereals lead all other types of food advertised; presweetened cereals are most heavily promoted. Candy, gum, and snack foods are also frequently advertised. Rarely is attention paid to vegetables, milk (with the exception of sweet things to add to milk), meat, or fruit. Advertisements for crunchy, chocolate flavored, crackly,

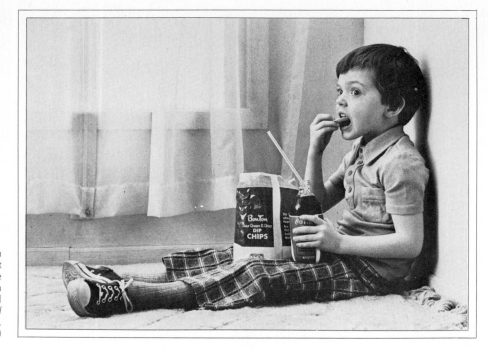

Routine snacking on foods of low nutrient density, often those advertised on TV, can rob the child of needed nutrients. (© 1982 Ed Lettau/Photo Researchers, Inc.)

sweet, sticky foods influence a child's preference for non-nutritious foods. As a result, children often ask their parents to buy these foods, and they often comply.

Children change their food likes and dislikes frequently during their middle years. Often they look up to their parents and teachers as authorities on many things, including what is nutritious food. Parents and teachers can thus become important nutrition educators, and can influence positive food habits by example. Children should be encouraged to experiment with new foods, to engage in food preparation, and to help plan menus.

While few U.S. children demonstrate clinical nutritional deficiency, some children evidence problems which may be related to diet. An increasingly publicized problem affecting many children is hyperactivity. The possible relationship between diet and hyperactivity is discussed in Box 15-2.

PHYSICAL GROWTH AND DEVELOPMENT IN ADOLESCENCE

Adolescence is that period of time bridging childhood and adulthood. The word adolescence, from the Latin word meaning "to grow into maturity," covers, roughly, the years from 12 or 13 to 20. Adolescents begin to take on an appearance different from that of children as their bodies develop due to hormonal changes. They think differently than they did as children, and their feelings about almost everything change. Since adolescence is the period in

Diet and Hyperactivity

According to some estimates, as many as 20 percent of U.S. children may be hyperactive, but others suggest that a much smaller number have this disorder. One of the difficulties in establishing a precise percentage stems from the fact that we don't have precise criteria by which to diagnose the syndrome. Basically, hyperactivity is neither a disease nor an emotional disorder. Both *hyperactivity* and *hyperkinesis* are used to describe a behavioral pattern characterized by abnormally increased activity, short attention span, excessive and purposeless activity, irrational actions, hostility, destructiveness, inability to get along well with others, and difficulty in sleeping. Hyperactivity appears to affect boys about six times as often as it does girls.

The most frequently used treatment in the past has been drugs which help hyperactive children calm down, focus their attention, and concentrate better. These drugs are not always successful, however, in helping children improve their performance in school. Even when they are helpful, risks must be considered. Of concern is the fact that the drugs diminish the appetite and consequently slow the growth rate of children. Furthermore, the long-term effects of these drugs on personality development of children is unknown. Because of these and other unanswered questions about drug use in cases of hyperactivity, many parents of hyperactive children are reluctant to have their children treated with drugs.

Little wonder, then, that parents of hyperactive children responded with great enthusiasm to a book published in the early 1970s by a California physician, Dr. Benjamin Feingold, called *Why Your Child Is Hyperactive* [21]. Dr. Feingold believed, on the basis of clinical observations he made on patients, that hyperactivity is due to a sensitivity to artificial food dyes and flavoring agents, to BHA and BHT (food preservatives), and in some cases to salicylates in aspirin or in certain fruits (such as tomatoes, apples, oranges, peaches, and grapes). As a result of Feingold's book and his frequent public appearances, Feingold Associations sprang up throughout the country to help parents learn how to rid the diet of the substances that, according to Feingold's hypothesis, were the cause of hyperactivity.

Dr. Feingold realized, however, that carefully executed studies were required to substantiate his hypothesis, studies he had been unable to perform on his own. Many parents reported that their children's behavior improved when on the diet, but scientists pointed out that these observations were largely subjective. Most children receive an increased amount of attention when they are on the diet, since generally the entire family diet changes and the family works together to prepare the food. This unaccustomed attention may account in part for improved behavior. Furthermore, just the knowledge on the part of child and parents that "something is being done to help" could account for improved behavior.

Scientists consequently set out to study whether or not the diet does, in fact, improve the behavior of at least 50 percent of hyperactive children, as Feingold claimed. Two types of studies have been conducted. In one, researchers put a group of hyperactive children on the diet and then studied their behavior over a period of time. At the same time, a second group of hyperactive children (the control group) continued to eat their usual diet, while their behavior was examined in the same way as the first group.

In the second type of study, children were put on the Feingold diet, and then were given foods or concentrates of food additives which were thought to be the offending ones to see if these resulted in a return of the symptoms of hyperactivity. A second group (or sometimes the same group at a different time) followed the same procedure, but a placebo was given in place of the test food or concentrate. The placebo looked, tasted, and smelled like the test substance, but did not contain the additives. This kind of study, called a challenge study, prevented the children or their parents or teachers from knowing exactly when the food additives were given to the child. This technique results in greater objectivity in observations of the child's behavior, as discussed in Chapter 5.

In both kinds of studies, the results have proved similar. The hyperactive children really fared no better on the Feingold diet than they did after eating foods containing artificial flavors and colors. Researchers now conclude that a very small percentage (1 or 2 percent) of very young hyperactive children appear to be sensitive to the substances Feingold believed to cause hyperactivity.

Investigators do not believe, however, that parents should be discouraged from following the Feingold diet. The diet may be a better balanced, more nutritious diet than families consumed previously, particularly if fruits are not excluded. Furthermore, family cohesiveness around the hyperactive child may be a great benefit for all. In the meantime, further research should help us gain insights into possible interactions among artificial flavors, colors, and preservatives and their combined effects on behavior.

which identity as an adult is established, this task is accompanied by evolving value orientations, by changing emotions as well as by physiological development, all of which affect nutritional status and food behavior.

During the period of rapid growth, sometimes referred to as the adolescent growth spurt, gains in height are more rapid than at any period since infancy. Teenagers may grow 4 or 5 in in 1 year. This growth usually occurs earlier in girls than in boys. On the average, girls begin puberty and experience the adolescent growth spurt between the ages of 8 to 10 years and reach maximal growth rates at about 12 years of age. Boys experience it between the ages of 12½ to 15½, with the greatest growth rate occurring about the age of 14. An average of 15 percent of adult height and approximately 48 percent of adult skeletal mass is attained during the adolescent growth period [22].

Growth in height is not the only evidence of physical development. Other significant changes occur in the reproductive organs as hormones signal the transition from childhood to adulthood. Both males and females gain an appreciable amount of weight during adolescence but the rate, the amount, and the different types of tissue gained vary between boys and girls.

Boys gain weight at a faster rate than do girls. They tend to increase muscle mass while their total body fat actually decreases. Girls increase both the amount of muscle and adipose tissue. On the average, by the age of 20, girls generally have twice the amount of total adipose tissue as boys, and about two-thirds as much lean body tissue [22]. These differences account for differences in protein and energy requirements between boys and girls during adolescence.

NUTRIENT REQUIREMENTS

Kilocalories

Nutrient requirements of adolescents closely follow physiological changes. Kilocalorie requirements are high because of rapid growth. During the adolescent growth spurt, appetites often greatly increase. The reference to a child as a "bottomless pit" or the saying that the teenager has a "hollow leg" attests to the large food intakes of teenagers. There is a considerable difference in the kilocalorie needs of boys and girls during the adolescent period. Girls require an average daily kilocalorie intake of 2100 or 2200, with a range of 1500 to 3000, while boys need about 2700 to 2800, with a range of 2000 to 3900. Actual needs vary with rate of growth and amount of physical activity.

Protein

Through childhood as well as adolescence, protein allowances are approximately 12 to 14 percent of total energy intake. As energy requirements increase to support the growth spurt, so do protein needs. Since protein is known to be important in supporting growth, adequate protein intakes during adolescence should be maintained. The RDAs for adolescence are given in Appendix A. During the growth spurt itself, the RDA is about 1 g per kilogram of body weight. While this is lower than the 2.2 g per kilogram of protein recommended for the infant or the slightly more than 1 g per kilogram of protein suggested for school-aged children, it is more than the 0.8 g per kilogram recommended for the adult.

Minerals and Vitamins

The minerals of greatest concern during adolescence are calcium, zinc, and iron, as these are more often limited in the adolescent diet than others. Needs for these nutrients parallel the adolescent growth spurt. Calcium is needed for skeletal development, iron for the increase in muscle mass and blood volume, and zinc for the increase in skeletal and muscle tissue.

The calcium recommendation for both boys and girls is 1200 mg/day until the age of 18, then 800 mg thereafter (Appendix A). To meet this high level large amounts of milk are usually required; as many as four cups a day may be needed. Boys are usually more likely to consume the types of foods that meet this requirement than girls [23]. Surveys show that perhaps half of all adolescent girls consume less than 70 percent of the RDA for calcium [22].

Requirements for iron vary considerably during the years from 10 to 20. Each kilogram of fat-free body weight contains a significant amount of iron—thus, increased weight of lean tissue during adolescence explains some of the increased iron need. Increases in blood volume and hemoglobin during this period of life also contribute significantly to the increased need for iron [24]. Low iron intakes are reflected in the large incidence of iron-deficiency anemia among teenage boys and girls. Both the Ten State Survey and HANES identified anemia among adolescents. Boys increase the number of red blood cells, expand their blood volume, and increase muscle mass to a greater extent than do girls, and thus require large iron intakes [25]. However, once menstruation begins, girls also have high iron requirements. Thus the RDA for both adolescent boys and girls is 18 mg/day. The Ten State Survey reported that intakes of iron were lower than for any other nutrient relative to the RDA. More than 80 percent of adolescent females consumed less than 18 mg/day. It is difficult to achieve this high iron intake on the average American diet. Teenagers should be encouraged to consume iron-rich foods such as iron-fortified breads and cereals, dried fruits, red meats, and leafy green vegetables.

Zinc is essential for growth as well as for sexual maturity of young adults. Severe lack of zinc has been shown to cause anemia, dwarfing, and lack of maturity of sexual organs. Even mild zinc deficiency may delay sexual maturation and retard growth. Foods rich in zinc include meats, eggs, seafood, and whole-grain cereal products. The RDA for both adolescent boys and girls is 15 mg/day (Appendix A).

Common adolescent nutrition-related problems include dental caries, obesity, and iron-deficiency anemia. Other problems identified in surveys of the nutritional status of adolescents include low intakes of vitamins A and C [26,27].

The HANES found that, for all age groups studied, youngsters aged 10 to 16 had the greatest incidence of unsatisfactory nutritional status. Average kilocalorie intakes of boys and girls in all income groups were low, as were average iron intakes. Findings from the Ten State Survey were similar.

PSYCHOSOCIAL CHARACTERISTICS AND FOOD HABITS

Most adolescents experience a growing sense of independence which often affects their eating habits. During adolescence, the individual begins to feel that adult privileges and rights are due, but are not granted; the adolescent period ends when society accords full responsibility and social status to the new adult. This view of adolescence can shed some light on factors that often influence the teenager's eating habits. As teenagers attempt to establish their independence, their attitudes, behavior, and interests change. They often attempt to express their increasing desire for independence from their parents and other adults in ways that may promote poor food habits. For example, they may refuse to eat meals prepared at home by Mom. Moreover, they may reject all advice on the need for a balanced diet and instead develop eating patterns which fully contradict what those in authority suggest should be eaten. Peers' food preferences are often adopted and much preferred over those of one's family, since adolescents generally are dependent on peer-group acceptance, standards, and values. Peer-group conformity is the rule and this extends to tastes in foods and food habits. As a result, unusual or bizarre food habits may result. Crash diets, missed meals, and unusual food preferences are not uncommon during the adolescence years.

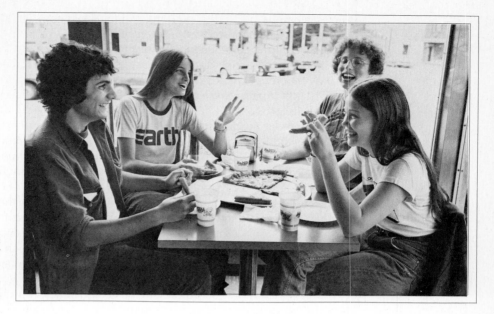

Teenagers enjoying a
snack in one of their
favorite places, a
fast-food restaurant.
*(Sybil
Shelton/Monkmeyer)*

A common stereotype about college students and their eating habits suggests that students are so involved in their studies or with extracurricular activities and that they are on such limited budgets that they have neither the time nor the money to plan and eat adequate diets. Is this true? Are college students especially poorly nourished? One group of investigators studied 195 college women in an attempt to answer this question [28]. Results showed that mean intakes of the group for all nutrients studied met or exceeded the RDAs except for energy, thiamine, and iron. About one-third of the group took nutrient supplements. There were a few very low intakes of nutrients. There seemed to be no relationship between the money spent on food and nutritional adequacy. Also, living in a dormitory did not appear to affect dietary adequacy.

Research indicates that perhaps one-quarter of American adolescents skip breakfast. What is the nutritional importance of breakfast in the total adolescent diet? Adolescents who eat breakfast generally have more adequate total daily nutrient intakes than those who do not. The other meals do not seem to make up for nutrients missed at breakfast [29].

Snacking is another common adolescent food habit. Most adolescents snack at least once a day [30]. Foods most often eaten as snacks include carbonated beverages, milk, candy, fruit, and ice cream. Snacks may contribute almost one-fifth of total daily nutrient intake for adolescents [31], and undoubtedly could provide more if they were always well chosen.

Concerns about physical appearance often have a significant influence on food habits. Generally speaking, boys want to be tall, muscular, and broad-shouldered, while girls want to be slim and sleek, but bosomy. Because adolescent self-concepts are greatly related to how attractive they feel, those who consider themselves attractive are likely to be happier and have more self-esteem even into adulthood. To this end, many adolescent girls diet to extreme and may fall victim to anorexia nervosa (Chapter 8).

Most teenagers are healthy; the greatest health threats in this age group result from those they inflict upon themselves. The principal causes of death for 15-to-24-year-olds are accidents, murder, and suicide [18]. Other health threats that are not usually immediately fatal include drug and alcohol abuse, and venereal disease.

Throughout history, humans have tried to alleviate physical and emotional discomfort through drugs. Although drug use is common among adolescents, a 1980 survey of 17,000 teens showed a slight decline in the number who said they had tried marijuana, as well as inhalants, barbiturates, tranquilizers, and hallucinogens such as PCP (phenocyclidine hydrochloride). The use of cocaine, heroin, and LSD had apparently stabilized [32]. Some of these drugs, such as marijuana, stimulate the appetite, so that for those who use them often, obesity may develop. The problem is compounded since the drug user may have decreased control over his or her actions. Other drugs, such as amphetamines, and narcotics such as morphine, heroin, and codeine, may cause loss of appetite with a resulting decreased food intake.

Alcohol, the most abused drug in the United States, is used to some extent by most adolescents. According to nationwide surveys by the National Institute on Alcohol Abuse and Alcoholism (NIAAA), nine out of ten high school students drink; more than one in four have at least one drink a week [33]. While many adolescents drink rarely and have no problem, some youths cannot handle alcohol and get into trouble with school authorities, friends, or police. Heavy use of alcohol may adversely affect nutritional status; as a large proportion of kilocalories comes from alcohol, food and nutrient intake may decline. In addition, alcohol increases the excretion of some nutrients from the body, decreases the absorption of others, and can damage body tissues, including the liver (see Chapter 13).

Complexion Problems and Diet

Skin blemishes and acne are common and upsetting problems for many adolescents. In an attempt to correct complexion problems, teenagers may change their diet in an unhealthful way. For instance, they may stop drinking milk, believing milk is the cause of the skin problem.

Most adolescents experience some acne between the ages of 16 and 20 [22]. Complexion problems are common during adolescence because the hormones which control the skin glands' production of oil become very active during the teen years and often cause oily skin, blackheads, and acne. Stress and emotional upsets may contribute to the problem. While a balanced diet is important for healthy skin, a poor diet is not usually the cause of teenage acne. A common myth holds that certain foods such as chocolate and greasy foods cause acne, but recent research fails to confirm such a relationship [1].

Food allergies may play a role in causing acne, however. In such instances, the offending food should be eliminated. Box 15-3 discusses food allergies in greater detail. Vitamin A and zinc sulfate in large doses may sometimes be helpful

Food Allergies

Food allergies can cause much discomfort and in some cases are dangerous. There are two different kinds of food allergy: the immediate and the delayed. The immediate reaction, which constitutes about 5 percent of food allergies, occurs within 4 h of exposure to the offending food; it is very intense and may be fatal. In contrast, the delayed reaction occurs up to 72 h after exposure to food; it is less intense than the immediate reaction, is rarely fatal, and is due to an allergic reaction to the digestive products of the offending food.

While a variety of foods can cause allergies in different people, the most common offenders include eggs, milk, and wheat, followed by corn, chocolate, nuts, and fish. Other foods to which some people are allergic include citrus fruits, strawberries, and tomatoes.

What causes food allergies? Usually genetic factors are involved. Children whose parents have allergies are more likely to develop them than those whose parents have none.

How are food allergies identified? Determining the cause of an allergy is often a long and frustrating process. Usually it is necessary to keep a careful history of foods eaten, the times foods are eaten, and the times any unusu-

al symptoms occur. It may be possible to observe a relationship between the cause and the reaction from this history.

Frequently an elimination diet is necessary. This involves eliminating a group of foods for a period of time, often a week. If the symptoms of food allergy disappear, then foods are added back, one at a time, to identify the offending foods.

Skin tests, in which the surface of the skin is scratched and extracts of possible offending foods are placed onto the scratches to observe a reaction, are not accurate in diagnosing food allergies.

Treatment How are food allergies best treated? At present the best treatment is avoiding the offending food. If the offending foods are common ones such as eggs, milk, or wheat this may present a problem. It is very difficult to buy prepared foods free of wheat, eggs, and milk. The next time you shop for food, examine food labels. What kind of a varied diet is possible avoiding these foods? Such a diet would have to consist primarily of minimally processed foods, with breads and cereals being prepared according to special recipes.

in treating acne. Lower levels of tissue zinc and serum vitamin A have been found in some patients suffering from acne [34] (see Box 11-1, Chapter 11).

FOOD PROGRAMS FOR CHILDREN AND ADOLESCENTS

Recognizing the special nutritional needs of infants and children, the federal government sponsors a variety of food and nutrition programs that aim to improve the nutrition of eligible young people. These programs may be aimed at the individual, or the entire family.

Table 15-7 summarizes some of the most important of these programs that are

TABLE 15-7. CHILD NUTRITION PROGRAMS. A NUMBER OF FEDERALLY FUNDED FOOD PROGRAMS CAN HELP PROVIDE FOOD AND NUTRITION TO ELIGIBLE YOUNGSTERS.

NAME OF PROGRAM	BRIEF DESCRIPTION
Food stamp	Varying amounts of coupons exchangeable for nonimported foodstuffs. Value of coupons issued depends upon household income.
Women, Infants and Children (WIC)	Distribution of special foods to pregnant and lactating women and small children who are nutritionally at risk. Foods include milk, infant formula, iron-fortified cereal, fruit juice, dairy products, and eggs.
School lunch	Purpose is to provide nutritionally adequate lunches and to educate children during the formative years about good food practices.
School breakfast	Cash assistance is provided for breakfasts in schools drawing attendance from low-income areas.
Head Start	Comprehensive educational-nutritional services are provided for poor children below compulsory school attendance ages.

designed to improve the nutritional status of infants, children, teenagers, or their families. Meeting nutrient needs throughout the life cycle is a complex process. Physical needs, social relationships, and psychological factors all have a bearing on nutritional status. While nutrition is important throughout life, infants, children, and adolescents have unique requirements because they are growing and developing so rapidly.

There is still much we don't know about nutritional requirements. Most of the available information relates nutrient needs to chronological age. But each person has individual needs and is at a unique developmental stage at a given age. More research is needed to relate nutritional needs to growth and developmental stages throughout childhood and adolescence.

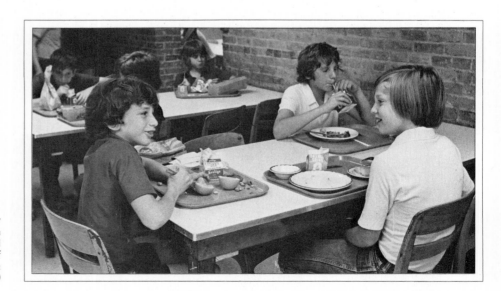

An orderly and friendly atmosphere along with well-prepared food enhances acceptance of the school lunch. *(Erika Stone/Peter Arnold, Inc.)*

SUMMARY

1 The growth process is very complex; processes of growth and differences in the rate of development lead to differences in nutritional needs.

2 During a critical growth period, malnutrition may have irreversible harmful effects.

3 Energy and protein needs of the infant are much higher per unit of body weight than they are for the older child or adult.

4 Breast-feeding is, in most cases, the preferable infant feeding method. Advantages of breast milk include the fact that its nutrient supply is tailor-made to the needs of the human infant, it has important anti-infective properties, and it can facilitate a favorable emotional climate between infant and mother. However, a child can also grow and thrive on appropriate bottle-feeding.

5 The age of weaning varies from infant to infant, but the majority of infants begin to consume some solid food by 5 months and to drink from a cup by 9 months. The introduction of solid food is best delayed until the baby weighs 6 to 7 kg, and should not occur before the baby is 3 months old.

6 During the middle years of childhood, peer pressures exert an increasingly stronger influence on food habits. Other factors affecting dietary intake include food preparation methods, parents' likes and dislikes, television advertising, and education and examples set by teachers relative to food and nutrition.

7 Rapid growth and physiological development during adolescence parallel high nutrient needs.

8 Many adolescents desire growing independence from parental and school authority and are quite dependent on peer-group influences. This may adversely affect their diets; unusual food habits, crash diets, and missed meals are not uncommon during adolescence.

FOR DISCUSSION AND APPLICATION

1 Foods of low nutrient density and vending machines often seem to go hand in hand. Conduct a mini-survey of the contents of vending machines in five different locations. What foods are commonly offered? Which selections are most frequently sold out? Question 10 people who use these machines to see if they would appreciate a greater selection of more nutritious foods. What foods would you suggest vending purveyors sell? How might you get them to put more nutritious foods into vending machines?

2 Some high school students feel they should be free to eat what they want—and their food preferences usually include confections and salty snacks. Visit a local high school and observe students at lunch. Are they purchasing a school lunch, or bringing their own? Are there facilities on the school grounds for purchasing candy? How do the packed lunches compare with the school lunches? What foods are commonly thrown away? What suggestions would you offer these adolescents for improving their diets?

3 Prepare homemade baby food—be sure to avoid the use of salt, sugar, and spices. Compare your products with commercial products. Which are most nutritious? Which are most expensive? Most convenient? Most appealing? How do they compare in flavor and texture?

SUGGESTED READINGS

Pipes, P., *Nutrition in Infancy and Childhood*, 2d ed., St. Louis: The C. V. Mosby Co., 1981. This is a good reference book on nutrition in infants and children.

Wanemaker, N., K. Hearn, and S. Richary, *More Than Graham Crackers: Nutrition Education and Food Preparation with Young Children*, Washington, D.C.: National Association for the Education of Young Children, 1979. This is a compilation of recipes, activities, and nutrition information. It makes suggestions for involving children in food preparation.

Goodwin, M. T., and G. Pollen, *Creative Food Experiences for Children*, from Center for Science in the Public Interest, 1955 South Street, N.W., Washington, D.C., 20009, rev. 1980. A fascinating collection of recipes, games, and ideas about food and nutrition for children. It also includes resources and teaching materials.

What's to Eat? And Other Questions Kids Ask About Food, U.S. Department of Agriculture, 1979. This 1979 Yearbook of Agriculture covers all aspects of food production, marketing, and nutrition. It includes activities for upper elementary school children.

Infant Nutrition and Feeding, Berkeley, Calif.: Society for Nutrition Education, 1980. An annotated bibliography of books, articles, and audiovisual materals pertaining to infant nutrition.

Endres, Jeannette B., and R. E. Rockwell, *Food, Nutrition, and the Young Child*, St. Louis: The C. V. Mosby Co., 1980. A paperback book covering aspects of feeding infants and small children including group feeding programs.

Cohen, Stanley A., *Healthy Babies, Happy Kids*, New York: Delilah Books, 1982. A paperback book by a physician providing commonsense guidance for feeding infants and small children.

16

THE LATER YEARS

Given reasonably good health and income, the older person has reached a point when he or she is free to set the life-pattern desired. You probably know older people who are active and energetic. The following headlines clipped from *The New York Times* and *The Chicago Sun-Times* give you an idea of the number of older people who continue to pursue education [1]:

> Ft. Myers, Florida: "Florida businessman, 57, starts work on a law degree."
> Brooklyn, N.Y.: "Life begins at 75." (This is the story of a freshman enrollee at Kingsborough Community College.)
> Salt Lake City: "New co-ed, 82."
> Fresno, California: "Woman, 81, seeking a college degree."

Many older people are active and successful well into their seventies and eighties. You are probably familiar with many in the art world who have remained active into old age. Aaron Copland, one of America's foremost composers, continued to conduct symphony concerts after his eightieth birthday. Lena Horne was a smash hit on Broadway after she reached sixty-five. Dumas Malone, one of America's most distinguished historians, published the last of his six-volume biography of Thomas Jefferson when he was almost 90. Robert Penn Warren, author of *All The King's Men*, a Pulitzer Prize-winning poet and novelist, continued to write when he was close to 80 [2]. Alberta Hunter, a singer, and a former nurse who was forced to retire because of "old age," is 88 at this writing and continues to sing four nights a week at a Greenwich Village nightspot. Eubie Blake, composer and pianist, continued to perform until he was almost 100. Although those in the arts are more likely to be "household names," they by no means exhaust the career options of older people. Jack Dempsey, former heavyweight boxing champion, was a successful restauranteur until his recent death at 87. Representative Claude Pepper, at 83 the oldest member of the United States Congress, is a member of the House Select Committee on Aging and president of the U.S. 98th Congress group of officers to the Interparliamentary Union which was founded in 1889 to promote personal contacts among members of the world's parliaments.

There are many myths about old age. A frequent misconception is that *all* older individuals experience serious degenerative diseases, are senile and confused, and hence, doomed to a tragic existence. However, as Maggie Kuhn, founder of the Gray Panthers and author of the material in Box 16-1 points out, this need not be the case [3].

At all phases throughout the life cycle, individuals have unique nutrient needs, and the later years are no exception. Older individuals also experience different situations which may influence their food habits; frequently their social and economic status changes somewhat and this in turn may affect their diets. An understanding of the special needs of older people can underline the importance of proper nutrition throughout life. This is the focus of the present chapter.

Experts in *gerontology* (the study of aging) view the aging process as a lifelong experience that begins at birth. By understanding nutritional needs at various stages of development, one may gain a perspective of the interrelated nature of these needs throughout the life span. The study of nutrition in older people is important, not only as a means to discover ways to improve their health and the overall quality of their lives, but also as a possible way to slow down or alter the process of aging.

AMERICA'S FASTEST-GROWING MINORITY

America's elderly, generally considered to be those over 65, have been called our "fastest-growing minority." The elderly population is growing much faster than the general U.S. population, and if current Census Bureau projections are correct, the elderly population will continue to grow much faster than the total population into the twenty-first century. Between 1985 and 2010 the over-65-year-old population is expected to increase from 27 to 34 million individuals. The total

This is indeed a New Age—an age of liberation and self-determination. I'm glad to have reached seniority at this time. I feel free to speak out and act in ways that I was not able to when I was younger. I'm seventy-three years old, and I haven't dyed my hair and I can't afford a face lift. I enjoy my wrinkles and regard them as badges of distinction—I've worked hard for them!

I guess that when I think about it, there are three things in particular that I like about getting old. First, you can speak your mind, as I certainly try to do—but you have to do your homework first; otherwise you'll quickly be dismissed as a doddering old fool. The second thing I have liked about getting old is that I have successfully outlived a great deal of my opposition: many of the people who were my detractors before are not around anymore! And then the third thing I've especially liked about getting old is that it's really kind of a miracle to be able to tap into the incredible energy of the young, while making use of the knowledge and experience that comes after living a long, full life. Having the power and energy of these two worlds is an enormously vitalizing and inspiring experience.

I think of age as a great universalizing force. It's the one thing that we all have in common. It doesn't begin when you collect your social security benefits. Aging begins with the moment of birth, and it ends only when life itself has ended. Life is a continuum; only, we—in our stupidity and blindness—have chopped it up into little pieces and kept all those little pieces separate. I feel that the goal of successful aging is to keep on growing and learning and becoming a mature, responsible adult.

Old age is not a disease—it is strength and survivorship, triumph over all kinds of vicissitudes and disappointments, trials and illnesses.

Source: Reprinted by permission of Margaret E. Kuhn.

population is expected to increase from 228 million to 250 million [4]. The 1980 census noted that the number of elderly 85 and older increased by 56.6 percent in the last 10 years.

Although the average number of years a newborn American infant can expect to live has increased by about 26 years since 1908, this improvement is due primarily to success in controlling diseases and disorders that formerly led to death in infancy and early childhood. There has been no increase, however, in the maximum length of life during the twentieth century. To illustrate this, consider how long many of our U.S. presidents lived: George Washington lived to the age of 67, John Adams to 91, Thomas Jefferson to 83, James Madison to 85, James Monroe to 73, and John Quincy Adams to 81. While the average life expectancy for people at age 60 has not greatly increased, many more people now live to this age [5]. As our control of bacterial and infectious diseases has allowed more infants to reach adulthood, the death rate from other diseases such as cancer and heart disease has increased.

THEORIES OF AGING

Despite innumerable attempts to solve the riddles of aging, the process remains a mystery. There are many hypotheses, but these have often been based on limited information, and none can answer all our queries about aging. We now realize that the aging process is probably the result of many different factors operating together.

Almost every theory of aging is based on changes in cells and molecules that take place over time. These theories can be broadly classified into two groups. The first holds that we age because we are genetically programmed to do so. The second contends that aging occurs because the body is gradually damaged until it finally ages and dies.

Genetic Theories

The "genetic clock" theory holds that our cells are pre-programmed to divide for just so long; after that time they simply fail to divide as they did in younger years. One writer has suggested that this process is similar to photocopying, in which copies are made from other copies—after awhile the copies are merely blurred images of the original [6]. If genetic factors do, in fact, determine how we age, an individual has a better chance of living a long life if his or her ancestors were long-lived.

There may be some type of a "biologic clock" which determines the time at which body cells self-destruct. The genetic material (DNA) may not contain a schedule for aging, but may simply deteriorate with time, losing accurate genetic information. The biologic clock, in other words, gradually slows down. This may lead to the synthesis of abnormal protein molecules that impair normal body functioning [7].

Cross-Linking of Collagen Molecules

Some researchers believe that the most important factor in aging is the cross-linking of molecules of *collagen*, the protein present in bones, tendons, and connective tissue. Cross-linking results in the formation of huge protein molecules that enzyme systems cannot metabolize. These abnormally large proteins may then accumulate in cells, and eventually promote hypertension, impaired passage of gases, nutrients, antibodies, and other metabolites, as well as toxins that could explain increased susceptibility to illness and injury [8].

Immunological Breakdown

Aging may also be part of a breakdown in the immunological capacities of the body. The normal individual produces antibodies which are proteins manufactured by cells to protect against bacteria, viruses, and other hazardous substances. According to this theory, antibody synthesis is impaired with aging; consequently, natural and desirable substances in the cells are attacked by antibodies and destroyed, and aging results [7].

Free Radical Theory

The *free radical* theory of aging suggests that free radicals, which are highly reactive, unstable components of cells, can change other essential molecules, causing cellular dysfunctions that accumulate during the life span. Free radical reactions may be especially damaging if they destroy polyunsaturated fatty acids in the membranes of cells, resulting in the deterioration of lipids, collagen, and other substances in the body. These membrane changes may alter the ease of entry of nutrients into or out of cells and eventually result in increased cell death, a process associated with aging [7].

Vitamin E is of interest here. Some investigators hypothesize that Vitamin E, because of its properties as an antioxidant, provides protection against excessive oxidation of lipids in the cell. Those who support this theory stress the importance of including adequate vitamin E in the diet, especially when large amounts of polyunsaturated fatty acids are consumed (see Chapter 11). Vitamin C acts in concert with vitamin E in its antioxidant role and may also play a role as a trap for free radicals. Both vitamin E and vitamin C deserve further study in relation to this theory [7].

Whether or not large intakes of either vitamin E or vitamin C can prevent any aspect of aging is not known at present. So far, animal experiments indicate that large doses of these vitamins do not prevent aging.

Environmental Factors

Environmental factors may also contribute to the aging process. One's diet, lifestyle, degree of stress, and physical exercise may all influence aging. Much research currently centers around the relationship between diet and the aging process. Early studies at Cornell University indicated that feeding young rats a reduced kilocalorie but nutritious diet resulted in an increased life span [9]. Followup studies have found that diet can affect the onset of some age-related illnesses in rats [8,10]. Diet appears to be a factor in the development of some of the degenerative diseases such as cancer and heart disease that often accompany old age (see Chapter 5).

Regular habits of caring for one's health contribute to longer lives. These include controlling one's weight, getting regular exercise, having regular meals, including breakfast, avoiding smoking, and consuming alcohol only in moderation (see Introduction).

Box 16-2 discusses some of the claims made in popular books and articles about people who reportedly live to well beyond 100 years of age.

NUTRITIONAL NEEDS OF THE OLDER PERSON

In general, the nutrient needs of the healthy older person do not greatly differ from those of the healthy younger adult. However, kilocalorie requirements decrease. Moreover, the many physiological changes that occur with aging may significantly increase certain nutrient requirements for a given individual, and may signal

NUTRITION IN THE NEWS

EATING LESS MAY BE THE KEY TO LIVING BEYOND 100 YEARS

Jane E. Brody, *The New York Times*, June 8, 1982

In searching for ways to extend the human life span and to ward off the diseases of old age, some scientists find themselves focusing not on enhancing diet but rather on limiting it.

Their approach grows out of increasingly convincing evidence that longevity can be significantly increased by "undernutrition"—a diet that contains all the required nutrients but about a third fewer calories than are needed to maintain "normal" body weight.

Eating less, their animal studies indicate, can add the human equivalent of 40 years to a mammal's life. It can also delay age-related declines in immune responses and diminish the risk of developing diseases associated with aging such as heart ailments, cancer, kidney disease and arthritis. Instead of becoming ill, many of the animals on restricted diets eventually simply die of old age. . . .

According to recent studies, merely reducing the protein content of the diet without lowering calories may be an effective technique to delay aging. Dr. Edward J. Masoro, chairman of the department of physiology at the University of Texas Health Sciences Center at San Antonio, showed that cutting protein intake in half significantly lengthened the lives of laboratory rats, though not as much as when their calorie intake was reduced to 60 percent of normal.

Furthermore, Dr. Masoro and Dr. Roy Walford have recently shown that the benefits of "undernutrition without malnutrition" apparently can be reaped even if food restriction does not begin until middle age. Dr. Walford, a pathologist and expert on aging at the School of Medicine at the University of California at Los Angeles, reported earlier this year that reduction of food intake starting in "middle age" in two long-lived species of mice resulted in a 10 to 20 percent increase in the animal's life span.

Dr. Walford's earlier studies showed that feeding mice from birth a diet containing 60 percent of the usual calories delayed the age-related decline in the animals' ability to ward off infections and reject foreign tissues. The restricted diet also delayed the appearance of immunological "errors"—autoimmune disorders in which the body attacks itself.

Studies in mice conducted at Memorial Sloan-Kettering Cancer Center in New York by Dr. Gabriel Fernandes, an immunologist who has just moved to the University of Texas, where he will collaborate with Dr. Masoro, showed that lowering the fat composition of the diet had reduced the animals' risk of developing immunological deficiency diseases and cancer. When the same strain of mice was placed on a low-protein diet, age-related declines in immune responses were inhibited. . . .

"Long-term undernutrition is thus far the only method we know of that retards aging and extends the maximum life span of warm-blooded animals," Dr. Walford said in a telephone interview. "The finding is undoubtedly applicable to humans because it works in every animal species thus far studied."

According to Dr. Masoro, "If we can manipulate aging in the rat by nutrition, we probably can do it in any mammal." . . .

Dr. Masoro emphasized that he was not advocating malnutrition as a means of extending life. "Our animals are not malnourished—their diets are not below the recommended limits for any food substance. Our studies do not mean that cuts should be made in Government feeding programs." . . .

ASK YOURSELF:

Why aren't human studies conducted in a manner similar to the animal studies described here? What appears to be the ideal "longevity" diet? Is this one that might be recommended for humans? What are the practical applications for this type of research? Do you think that readers could misinterpret this news story? Why do you think these researchers felt it necessary to make a statement that their studies did not justify cuts in government food programs?

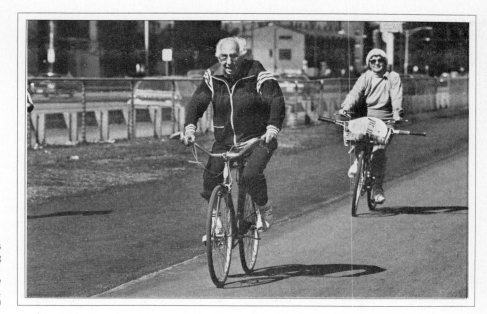

Exercise throughout life is important for maintaining good health. *(© Jean-Claude Lejeune/Stock, Boston, Inc.)*

the need to increase the quantity of certain nutrients to maintain optimal nutritional status.

The Recommended Dietary Allowances [13] are often the guidelines used in discussing the nutritional needs of the elderly. They were intended to be guidelines for sound nutrition, but they were designed for groups of healthy Americans. Because many older persons have chronic illnesses, their nutrient needs under these circumstances are not considered within the framework of the RDAs. This does not mean that the RDAs should be rejected in terms of planning diets for healthy elderly people, but they are not meant to apply to groups of older persons with diseases. It is important to consider the older person's specific health status in relation to his or her nutrient needs.

Kilocalories

With aging there is a decrease in basal metabolic rate (BMR), and hence a reduced need for kilocalories. The gradually declining BMR characteristic of older people is due to a decrease in lean body mass, chiefly muscle and organ tissues. The healthy 20-year-old is very different from the healthy 70-year-old in body composition. With age, an increased proportion of the body weight is adipose tissue, and a lesser proportion is lean body mass. There is also a tendency for older people in this country to reduce their physical activity, due to our sedentary lifestyle. Exercise and sports can increase muscle mass and bone mass in elderly people [14]. Regular exercise throughout one's life is therefore recommended by most health care professionals. Apparently the effect of the stress of exercise on both bone and muscle stimulates the formation of new tissue, while inactivity clearly contributes to bone loss [15].

Shangri-La and the Fountain of Youth

There are some places in the world where people have been reported to live well into very old age, beyond 100 years, and who continue to remain healthy, vigorous, and active. Such areas include the Andean area of Ecuador, the Caucasus Mountains of Russia, and the State of Hunza in Pakistan. In the early 1970s word spread that the people who lived in these remote mountainous regions had really found the secret of longevity. Interest developed in the diets of these populations, and some even claimed that the key to longevity was the Vilcabamba and the Hunza diets. The diets of these peoples are low in animal fats, low in calories, and rather low in protein, with most of the protein coming from plant sources. Obesity was rare, and vigorous physical work and activity was the rule of life. However, the equally old Abkhazia people in Russia consumed a decidedly different diet. Their diet was high in sweets, milk, meat, and alcoholic beverages. Specific dietary factors which might account for the old ages reached by these various people have not been identified [11].

Closer investigation of these populations in 1978 revealed that many of these elderly people were not as old as they stated. Exaggeration of age often began at about the age of 70 and sometimes was as much as a 20-to-40-year exaggeration. Individuals who had said in the early 1970s that they were over 100 often turned out to be less than 90. While there does seem to be a higher-than-average percentage of people over the age of 60 in these remote regions, this may be partially due to a tendency for older people to gather together from surrounding villages—a situation similar to that of St. Petersburg, Florida, where many older people have gathered from different areas of the United States [12].

Another possibility is that the prestige enjoyed by these elderly people in their communities actually prolongs their lives. In these cultures, they are admired and revered by younger people and do not suffer the trauma of retirement characteristic of affluent western countries. Whatever the explanation for continued vigor in the later years in these cultures, it is clear that we have yet to find the Fountain of Youth.

Studies of human longevity point up the importance of investigating beyond superficial answers to questions. Careful study of a broad range of possible contributing factors is essential before real answers to complex questions can be found.

One investigator determined the number of kilocalories needed to keep weight constant in people of different ages. The study showed that with age fewer kilocalories were needed to maintain constant weight. A daily 43-kcal reduction in males with each decade after the thirties, and a daily 27-kcal reduction per decade in females allowed for maintenance of body weight with increasing age [16]. The Food and Nutrition Board suggests that to estimate the kilocalorie needs of a large group of persons aged 51 to 75 years of age, kilocalories should be reduced to about 90 percent of the amount recommended for a group of young adults. For those over the age of 75, kilocalorie recommendations are reduced to 75 to 80 percent of those of the 51-to-75-year group [13]. For an individual, however, the kilocalorie intake that allows the person to maintain desirable body weight is the right amount.

In spite of a declining kilocalorie need, many middle-aged and older people continue to eat as they did in their younger years and consequently become obese. The Ten State Survey found that 50 percent of the women and 18 percent of the men over age 60 were obese. For persons over the age of 80, this prevalence was reduced to 25 percent for women and 17 percent for men [17]. Because obesity is related to many metabolic disorders, care should be taken to prevent it. Individuals should watch their weight as they get older, and when they observe an increase in weight, even by 4 or 5 lb, they should cut down on food intake or increase exercise to lose those pounds. Preventing obesity is much easier than curing it.

Another practical aspect of the decreased kilocalorie need with aging is that all the nutrient needs must be obtained from a lower kilocalorie diet; this means there is less room for foods of low nutrient density. A practical way to prevent middle-aged spread is to cut down or eliminate foods high in fat and sugar.

Protein

Inadequate protein intake when it occurs among the elderly may be the result of economic factors limiting the purchase of often expensive protein-rich foods, or of illnesses which increase protein needs or decrease the intake. Many recent studies have attempted to determine the protein requirements of elderly people.

The Food and Nutrition Board, in the RDAs, recommends a daily allowance of 0.8 g of mixed protein per kilogram of body weight to cover protein needs of most healthy U.S. individuals, including the elderly [13]. However, several studies have recommended either higher or lower protein intakes for older persons [18,19]. Because of reduced lean body mass and consequent reduced body protein synthesis, protein needs may be somewhat reduced. On the other hand, those older persons who have frequent illnesses may consequently have increased protein requirements, suggesting that protein allowances be increased to provide a protective safety margin.

In view of the limited information on the protein requirements of the elderly, to ensure adequate nutrition it is probably wise for older individuals to receive at least 12 percent or more of their kilocalories from protein [13].

Carbohydrates and Fat

Although need for dietary fat changes little with age, malabsorption disorders, diseases of organs such as the gallbladder and liver, chronic degenerative diseases such as heart disease that are frequent among the elderly, and the increased tendency toward weight gain suggest that intakes of dietary fat be controlled. (Recommendations for controlling dietary fat intake are discussed in Chapter 5).

A carbohydrate intake making up 55 to 60 percent of total kilocalorie intake, and a fat intake accounting for no more than 30 to 35 percent of total daily kilocalorie intake is probably a wise recommendation for older people, as well as for younger adults. The majority of carbohydrate kilocalories should come from complex carbohydrates, while consumption of foods high in sugars and refined carbohydrates should be limited because they tend to be of low nutrient density.

Vitamins

While low intakes of some *fat-soluble vitamins* have been noted among the elderly, deficiencies can also result from drug–nutrient interactions. For example, mineral oil, often used as a laxative by older people, may interfere with absorption of fat-soluble vitamins. Conditions such as liver diseases, kidney problems, and malabsorption disorders may also contribute to a deficiency of fat-soluble vitamins.

Ingestion of large amounts of polyunsaturated fatty acids may increase the need for vitamin E; fortunately, most foods rich in polyunsaturated fatty acids also contain vitamin E.

Vitamin D is especially important for proper calcium absorption and bone health. Individuals who are rarely exposed to sunlight or who suffer from malabsorption disorders should make an effort to consume vitamin D–fortified milk.

Diets of older persons are often low in some of the *B complex vitamins*. Many drug therapies may interfere with absorption and utilization of these vitamins or may increase requirements for them. For example, digitalis, used for certain heart conditions, may increase thiamine requirements. Some drugs used to treat hypertension can lead to vitamin B_6 deficiency, and drugs used to lower blood sugar in diabetes may impair vitamin B_{12} absorption [20].

Digestive changes, such as reduced gastric acid secretion and resulting changes in intestinal flora, may result in a reduced utilization of thiamine. Reduced secretion of intrinsic factor by the stomach due to a genetic defect may show up in certain people over age 50, and prevent absorption of vitamin B_{12}, leading to pernicious anemia. Illnesses common to older persons, such as cancer, may also increase needs for the B vitamins. Prolonged elevated body temperature which accompanies some illnesses will also increase the needs for water-soluble vitamins.

Deficiency of some of the B vitamins may account for mental confusion sometimes seen in the elderly. A deficiency of folate and vitamin B_{12}, for example, is a known cause of mental confusion [8].

There is a need to more fully understand the complex functions of *ascorbic acid*. We know that only small amounts (10 mg/day) prevent frank deficiency symptoms. We are still unsure, however, of the optimal amounts of vitamin C needed for other functions, and whether or not vitamin C can retard the cellular aging process. Vitamin C, because it acts as a synergist in the antioxidation functions of vitamin E, may play a protective role in cellular function. Tissue depletion of vitamin C may result from drugs such as aspirin, alcohol, and those used to reduce the appetite, commonly used by many older persons [8]. There is no evidence, however, that large doses of vitamin C actually prevent aging. Much more research is needed before scientists understand to what extent, if any, vitamins are related to the aging process.

Minerals

Although minerals are essential for good health for persons of all ages, calcium, phosphorus, iron, potassium, and sodium represent special concerns for older people. Other minerals of particular interest in relation to the nutritional status of older persons include fluoride, magnesium, zinc, and chromium.

Calcium and *phosphorus* have many metabolic and nutritional functions closely related to bone structure and possibly to the prevention of bone disorders. One bone disorder frequently found in elderly people is *osteoporosis*. Osteoporosis is a disorder in which the amount of bone is diminished because the rate at which bone is torn down (resorbed) exceeds the rate at which new bone is synthesized. Surveys indicate that perhaps 30 percent of women over the age of 55 and of men over the age of 60 have suffered enough loss of bone mineral to result in spontaneous fractures. An estimated 12 million American women, most of them postmenopausal, suffer osteoporosis to the extent that it results in a vertebral fracture [15].

We still are not sure of the cause of osteoporosis. A deficiency of the hormone, estrogen, or physical inactivity may contribute to loss of bone, but a very important factor may be nutrition.

Controversy exists as to whether patients with osteoporosis have routinely consumed low amounts of dietary calcium. These patients often excrete large amounts of urinary calcium, and the calcium needed to maintain normal blood levels of calcium is removed from bone [21]. Lutwak believes that osteoporosis develops as a result of this process. However, other studies have found no relation between loss of bone and calcium intake, and suggest that by the age of 50 some bone loss is normal [22].

Some researchers suggest that changes in the jaw bones and periodontal disease may be early indications of generalized osteoporosis [23]. There are two different schools of thought on this topic. One suggests that osteoporosis and periodontal disease are unrelated disorders. Osteoporosis is viewed as a slowly developing degenerative bone disorder, while periodontal disease is seen as a chronic gum infection leading to erosion, loosening, and loss of teeth. The other school believes both diseases are of similar causation, originating from a long-term deficiency of dietary calcium which leads to both bone fractures and changes in the bones in the jaw, resulting ultimately in loosening of teeth.

The latter concept suggests that supplementing the diet with calcium before the development of osteoporosis may retard the disorder. Those holding this theory recommend high intakes of calcium, in the range of 1000 mg or more of calcium daily, amounts higher than the RDA. They also suggest that the ratio of calcium to phosphorus in the diet should be greater than 1 [21,23]. The other school of thought maintains that low calcium intake in early life has no causative relationship to osteoporosis, and calcium treatment therefore will not be effective in treating osteoporosis or in preventing periodontal disease [24].

Some investigators believe that excessive intakes of phosphates, especially phosphate additives, may increase bone loss. Many foods commonly eaten by Americans, such as meat, bread, snack foods, and many processed foods contain

A CLOSER LOOK

Many investigators now suggest that postmenopausal bone loss can be effectively decreased by combining a high calcium intake with weight-bearing exercise such as walking or jogging [25]. The suggested calcium intake is 1000 to 1500 mg/day (many women consume 500 mg or less). Three cups of skim milk per day provide 900 mg of calcium; the remainder might be supplied as supplements of calcium lactate or gluconate. Once calcium is absorbed, it tends to suppress the action of PTH (parathyroid hormone) which otherwise triggers release of calcium from the bone. Postmenopausal women often absorb calcium less well than younger women, apparently because their kidneys are sluggish in secreting the active form of vitamin D, required for calcium absorption [26]. Increased intakes of calcium are therefore needed for sufficient amounts to be absorbed. Routine walking, running, or jogging decreases losses of urinary calcium and aids in the building up or repair of bones [26]. Several researchers now recommend large calcium intakes and appropriate exercise in efforts to prevent osteoporosis.

much phosphorus but little calcium. It has been suggested that the current American diet, which is higher in phosphorus than calcium, may contribute to the development of osteoporosis [15].

Recently, researchers have speculated that osteoporosis may be related to consumption over many years of a diet relatively low in calcium but high in protein. Such a diet has been shown to induce increased urinary calcium excretion in experimental human subjects, presumably by withdrawing calcium from bones [27]. However, when intakes of both protein and phosphorus are high, the increase in calcium excretion is markedly less, although there is still an increase [28]. Since most high-protein foods are also high in phosphorus, the overall effect of a high-protein diet on urinary calcium losses may not be very great. Only further research can tell us whether or not a high-protein diet has any relationship to osteoporosis. Clearly, the possible relationships of diet to development of osteoporosis are highly complex.

In general, in view of the available information, it seems wise to include generous amounts of calcium-rich foods in the diet throughout life, beginning in infancy, while maintaining an adequate exercise program. Although experts are not certain that this plan will prevent osteoporosis or periodontal disease, its benefits may be significant, while there is no indication of harm.

Fluoride is being investigated as a possible means of preventing or treating osteoporosis. Theoretically, fluoride may help to protect against osteoporosis by stabilizing the bone minerals, preventing their loss. Experimental treatment with fluoride depends on sufficient calcium in the diet, and requires high levels of fluoride. Toxic effects of excessive fluoride constitute a problem in its use. At present, however, the effectiveness of fluoride as a treatment is still open to further investigation [15]. Part of the inconsistent results reported in the use of fluoride in the treatment of osteoporosis may be due to failure to include a control for an adequate amount of vitamin D in the diet.

Iron deficiency is a common problem among elderly people from low-income groups or among those suffering from chronic illnesses. In cases of certain gastrointestinal difficulties, dietary iron may be poorly absorbed. In such cases, it is important to include in the diet sufficient amounts of iron-rich foods such as meat, legumes, and leafy green vegetables. Plant sources of iron should be consumed with a source of vitamin C to increase iron absorption. The RDAs suggest a daily allowance of 10 mg of iron for individuals over 50 years of age who are in good health. Higher intakes should benefit older people who have specific disease states that interfere with absorption.

Potassium deficiency may pose a significant problem for many elderly people. Although dietary deficiency of potassium is not common in younger adults, it becomes more frequent with increased age. Many older persons are more likely to develop potassium deficiency because of restricted diets, diuretic therapy, diarrhea, diabetes, or kidney disorders. In a study of elderly persons with symptoms of weakness, slight confusion, and urinary incontinence, 86 percent improved in at least one symptom when treated with potassium supplements [29]. Many fruits are good sources of potassium. Supplements of potassium in pill form should be taken only under a physician's supervision.

High intakes of *sodium* should be avoided because of its relationship to congestive heart failure, excessive fluid retention, and hypertension.

Magnesium deficiency, while uncommon, may result from long-term treatment with diuretics used to treat various diseases common in the elderly, or from alcoholism. Diuretic therapy may also decrease serum *zinc* levels.

Chromium levels in body tissues have been noted to be low in the general American population, but they decline even more with age. Conditions associated with chromium deficiency, such as elevated serum cholesterol levels, glucose intolerance, and lipid deposition in the aorta, also increase with age. Older persons have also been successfully treated for elevated serum cholesterol levels with chromium supplementation [30], but further work is needed. Currently, there is interest in whether or not adult-onset diabetes is related to a chromium deficiency.

Water

Dehydration is a common condition found in the elderly. Serious protein, vitamin, and mineral deficiencies may accompany severe dehydration. Chronic constipation is another frequent problem among older people. Large intakes of water, six to seven glasses daily, along with adequate amounts of dietary fiber, may prevent both these conditions.

Dietary Fiber

While there is no RDA for dietary fiber, the diet should include adequate amounts because of its possible preventive and therapeutic value in many gastrointestinal health problems. Fiber not only aids the motility of the gastrointestinal tract, preventing constipation, but may possibly help prevent diverticulitis (see Chapter 3). At the same time, it is important to recognize possible adverse physiological results of large intakes of dietary fiber, such as poorer absorption of certain minerals. Moderate increases in dietary fiber can be achieved by consuming more vegetables, fruits, and whole-grain cereals. (Dietary fiber is discussed in greater detail in Chapters 3 and 5).

How difficult is it for the older person to meet these nutritional needs? What factors determine the adequacy of the diets of older individuals? Does the older person experience special situations which make it especially difficult to meet nutritional needs?

FACTORS INFLUENCING NUTRITIONAL STATUS

The nutritional status of the elderly is influenced by the same factors which influence nutritional status of other age groups such as food habits, health, and socioeconomic status. Additional factors may influence the nutritional status of the elderly in particular. These factors, with special reference to their impact on the elderly person, will be reviewed in this section.

The Ten State Survey summarized factors related to food habits of older people: ". . . older persons often have poor food habits because of physical disabilities, lack of mobility necessary for food purchasing, and decreased interest in preparing food. Because of these factors, this group is often considered to be at high nutritional risk" [17].

Physiological Changes

Older people are often spoken of as a group, but they are a very heterogeneous group. As noted earlier, many older persons are mentally and physically healthy and actively involved in work and leisure. People vary in the rate at which they age; nevertheless, when physiological changes *do* occur, they may be related to reduced ability to obtain an adequate diet, as the following discussion indicates.

Gradual changes in posture are common and are attributed to structural alterations in ligaments, bones, and joints. These changes are often accelerated by lack of physical activity, and may be influenced by diet and nutrition throughout life. Often the skeletal changes limit the mobility and activity of older people, making it more difficult for them to carry out the normal activities of daily living. Shopping for and preparing food may pose difficulties which are likely to have a negative impact on the diet.

Neuromuscular problems may also result in reduced ability to prepare food, or to handle eating utensils. Psychological changes may interfere with nutritional status as well—for example, the older person may forget to eat at regular times, or become very set in certain food habits and not want to eat a varied diet. Tea and toast may be the norm for one or more meals a day, and any suggestion that a more balanced diet might be desirable may be scoffed at.

Digestive and intestinal difficulties are often problems. Changes in the digestive system may include reduced secretion of stomach acid and certain enzymes, as well as decreased motility of the stomach. Peristalsis in all areas of the gastrointestinal tract may diminish, which may be partly responsible for the constipation so often experienced by the elderly. Frequently they experience discomfort after eating, and consequently may modify their diet in such a way that it becomes nutritionally inadequate. Many have been put on very restricted diets for gastrointestinal problems by physicians who were unaware that the patients believed they must remain on these diets indefinitely. Such patients may believe, for example, that they can never again eat fresh fruits and vegetables since they believe these foods contain so much "roughage" that irritation of the intestinal wall results. Health professionals must be sure that elderly persons understand their instructions.

Dental changes such as loss of teeth, poorly fitting dentures, and irritations or sores in the mouth can lead to poor eating habits. An estimated 50 percent of the American population have lost a majority of their teeth by the time they are 65 years old, while 75 percent have lost all their teeth by the age of 75. Loss of one molar may reduce chewing efficiency by 33 percent, while loss of three molars results in a 66 percent decrease in the efficiency of mastication [31]. These circumstances may result in selection of a soft, easy-to-chew diet. Some older people may buy baby foods under the pretense that they are shopping for their grandchildren, but actually eat these foods themselves. Such a diet, because of its reduced bulk, may lead to problems of the colon. Furthermore, limiting one's diet to soft foods may result in a low intake of certain nutrients.

Taste, smell, vision, and hearing often decline with age and greatly influence food habits and intake. Some researchers believe that with increasing age there is also a loss of taste buds [32]. There may also be a reduced ability to distinguish between subtle differences in the four tastes (sweet, sour, bitter, salty). Such changes in taste perception may lead the older individual to use more spices or seasonings, and may also lead to a reduced appetite which in turn directly affects nutritional status. Loss of the sense of smell may also cause changes in food intake, since the smell of food plays a great role in enhancing appetite.

Visual impairment may make it very difficult for the older person to obtain an adequate diet. Reading nutrition labels to compare food quality while shopping, and cooking or preparing food may be difficult. Actual enjoyment gained from eating can diminish in an individual with vision problems. To experience some of the effects of a visual handicap yourself, try to eat while blindfolded. What problems do you experience that interfere with the normal eating process? You may find that even if someone feeds you, the normal pleasure of eating diminishes.

Hearing impairment may cause an individual to withdraw from others, or to feel isolated from family or friends. Isolation and social withdrawal, in turn, are often related to reduced food intake.

Disabilities and chronic diseases that often afflict older people, together with restricted physical activity resulting from them, may also limit food intake. Some of these conditions also influence the need for nutrients. Illness may lead to nutritional problems by interfering with utilization of nutrients, increasing their excretion, or increasing their requirements. For example, if an individual is confined to bed for a long period of time, significant losses of calcium and nitrogen result. Frequently, sick patients have no desire to eat and may actually be repulsed by the sight or smell of food. Sometimes an older person may experience loss of appetite when placed on a special diet. A person accustomed to highly seasoned food may lose a desire for food if all the food has to be salt-free. On the other hand, some elderly people focus on food as one of their few remaining pleasures, and may gain weight to the detriment of health.

Drug–Nutrient Interactions

When your doctor prescribes medication for you, does he or she tell you when to take it, and what food or drinks to avoid while taking it? Do you realize that you shouldn't take milk with the antibiotic tetracycline? The issue of drug–nutrient interaction concerns everyone, but is of particular significance to older adults who are often ill or subject to chronic disorders.

For the person taking medication, food and drink might interact with the drugs; the result influences the actions of the drug, or the absorption and utilization of food and nutrients.

Changes in Drug Responses Caused by Food or Nutrients   Food may alter drug absorption, metabolism, rate of excretion, or drug response. Generally speaking, food changes the effectiveness of the drug by increasing or decreasing the time it takes the drug to pass through the gastrointestinal tract to the area in the body where it must work. Food and drink decrease the absorption of many drugs. For example, when the antibiotic tetracycline is taken with dairy products containing large amounts of calcium or foods rich in iron, the drug combines with the metal ions to form complexes which are poorly absorbed. But some drugs, such as griseofulvin, used to treat fungus infections, are absorbed faster if fatty foods are eaten before the drug is taken [33,34]. On the other hand, an excess of some nutrients may interfere with the effects of certain drugs.

Alcohol, itself a drug, greatly influences the response to antihistamines, barbiturates, tranquilizers, antidepressants, and other substances affecting the central nervous system. Alcohol, when taken with antihistamines, sedatives, or antidepressants, often causes excessive drowsiness that can be very dangerous to an individual who is driving, operating machinery, or performing other activities that demand an alert mind. Many deaths have resulted from combinations of alcohol and tranquilizers. In general, it is wise to avoid drinking alcoholic beverages when taking any prescribed or over-the-counter medication [35].

Many drugs affect the stomach and intestines and influence nutrient utilization. Mineral oil and laxatives, often used by older people, reduce absorption of fat-soluble vitamins. Chronic and excessive use of antacids can lead to deficiencies of thiamine, phosphorus, and fluoride. Other drugs such as anticonvulsants and antibiotics impair the activity of some of the B vitamins. Drugs may also interfere with enzyme activity. Diuretics, commonly called "water pills," can cause deficiencies of potassium, magnesium, and zinc by increasing their excretion.

Drugs may also affect nutritional status by suppressing appetite, or interfering with taste, smell, or production of saliva. They may also cause nausea, vomiting, or diarrhea, causing a reduction in food intake. This is often seen in cancer patients undergoing chemotherapy.

Who is Most Likely to Suffer Drug-Induced Nutritional Problems?   At greatest risk are individuals who are long-term drug users and who also have a poor diet, a chronic disease, or excessive alcohol intake. Such individuals include the elderly, especially those who receive a combination of many different drugs. It is not uncommon, for example, to find that some elderly patients in nursing homes are taking as many as 9 or 10 different drugs in combination [36].

What Can Be Done to Prevent Undesirable Drug-Food Interactions?   FDA regulations require drug manufacturers to state on the package inserts known adverse interactions between food and drugs or between different prescribed drugs. However, package inserts are included with prescription drugs only if patients request them. Drug manufacturers are also required to provide physicians with information about interactions. Some manufacturers are voluntarily providing information [35].

What action can consumers take to avoid harmful drug–food interactions? Consumers should carefully read labels or ask the druggist for package inserts to learn as much as possible about the drugs prescribed. This is especially important for the older person who is taking a number of medications. If the physician fails to volunteer information, the consumer should ask whether the drug should be taken before, with, or between meals, or on an empty stomach, and then follow the recommendations. The physician should be kept informed about other drugs being taken in addition to the one he or she is giving.

Pharmacists can also provide information about precautions or possible side effects. A helpful reference on medications is the *Physicians' Desk Reference*, available in libraries, often referred to as the PDR [37]. It explains prescription procedures and drugs, but is too technical for most laypersons.

In addition, the older person should be counseled to eat nutritious, well-balanced meals. If he or she is in good nutritional health, a needed medication is less apt to cause problems with nutritional status.

Drugs prescribed for the elderly may also affect nutritional status. They frequently affect appetite, may cause nausea and stomach upset, or may interfere with the utilization, excretion, or requirements of certain nutrients (see Box 16-3).

Socioeconomic Factors

Poverty exerts a major influence on food patterns. Older individuals in the United States have significantly lower incomes than the median for the total U.S. population, as indicated in Table 16-1. The incidence of poverty is estimated to be twice as high among older, as compared to younger persons. Twenty-five percent of America's elderly people have incomes below the official poverty line, while only one in nine is considered poor among the younger population. Many of these elderly poor become so only during their later years [31]. Restricted or fixed incomes reduce their ability to purchase needed foods.

One study of 234 adults over the age of 60 in Akron, Ohio, found that the most important influence on food habits was income, followed by nutrition knowledge, eating of convenience foods, poor dental health, and eating alone. Many older people were concerned with maintaining good food habits, but were unable to do so because they lacked sufficient income [38].

Many older people live alone. Living alone in itself doesn't automatically promote loneliness and isolation, but many elderly are lonely and isolated. Because of the difficulty in getting out to the supermarket to buy food, or because of dislike of preparing a meal for one, they may pay little attention to planning a well-balanced meal. Those who are more socially active and who can participate in different civic, community, recreational, or family activities tend to have better diets than those who remain alone and isolated from others.

TABLE 16-1. MEDIAN TOTAL MONEY INCOME FOR ELDERLY POPULATION BY COUPLES, AND SINGLES UNITS

AGE	ALL UNITS	COUPLES	NONMARRIED UNITS
55–61	$12,100	$16,490	$5,260
62–64	8,830	12,750	4,450
65–67	6,250	9,710	3,770
68–69	5,630	8,620	3,740
70–72	5,110	8,140	3,500
73 and over	3,920	6,780	3,130

Income for most aged persons is lower as age increases.
Median total income is lower among the nonmarried than among couples.
SOURCE: *Income and Resources of the Aged*, USDHEW,
SSA Publ. No. 13–11727, January 1980.

Location or place of residency may also affect food habits. The older person living in a rural area is more likely to have an adequate kilocalorie intake than the older person living in an urban area. One reason for this may be the increased availability of food. Rural residents are more likely to have established habits of growing, canning, and freezing their own food. Another reason may be that those living in rural areas remain more physically active than those in urban areas. Increased physical activity is apt to result in increased food consumption [39]. The urban elderly face many difficulties in obtaining foods. In poor sections of cities, stores often set higher prices than in affluent sections, despite the fact that the food quality is frequently inferior. Supermarkets often move out of inner-city areas, leaving only "mom and pop" grocery stores, with their high prices. Limited mobility, or fear of getting out and about in the city may also restrict food purchases and reduce the dietary quality of the urban elderly.

As a group then, elderly people are vulnerable to poor food habits on many counts. Physiological ailments, limited incomes, limited social contacts, and loneliness and isolation are all factors that combine to affect the diets of many older people. Because of physical and socioeconomic problems, and because of a great hope that these problems can be solved by food and nutrition, they are likely to fall prey to fraudulent claims, food faddism, and health swindles. This points up the need for nutrition education, not only to teach older people about food, but to encourage wise consumer practices, to help them plan diets to meet changing needs, and to help them make sound, economical food selections.

How Well Nourished Are Older Adults?

Various research studies have reported that many older persons have poor dietary intakes. Frequently reported nutritional problems among older individuals include low intakes of dietary iron, vitamins A and C, and calcium [40]. However, the nutritional status of the elderly is not as poor as is often believed. In general we can conclude that there is little real malnutrition among the elderly, but certain groups within the elderly population, such as minorities, have less-than-adequate diets in terms of certain nutrients.

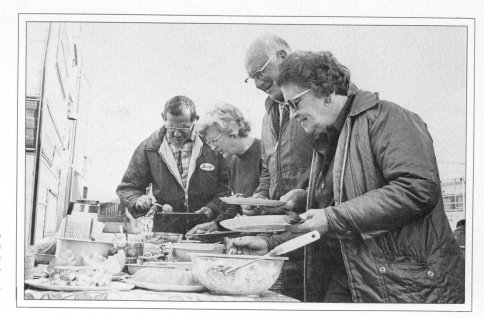

Older individuals who are socially active are more apt to have adequate diets than those who are socially isolated. (© Bob Krueger/Rapho/ Photo Researchers, Inc.)

DIETARY PLANNING

Nutritionists are frequently involved in dietary planning for older people. They may work as consultants or do individual dietary counseling, or they may direct nutrition programs for senior citizens. How do nutritionists go about creating menu plans for older people?

Basically, considerations for dietary planning for older individuals are the same as for younger ones. One needs to take into account specific nutrient needs, cultural background, lifestyle, food preferences, economic status, and skills in food preparation.

Generally, the kilocalorie need is less for the healthy older person than for the same individual 30 or 40 years earlier. Otherwise, nutrient needs are about the same after age 60 or 65 as before. In cases of disease or declining ability to absorb or utilize nutrients, the nutritionist modifies recommendations for nutrient intake on an individual basis. Many older women probably need larger calcium intakes than in their youth.

Since the kilocalorie need is lower but needs for other nutrients are mostly unchanged, the diet should have high nutrient density. Weight, for optimal health, should be maintained within the desirable or ideal range. Guidelines for dietary planning for the elderly therefore are like those discussed in Chapter 3 for younger adults. These include: (1) choosing a wide variety of foods to ensure that all needed nutrients are obtained; (2) practicing moderation—avoiding excesses of any one food or food group; (3) choosing nutrient-dense foods, by avoiding foods that are excessively high in fat and sugar; (4) adding little, if any, salt to food in cooking, and limiting foods high in salt; (5) including whole-grain breads and cereals, legumes, seeds, fruits, and vegetables for dietary fiber and for their wide

TABLE 16-2. PRACTICAL HINTS FOR OLDER ADULTS IN PLANNING HEALTHFUL DIETS

CHOOSE MORE OF THESE	SUGGESTED NUMBER OF SERVINGS	LIMIT THESE
BREADS, CEREALS, AND STARCHY VEGETABLES Whole-grain breads, cereals, crackers Plain ready-to-eat cereals Potatoes, served without added fat Pasta (macaroni, spaghetti), whole wheat if desired	3 to 4	Presweetened ready-to-eat cereals Refined breads, cereals, crackers, especially if unenriched Danish pastries, doughnuts Pretzels, potato chips and other salty, fatty snack items Cookies, cakes, pies
VEGETABLES (Think dark green and deep yellow or orange) Choose frequently from: cabbage, broccoli, cauliflower, brussels sprouts, carrots, sweet potatoes, orange and yellow squash, dark-green leafy vegetables (spinach, kale, collards, mustard and turnip greens) Use fresh vegetables when possible. Choose plain frozen vegetables (not with sauces). Season with herbs, not with salt Include raw vegetables for crisp texture and ease of preparation	2	Fried vegetables Overcooked vegetables Canned vegetables if high in salt Frozen vegetables in rich sauces
FRUITS Choose frequently from those high in vitamin C (oranges, grapefruit, melons)—but remember that dark-green vegetables are also good vitamin C sources Canned fruits should be water-packed or in own juice	2	Fruits canned in sugar syrup Fruit drinks containing little if any real fruit juice. These products are lower in many nutrients than are real fruits or fruit juices
MILK AND MILK PRODUCTS Choose skim or 1 to 2% fat milk, low-fat yogurt, low-fat cottage cheese, cheddar cheese	2	Full-fat cheddar cheese and cottage cheese Whole milk Cream, half-and-half Ice cream Cream cheese Rich custards or puddings
LEGUMES, SEEDS, NUTS Choose from a wide variety of legumes—pinto, kidney, black, navy, lima, and garbanzo beans (chickpeas); black-eyed peas, split peas, lentils, etc. A serving a day of legumes contributes many nutrients and can be inexpensive and delicious Choose from a variety of seeds—sunflower, sesame, and others (these can be expensive, but can be used in small amounts) Nuts can add variety in texture and flavor, and many nutrients to the diet. Peanut butter is a great favorite.	1	Use nuts and seeds in small amounts because of their high kilocalorie and fat content. Nuts and seeds are preferable to cakes and cookies as snack items

TABLE 16-2. PRACTICAL HINTS FOR OLDER ADULTS IN PLANNING HEALTHFUL DIETS *(Continued)*

CHOOSE MORE OF THESE	SUGGESTED NUMBER OF SERVINGS	LIMIT THESE
MEATS, POULTRY, FISH Choose lean fresh or frozen meats, poultry, or fish, and bake or broil rather than fry them Choose canned tuna packed in water rather than oil Trim fat off meat	1	Fried meats, poultry, or fish Fatty meats Bacon, corned beef, and other cured meats (these are high in salt and fat)
OIL Include 1 tbsp of polyunsaturated oil or margarine daily	1 tbsp	Coconut or palm oil Lard, butter, hydrogenated shortenings
EGGS Include in baked products, or cook without fat	3–4 per week	Fried eggs
BEVERAGES Water, milk, and fruit juices are preferable	6–8 glasses day	Sodas Large amounts of coffee or tea Herbal teas, since little is known about their composition

range of nutrients; (6) including at least 1 tbsp of polyunsaturated fat or oil daily for vitamin E and linoleic acid.

Practical hints for making choices are given in Table 16-2.

Older people frequently profit from guidance on how to shop wisely for only one or two people, and how to prepare or store food.

Knowledge about programs available to help older adults meet their nutritional needs is also valuable, and some of these are discussed below.

NUTRITION PROGRAMS FOR OLDER ADULTS

Partly as a result of the increasing numbers of older people and partly as a result of publicity about programs for the elderly, there has been an increased social concern for the plight of older Americans. The increased visibility of the needs of older people through political organizations has increased society's awareness of its social responsibilities to improve the quality of life for the elderly. With this growing awareness has come a growth in nutritional services available to older people.

In 1965 Congress passed the Older Americans Act which provided for various programs designed to improve the quality of life for the elderly. One of the programs provided for under this legislation was the National Nutrition Program for the Elderly, currently referred to as the Title III Meal Program.

The program is designed to provide inexpensive, nutritionally balanced meals for older persons. Low-cost meals are served in congregate settings to individuals who are 60 years of age or older and to their spouses. Meals are

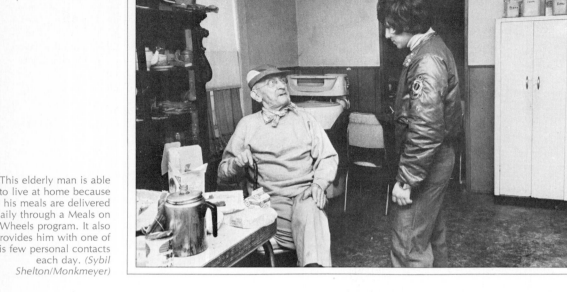

This elderly man is able to live at home because his meals are delivered daily through a Meals on Wheels program. It also provides him with one of his few personal contacts each day. *(Sybil Shelton/Monkmeyer)*

designed to provide at least one-third of the RDAs for older persons. The elderly are not required to pay, but may voluntarily contribute toward the meals.

In addition to food, various supportive services are also provided as part of the program. Transportation to the meal and back home, information and help for other services, health counseling, nutrition education, and recreation activities are some of these other services. Outreach, or information for eligible older people about the program and how to participate in it, are also provided.

Another program that helps to meet the nutritional needs of many elderly is the Meals on Wheels program, operated on a private, nonprofit volunteer basis. Often, church groups organize these programs, through which hot meals are delivered to homebound elderly, infirm, or handicapped individuals. Usually hot noon meals are delivered, and sometimes a cold supper may also be left for those who are unable to prepare their own meals.

To recap, changes in physiology, health status, environment, and lifestyles of the elderly significantly influence their diets. These changes may appear tragic and overwhelming to the young, but most of them take place so gradually that an individual is able to adapt and cope with them.

Despite the "gloom and doom" commonly associated with old age, many older people live happy and contented lives. "Aging truly can be a jewel in the mosaic of life" [41]. Our concern should be for the ways nutrition throughout life can improve the quality of life for the elderly.

SUMMARY

1 Good nutrition throughout life is important, not only to improve health and the general quality of life, but also as a possible way to slow down the aging process. Future research should focus on delineating how this might be accomplished.

2 Numerous theories have been proposed to explain the process of aging. Genetic as well as environmental factors play a role.

3 Good food habits of the elderly are influenced by changes in their physical, mental, and environmental circumstances.

4 Basic nutrient needs of the older person do not greatly differ from those of younger people. However, kilocalorie requirements decrease and some of the physiological changes that accompany aging may increase needs for particular nutrients.

5 A number of surveys have focused on the nutritional status of the elderly. These studies suggest that the nutrients most often limited in the diets of older people are iron, vitamin A and C, and calcium. In general, however, gross evidences of malnutrition among the elderly seem to be infrequent.

6 In planning diets for older individuals, one must pay special attention to their cultural backgrounds, lifestyles, and food preferences. It is essential that they be informed about wise consumer buying practices, nutrition basics, and programs available to help them meet their nutritional needs.

7 An important nutrition service for older people is provided by the National Nutrition Program for the Elderly. This program is designed to provide inexpensive, nutritionally balanced meals for older individuals.

FOR DISCUSSION AND APPLICATION

1 Visit a center that serves Title III meals. Get acquainted with some of the elderly participants. Among things you might want to find out are: (a) How did they find out about the program? (b) Is there any nutrition education in the program? What would participants like to learn about food or nutrition? (c) Do they cook at home? If so, for how many? Do they find it difficult to cook for only one or for two? Do they have any ideas to pass on about cooking for only one or two? (d) Are there any foods they cannot eat? If so, why? Does this cause any problem? (e) What aspects of the Title III program do they appreciate most?

2 Volunteer for a Meals on Wheels project. Find out what you can about problems in managing the program. Visit elderly participants in the program and learn all you can about practical problems they face that affect what foods they eat, when they eat, and how much they eat.

3 Ask your grandparents or other older relatives or friends about meanings that foods hold for them. How do their current food habits relate to their food habits when they were younger? If their food preferences have changed over the years, what factors brought about the change? Did they grow any of their own food in early years? Do they now? What foods were celebration foods in their youth? Your objective should be to stimulate a rich discussion of associations that people have with food.

SUGGESTED READINGS

The Fitness Challenge in the Later Years. It is important for older people to try to stay fit. This publication from the President's Council on Physical Fitness and Sports, and the Administration on Aging points out the importance of physical fitness in the later years. It can be ordered for $2.25 from Consumer Information Center, Department 145J, Pueblo, Colo., 81009.

Eating Right for Less, New York: Consumer Report Books, 1977. This booklet, printed in large type to aid the older person, discusses diet plans, shopping, and questions about health and nutrition.

Food and Drug Interactions, FDA Consumer, 1978. From Consumer Communications, HFJ-10, Food and Drug Administration, 5600 Fishers Lane, Rockville, Md., 20857. This reprint covers interactions between food and drugs and suggests ways to avoid harmful interactions.

A Guide for Food and Nutrition in the Later Years, Berkeley, Calif.: Society for Nutrition Education, 94704, revised 1980. This publication discusses wise nutrition for older people. Resources and organizations are listed.

Aging and Nutrition, Berkeley, Calif.: Society for Nutrition Education, 94704, revised January 1980. An annotated bibliography of resources related to nutrition and aging.

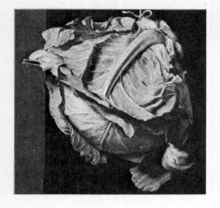

PART V

FOOD SAFETY
AND ADEQUACY:
AT HOME
AND ABROAD

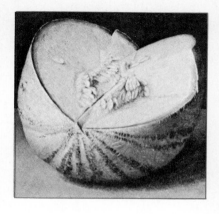

Americans are indefatigable consumers. Think of the number of times you got over a period of boredom by buying something; something to wear or read or listen to—or eat. Notice how, for many schoolchildren, the accepted afterschool activity is to head for nearby stores to buy candy, ice cream, or sodas. Large shopping malls are recreational centers for teenagers in the United States. In a country in which consuming is a favorite pastime, people find it difficult to imagine being without money to purchase food. Yet, in recent years, as downturns in the U.S. industrial productivity and consequent unemployment have spread, many family heads, who never before had to do so, now must worry about obtaining enough food to feed their families. For the first time in their lives, they have had to face a fundamental problem of existence: how to get enough food. This is an all-too-familiar problem for millions living in the developing or third world countries.

Most Americans are fortunate in having plenty to eat. At the same time, many need and want to make their food dollar go as far as possible. Additionally, they want to know what is in the food they consume. Is it safe? Are additives or toxicants present that might be harmful? What nutrients are present? What can they learn from food labels? Chapter 17 is devoted to supplying answers to these questions.

Ironically, there is a connection between the American propensity for consumption and hunger in developing countries. Land that might otherwise be used to produce food for people in a developing country is frequently used, instead, to grow food for export to the United States. Chapter 18 provides some examples of this economic situation as part of a larger discussion of the causes and consequences of poor nutrition in developing countries.

These two chapters should expand your awareness of (1) what, if anything, Americans need to worry about regarding their food supply; (2) why poor nutrition is prevalent in many countries; and (3) what the affluent countries, particularly the United States, might do to remedy this serious problem.

17

CONSUMER ISSUES: FOOD LABELING, ADDITIVES, AND TOXICANTS

In our complex society, consumer food choices are influenced by many diverse factors, as pointed out in Chapter 1. Although American consumers are better informed today about foods than they once were, their choices are complicated because, in most supermarkets, they must choose among more than 10,000 items. Most consumers take into account the amount of money they have to spend and the food preferences of family members when deciding which foods to buy, but for an increasing number of consumers the nutritional value of foods is also an important consideration. Other factors that may influence decisions include convenience, safety, health, and advertising.

As an example of the complexity of decision making, consider the choice of orange juice or orange drink for breakfast: Choices include fresh fruit, bottled fresh juice, frozen or canned juice, or a variety of imitation juices or drinks, some of which contain some orange juice while others contain none. Some imitation products are frozen while others are powdered. How does each of these products compare with fresh orange juice in convenience, cost, nutritive value, and presence of additives? This chapter provides guidance for finding answers to such questions by increasing your skills in interpreting information on food labels, including nutrition labeling.

Fabricated or *engineered foods*, such as cookie-like breakfast substitutes, have grown in numbers in recent years. Many such foods contain food additives. Are there risks associated with consuming food additives? Do the benefits of food additives outweigh any risks? To what extent do natural toxicants in foods constitute a safety problem? Some foods are fortified with a wide range of vitamins and minerals. Is fortification desirable? These important consumer issues are the focus of this chapter.

FOOD LABELING

Before 1938, when the Food, Drug and Cosmetic Act was enacted by Congress, food manufacturers were not required to inform consumers of specific ingredients in foods. Because manufacturers sometimes replaced some ingredients with less expensive and often inferior ones, Congress empowered the Food and Drug Administration (FDA) to establish *standards of identity* for more than 300 food products. At that time, many consumers still prepared at home such foods as ice cream, mayonnaise and other salad dressings, canned fruits and vegetables, and jellies and jams. Standards of identity specify the proportion of ingredients that must be used in such foods, ensuring that the consumer obtains a product containing the expected ingredients. For example, the standard of identity for fruit jellies specifies that these must contain at least 45 percent by weight of fruit or fruit juice and 55 percent of sugar or other sweeteners. The manufacturer is not required to list on the label all the ingredients of foods having standards of identity, since the standards define what these must be. Any optional ingredients used must be listed on the label, however. Since consumers do not have easy access to standards of identity, some manufacturers voluntarily list on the label all ingredients used, even for foods having standards of identity.

Food labeling is regulated by various federal agencies. The United States Department of Agriculture (USDA) regulates the labeling of fresh and processed meat, poultry, and dairy products. The Food and Drug Administration regulates the labeling of processed foods that cross state lines, with the exception of foods containing meat or poultry. The Federal Trade Commission (FTC) oversees false or misleading advertising claims. Foods that do not cross state lines but are grown and shipped within one state (intrastate commerce) are, with the exception of meat and poultry, regulated by state laws.

According to the Fair Packaging and Labeling Act, passed by Congress in 1966, all food labels must contain the following basic information:

1. Product name, in clearly legible form as well as the product form or style and the packing medium. For example, a can of pineapple must indicate "sliced"; "in heavy syrup."
2. Net weight. If a package contains between 1 and 4 lb, its contents must be stated both in terms of total weight in ounces and in pounds and ounces. For example, "Net Wt: 32 ounces (2 pounds)." This weight includes any liquid present and is different from *drained* weight, which is the weight of a food after any liquid is drained off.

3. Name, address, and zip code of manufacturer, distributor, or packer.
4. A list of ingredients, for those foods having no standard of identity. This list must present ingredients in order of decreasing weight. In other words, if the product contains more water than any other ingredient, water must be listed first.
5. A statement about any artificial color, flavor, or preservative that is added, or about other special treatment the food has received (e.g., concentrated, enriched, fortified). The statement can say simply "artificial color" and does not need to specify what coloring agent is used. Some dairy products such as cheese and butter are exempted from the general requirement of disclosing information about artificial colors except when there is a question of safety.
6. "USDA Inspected and Passed" is mandatory on all processed meats and poultry products. This tells the consumer that USDA inspections have certified that the processing procedures meet requirements.

Nutrition Labeling

Ingredient labels provide useful information about the food product, but tell little about the nutritive value of the food. Nutrition labels, on the other hand, provide information about the number of kilocalories and amounts of protein, carbohydrate, fat, and certain other nutrients in a food. Not all foods have a nutrition label, however.

Nutrition labeling is required if: (1) a nutrient has been added to a food by the manufacturer; (2) the manufacturer makes a nutritional claim about the foods, either in advertisements or on the label; or (3) the food is for special dietary use. Labeling of other foods may be done on a voluntary basis; increased consumer awareness and competition among manufacturers has brought about voluntary nutrition labeling of many foods.

Products most frequently carrying nutrition labeling are cereals, margarine, powdered soft drinks, flour, dry pasta, canned and powdered milk, frozen toppings, canned seafood, baby foods, and frozen fruit juices. Products least likely to bear nutrient labels are coffee, sugar, condiments, pickles, spices and seasonings, canned sauces, and miscellaneous refrigerated products such as salads and seafoods [1].

The nutrition information panel of the food label must be standard in design and placed at the right of the package front or display panel. Information on the label must always be presented in the same order as that shown in Figure 17-1.

U.S. Recommended Daily Allowances   The standards used for nutrition labeling are called the *U.S. Recommended Daily Allowances*, or *U.S. RDAs*. The U.S. RDAs are different from, and should not be confused with, the RDAs. The U.S. RDAs were developed by the FDA to be used as legal standards for labeling the nutritional content of foods, and to provide consumers with accurate and reliable information. They were developed on the basis of the 1968 RDAs. The 26 age/sex categories of the RDAs were condensed into four categories comprising the U.S. RDAs. The four categories include: (1) infants, (2) children under 4, (3) adults and

```
                    GREEN BEANS
              NET WEIGHT 16 OZ. (1 LB)
               WT. OF BEANS 9.2 OZ.*
   *Weight of beans means weight before addition of liquid necessary for
    processing.
              Ingredients: 1/2-in. Diagonal Cut
                 Green Beans, Water, Salt.
              NUTRITION INFORMATION
   Serving Size......1 Cup
   Servings per Container......... 2 (or 4-½c Servings)
   Per One-Cup Serving:
   Calories...........40        Carbohydrate ...7 grams
   Protein ........2 grams      Fat ..........0 grams
          PERCENTAGE OF U.S. RECOMMENDED
            DAILY ALLOWANCE (U.S. RDA)
   Protein...... 2    Thiamine ...2    Calcium ....4
   Vitamin A ...10    Riboflavin ..1   Iron .......8
   Vitamin C ...10    Niacin .....*
   *Contains less than 2% of the U.S. RDA of this nutrient.

                    DISTRIBUTED BY
                 XYZ FOOD COMPANY
                 ANYTOWN, U.S.A. 99999

        Packed in U.S.A.          Printed in U.S.A.
```

FIGURE 17-1. An example of a food label. The list of ingredients, net weight, name and address of the distributor, and nutrition information all are shown.

children over 4, and (4) pregnant and lactating women. The U.S. RDAs used for food labeling can be found in Appendix N.

Except for calcium and phosphorus, the highest values in the 1968 RDA table were selected for use within each U.S. RDA category, as an added safety measure. For example, 18 mg/day is the standard set for iron. The U.S. RDAs for calcium and phosphorus are not quite the highest values in the RDA table, but are set at 1 g each, which is still higher than the 800 mg/day RDA set for adults. The U.S. RDAs therefore are often higher than the nutrient needs of many individuals.

The U.S. RDAs set two different protein standards. If the quality of a food protein is less than that of casein, the U.S. RDA for adults is 65 g. (Recall from Chapter 6 that the quality of a protein depends upon how closely its amino acid pattern resembles that of body proteins.) If the quality is equal to or greater than that of casein, the U.S. RDA for adults is 45 g. If the protein quality is less than 20 percent that of casein, it cannot be considered as contributing protein. For example, the protein in gelatin cannot be considered to be a contributor to the total protein value of a gelatin cream pie.

What's On A Nutritional Label?   For those foods for which nutrition labeling is required, the following must be included on the nutrition information panel:

1. Serving size. The label states the size of a serving, for example, "one-half cup," and also how many servings the container holds. Nutrition information is given for one serving amount.
2. Kilocalories per serving are listed first, followed by amounts in grams of protein, carbohydrates, and fat.
3. Protein is listed in grams per serving and also as a percentage of the U.S. RDA.

4. The following nutrients as percentages of the U.S. RDA must be listed: protein, vitamin A, thiamine, riboflavin, vitamin C, niacin, calcium, and iron. Additional nutrients, shown in Appendix N, may be listed if the manufacturer wishes.

   At present, sodium content need not be listed on a nutrition label. However, the FDA is currently working on proposed regulations that would require the mandatory listing of sodium content of any food for which a nutrition label is used [2].

5. If a product claims to be a significant source of a nutrient, this nutrient must be present in an amount at least 10 percent of the U.S. RDA per serving. If the label claims a food is nutritionally superior to another food, the nutrient in question must be present in at least 10 percent more of the U.S. RDA per serving than the food of comparison.

6. If the product contains less than 2 percent of the U.S. RDA for any of the nutrients for which labeling is required, zeroes or asterisks can be used to refer to a footnote stating "less than 2 percent of these nutrients." If any vitamins or minerals are *added* to a product they *must* be listed.

7. The listing of fatty acids or cholesterol is optional. If stated, however, such information must be placed on the label adjacent to the statement on fat content.

Food manufacturers are required to have their products analyzed in a laboratory for nutrient composition in compliance with specific FDA regulations. Usually, products are required to fall within a range of nutrient values to provide for variation in nutrient content. For example, a naturally occurring nutrient must be present at 80 percent of the stated value. A manufacturer may tend to underestimate the nutrient values of products to be in compliance with the regulations. Therefore, values on labels indicate only approximate, not exact levels in the foods you buy.

Nutrition Labeling For Special Foods: Low-Kilocalorie Foods   There are special regulations for the labeling of low-kilocalorie or reduced kilocalorie foods, or foods for diabetic individuals. A so-called "low-calorie" food may contain no more than 40 kcal per serving, and no more than 0.4 kcal per gram. Thus, a food cannot be called "low-calorie" by the piece (for example, a cracker) if it is usually eaten in larger amounts. "Reduced calorie" foods must have kilocalorie contents at least one-third less than the higher kilocalorie foods for which they are substituted. "Reduced calorie" foods must be labeled to describe the basis for the comparison. An example might be "artificially sweetened fruit cocktail packed in light syrup, 80 kilocalories per ½ cup serving, 30 percent less than brand X fruit cocktail packed in heavy syrup."

Foods normally low in kilocalories such as broccoli cannot be termed "low-calorie broccoli" because this implies that one type of broccoli is lower in kilocalories than another. The label can, however, state "broccoli, a low-calorie food."

A food may not be termed a "diabetic food" unless it is of use in the diabetic diet. A food labeled "sugar-free," "sugarless," or "no sugar" must also be labeled "low-calorie" or "reduced calorie" and conform to the above-mentioned regulations for those categories, or be labeled as "not a reduced calorie food" or "not for weight control."

Are Nutrition Labels Adequate?   Although labeling regulations satisfy the consumer's "right to know" to some extent, many people have voiced criticism of them. Some of the information that appears on labels is new "vocabulary" to many consumers. For example, nutrients such as vitamin B$_6$ are not commonly discussed in lay reading materials, and the average consumer may be unfamiliar with them. Many consumers don't understand the implications of nutrition labeling. For example, it is no help to know the carbohydrate content of a food if one believes that carbohydrates should be avoided because of the mistaken notion that they are more fattening than protein foods.

Other problems involve the time required to read labels and to use the information in comparison shopping. Results of surveys conducted to determine if consumers read and use labels indicate that:

1. Since the inception of nutrition labeling, its use has greatly increased [3].
2. In general, the nutrition information is used most by those who seem to need it the least—for example, the younger, more affluent, better-educated consumer is more likely to use labeling information than the older, poorer, less well educated consumer whose nutritional needs may be greater, and whose resources are lowest.
3. Slightly more than half the population uses food labels to help them avoid certain ingredients such as sugar, salt, fat, and preservatives.
4. Labels are more often used to compare different products than to provide help in menu planning.
5. Most consumers think they understand the information included on labels, but many really do not and so are unable to wisely apply it to food selection.
6. There is increasing desire among consumers for more simplified labeling information. Consumers would profit by a listing of all ingredients, simpler language, and the use of ingredients on labels of all food products.

Improvements suggested include: (1) use of a graph to display the amounts of fat, sugar, complex carbohydrates, and protein; (2) listing polyunsaturated, monounsaturated, and saturated fats; cholesterol, sodium, and dietary fiber; and (3) making a distinction between sugars present naturally in foods and refined sugars added to foods.

Using Labels Wisely: A Guide for Consumers

Since the U.S. RDA standards are based on the age/sex group whose needs are the highest, "average" adults do not necessarily need to include 100 percent of the U.S. RDA for each nutrient in their diets on a daily basis in order to consume a balanced diet. With this in mind, how can consumers use the information on nutrition labels to make wise food choices? How can parents select food for

A CLOSER LOOK

Sometimes labeling information may be misleading. Take the label of an orange-flavored instant breakfast drink, for example. The label states that the product contains no fruit juice, and specifies that a serving contains a "full day's supply of vitamin C." The average consumer is likely to feel comfortable substituting a glass of this drink for a glass of orange juice. In reality, the product is largely sugar, orange flavors, and added vitamin C. It does not contain other nutrients such as potassium and folacin that are present in orange juice.

Food labels may mislead in other ways. A 12-oz cola beverage may boast, for example, that it contains the same percentage of sugar as an apple—only 11 percent. But if you consider the *amount* of sugar present in *one serving*, the cola contains 39 g of sugar while the apple contains only 16 g. On the other hand, an ounce of sugar-frosted cereal corn flakes contains only 12 g of sugar, although it is 39 percent sugar. Clearly, providing the *grams per serving* of sugar content is more informative to the consumer than the percentage by weight [4].

family members of different ages, sex, and nutritional needs? It would be both impractical and misleading to add up all the percentages of the U.S. RDAs supplied by each food and compare this to the RDAs for each age/sex group. Many essential nutrients do not appear on nutrition labels, so this practice would lead to erroneous conclusions. In addition, the RDAs were not meant to form the basis for planning or evaluating diets of individuals, but rather to serve as guidelines for planning the diets of groups of people. Of what practical use, then, is nutrition labeling to the consumer? Box 17-1 points out how consumers can compare the nutritive value of products relative to their costs by using nutrition labeling.

To summarize, nutrition labeling is a useful aid for helping consumers:

1. Determine major food sources of some important nutrients.
2. Compare nutritional values of different foods for some, but not all, nutrients.
3. Select the most economical sources of certain nutrients.
4. Select the most nutritious foods for the kilocalories eaten.
5. Appraise a day's nutritional adequacy for some nutrients.
6. Choose foods for special modified diets, such as for a low-fat diet.

Food Grading

In addition to nutrition labeling, other types of information may appear on the food package. Food grading is unrelated to nutritional quality but, rather, relates to texture, appearance, or "eating quality" characteristics. "Eating quality" refers to various aspects of the food that affect flavor, texture, or juiciness as discussed below regarding beef. The USDA has established grades for eggs, meats, and canned, frozen, or fresh vegetables, and fruits. The consumer can compare prices for products of the same grade when deciding what to buy. Manufacturers are not required to use USDA grading, but many elect to do so because higher grades can be sold at higher prices.

Interpreting Information on Food Labels

Food labels can help you compare the nutritive value of products relative to their cost.

Suppose you want to compare the nutritional value and cost of ready-to-eat breakfast cereals. Here is the information on the labels of three such cereals:

1   Granola. INGREDIENTS: rolled oats, brown sugar, vegetable oil (coconut, peanut, or palm oil), raisins, honey, sesame seeds, salt, cinnamon, and soy lecithin.

NUTRITION INFORMATION PER SERVING

Serving size:

1 oz = ⅓ cup	Carbohydrates, g. . .19 (12 g starch; 7 g sugars)
Calories 130	Fat, g. 5
Protein, g. 3	Sodium, mg 45

Percentage of U.S. RDA

Protein.	4	Iron	6
Vitamin A	*	Phosphorus	8
Vitamin C	*	Magnesium	6
Thiamine	6	Zinc	4
Riboflavin.	*	Copper	4
Calcium	*		

*Contains less than 2% of U.S. RDA of these nutrients.

Cost: $1.69 per lb or 10.5¢ per serving.

2   Puffed wheat. INGREDIENTS: puffed wheat, ferrous sulfate (iron), niacin, citric acid, and thiamine mononitrate.

NUTRITION INFORMATION PER SERVING

Serving size:

0.5 oz = 1 cup (heaping)	Carbohydrates, g. . .11 (all starch, no sugar)
Calories 50	Fat, g. 0
Protein, g. 2	Sodium, mg 10

Percentage of U.S. RDA

One serving contains less than 2% of U.S. RDA for protein, vitamin A, vitamin C, thiamine, riboflavin, calcium, and iron.

Cost: $3.07 per lb. or 9.5¢ per serving.

3   Sugared cereal. INGREDIENTS: sugar, oat flour, degermed yellow corn meal, corn syrup, cocoa, cornstarch, wheat starch, dextrose, salt, gelatin, calcium carbonate, trisodium phosphate, sodium ascorbate (vitamin C), artificial flavors, niacin, iron, vitamin A palmitate, pyridoxine (vitamin B_6), riboflavin, thiamine, vitamin B_{12}, vitamin D_2.

NUTRITION INFORMATION PER SERVING

Serving size:

1 oz = 1 cup	Carbohydrates, g. . .24 (11 g starch; 13 g sugars)
Calories 110	Fat, g. 1
Protein, g. 2	Sodium, mg 205

Percentage of U.S. RDA

Protein.	2	Vitamin D	.10
Vitamin A	.25	Vitamin B_6	.25
Vitamin C	.25	Vitamin B_{12}	.25
Thiamine	.25	Phosphorus	6
Riboflavin.	.25	Magnesium	6
Calcium	2	Zinc	2
Iron.	.25	Copper	4

Cost: $2.33 per lb or 14.5¢ per serving.

The lists of ingredients tell you that the sugared cereal has more sugar in it than it has cereal, while sugar is the second most prevalent ingredient in the Granola. The puffed wheat, on the other hand, has no sugar added. The ingredient lists fail to tell you *how much* sugar is present in any product, however. Let's look further to see if nutrition information tells us more about the amount of sugar present. We find that it does for these foods, but only because the manufacturer volunteered to put the amount of sugar on the label; labeling regulations so far do not require the manufacturer to do so. We see that more than one-half the carbohydrate in the sugared cereal is from sugars, while about one-third of the carbohydrate in the Granola comes from sugars.

The labels tell you that the Granola is the

most concentrated source of kilocalories of the three, and more kilocalories come from saturated fat in the Granola than in the other cereals. Since there are only 50 kcal in one heaping cup of puffed wheat, you would need to eat about 2⅔ cups of this cereal to obtain the same number of kilocalories as in ⅓ cup of Granola.

How do these two cereals compare in nutrients other than fat and carbohydrates? In percentage of the U.S. RDA, the Granola is higher in protein, thiamine, and iron than the puffed wheat. Do not be misled by the fact that iron (ferrous sulfate) is the second ingredient in the list of ingredients for puffed wheat; the amount is insignificant *as a percentage of the U.S. RDA*. The mere listing of an ingredient with no mention of the amount is a major disadvantage of current ingredient listing practices.

Using the percent of the U.S. RDA for vitamins and minerals on the label, you can quickly calculate the amount of these nutrients in a serving. Refer to the U.S. RDA standards in Appendix N to find the standard for the nutrient in question. For example, the standard for iron is 18 mg. The Granola contains 6 percent of the U.S. RDA for iron; therefore it contains 18 mg × 0.06 = 1.08 mg of iron per serving. The sugared cereal contains 18 mg × 0.25 = 4.5 mg of iron per serving.

Now, let's take a look at the sugared cereal. The cereal ingredients, oat flour and yellow corn meal (with the germ removed), are the second and third ingredients, respectively. Three ingredients are sugars: the first one, the fourth one (corn syrup), and the eighth one (dextrose). The remaining ingredients are purified starches, cocoa, gelatin, artificial flavors, and vitamins and minerals. This cereal is much higher than the other two in certain vitamins and minerals—those that were added. Notice that it is not higher than the Granola in phosphorus, zinc, magnesium, and copper—nutrients that were naturally present in the cereals. The sugared cereal is much higher than the other two in sodium, and costs from 4 to 5 cents more per serving than the other two.

This sugared cereal is one of many on the market. Are they good choices nutritionally? Does the addition of several vitamins and minerals to a high-sugar food make it a nutritious food? Why or why not? What arguments for and against such a practice can you make? Would it be cheaper to consume a basic unfortified cereal plus a vitamin pill to obtain the same nutrients? Do you need the nutrients that are added to cereals, if your total diet is well chosen? Which of the three cereals described here is the best choice you could make? What is the basis for making this decision? Examine ready-to-eat cereal packages in the grocery store, and decide which ones are the best choices nutritionally for you.

Except for meats, a higher grade product does not differ in nutritive value from that of a lower grade product. For example, eggs are graded by the USDA according to a standard that takes into account their physical characteristics. Grade AA eggs have firm yolks and thick whites which spread out very little when the eggs are removed from the shell. Grade A eggs have thinner whites that spread out moderately when broken out of the shell. While Grade A eggs are no less nutritious than Grade AA eggs, they usually cost less.

On the other hand, the highest USDA grade of beef, Prime, when compared with the next grade, Choice, has more fat on the exterior of the cut and a greater degree of fatty streaks throughout the lean meat (called marbling). The next lower grade, Good, contains even less fat. The higher the amount of marbling in beef, the greater the tenderness, juiciness, and flavorfulness. USDA grading of meats is therefore based upon these ''eating quality'' characteristics. Nutritionally, however, it is questionable whether or not large amounts of beef fat are desirable. Lower grades of beef therefore are not only less expensive than higher grades, but can be flavorful and tender with proper use of slow, moist cooking techniques, and contribute less fat to the diet than higher grades.

Grades for fresh, canned, or frozen vegetables or fruits are based on color, size, and texture characteristics, not on nutritional value. Milk products may also be graded, based on the bacterial count. Most fluid milk on the market is Grade A—that grade having the lowest bacterial count.

Product Dating

In addition to ingredient, nutrition information, and grades, product labels may also feature "open dating" information. This date may mean a number of things. It may be:

- The "pack date," meaning the date of product packaging
- The "pull date," meaning the day the product should be pulled from the shelves and not sold
- The date after which product quality declines

These dates can obviously provide you with much useful information, but there is no clear way to know which meaning to apply to the date you see listed on the package.

The food package may also feature a *universal product code*. This code is used by stores having computerized checkout stations. The computer reads the code to identify the product and the price. A universal product code is on the label shown in Figure 17-1 (the vertical lines of varying widths).

FOOD ADDITIVES

Knowing the ingredients in a food product is not always as helpful in evaluating the product as we might wish. A case in point is the subject of food additives. Knowing what is added to a product is not always sufficient to allow one to judge the benefits or possible risks involved in consuming it.

By bringing up the question of food additives with a group of people, you will almost certainly spark controversy and lively debate. On the one hand are those who fear that any additive will cause "eating to be hazardous to your health." At the other extreme are staunch additive supporters who take any criticism of additives as a direct attack on "science, technology, and the food industry." Others occupy a middle ground somewhere between these extremes.

How can one determine what attitude to take toward additives in view of the controversies they evoke? Knowing the facts about food additives will help you select foods to avoid certain additives if you wish. In addition, individuals can decide the extent to which, as consumers, they wish to become involved in legislative or regulatory decisions regarding food additives.

Food additives are substances directly added to foods to obtain a specific effect, such as enhancing color, texture, flavor, stability, shelf life, or nutritional quality. Additives also include substances that become part of food because of contact through equipment or packaging. For example, radiation used in food processing may affect food without actually becoming part of it, or a chemical substance may become part of a food through contact with equipment or packaging materials [5].

Additives have been around for a long time. When prehistoric peoples discovered that salt could preserve meat, they started to use an additive. Ancient Egyptians made food colors from vegetables. Merchants in the Middle Ages sometimes disguised spoiled food with heavy doses of saffron. Colonial Americans often used salt or brine to preserve meat and vegetables, and packed fruit in heavy syrup to preserve it, a practice which continues today [6].

Highly processed foods, so common in the American diet, often contain many food additives. Some people consume large quantities of such foods. Before processed foods became so readily available, our chief concern regarding food safety was microbial contamination. Now that food-borne infections are better controlled through wide use of refrigeration and sanitary methods of food handling, the concern is now about substances we add to our food supply, and that enter food during processing or packaging.

Today there are more than 3000 intentionally used food additives. As many as 10,000 substances may find their way into processed foods during the processing, packaging, or storage process [7]. The total consumption of food additives by a population is difficult to estimate. In 1973 the President's Science Advisory Committee estimated that somewhat more than 9 lb per person per year were consumed. This estimate did not include added sugars, salt, and fat [8]. But how important are food additives as a possible cause of harm relative to other food-borne problems? The Food and Drug Administration, the agency charged with monitoring food additives, noted in 1972 that it ranked the dangers of food additives relative to other dangers from foods as follows (in order of descending importance) [9].

1. Food-borne disease
2. Malnutrition
3. Environmental contaminants (nonintentional additives)
4. Naturally occurring toxins
5. Pesticide residues (nonintentional additives)
6. Intentional food additives

The agency consequently considered intentional food additives to be less of a danger than other substances in or other characteristics of foods.

There are many benefits of food additives. They have reduced the incidence of food-borne disease; they have increased the shelf life of many packaged goods; they have made possible a wide and varied food supply. We enjoy a year-round variety of fruits, vegetables, meat, poultry, and other foods that our grandparents never dreamed was possible—in part because of food additives. In addition, food additives have made possible a wealth of convenience foods that save hours of time in the kitchen.

But there are also risks. There are disadvantages to some of the foods made

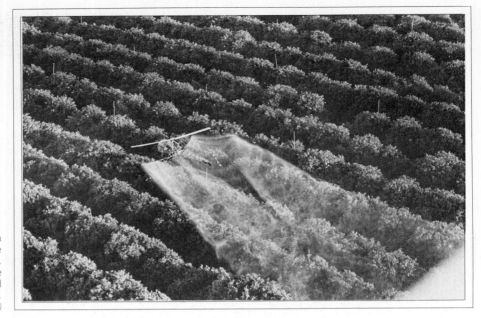

Spraying pesticides on
crops may result in some
residues on foods,
amounts of which are
monitored by state and
federal officials.
(USDA Photo)

possible by food additives—such foods are frequently high in salt, fat, sugar, and kilocalories. Sugar is the most often used additive, while salt is the second most widely used. Additives such as artificial flavorings and colorings are often found in largest amounts in foods of low nutrient density. Food made attractive by food additives may convince consumers that the food itself is highly nutritious. An example is a fruit punch advertised as "high in vitamin C," but which contains only 10 percent real fruit juice. The consumer may believe it has all the nutrients furnished by full-strength fruit juice, but in fact it furnishes only added vitamin C.

There are other risks to certain food additives too. The most highly publicized are those thought to have a possible association with cancer, such as nitrites, and some artificial sweeteners which will be discussed in some detail shortly. Some additives, such as red dye no. 2, an artificial coloring agent, have been found to cause cancer in animal studies, and thus have been prohibited from being added to food.

Intentional and Unintentional Use

Food additives may be classified as either *unintentional* or *intentional*. Unintentional additives are those that become part of the food by coming into contact with it through packaging materials or other indirect routes. *Pesticides*, which may be sprayed on fresh produce or applied to the ground where plants are growing, are examples of unintentional additives. Residues may remain on the plants or enter the plants through their roots. The Environmental Protection Agency sets tolerance levels for pesticides based on product toxicity. Legal residues on food must be no more than 1/100 of the smallest amount known to cause harm to laboratory animals. Foods are routinely sampled and tested for pesticide levels by state and federal officials as they are harvested, processed, and marketed. Foods containing more than the allowed tolerance level are not supposed to be sold.

A guide to intentional food additives is presented in Table 17-1. Intentional food additives are substances which manufacturers purposely add for one or more of the following general reasons [7]:

1. To maintain or improve the nutritive content of foods. The addition of vitamins and minerals to certain foods has been an important public health measure.
2. To ensure freshness. Ascorbic acid prevents certain frozen fruits from turning brown. BHA (butylated hydroxyanisole), and BHT (butylated hydroxytoluene) are antioxidants which stop undesirable changes in color or flavor that may occur when foods are exposed to oxygen. Some preservatives, such as benzoates and sulfites, prevent the growth of microorganisms, reducing spoilage and spread of disease.
3. To aid in preparation or processing. Some additives, such as emulsifiers, prevent oil from separating out of foods like peanut butter and mayonnaise. Thickeners improve the texture of ice cream. Leavening agents are needed to allow breads, cakes, and other baked goods to rise properly for good texture.
4. To enhance consumer acceptance. Colorings, flavorings, sugar, salt, and corn syrup all help to make foods either look or taste the way many consumers accept as being "better." The Food, Drug and Cosmetic Act prohibits the use of a color additive if it will deceive the consumer in any way. For example, a manufacturer is prohibited from using a color additive to conceal damage or inferiority in a food.
5. To decrease production costs for the manufacturer, resulting in lower consumer prices. Additives in bread, for example, prolong shelf life and diminish the number of deliveries needed to stores.

Are Additives Safe? Weighing the Risks and Benefits

In considering this question we should make a distinction between *toxicity* and *hazard*. A substance may be toxic if it is capable of causing injury under specific conditions; toxicity is a general property of matter. Water, if taken in huge amounts, for example, can be toxic but under conditions of normal use is not toxic. Hazard, on the other hand, is the ability of a substance to cause injury under normal use. Both the level of toxicity as well as the amount of a substance consumed influence possible risk. "All substances are potentially *toxic*, but are *hazardous* only if consumed in sufficiently large quantities" [10].

As testing methods for additives safety become more sophisticated, scientists are discovering, and the media are publicizing, more and more hazards associated with food additives. Many people are rapidly coming to the point of wanting to ignore all warnings—they feel it is pointless to be concerned when it is virtually impossible to eat anything not in some way associated with hazards. So they throw their hands up in dismay. Others react by concluding that *all* food additives should be avoided. What is a person to do? Let's take a look at some of the considerations involved in making judgments about the safety of food additives.

TABLE 17-1. GUIDE TO FOOD ADDITIVES

FUNCTION OF ADDITIVE	DESCRIPTION
Acid-base control	Used to alter pH of food medium or to impart flavor to food. Examples include sodium bicarbonate and potassium carbonate used in baking powders; tartaric, citric, or lactic acids in fruits, jams, and jellies. Other typical additives include hydrogen chloride, sulfuric acid, sodium hydroxide, and calcium oxide.
Antioxidants	Used to prevent fats and oils from combining with oxygen and turning rancid. Used to preserve the flavor of fats and to prevent destruction of fat-soluble vitamins in such foods as packaged mixes, dehydrated foods, frozen fruits, vegetable oils, and bakery products. Typical additives include sodium bisulfite, sulfur dioxide, ascorbic acid, tocopherols, butylated hydroxyanisole (BHA) and butylated hydroxytoluene (BHT).
Artificial sweeteners	Used to make food taste sweeter without contributing kilocalories. Sweeteners currently in use include saccharin and aspartame. Cyclamates were withdrawn from use in 1970.
Bleaching agents	Used to give a white color to foods such as flour and cheese. Typical additives include chlorine dioxide, potassium bromate, and potassium iodate.
Colors	Used to enhance the colors of foods which may have lost their natural color in food processing. Typical additives include annatto extract, beta carotene, canthaxanthin, caramel, carrot oil, citrus red no. 2, blue no. 1, red no. 3 and 40, and yellow no. 5.
Flavoring agents	Used to supplement, enhance, or modify original taste and/or aroma of a food, heighten natural flavor or restore flavors lost in processing. Typical additives include natural oils, fruit juices, disodium guanylate, disodium inosinate, hydrolyzed vegetable protein, and monosodium glutamate (MSG).
Jelling agents, stabilizers, and emulsifiers	Used to keep foods such as baby foods and jellies in a set state and prevent ingredients from settling out; used to keep products such as ice cream creamy, or to improve texture of fish cakes and sausages. Emulsifiers are used to keep oil and water in products such as mayonnaise properly mixed. Typical additives include pectin, alginate, vegetable gums, agar, methylcellulose, sodium caseinate, sodium triphosphate, disodium pyrophosphate, calcium lactate, mono- and diglycerides, polysorbate, and sorbitan monostearate.
Improving agents	Used for various purposes. They include compounds used for glazing candies; enzyme materials used in meat and baked products; foaming agents used in whipped toppings; antifoaming agents to prevent certain juices from bubbling over when containers are filled; anticaking agents to keep products such as salt from caking; firming agents to keep processed produce crisp.
Nutrients for enrichment and fortification	Examples include the B vitamins and iron used to enrich baked products; vitamin A and D used for fortifying milk; and iodine used in salt.
Preservatives	Used to prevent food spoilages. Typical additives include ascorbic acid, benzoic acid, butylparaben, calcium lactate, calcium propionate, calcium sorbate, citric acid, and propylparaben.

This guide will help you sort out the facts about important additives found in our food supply.
SOURCES: 1. Mayer, J., "Experts are Divided about Food Additives," *Family Health/Today's Health,* July 1976, p. 38.

2. "More Than You Ever Thought You Would Know about Food Additives," reprint from *FDA Consumer,* April 1979. HEW Publication No. (FDA) 79–2115,

Testing for Safety   Rigorous testing requirements for food additives help enhance the safety of our food supply. Manufacturers must receive approval from the FDA to use any *new* additives. Before this approval can be granted manufacturers must supply convincing evidence that the additive is safe and that it will play a useful role in the food supply. Because of the difficulty in proving that an additive is safe, at least three types of toxicity tests must be conducted with laboratory animals [11]. Animals, rather than human subjects, are used for ethical reasons.

1. An acute toxicity test must show the effects of one dose of the additive given to a minimum of two different species of animals.
2. Short-term toxicity tests determine the effects of feeding diets containing varying levels of the additive to at least two different animal species over a period of 30 to 180 days.
3. Long-term tests determine the extent to which the additive produces diseased or harmful states, such as chronic diseases. Where possible, tests to determine birth defects, mutations, or genetic changes should also be carried out.

The testing procedures often involve determining the "no-effect" dose—that level of intake that produces no harmful effects. For example, we might give animals 100 mg of a particular additive and see no harmful effects. We might increase the dose to 200, 500, and 800 mg and still see no harmful effects, but find that giving 900 mg resulted in, let's say, nervous system damage. Thus, we have found the "no-effect" dose, and the dose that results in a noticeable and harmful effect.

An additive is not usually approved by the FDA for human use unless the dose that results in a harmful effect is more than 100 times the amount that humans would normally use—in other words there must be a 100-fold safety factor. This safety factor does not apply in the case of cancer-causing substances, however. Substances that cause cancer when fed to animals *in any amount* are prohibited from use in foods.

Critics of animal studies sometimes take issue with the quantity of an additive used in a test, comparing this amount, relative to the size of the animal, to the amounts a human would ingest. For example, a typical remark might be, "Dosages of additive X fed rats in the study were more than the amount a human would consume by eating 500 hot dogs a day over a lifetime." The critics might say that the animal studies used to test the safety of additive X could not be applied to humans because of the extremely large doses used. Is this a legitimate criticism?

Why are such large doses of additives used in animal studies? One reason is to compensate for the rapid metabolism and excretion of additives by animals, in contrast to the slower rate of metabolism in humans. A slower metabolism means that chemicals stay in the human body longer, thus exerting possible harmful effects for a longer time period. Another reason is to compensate for the very short life span of animals—many animals used in testing food additives, such as small rodents, live an average of only 2 years. There is also a statistical reason. If we tested only low amounts, we might have to use as many as a million animals per study to find a significant effect. Such a study would be physically and economically impossible to carry out. Another consideration is that the harmful effects of food additives may accumulate over a period of years. In addition, some forms of cancer may take 20, 30, or even 50 years to develop in humans. It is possible that extremely large doses may shorten the time it takes for cancer to first appear in animals.

Critics of some of the animal studies suggest that as long as humans don't eat huge quantities of the additive-containing food each day, we don't have to worry about cancer. But others are convinced that there is no safe level of intake of a carcinogen. The present assumption is that if a large amount of a substance causes cancer in animals, there may be some risk when humans eat only a small amount. What we don't know is exactly what the level of risk is. The risk may be very small, but it is *not* zero. While a chemical that causes cancer in animals may not necessarily be carcinogenic in humans, many experts agree that animal studies are valid for determining those substances likely to cause human cancer.

With any testing for food hazard we run into the problem that our methods of testing are not good enough to ever prove *absolute* safety. The National Academy of Sciences' Food Protection Committee stated it this way: "No method is at hand—and none is in sight—for establishing, with absolute certainty, the safety of a food chemical under all conditions of use. Experience has shown, however, that properly conducted and interpreted animal experiments can provide that degree of assurance of safety reasonably expected in the evaluation of chemicals for use in human food " [12].

Regulation of Additives

Food additives are more closely regulated now than ever before. The 1906 Food and Drug Act, and the 1938 Food, Drug and Cosmetic Act provided federal authority for removing poisonous and adulterated food from the market [11]. The 1958 Food Additives Amendment to the Food, Drug and Cosmetic Act provided that the manufacturer had to put new additives through the battery of animal tests previously described *before* they could be added to foods. Prior to 1958, the *FDA* had to test additives for safety *after* they had been added to foods [13].

The 1958 law exempted certain additives from testing. These included about 600 additives that scientific experts judged to be safe, and included sugar, salt, spices, and baking powder. These additives were "generally recognized as safe," and are referred to as *GRAS* substances. In 1969, however, the cyclamate sweeteners, classified as GRAS, were found to produce bladder cancer in animals. Public confidence in the safety of the GRAS list of additives was shaken, and a review of these additives began [14]. The FDA called upon the Federation of American Societies for Experimental Biology (FASEB) to conduct the review [15]. This group classified additives as follows:

Additives such as vegetable oils, casein, and certain aluminum compounds are given *Class 1* status, meaning that they are considered to be safe for use at current levels.

Class 2 substances, including certain iron and zinc salts, are considered safe for use at current levels, but should be studied to determine *if* a large increase in consumption would be hazardous.

Class 3 substances, such as caffeine, BHA, and BHT, are recommended for further study because their safety is not clearly resolved.

For *Class 4* substances, including salt and some modified starches, it is recommended that the FDA establish safer conditions for use or prohibit their addition to food.

Class 5 substances, including some glycerides and certain iron salts, are recommended for removal from the GRAS list unless additional data become available to allow adequate evaluation of their safety [15].

The *Delaney Clause* of the 1958 Food Additive Amendment forbids the use of any additive found to induce cancer in either humans or animals [11]. This amendment pertains to food and color additives but not to substances used in animal feed that do not harm the animal or appear in edible meat.

While the objectives of the Delaney Clause are admirable, it has been the source of much controversy. Basic to the controversy are several unanswered questions. Is there a threshold level below which a substance will not cause cancer? Modern technology can detect substances in foods at extremely low levels. Must even the tiniest trace be regarded as cancer-causing? Are there cumulative effects of additives? Might a substance be harmful to humans but not to animals? Or harmful to some, but not all humans?

Much of the current debate centers around saccharin and nitrites. Let's explore some of the issues involved in the debate over these two additives. The nitrate controversy is discussed in Box 17-2.

The Saccharin Controversy

Artificially sweetened products constitute a $2 billion market in the United States. An estimated 50 to 70 million Americans, including up to one-third of American children under the age of 10, consume saccharin regularly [23]. Some 6 million lb of saccharin are consumed each year—three-fourths of this is in soft drinks, while the rest is in tea, coffee, and dietetic foods. Saccharin, discovered in 1879, was initially used as an antiseptic and as a food preservative. Later it began to be used as a noncalorie dietary sweetener [23]. Before 1900, European tests reported its safety, but in 1912 President Roosevelt ordered saccharin to be reviewed for safety. The review board reported that an intake of 300 mg daily was safe but more than 1000 mg was likely to cause digestive disturbances. It was banned from food, but allowed again in food during World War I when sugar became scarce. Saccharin has been frequently reviewed—no less than five expert committees of the National Academy of Sciences have reviewed its safety [24].

The event that led to much of the current controversy was the demonstration, in Canadian studies, that saccharin was associated with an increased incidence of bladder cancer in rats [25]. The experiment was conducted on two generations of rats. One group of 100 rats was given a standard diet containing 5 percent saccharin while another group, the controls, received the same diet without the saccharin. The study continued through the entire lives of these rats, and through the lives of their offspring. The offspring of the saccharin group were therefore exposed to saccharin not only in their diet but also in utero.

The results showed a significant increase in bladder cancer in the parents and

The Nitrate-Nitrite Controversy

The nitrate controversy is largely focused on whether or not nitrates and nitrites should be permitted in cured meats such as bacon, ham, and cold cuts. Concern escalated when it was found that nitrites can combine with substances in food or drugs, called secondary amines, to yield *nitrosamines*, which have been found to cause cancer in animals. Nitrosamines have been found in cigarette smoke, cooked bacon, and in certain beers [16]. In the United States about 1.1 μg per day of nitrosamines are estimated to be consumed daily [17].

Nitrates occur naturally in vegetables, soil, and water, and have been used to cure meats for thousands of years. In the United States, about 80 percent of our nitrate intake comes from vegetables [18]. Nitrite is a chemical derivative of nitrate. The conversion of nitrate to nitrite occurs during storage of food at room temperature, and also, at a slower rate, under refrigeration. The average U.S. diet furnishes about 75 mg of nitrate and 0.8 mg of nitrite per day [19].

Although it has been assumed that decreasing the use of nitrates and nitrites as preservatives in meats and cheese and limiting the amount of nitrosamines allowed in foods would diminish the risk of cancer, recent research indicates that the picture is more complex than it seemed at first. Researchers have demonstrated that bacteria in the mouth convert nitrates entering the mouth via saliva to nitrites. Furthermore, bacteria in the intestinal tract also produce nitrite, which may be absorbed into the blood and converted to nitrate. This is one of the sources of the nitrate found in saliva [20].

The nitrite formed from the nitrate in saliva can form nitrosamines if it encounters amines in the stomach or intestines. Therefore nitrosamine formation in the human body does not result solely from dietary intake of nitrites or nitrosamines. These observations have prompted the meat industry to argue that banning the use of nitrates and nitrites in cured meat would result in only a very small reduction in risk of cancer.

Let's consider the nitrite controversy from a risk-benefit standpoint. The meat industry argues that nitrite benefits the public because it is essential in cured meats to [21]:

Sausages are among many meat products treated with nitrates and nitrites to prevent spoilage and impart a characteristic color and flavor. (© *John Coletti/Stock, Boston, Inc.*)

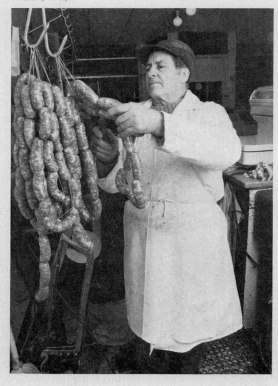

- Prevent botulism, a serious form of food poisoning
- Give cured meat a special flavor and appearance which many consumers now expect and like
- Reduce oxidation in cured meats which otherwise results in an undesirable, warmed-over flavor.

The long-term risk of cancer if nitrite use in cured meats continues must therefore be weighed against the immediate risk of botulism if nitrite use is discontinued. Banning nitrates and nitrites would also result in tremendous economic losses for the meat industry, adversely affecting meat prices for the consumer.

The problem's solution lies in documenting through further research the extent to which cured meats contribute to cancer risks. While products such as nitrate- and nitrite-free sausages and bacon have been developed and marketed, the industry maintains that consumer acceptance of such products is less than for products treated with nitrate [21]. Currently, the use of vitamin C to prevent formation of nitrosamines in foods is under study [22].

In the meantime, research is needed to establish whether or not foods high in vitamin C and vitamin E effectively block nitrosamine formation in the human body [20]. Consumers themselves must decide whether the benefits of consuming cured meats outweigh the risks. Two recent reports of the National Academy of Sciences recommended that exposure to nitrites and nitrosamines should be minimized [17,19]. In deciding whether or not to moderate consumption of cured meats, consumers may wish to take into account the fact that these products also tend to be high in fat and salt.

offspring fed saccharin, but no significant increase in bladder cancer in the control rats. Consequently, the Food and Drug Administration proposed to ban saccharin [26]. The FDA maintained that it was imposing this ban under the Delaney Amendment anticancer clause, as well as under the provisions of the Food, Drug and Cosmetic Act.

As a result of the proposed ban, the FDA reported that it received more telephone calls than about any other issue in its history. The Calorie Control Council, representing the diet food industry, encouraged consumer protest.

In view of consumer protest, and because saccharin was the last available nonnutritive sweetener permitted in food, Congress directed that the ban be delayed while further study of its safety was conducted. At present, researchers continue to search for a safe noncalorie sweetener acceptable to the American public. Since the proposal to ban saccharin, aspartame has been approved as a sweetener by the Food and Drug Administration [23]. A low-calorie synthetic sweetener 180 times sweeter than sugar, aspartame can be used as a dry table-top sugar substitute, but is not suitable for cooking or baking since heat causes it to lose its sweetness. Aspartame provides 4 kcal/g; the sweetener equivalent of 1 tsp of sugar will contain only $\frac{1}{10}$ of a kilocalorie.

Risks and Benefits of Saccharin The National Academy of Sciences (NAS) studied both the benefits and risks of saccharin [27]. The Academy concluded that saccharin is a carcinogen, but of low potency compared to other carcinogens. In other words, a much larger dose of saccharin is needed to cause cancer than is needed for other, stronger carcinogens, such as some of the artificial colors now banned from our food supply.

The NAS also found that saccharin can promote the action of other carcinogens—when animals previously exposed to other substances that cause bladder cancer consume saccharin, the incidence of cancer is increased. Since saccharin is widely used in the American food supply, even a small risk might result in anywhere from 0 to 3000 cases of bladder cancer a year.

Saccharin is particularly dangerous to, and should not be used by pregnant women and young children, who may consume great amounts of saccharin in soft drinks, toothpaste, and sugarless gum over long periods of time [27]. Children are at greater risk than adults for any harmful substances because a smaller dose can be more damaging to their small bodies than for adults. They are also at greater risk because of possible long-term effects of consuming a harmful substance.

Many argue that a benefit of saccharin is that if substituted for sugar, it may reduce the incidence of obesity and dental caries. Saccharin use also allows an individual with diabetes to enjoy a sweet taste while still avoiding sugar. The NAS reviewed studies on the benefits of saccharin in weight control, in decreasing dental caries, and in the control of diabetes and found insufficient information on the effects of saccharin on food habits to be certain that banning it would increase sugar consumption, which in turn might lead to detrimental health effects. However, the possible increase in sugar intake would probably be small, since saccharin represents only about 6 percent of the total sweeteners used in the American diet.

For many weight watchers and diabetic patients saccharin may be of psychological value, since it allows them to feel less deprived. But is this a real benefit? Should the craving for sweetness be encouraged by a product that entails health risks? Does saccharin merely allow us to cater to the sweet tooth syndrome? Instead, should we be trying to retrain our eating habits, to require less "sweetness"?

Many Canadian scientists believe that the original decision to limit saccharin was a wise one [28]. But because the saccharin controversy has become a compelling symbol for different causes, it will not be easily resolved. Some hail it as an issue of safeguarding the right of individual freedom of choice, believing that each individual should be allowed to decide whether or not to use saccharin. Others see the issue as one of safeguarding our food supply, believing it necessary to ban saccharin to keep our food supply as safe as possible. Meanwhile, by reading labels carefully, one can avoid products containing saccharin if one desires.

Weighing Risks Against Benefits

People in modern industrialized societies encounter a great many risks. The risk of death in a car accident is about 170 per million persons per year, while that from smoking a package of cigarettes per day is about 5000 per million persons per year [29]. Yet people continue to drive cars and smoke cigarettes. Obviously, for many people, the benefits they receive from automobile use and cigarette smoking outweigh the risks.

When we try to weigh risks against benefits for food additives, many problems need to be understood. Most authorities tend to agree that we cannot have an absolutely risk-free food supply. Modern technology allows us to detect chemical contaminants or additives in foods at levels as low as one part per billion, and, for some, even as low as one part per trillion. If such minute amounts of possibly harmful substances were required by law to be eliminated from foods, we would be unable to feed our population. A major problem is the great difficulty we face in determining scientifically to what extent a substance is harmful in the food supply. Unfortunately, our scientific methods for trying to assess risk are far from perfect. Despite such imperfections, however, policy makers must make decisions about the safety of the food supply.

The NAS has suggested that the FDA should categorize food additives into those of high, moderate, or low risk [27]. Foods or ingredients categorized as *high-risk* would be those implicated in causing severe damage with great frequency. These would be banned from the food supply. *Moderate-risk* foods or ingredients would be those causing harm with enough frequency to justify regulation of their use. The FDA would endeavor to reduce the public's consumption of such additives. Products containing them might be labeled as to the nature and magnitude of the risk involved. Alternatives to these additives might be sought, with a view toward a gradual phaseout of such additives. *Low-risk* additives would be those having apparently little or no risk. These would be permitted in the food supply with no restrictions.

Unfortunately, this system would depend upon the ability of science to properly categorize additives. Consumers still could become cynical about the safety of the food supply if several additives, originally categorized as low risk, were later found to be of moderate or high risk.

Dr. Sanford Miller, head of the FDA's Bureau of Foods, has maintained that it would be impractical for his agency to attempt to weigh the risks of an additive against the benefits. As he pointed out, it would be impossible to quantify the benefits in terms of economic gain, convenience, palatability, and aesthetic appeal against the risks, which are often of uncertain probability [30]. Many writers in the field believe that only the public can decide the *benefits* of additives, while the health risks must be scientifically assessed. The public, however, can assess other practical disadvantages of food additives. Some of these become apparent in examining fortified and enriched foods.

Fortification of Foods   *Fortified foods* are those to which nutrients are added, many of which may never have been present in the original food. Vitamins A and B_{12} may be added to breakfast cereals, for example. *Enrichment* is a specific form of fortification in which certain nutrients, removed in processing, are added back. The best-known example is that of enriched breads, cereals, and flour to which thiamine, riboflavin, niacin, and iron are added. This procedure has been an important public health measure to combat pellagra, beriberi, and iron-deficiency anemia. Fortification of milk with vitamin D has prevented rickets, and

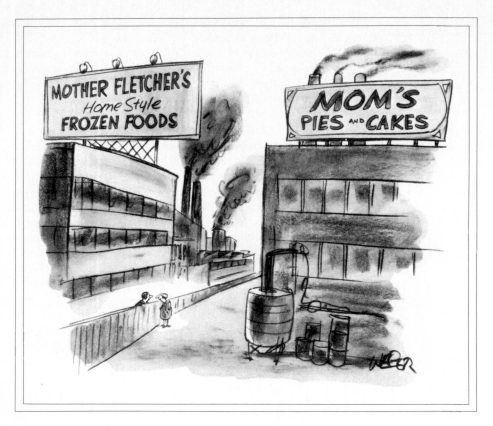

the addition of iodine to salt was effective in eradicating goiter in many areas. The addition of vitamin A to sugar has been an effective means of preventing serious vitamin A deficiency and resulting blindness in some developing countries.

The use of sugar as a carrier for vitamin A fortification brings to light some of the problems with fortification, however. Some have argued that fortification is advantageous because it allows people to continue with their usual food habits, rather than learning to eat new foods, or foods they like less well. But adding one or a few nutrients to foods such as sugar or sodas can never be regarded as a long-term solution to nutritional problems. Long-term solutions involve finding means to provide people with a variety of foods furnishing all the nutrients needed. Educational programs aimed at changing food habits constitute an important part of such an endeavor.

In the industrialized countries, many highly fortified foods are high in kilocalories, fat, sugar, and salt. Unsuspecting consumers may be misled by the long list of nutrients on the wrapper or package, and believe they are nourishing themselves well. They may be unaware that the cost of fortification to the manufacturer is extremely low, and that the product they are consuming is made up entirely of very inexpensive ingredients. Yet they have paid a premium because the markup is usually high on fortified foods.

IRRADIATED FOOD: PROMISE AND CONTROVERSY

James P. Sterba, *The New York Times*, June 30, 1982

When Mona Doyle, a marketing pollster, asks people if they want alternatives to the chemical preservatives in their food, most of them say yes. When she asks if they want fruits, vegetables and meat that stay fresher longer, they say yes.

But when she mentions a preservation technique that promises to make those things possible, they respond, she says, by asking such half-serious questions as "Does it make you glow in the dark?"

The technique is irradiation—exposing foods to gamma rays or electrons emitted by radioactive materials— . . .

. . . In this country, where the technology was pioneered, food preservation through irradiation has remained, with minor exceptions, illegal. Its only authorized uses are for potatoes, wheat, and wheat flour—all products cheap and abundant enough to make irradiating them uneconomical. Otherwise, only nonpublic, experimental uses have been allowed. For example, during the Apollo space program, men on the moon ate ham sterilized by irradiation. . . .

Dr. Sanford A. Miller, director of the Food and Drug Administration's Bureau of Foods, predicted in an interview last month that rule changes allowing low-level radiation doses would be completed sometime this year. He said medium-level doses of up to one megarad would probably be approved "within a year or so." A rad is a measure of absorbed radiation; a kilorad equals 1,000 rads, and a megarad equals 1,000 kilorads. Many scientists, in and out of the Government, contend that years of United States Army research have shown that some chemicals currently in use may pose greater problems than irradiation. They also argue that in relatively low doses, radiation changes food chemically far less than does canning or cooking in conventional or microwave ovens.

On the other hand, a proliferation of plants using the irradiation process might face opposition from nearby property owners and others concerned about the transport of radioactive materials, disposal of wastes and employee health and safety.

Opponents . . . say research on irradiation to date remains inadequate. They argue . . . that the rays or electrons can result, at least in theory, in chemical changes that do not occur in other forms of processing and that might be dangerous. . . . They urge more study to determine the nature of these chemicals, the quantities in which they are created, whether or not they are found in other foods or in nature, and whether human digestive processes are capable of rendering them harmless.

Charles Merritt Jr., a researcher at the Army's food engineering laboratory at Natick, Mass., said long-term animal feeding studies to answer the above questions have turned up "no red flags" or harmful signs. Those results are now being turned over to an independent laboratory for verification. . . .

In explaining the process, Dr. Jack Schubert, professor of chemistry at the University of Maryland . . . said that the gamma rays, which are shorter and more penetrating than X-rays or microwave radiation, kill bacteria by disturbing their metabolism, making them unable to divide and grow. Irradiation slows down the ripening of fruit and vegetables by slowing down cell division.

The F.D.A. served notice in the March 27, 1981, Federal Register of its intention to allow irradiation up to 100 kilorads for normal foods and up to five megarads for foods that comprise only a small portion of the human diet, namely spices.

Applications within the 100-kilorad range include slowing down sprouting of potatoes, onions, garlic, ginger, carrots, sweet potatoes and yams, killing off fruit-fly infestations, and slowing down ripening in tropical fruits. . . .

. . . Mona Doyle, who is president of Consumer Network Inc. in Philadelphia . . . told

Fortified foods do not and cannot contain all the nutrients the body needs in the proportions needed. Human beings evolved consuming a variety of minimally processed foods, and so far no fortified or "engineered" food or group of foods has been shown to equal a mixture of minimally processed, traditional foods in nutritive value. The public, therefore, can assess the risks of consuming large amounts of fortified foods relative to the objective of obtaining a diet furnishing all the needed nutrients without being high in kilocalories, fat, sugar, or salt.

How can we answer our original question, "Are food additives safe?" As it turns out, we can't give a definite answer. We simply don't know the effects of many additives as they interact with each other and with other food ingredients, and sometimes we can't be sure of the effects of single additives. A wide variety of foods helps ensure that if some dangerous substances are eaten they will be eaten in relatively small amounts. There is probably a much greater health risk in consuming too much food in general, or in consuming a diet too high in fat, sugar, or salt than there is from food additives (see Chapter 5). The prudent course to follow is to eat a wide variety of foods, and to be moderate in the consumption of any one food. Choosing minimally processed foods also helps lower one's intake of additives. These practices limit the dangers of overconsumption of any one additive, as well as provide the consumer with a healthy range of essential nutrients.

NATURALLY OCCURRING TOXICANTS IN FOOD

While much of the concern about food hazards centers on food additives, some toxins occur naturally in foods. Some foods contain substances that interfere with the utilization of nutrients, for example. Oxalates, commonly found in spinach, Swiss chard, beet tops, and rhubarb, interfere with the absorption of calcium. Rhubarb leaves contain a large concentration of oxalic acid and can result in poisoning. Symptoms include abdominal pain, diarrhea, and vomiting.

Some foods are toxic under special circumstances. For example, people eating substances to which they are allergic may develop toxic reactions. Table 17-2 presents additional information about other toxicants that occur naturally in foods. Although the amount of these toxic substances found in particular foods is important in determining how toxic they will be to humans, other factors must be considered also. These include the size of the subject (children are more vulnerable than adults), the speed of ingestion, other foods eaten with the toxicant, the amount of food ingested at one time, and the individual's ability to detoxify the toxin.

What is the prudent approach to take to avoid danger from naturally occurring toxicants? The advice is similar to that given regarding food additives. Avoid, to the extent possible, foods likely to contain toxicants. Avoid fad diets relying heavily on one particular food. By eating a wide variety of different kinds of foods, it is unlikely that you will consume an excessive amount of a food.

ANTIBIOTICS IN ANIMAL FEED

Antibiotics such as penicillin and tetracycline are widely added to animal feed. In fact, such drugs have revolutionized agriculture. Almost all American poultry,

TABLE 17-2. NATURALLY OCCURRING TOXINS IN FOOD

TOXIC SUBSTANCES	MOST OFTEN FOUND IN	COMMENTS
Aflatoxins	Peanuts, corn, rice, soybeans, wheat, sorghum seed and ground nuts. These foods are monitored for aflatoxins.	Aflatoxins, produced by fungi, may grow on nuts, cereals, and legumes during storage and drying. Toxicity results in degenerative changes in kidney and liver, hemorrhages, and cancer.
Citral	Uncooked orange peel.	Acts as an antagonist to vitamin A. Large doses may result in a deficiency of vitamin A.
Oxalates	Spinach, swiss chard, beet tops, rhubarb, tea, cocoa.	Decreases absorption of calcium. Consumption of large amounts results in human poisoning.
Safrole	Occurs in several spices, including mace, nutmeg, ginger, anise, black pepper, also in cocoa. Also in sassafras tea.	Causes cancer in animals.
Solanine	Primarily in potatoes; smaller amounts in apples and eggplant, in roots and leaves of tomatoes, and in sugar beet roots. Potatoes are now monitored for solanine.	Gastrointestinal upset and neurological disorders, hemorrhaging and comas and eventually death may result from toxic dosages.
Cyanogenetic glycosides	Pits of peaches and apricots, choke cherries; cassava, lima beans.	Results in hydrogen cyanide (HCN) production or release when treated with acid. HCN inhibits respiration, and hence poisons humans.

SOURCE: Committee on Food Protection, Food and Nutrition Board, *Toxicants Occurring Naturally in Foods*, Washington, D.C.: National Academy of Sciences, 1973.

hogs, and veal calves and more than half our cattle receive antibiotics in their feed. Forty percent of the antibiotics used in the United States are used in animal feeds. These drugs not only help keep the livestock in good health, but allow them to grow faster while eating less food [31].

Evidence is now beginning to show that widespread use of antibiotics in animal feed may cause human health problems, however. As disease-causing bacteria are exposed to increasing amounts of antibiotics, they begin to become resistant to the action of the antibiotic. For example, penicillin, once an easy cure for many diseases, has become increasingly ineffective. Many scientists believe that the resistance to antibiotics shown by some bacteria in humans may originate from the use of antibiotics in animal feed. When bacteria in animals are exposed to antibiotics over a long period, the bacteria evolve into strains that are resistant to the antibiotics. The resistant bacteria grow and multiply. Some strains of bacteria exist in both animals and humans, and resistance to antibiotics can be passed from animals to humans [31]. Slaughterhouse and farm workers who frequently work with antibiotic-containing feed or raw meat have more drug-resistant bacteria in their intestines than do other workers [32].

The FDA has tried, unsuccessfully, to limit the amounts of antibiotics added

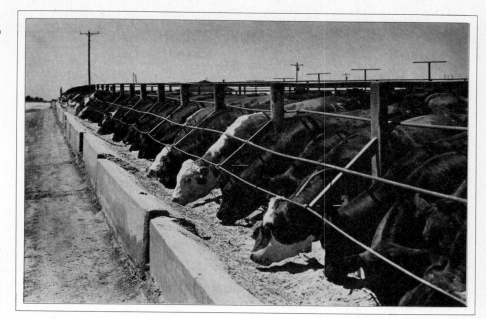

Antibiotics used in animal feeds to increase their growth rate and to keep them healthy may result in some human health problems. *(USDA Photo by Fred S. Witte)*

to animal feed. Those who manufacture such drugs, as well as many farmers, have convinced Congress to prevent action by the FDA. These special-interest groups maintain that limiting antibiotics in animal feed could result in up to 25 percent increased cost of meat and poultry production. Animals can reach optimum weight without the addition of antibiotics to feed. However, the rate of gain is slower and more food is needed to reach the same weight than is the case for animals fed antibiotics. Feeding efficiency is increased with the use of antibiotics, so that the use of antibiotics in animal feed improves the utilization of nutrients. The economic advantage for the producer is obvious.

Proponents of antibiotics in animal feed say that it is impossible to tell if one specific case of a resistant disease in humans is the result of the use of antibiotics in animal feed, or if, instead, it is the result of too heavy use of antibiotics in human therapy. However, many scientists point out that because feeding animals antibiotics increases the earth's population of resistant bacteria, such a practice should be banned. While the controversy will probably rage on, many concerned individuals are calling on livestock producers to voluntarily stop using antibiotics, and to search for practical alternatives.

SUMMARY

1 All food labels must contain certain basic information including product name, net weight of the product, and a list of ingredients presented in the order of ingredients' decreasing weight.

2 Nutrition labeling is required on foods if a nutrient has been added, if a nutritional claim is made about the food, or if the food is intended for special dietary use. The U.S. RDAs are the legal standards for labeling foods according to their nutritive content.

3 Food additives may be either intentional or uninten-

tional. Additives are used for a variety of reasons, including to improve nutritive content, to ensure freshness, to aid in processing, and to improve consumer acceptance.

4 There are benefits as well as risks involved in consuming foods with additives. In considering the question of food additive safety, both need to be weighed.

5 Before manufacturers can use a new food additive they must receive approval from the Food and Drug Administration by providing evidence that the additive is safe and useful. Among additives that do not have to be approved are those on the GRAS (generally recognized as safe) list.

6 Examples of controversial additives include saccharin, nitrite, artificial colors, pesticides, and antibiotics used in animal feed. The National Academy of Sciences has suggested that the risk involved in using an additive should be defined as low, moderate, or high. Regulatory action to be taken would depend upon the degree of risk involved in using the additive.

7 Certain substances which occur naturally may be toxic. Examples include substances that interfere with nutrient utilization, such as oxalates, and some foods that are toxic under certain circumstances, such as potatoes containing solanine, if eaten in large quantities.

8 Consumption of a wide variety of minimally processed foods coupled with moderation in consumption of any one food helps minimize the intake of food additives and of toxicants occurring naturally in food.

FOR DISCUSSION AND APPLICATION

1 Nutrition labeling
   a. Compare the amounts of protein, kilocalories, fat, calcium, and vitamin A and D in whole fluid milk, low-fat milk, skim milk, and reconstituted nonfat dry milk. Which is the most economical buy? How did you decide? Which is the lowest in kilocalories? In fat? In calcium? Which type of milk would you choose? Why?
   b. Read the label of a frozen beef pie. Compare the amount of protein in the entire dinner with the protein content of a serving of hamburger; of chicken. Compare the costs per serving.
   c. Compare the amount of vitamin C and of added sugar (if on the label) in a fruit drink and in bottled orange juice. Which drink has the highest vitamin C content? The highest kilocalorie content? The highest sugar content? Compare the cost per serving of the various products. Which is the best food buy, in light of these factors?
   d. Select a food product that comes in a variety of different brands and forms. For example: raw potatoes, french fries, potato chips, creamed frozen potatoes, instant mashed potatoes, etc. Study the ingredient and nutrition labels of these foods. Evaluate the nutritional advantages and disadvantages of each. Also, identify other advantages and disadvantages of each, such as taste, convenience, cost, etc. Select the best buy and justify your choice.

2 Food cooperative assignment

Many small food cooperatives have the objective of providing their members and other patrons with nutritious foods at low cost. Often, such stores operate using volunteer help from their members and make little if any profit.

Visit a food cooperative (not a health food store, since these exist for profit) and answer the following questions about the store.
   a. Describe briefly the neighborhood in which the store is located.
   b. Describe the physical appearance of the store. How does it differ from a supermarket?
   c. What items are for sale that are not commonly seen in supermarkets?
   d. What items commonly available in supermarkets are not available in this store?
   e. Are vitamin and mineral supplements sold here? If so, how much space is devoted to them?
   f. Are most foods sold already packaged, or are they available in bulk so that the consumer sacks his or her own purchase?
   g. Are fresh fruits and vegetables available? If so, do they look fresh? How are they displayed?
   h. Are fresh meats available? Dairy products?
   i. Are any nutrition books or pamphlets available? If so, what are some of the authors and titles?
   j. If you have the opportunity, speak with someone in charge about the basic philosophy behind the store. Alternatively, interview a customer about the extent to which his or her food

purchases are made at this store, and why he or
she has chosen to shop here.

k. Get the lowest prices on:

1 lb brown rice
1 lb kidney beans
1 lb navy beans
1 lb whole wheat flour
1 lb whole wheat bread
1 lb oatmeal
1 lb cheddar cheese

l. In class, (1) compare prices obtained with those
in local supermarkets, (2) have a discussion,
bringing out each student's observations.

SUGGESTED READINGS

Consumer's Resource Handbook. This is a "what-to-do,
where-to-go" manual for resolving consumer problems. Published by the White House Office of the
Special Assistant for Consumer Affairs, it may be
obtained by writing to: The Consumer Information
Center, Department 532G, Pueblo, Colo., 81009.

Consumer Information Catalog lists over 200 publications from the federal government. Many of these
relate to food and nutrition and health care. To
receive a free copy, write to: The Consumer Information Center, Department 52, Pueblo, Colo.,
81009.

Wurtman, J. J., *Eating Your Way Through Life: A No-
Nonsense Guide to Good Nutrition for All Ages and
All Eating Styles*, New York: Raven Press, 1979. An
interesting book offering a practical approach to
food and nutrition for people with various needs.
Consumer issues are discussed.

Black, J., ed., *The Berkeley Co-op Food Book*, Palo
Alto, Calif.: Bull Publishing Co., 1980. This book
shows the way to "eat better and spend less." It
compiles 25 years of articles, recipes, and consumer resources.

18 WORLD FOOD PROBLEMS

The importance of good nutrition and the problems associated with both over- and undernutrition in the United States have been discussed in earlier chapters. This chapter will focus on the causes and consequences of malnutrition in developing countries. It will discuss the crisis proportions of the problem and describe strategies that have been proposed or implemented to solve the problems of hunger and malnutrition.

Most of you probably have not directly experienced hunger and nutritional deprivation yourself, and it would be highly impractical to try to directly experience hunger. What is it like to be hungry? Arthur Hopcraft, who studied worldwide hunger, provides a moving description of his observations on visiting a famine area in India where a mass of 300 to 400 people gathered in a church courtyard, where each received a bowl of watery gruel. In his report, *Born To Hunger* he writes [1]:

> They were emaciated, dirty and in rags. They were keeping up a shrill clamour of pleading, harsh and feeble at the same time, and the most chilling sound I have ever heard. Bony fingers, with the skin peeling off them, clutched the railing. More hands reached through, holding out bowls. Every face had the same glazed desperation. At the front of the crowd were several children. One little boy with wasted, dangling arms had a particularly grey look about his skin. I reached out to touch him, and felt a dry, rough texture, not like skin at all but more like matting. It seemed to me that at least one-third of these people had fallen so far below the stage of mere hunger that they needed hospital attention, as well as food. There was not the slightest chance that they would get it.

While it is helpful to gain some understanding of what it is like to be hungry, we need also to know the facts about world food problems.

KINDS AND EXTENT OF MALNUTRITION

Malnutrition is a state that adversely affects growth and development of body functioning as a result of either an inadequate or an overabundant supply of kilocalories or nutrients to body tissues. (The prefix *mal* means bad.) We have noted that overabundance is an important factor in many diseases of affluent countries (Chapter 5). *Undernutrition* or inadequate nutrition, on the other hand, is more common in developing countries. In this chapter, the term malnutrition is used to denote undernutrition.

Consequences of Malnutrition

Malnutrition may take forms other than that of protein-calorie deprivation discussed in Chapter 6. Numerous vitamin and/or mineral deficiencies frequently occur along with or in the absence of protein or kilocalorie deficiencies (Chapters 9–12). Table 18-1 presents a summary of these nutritional disorders. A possible consequence of malnutrition is its effect on mental development. Is severe malnutrition suffered throughout much of childhood a causative factor in retarded mental development?

If we had asked this question in the 1960s we might have received a "yes" answer from the nutrition experts. In 1969, for example, an editorial in *Science* summarized current thinking on the relationship between malnutrition and mental development by stating that it seemed likely that millions of poor children experienced some retardation in learning as a result of inadequate nutrition [2].

But our thinking on the subject has greatly changed. We now have a greater appreciation for the complexity of the relationships among environmental factors and mental development. We now realize that the human brain does not live by bread alone. Malnutrition causes children to become listless and apathetic. Because they are less curious, they explore less, and respond less to their surroundings than do well-nourished children. Consequently, adults and other sources of stimulation are often less responsive to the child. Reduced learning

TABLE 18-1. NUTRIENT DEFICIENCY DISEASES

DISEASE	NUTRIENT DEFICIENCY	CHARACTERISTICS	POPULATION GROUPS AT HIGH RISK
Anemia	Iron, folic acid, B_{12}	Lethargy, pallor, low hemoglobin and hematocrit	Women before menopause, infants, children
Beriberi	Thiamine	Heart failure, brain, muscle damage	Pregnant women, young infants, adults
Fluorine deficiency	Fluorine	Dental caries	Risk begins in childhood
Goiter	Iodine	Enlarged thyroid gland	Adults, adolescents
Endemic cretinism	Iodine	Mental retardation, deafness, retarded growth	Infants
Pellagra	Niacin	Skin inflammation, diarrhea, dementia	Adults, adolescents
Protein-calorie malnutrition	Protein, kilocalories	Lethargy, wasted bodies, stunting, impaired organ development, death in severe cases	Infants, young children; less often in adults
Rickets	Vitamin D	Softened bones, deformities	Infants, young children
Osteomalacia	Vitamin D	Softened bones, deformities	Pregnant women, elderly
Scurvy	Vitamin C	Pinpoint hemorrhages, poor wound healing, spongy, bleeding gums, spontaneous bruises	Infants, elderly
Pernicious anemia	Vitamin B_{12}	Anemia, spinal cord degeneration	Adults with genetic predisposition
Xerophthalmia	Vitamin A	Blindness	Children

aptitude may be a result of reduced environmental stimulation, rather than of malnutrition itself.

Studies of Korean orphans adopted by U.S. families after they were 2 years old have shown that those children who were malnourished before adoption evidenced some degree of retardation in learning. After these children were adopted and, consequently, received adequate nutrition as well as greatly increased environmental stimulation, however, they were able to score higher than the average on school performance tests. Researchers who studied this found that the effect was the result of the special environmental stimulation, rather than the improved nutrition alone [3]. Thus, mental retardation, once attributed to "brain damage" that resulted from malnutrition, had been overcome by an enriched learning environment, in combination with an improved diet and/or by other types of medical care [4].

Although more research is needed on the effects of malnutrition on mental development, it is clear that malnutrition rarely occurs in isolation from other poor environmental factors. It usually occurs along with poor housing, poor sanitation, poor health, low levels of education, ignorance, apathy, and despair.

Thus, to improve the diet alone will not eliminate the whole syndrome of deprivation associated with retardation in intellectual development.

Extent of World Hunger

What is the extent of world hunger? The answers to this question vary widely depending on the source of information used. Many estimates are based on studies conducted by the Food and Agriculture Organization of the United Nations (FAO), the United States Department of Agriculture (USDA), and the World Bank. Thomas Poleman, an agricultural economist, reviewed these studies and pointed out that, depending on the source, the number of people estimated to be suffering from malnutrition range from 400 million to two-thirds of the world's population [5,6]. Part of the reason for the different conclusions arises from the methods used in making estimates. The statistics used to estimate the extent of world hunger are discussed in Nutrition In The News.

Most of the estimates rely on food balance sheets to determine the food available in a region or country. Food balance sheets often tend to underestimate the actual food availability for a number of reasons. A primary difficulty is that food produced locally, or by small farmers, is usually not taken into account by those doing the analysis, and thus is not included in the estimate.

Once food availability to the entire population is estimated, the amount of food available per person is calculated by dividing by the number in the population, and this amount is then compared with standard nutritional allowances. Because nutrition is still a young science, our methods of determining amounts of nutrients absolutely required for good health may pose problems. Remember from earlier chapters that if a person's diet does not meet the nutrient allowances (the RDAs), this does not mean that the individual is malnourished. His or her requirements may be less than that of other individuals. A source of uncertainty and error, therefore, resides in the use of allowances as if they were absolute requirements below which individuals develop malnutrition.

The areas of the world where the largest concentration of malnourished people live are in the developing countries. In many of these areas, the diets contain relatively small amounts of protein (compared with developed countries) but large amounts of carbohydrate foods such as millet and sorghum or roots and tubers. Figure 18-1 illustrates the diet patterns and the food resources prevalent throughout the earth's population groups.

WHAT ARE THE CAUSES OF MALNUTRITION AND THE WORLD FOOD CRISIS?

Despite the fact that previous estimates of the extent of real hunger in the world may have been too high, from a humanitarian view the existence of serious malnutrition anywhere is intolerable. Does the world presently produce enough food to feed its population? If so, why are so many people hungry? What factors limit food production? A consideration of answers to these questions will help us to better understand how to deal with the problems of hunger and malnutrition.

NUTRITION IN THE NEWS

FOOD AND HUNGER STATISTICS QUESTIONED

Ann Crittenden, *The New York Times,* Oct. 5, 1981

. . . The United Nations Food and Agriculture Organization is disseminating statistics purporting to show the dimensions of the world hunger program.

"In 1981 at least 420 million people do not have enough to eat," the agency's literature says.

Increasingly, however, the unqualified assertion of such statistics is being challenged. Indeed, a vocal minority of critics maintain that the world hunger problem has been vastly exaggerated. . . . As Prof. Thomas T. Poleman of Cornell University put it in a recent interview: "We simply don't have sufficient evidence to estimate the numbers of hungry people. There is no basis for coming up with concrete estimates."

According to Professor Poleman, there are "three great unknowns" in trying to estimate the extent of hunger. These are the actual availability of food, the exact amount of food people need for nourishment and how access to food varies among different income groups within a country.

Because of these uncertainties, predictions of future global famines, or of the numbers of starvation deaths that will occur by the year 2000, are widely viewed as meaningless. Even the figures on existing hunger and malnutrition vary widely.

In a recent issue of *Commentary* magazine, for example, Nick Eberstadt of the Harvard Center for Population Studies guessed that at most about 100 million people—or less than one-quarter the number estimated by the FAO —were "desperately hungry." This is "a lower fraction, in all likelihood, than for any previous generation in man's recorded history," Mr. Eberstadt wrote. . . .

Even greater discrepancies surround the estimates of the numbers of malnourished.

The Food and Agriculture Organization's estimate of roughly half a billion people suffering from acute malnutrition in the developing countries—excluding China—was made in 1974.

Just before the World Food Conference in that year, a revision in methodology lifted the FAO estimate of the seriously malnourished from 350 million to 434 million—or 25 percent of the developing world. . . .

Professor Poleman . . . agrees that 100 million is a better figure than the FAO's half a billion. In his view, food production in developing countries tends to be understated because taxation is often based on production, and because so much backyard production is locally consumed and never counted.

A number of nutritionists have also noted that food needs vary from person to person by as much as 50 percent. Individual calorie requirements established by the FAO and the World Health Organization are based on the needs of Americans and Europeans and are exaggerated for individuals in the tropics, perhaps by as much as one-third, according to some nutritionists. . . .

On the other hand, other authorities insist that much hunger, especially in remote rural areas, is inadequately reported. Larry Minear of the Interreligious Task Force on United States Food Policy told an interviewer recently that "malnutrition is understated because there are a lot of people who don't show up in the planning nets, either because the censuses are bad or because they are not in the market economy, and their inability to purchase food isn't measured." . . .

Several hunger experts said in interviews that they were familiar with the efforts of some developing countries, such as Brazil, to suppress information on highly unequal income distribution, implying the existence of malnutrition among the poorest segments of their populations.

Those who believe that the incidence of

hunger has been overstated argue that the problem becomes more manageable if it is more carefully defined. By Professor Poleman's calculations, food aid of only three million tons of grain a year, if it could be channeled to the truly needy, would enable 100 million malnourished people to have an adequate diet. . . .

Walter Falcon, the head of the Food Research Institute at Stanford University, believes, however, that the debate over how many underfed there are does not affect public policy very much.

"It might focus more attention on Africa, where the most serious hunger exists, rather than on Southeast Asia, where the numbers are," Mr. Falcon said in a telephone interview. "But if only 100 million individuals are clinically malnourished, there are probably another 200 million to 400 million that go hungry part of the time. If they're not in the hospital, they're not doing too well."

"A lot of the argument is what do you do about those people who are simply inadequately fed," Mr. Falcon added. "That is one of the toughest questions."

Food Production

On a global basis the world produces more than twice the amount of food supplies needed to meet present human needs. Food production per capita (the amount of food produced for each person in the population per year) has greatly increased over the years in the developed industrialized nations; but in many of the developing, or poorer countries, it has increased only slightly or even declined [7].

If enough food is to be produced to feed the world, a number of resources, such as land, water, energy, fertilizer, and technology must be available and wisely used.

Land   Is it possible that land available for agriculture on a worldwide basis could limit food production in the near future? Most experts respond negatively to this question. While certain areas are experiencing or about to experience a shortage of arable land, on a global basis land shortage does not appear to be a problem. It has been estimated that, on a worldwide basis, over 4 billion hectares (1 hectare equals 2½ acres) are available for agriculture. Yet less than half this land is now used for growing food in a given year. If this land could be irrigated and if the soils could be properly treated there would be considerable room for increased agricultural production [8].

It has been estimated that using a hectare of new land for food production can yield 0.9 metric tons of cereal grain; if the land is well irrigated this can rise to

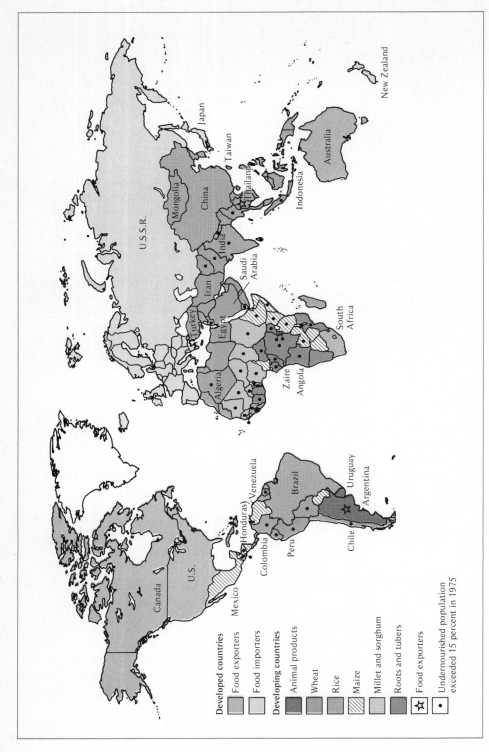

FIGURE 18-1. World Food Resources and Diet Patterns. The key shows the predominant source of food calories in 90 developing countries according to the most recent FAO classification. China and Mongolia, not included in the FAO list, are classified among the rice countries. A number of smaller countries, also omitted by the FAO, are assigned a diet similar to that of their neighbors. Black dots identify 52 developing countries where more than 15 percent of the population was undernourished by FAO standards in 1975. (The FAO defines a diet containing fewer than 1600 calories per day as inadequate; a typical "first world" diet averages about 3100 calories per day.) The "third world" countries where wheat and rice are the principal crops have been the most successful in meeting food demand. In 11 of the 17 countries where maize is the chief crop, more than 15 percent of the population was undernourished in 1975. In populations that subsist on millet and sorghum or roots and tubers some degree of malnutrition is virtually universal. (Source: Scrimshaw, N. S., and L. Taylor, "Food," *Scientific American*, 243:80–81, 1980.)

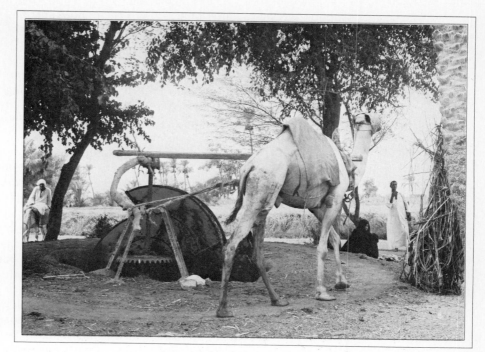

Land irrigation does not require modern equipment. Here, as late as 1965, a camel in the Nile Valley of Egypt pulls a waterwheel to irrigate nearby crops. *(United Nations)*

3.5 metric tons [8]. In the early 1970s, one hectare of land produced the food needed to feed approximately 2.6 persons. By the year 2000 it is estimated that one hectare of arable land will have to produce food to feed 4 persons [7].

Not all experts are so optimistic about land availability, however. On a per capita basis, there will be much less land available in the near future. Cultivation of farmland often results in soil erosion which will remove many inches of arable soil from croplands all over the world. In addition, because of soil erosion and loss of natural soil fertility, a significant part of the world's cropland will become desert land, unsuitable for most agriculture [7].

While the world does not face serious land shortages in the near future, there are difficult problems facing certain areas of Asia and northern Africa, where available land is nearly exhausted. Areas of India, Bangladesh, and Egypt, for instance, are confronted by such problems. Opportunities for increasing the world's cultivated land are mainly restricted to areas of Latin America and sub-Sahara Africa.

Water   Water, more so than land, may be a significant factor that limits world food supplies in future years. There is much land available throughout the world that could be productive farmland if water supplies were available. Irrigation is not without its problems, however. Intensive irrigation often results in the accumulation of salt deposits in the land, contributing to eventual loss of arable land.

Agriculture, irrigated or not, demands huge water supplies. If we include water needed in food processing, as much as 80 percent of a country's total water supplies may be required by the food system alone [9]. The FAO estimated that the irrigated areas of the world must be doubled by the year 2000 if widespread starvation is to be averted [8].

Energy Sources Energy is an extremely important factor in food production. It ranks with land and water as a critical variable in meeting world food needs. Energy is needed for a variety of agricultural purposes—to lift water for irrigation; to mechanize farm operations, such as planting and harvesting; to transport farm machinery and produce; and to manufacture fertilizers.

Sources of energy required to farm, process, and transport food are now exceedingly expensive. In 1980, the cost of oil was more than 10 times that of 1972. Energy prices continue to rise. Since energy sources are so expensive, energy ranks in importance with land, water, and other such factors in influencing food production [10]. Farm systems in industrialized nations use much more fuel than do traditional farm systems in which much of the mechanical energy is supplied by human labor. World energy demand is projected to increase by 58 percent by 1990, while petroleum production on a global basis is failing to keep up with demand. Engineers and geologists predict that world petroleum production will have reached its peak by the year 2000 [7].

The continued spread of modern agricultural technology to less developed areas of the world will lead to an increased demand for energy, thus worsening the energy crisis. In some cases, the technology used by traditional farming methods may actually be more efficient than modern agricultural methods. Focusing on basics such as proper crop spacing, weeding, use of promising seeds, and so forth can greatly increase food production without the high-energy use and cost that modernization would require.

Fertilizer Chemical fertilizer requires expensive oil or natural gas for its production. Fertilizer is an important agricultural resource, said to be responsible for about half the increased food production in recent years [8]. Although prices of fertilizer rose dramatically and there were global shortages in the mid-1970s, there has been more than an average 10 percent increase in fertilizer use each year since 1975. Continued growth in fertilizer application could yield crop surpluses in parts of the developing world by the early 1990s [8].

Climate No matter how traditional or how sophisticated, agriculture ultimately depends upon the weather. In recent years, we have seen many unusual climate patterns—persistent droughts, flooding, severe cold weather, and shifts in monsoons—forcing us to become concerned about long-term climatic influences on food production. Despite great technological breakthroughs, we still lack the skills required to control climate to a significant extent. While experts have speculated about future climate trends, advance knowledge of future climate is not available. Thus, agriculture must, to the extent possible, adapt to changing conditions.

Technology Technology can be used to greatly increase the food produced on a limited area of land. One widely publicized effort to increase food production by

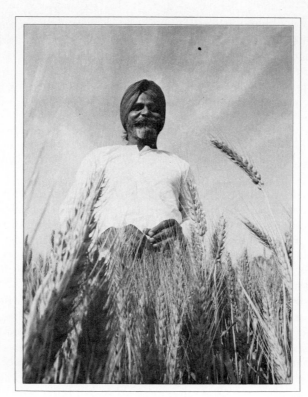

The Green Revolution: a well-to-do northern Indian farmer displays his miracle wheat field. (© Marc & Evelyne Bernheim 1980/Woodfin Camp & Assoc.)

exploiting modern technology has been termed the "Green Revolution." It involves the use of high-yielding varieties (HYV) of certain food grains such as wheat and rice. These high-yielding varieties were produced as a result of research efforts—they do not appear in nature on their own. They mature in less time and are more weather-resistant than traditional varieties. Their potential for increased food production is great. For example, the Green Revolution began in Mexico in the 1940s. By 1958 wheat yields doubled, then doubled again during the 1960s.

To many, the Green Revolution is a Pandora's box—opening the lid on more problems than it solves. Irrigation is necessary for the success of HYVs, but in many poor countries extensive irrigation is impossible. The marketing systems in many poor countries often are inadequate to handle increased loads from HYV, and much of the grain is often wasted and lost. The wealthy farmers who farm large acreage are usually the ones to profit from the Green Revolution—they can afford the fertilizer, the seeds, the sophisticated machinery, and the irrigation required. The small farmer cannot afford to invest in a new technology, and may become poorer than ever in the midst of the Green Revolution. Moreover, HYVs are very vulnerable to attacks by insects and diseases; since they are genetically uniform, a single pest can wipe out entire crops.

Another disturbing consequence of the Green Revolution is the decline in production of higher protein foods that often results. Because farmers want to double their yields, they may switch to HYVs in place of producing high-protein foods such as legumes, plants which often make up a large part of the diets of people in poor countries [11,12]. It is clear that we cannot transfer western technologies to developing countries without adapting these technologies to the special circumstances in these countries.

Food Distribution

As we saw earlier, the world as a whole currently produces more than twice as much food as is required to meet human needs, but large numbers of people still lack sufficient food [13]. Since the late 1970s, food production in the developing nations has been sufficient to meet the minimal nutritional requirements of the populations in these areas. Ironically, however, the number of undernourished people on earth appears to have increased. A large part of the problem is inequitable distribution of food supplies, both among nations and within nations [14]. Let's consider a few examples in which increases in a nation's food production have *not* led to improved diets for the poor.

Many nations in Central America have increased their beef production, but they have also increased their beef exports to the United States. Thus, the increased production actually resulted in lower beef consumption and higher local rates of malnutrition for many Central American poor. For many of the poorer nations, economic necessity dictates that they export large amounts of food. High prices paid for food exports are funneled back into the production of more food for export. The same food would not bring such high prices from the poor within the country.

As we have indicated, increased crop yields resulting from the Green Revolution usually benefit the larger, more prosperous farmer. In Mexico, for example, the techniques of the Green Revolution were used to produce large-scale agricultural production for export. The number of small farms and farmers declined in favor of an increased number of large modern farms. It is the wealthy who can afford to take a risk in the beginning, and profit in the end. The small, poor farmer may actually grow poorer, and be unable to afford food, even though the country's food supply has increased. There is a far greater proportion of small farmers than of prosperous ones. In Mexico, for example, less than 5 percent of the farms occupy approximately two-thirds of the irrigated arable land, and account for more than half the production. Approximately 85 percent of the farms contribute only 20 percent of the value of food produced [6].

Marketing and distribution systems in some countries are very inefficient— much food is lost during transportation, storage, and handling because of pests, mold, and spoilage. One estimate suggested that it would take a train 3000 miles long to pull away all the grain spoiled by rats in 1 year in India [13].

Trading and pricing policies also directly influence the distribution of food. For example, in Egypt the government controls the prices of cotton and wheat, but not the price of meat. As a result, producers tend to shift production of crops away from cotton and wheat to clover, a crop used in meat production. Only the wealthier consumers in Egypt can afford meat regularly [8].

Production of sufficient foods in the appropriate places greatly depends on markets and food prices. Schatan [15] has compared the food marketing and pricing system to the circulatory system in the human body. If the system is organized and effective, nutrients will flow smoothly to various areas of the body. Just as the human body suffers when there is a circulatory difficulty, so does the social body suffer when food marketing systems break down. As the extremities suffer most from a fault in the circulatory system so do the poorest suffer from problems in the pricing and marketing system. These problems are only small parts of the broader problems of poverty and underdevelopment in the poor nations of the world.

Poverty

It should now be apparent that a major cause of unequal food distribution is the result of inequitable income distribution. The World Bank estimated that in the early 1980s there were 780 million people who were too poor to afford an adequate diet [16]. Income bears an important relationship to the quality of diet. In general, as incomes increase, the kinds of foods purchased change. Those with very low incomes usually consume a diet very high in carbohydrates. As incomes increase, more kilocalories are derived from costlier animal and vegetable proteins. In terms of general nutritional effects the immediate impact of increased income for the very poor is usually positive; increased income allows for increased food consumption. Where kilocalories and protein were previously lacking, this change helps to overcome malnutrition.

A graphic illustration is the way large amounts of cereal grains are fed to animals. As their incomes increase, people usually tend to want more meat. Therefore, greater quantities of grain are fed to livestock. Producing 1 lb of meat requires between 3 lb of grain for poultry, and 10 lb for beef. In the mid-1970s 41 percent of the total world grain production, or 493 million tons, were fed to animals, compared with the 538 million tons of cereal grain eaten by the 3 billion people living in developing nations [16]. The typical American consumes about 1600 lb of grain a year; only 150 lb of this grain is consumed directly while the rest of it—1450 lb—is consumed indirectly in the form of livestock products such as eggs, milk, chicken, pork, and beef. In the poorer nations the average person consumes only about 360 lb of grain a year, and most of this grain is consumed directly [17].

Would people in underdeveloped countries have more to eat if Americans consumed less? If Americans reduced their beef consumption by 5 lb per person per year, the beef saved would not find its way overseas. But because beef cattle generally consume a great deal of grain, such a reduction in beef production could trigger a drop in grain prices worldwide. The grain saved by producing fewer cattle also might be contributed to a wheat reserve system. In late 1980, the United States guaranteed a modest 4 million metric ton wheat reserve. The purpose of this reserve is to help stabilize grain prices worldwide, and also to serve as emergency food aid in cases of famine or severe food shortages.

There are other consequences of poverty that influence malnutrition. For example, poverty is often accompanied by long periods of unemployment, or employment at low levels of skills. In addition, poverty is associated with low education levels, high rates of illness, poor environmental sanitation, and limited social and cultural alternatives. These factors may not only restrict the procurement of food, but may result in a high rate of infection and general poor health, which in turn can increase nutritional requirements, making it even more difficult to obtain adequate nourishment.

The Population Problem

We can look at food available to an individual as an equation which represents the food available to the total population divided by the number of people who must share it. In many areas of the world burgeoning populations mean little food for many people.

In 1975 the world population reached an ominous point—it passed the 4 billion mark. It may reach 6 billion by the year 2000. To appreciate the rapid growth in population, consider the time required at present for the population to double in size. In 600 B.C. the world population was about 5 million people—it had taken some 1 million years to reach this number from 2½ million. Until 1650 A.D. it took about 1000 years for the population to double—but from 1650 to 1850, 200 years, the population again doubled. The next doubling required only 80 years. Currently, the world population doubles in approximately 37 years, but in many of the poor countries, doubling times are much shorter. Latin America has an average doubling time of 25 years while Africa and the Near East double their populations every 27 years [18].

Can you imagine what it means for the population of a nation to double in 25 years? There is a need, not only for twice as much food, but for twice as many resources to grow the food, in addition to twice as many resources for housing, clothing, medical care, education, transportation, employment, and so on.

Just how are these population trends related to world food and malnutrition problems? Lester Brown, a noted expert on the subject, observed that if world population continues to increase at current rates, food production would have to almost double in little more than a generation just to maintain current food consumption levels, which are inadequate for some people [19].

While the worldwide population growth rate has stabilized in recent years, birth rates have not declined in many developing nations where the problems of providing sufficient food for the population are the greatest. Again the problem comes down to one of distribution—the greatest population growth occurs in the poor, "have-not" countries where food supplies are scarcest.

Is it realistic to expect that we can curb population growth? Part of the answer to this question involves looking at why people, especially those in developing nations, have so many children. One widely publicized theory, called the "child survival hypothesis," holds that parents want children as a form of security in old age; they also want more farmhands. With high infant mortality rates prevailing in developing nations, parents with more children have a better chance that some, especially sons, will survive into adulthood. If this hypothesis is valid, one way to stem population growth in the future is to provide health and

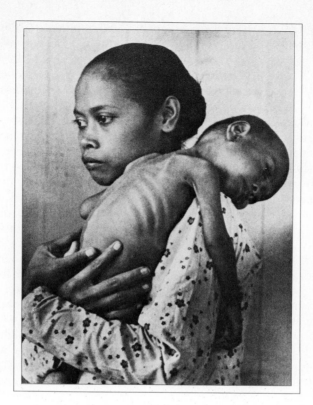

Malnutrition is common
among small children in
developing countries.
(WHO)

nutrition services in the present to mothers and their children, and to encourage economic development for the very poor. Increased income means children can be better fed; nutritional and health services mean they are likely to have a better chance of survival, thereby perhaps decreasing parents' motivation to produce more children.

Parents also need information about birth control. They need help in practicing modern methods of fertility control, and the right environment to enable them to make an informed and free choice about reproduction. Although such family planning programs are relatively new—in 1960 only India and Pakistan had national policies designed to curb population growth rates—more than 90 percent of the population in the developing world live in nations that offer family planning programs [20].

Cultural Factors

One of the saddest causes of malnutrition involves social or cultural beliefs that so restrict the diet that malnutrition is inevitable. As we pointed out in Chapter 1, nowhere in the world do people eat the full range of foods available to them. We all have individual food preferences and aversions to certain foods, and all societies have food taboos based on cultural or religious beliefs. Sometimes these cultural beliefs promote poor diets, even though foods for an adequate diet are readily available. How might this lead to inadequate diets? In areas such as Malaysia, vitamin A deficiency results in blindness for many children. Foods rich in vitamin A value, such as papaya and green leafy vegetables, are prevalent and inexpensive but often these foods are not given to young children because they are considered too "cold." In this belief system, the healthy body is viewed as temperate, with heat and cold kept in balance. Disease is thought to result from excess heat or cold. In South America the distinction between hot and cold foods leads to food avoidances and preferences that may influence work habits, the way children are brought up, the diagnosis and treatment of disease, and the rehabilitation of the soil [21].

Often a child suffering from malnutrition, infection, diarrhea, or fever is restricted from all foods except broth or diluted cereal with a bit of added fruit. This only aggravates malnutrition. In some areas of Jamaica, for example, fever, diarrhea, or respiratory problems are frequent among young children. These disorders are referred to as "marasmi cold" and are thought to result from a spirit or ghost which invades the child's body. Milk and high-protein foods, believed to "curdle the cold," are withheld while the child is treated chiefly with baths and herbal teas [22].

Many food taboos center around the restriction of high-protein foods and usually apply to pregnant women, lactating women, infants, and young children. The cultural values of modern industrialized nations may also play a role. Box 18-1 discusses how adopting western attitudes, values, and practices in developing countries has contributed to malnutrition among infants and small children.

CAN GLOBAL MALNUTRITION BE ALLEVIATED? PROGRAMS AND STRATEGIES

Malnutrition and nutritional deprivation are basically problems of poverty—of unequal and inequitable income distribution, not only among individuals, but among countries. Malnutrition won't disappear by simply producing more food, or by raising the overall economic levels of poor nations. An attack on malnutrition must involve an attempt to eliminate poverty. How can we solve the problem of poverty? Long-term solutions involve finding ways to provide the landless rural poor with plots of land and the means to produce food; to increase the productivity of poor agricultural land; to provide employment for those without jobs; to provide the poor with health services and educational services. All these approaches are intimately related to solving the problem of hunger and malnutrition.

The FAO [34] suggested that such a strategy to eliminate world hunger should include three elements:

1. Development strategies should promote improvements in food production and at the same time improve the distribution of income among populations.

The Bottle-Feeding Problem

Dr. Jesus T. De La Paz, an obstetrician and gynecologist in the Philippines, tells of visiting a friend in a rural area of Luzon in 1970. The friend had a newborn infant who was ill with fever, diarrhea, and dehydration. The mother had been feeding the baby infant formula given to her by the nurse in the hospital where the baby was born. The nurse had told the mother that her own milk was "inappropriate" for the baby [23].

In the view of many health professionals, this kind of promotion of infant formula has persuaded many mothers in developing countries that bottle-feeding is the best, most modern way to feed a baby [24]. But the problem is that many mothers in developing countries can't afford to buy sufficient formula to properly feed their babies. In Kenya, for example, the annual cost of a commercial formula which could provide adequate nutrition for an infant costs about half the money paid annually to the average road worker [25]. In fact, it has been estimated that the economic cost of bottle-feeding amounted to $11.5 million a year, which was equivalent to two-thirds of the health budget for Kenya, or one-fifth the average economic aid received by that country [26]. The average laborer in Uganda may spend 33 percent of his income to feed an infant with cow's milk; in Chile it would cost 20 percent of an average salary to feed a baby cow's milk. If more expensive commercial formula is used, the cost is considerably greater [27].

What often happens, then, is that a mother in a developing country who decides to buy formula dilutes it to make it last longer. The baby may eventually die of starvation. The mother may have no safe source of water, and may lack both the knowledge and the equipment needed to boil water to mix with formula, or to sterilize bottles or nipples. The baby is at very high risk for infections, diarrhea, and frequently death.

One example of the misuse of formulas comes from Jamaica. A grandmother, a mother, and a daughter each had an infant less than a year old. All lived in the same house—a 12-foot-square shack. All had been using one can of formula for 10 days and still had a third of the can left. The appropriate amount of formula would have been two cans a week for each of the babies. The mothers had severely diluted the formula, actually offering only whitened water [28].

Bottle-fed infants in developing countries have illnesses such as diarrhea more often and of greater severity than breast-fed babies. In Mexico, one study reported that diarrhea was 10 times more frequent among bottle- than breast-fed infants [29]. A study of childhood mortality in 10 countries in the Americas found that the most serious health problem was malnutrition, but that breast-feeding offered protection against both malnutrition and diarrhea [30]. A 1970 San Salvador study revealed that 75 percent of babies who died during the first 5 months of life had been breast-fed for less than 30 days [27].

With such evidence of the hazards of bottle-feeding in developing countries, why the drift away from breast-feeding, "the original convenience food, always on tap from its unbreakable containers that need no mixing, warming, sterilizing, or washing up afterwards" [28]?

The decline in breast-feeding is associated with the adoption of western values and attitudes, such as the change from viewing the breast as a source of nourishment to viewing it as a sex symbol. Another is the value placed on modern gadgets that seem to hold the magic of industrialization—such a gadget is the baby

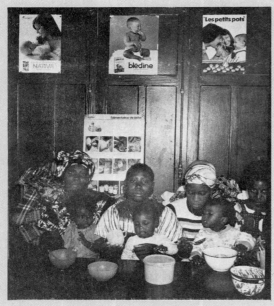

Many experts believe that advertising infant formulas in developing countries has influenced the preference for bottle-feeding over breast-feeding. (© Beryl Goldberg 1981)

bottle. This was vividly illustrated by the baby bottles strewn on infant graves in Zambia. Mothers wanted the magic of the bottle to go with their infants, even to their graves [23].

While some suggest that a primary reason for the decline in breast-feeding is urbanization which forces new mothers to seek jobs, this factor cannot account for the very low numbers of mothers breast-feeding their infants in the world at large. The low number of paying jobs for women in developing nations would seem to negate this as an influential factor [24]. The inability to nurse a child is a reason often cited by formula manufacturers, who insist that they are performing a truly generous action by liberally dispensing formula to those who haven't enough high-quality breast milk. Yet medical authorities working in developing countries find that few women are unable to nurse their infants [31].

Recently, advertising has been singled out as an important influence on the preference for bottle-feeding over breast-feeding. Multinational corporations and private manufacturers saw third world countries as an unexplored and potentially lucrative market for infant formulas. They promoted their products in a variety of ways, from radio ads, to posters, to providing hospitals with free samples. Doctors and nurses gave samples to new mothers and encouraged their use. Some companies employed either nurses or women who dressed like nurses to visit mothers and sell formulas. Outdoor billboards, company vans with public address systems, and baby contests sponsored by formula makers all were forms of promotion used in various countries.

In 1981, 118 nations overwhelmingly approved a voluntary international code, drawn up by the World Health Organization (WHO) that discouraged unnecessary distribution and use of infant formula and encouraged breast-feeding [32]. The code restricts advertising and promotion of infant formulas, but formulas would still be available in developing countries for those who could afford them. The United States, the only nation to vote against the code, did so on the grounds that it was antagonistic to free trade and in violation of American antitrust laws and the right to free speech.

In response to the code, some manufacturers of infant formulas developed new policies. For example, Nestlé, a major supplier of infant formulas, developed guidelines requiring that free samples of formula be given to mothers only on the request of a doctor or qualified medical professional. The company also undertook to rewrite printed educational materials and produced labels to conform with the principles of the code [33].

A serious dimension of the bottle-feeding problem is noted by Berg, who points out that breast milk is an important natural resource that is steadily declining in the poorest countries that need it most [27]. Comparable depletion of crude oil reserves in an oil-producing country would be regarded as a crisis, according to Berg; yet the loss of breast milk goes practically unnoticed.

2. Programs should influence the kinds of food produced and should improve the transportation, processing, and distribution of foods to all in the population.
3. Health and nutrition intervention measures should be implemented to directly improve the nutritional status of subgroups, such as mothers and young children, who are especially vulnerable to malnutrition.

Improving Food Production and Distribution

The greatest potential for improving food production lies in more intensive cultivation of the land currently used for crops. Improved methods of irrigation, fertilization, and technology can greatly increase food yields. The extent to which various ways of increasing food production are used will depend greatly upon numerous decisions made by millions of farmers, suppliers, governments, and consumers. Programs should be designed for regional and national situations. The objective should be not only to produce enough food, but also to see that individuals' needs for food are met. In other words, attention must be paid not only to food production, but also to food distribution, to alleviating poverty, to coping with the population problems, and to educating the population about sound nutritional practices. Box 18-2 illustrates one successful attempt to improve nutrition through improving food distribution and marketing.

Nutrition Intervention Measures

Nutrition intervention strategies by governments should be used only when it is impossible to reduce the basic *causes* of hunger and malnutrition. There are a number of different measures which can be taken to reduce malnutrition on a *short-term basis*; they include supplementary feeding programs, food fortification, food mixes, novel protein sources, health and nutrition education programs, and food aid.

Supplementary Feeding Programs   Supplementary feeding programs are probably the oldest and most common of nutrition intervention programs. They are designed to provide needed food to those most vulnerable to malnutrition. Early programs were started after World War II when aid programs were financed by modern developed nations in many poor areas of the world. These programs often relied upon surplus foods from affluent countries, such as dried skim milk, and thus served a dual purpose—they aided the poor and provided significant political benefits to the affluent countries.

Such programs serve not only to improve the nutritional quality of the diet, but can also improve family incomes by making more money available for other needs. Moreover, supplementary feeding programs can strengthen the work of clinics or schools that distribute food. For example, food given out at a clinic may provide an incentive for mothers to bring their children to the clinic for health care.

However, feeding programs are a very costly form of intervention—they consume more than 95 percent of all child nutrition budgets in developing nations. In addition they reach only limited numbers of people [27]. Often those

18-2
BOX

Improving Nutrition through Marketing and Distribution— An Example

In recent years there has been increased government involvement in the establishment of national distribution channels. Early attempts in Latin America, for example, were aimed at establishing food stores that offered basic foodstuffs at lower prices. The higher prices placed on luxury items were expected to compensate for these lower prices. However, in actual practice, it was found that this type of reduced-price outlet drew many customers from more wealthy buyers who desired the convenience of such stores. Because the poor often did not have money, transportation, or storage facilities, they were not equipped to take advantage of such opportunities.

Some governments have tried to overcome such difficulties by joining with commercial businesses to aid the poor consumer. A successful example of this government–commercial merger is the Mexican CONASUPO system (National Company for Popular Subsistencies), a major agency in the marketing of Mexican foodstuffs.

CONASUPO guarantees minimum prices for such foods as maize, beans, wheat, rice, soybeans, sorghum, sesame, and saffron. The activity that most directly touches consumers is the distribution of supplies at the retail level. More than 3000 different products are made available to consumers through approximately 3000 retail outlets. Outlets vary in size and type from supermarkets to small "popular" stores, mobile units, and concessions.

Administration of the stores is decentralized, allowing regions to meet the individual needs of their communities. The food-processing industry is also operated by CONASUPO, which not only supplies processors with necessary raw materials, such as wheat, maize, sorghum, barley, oilseeds, oils, and fats, but also directly participates in food-processing activities, such as the milling of wheat and maize into flour, and the processing of cooking oil.

The regulatory activities of CONASUPO have avoided excess speculation and profits from middlemen. Their greatest impact is in times of abundance, when crops are purchased from farmers, and in times of scarce supplies, when food is offered to consumers at fair prices. Thus, producers and consumers have benefited from the activities of this Mexican marketing system.

CONASUPO also operates the government's import and export program for grains and foodstuffs according to supplies of products in relation to consumption needs.

Estimates of the benefits of CONASUPO indicate that consumers have saved from 10 to 18 percent of the cost of food purchased. It is evident that the CONASUPO has aided lower-income groups to improve their diets and hence their nutrition. In addition to this indirect method of improving nutritional status, CONASUPO also conducts activities geared toward direct nutritional benefits, such as the fortification, reconstitution, and distribution of low-fat dried milk for low-income peoples at less than one third the commercial price.

CONASUPO also plays a role in the functions of the National Food Program (PRO-NATAL), a high government-level body created to investigate, plan, and recommend food supply and distribution policies.

CONASUPO is just one example of an innovative marketing scheme that can be designed and implemented to effectively improve food distribution, and hence, nutritional status of the population.

Source: Caliendo, M. A., *Nutrition and the World Food Crisis*, New York: Macmillan Publishing Co., 1979, pp. 151–152.

most in need of nutritional help fail to go to the sites where the food is being given out. In general, supplementary feeding programs should be seen only as a stopgap measure—they should not make it easier for governments to put off dealing with the real problems of malnutrition.

Food Fortification   The addition of needed nutrients to foods is an attractive way to improve the nutritional status of the population. Early programs involved the addition of iodine to salt to control goiter, a technique responsible for the low incidence of goiter in the United States. Vitamin A has frequently been added to food such as skim milk to prevent xerophthalmia, and vitamin D is added to milk to prevent rickets. Wheat flour is often fortified with vitamins or minerals in both developing and developed nations—in Israel and India, for example. The addition of niacin to corn meal and wheat flour was in part responsible for the control of pellagra in the southern United States. Rice has been fortified in countries where it is commonly used, such as in the Philippines, Japan, Thailand, Colombia, Venezuela, the Dominican Republic, Puerto Rico, and the United States. Other foods commonly fortified include tea, flavoring agents, and cooking oil.

There are many benefits to fortifying foods. There is usually no change in the taste or appearance of the food, no need to change eating, preparation, or purchasing habits. Fortification is relatively easy to do—the cost is usually minimal and benefits occur in a short period of time. But fortification is not possible for every food; only foods which are processed in a central place can be easily fortified. The rural poor who grow their own foods are missed by fortification programs. The benefits of fortification may be related to income— those who have more money and can buy more food will receive more fortification. Often, fortification may reach those who don't need it—and for certain nutrients such as vitamins A and D the excess may be hazardous. Other drawbacks of fortification are discussed in Chapter 17.

Food Mixes   Another type of nutrition intervention is the use of food mixes. Food mixes are made up of different foods combined in such a way as to complement the different amino acid patterns of single, often poor-quality protein foods. For example, cereals, roots, or tubers (such as sweet potato and cassava) may be combined with dried beans, or small amounts of dried milk in order to provide a complete mixture of amino acids. Diets in many developing nations are largely based on cereals or other foods which may be low in some amino acids. Legumes, cottonseed flour, or milk, on the other hand, can supply the needed amino acids to improve the protein quality. Other ingredients sometimes used in the food mixtures include defatted oilseed flours such as cottonseed, rapeseed, peanut, sesame, and sunflower. These foods are relatively inexpensive and often found in developing nations. Mothers can often be taught to take foods commonly available and mix them in such a way as to provide a complete food mix. Foods indigenous to the community are used where possible in order to increase the receptivity to the food mixes.

The typical formula for such a mix might include the staple of the diet, usually a cereal,

+ a small amount of animal protein such as milk or egg, or
+ a legume, or
+ a dark-green leafy vegetable that can provide needed vitamins and minerals, or
+ a compact source of calories, usually in the form of a fat [35].

Novel Food Sources Modern technology and research have led the search for new types of food that might help to solve some of the problems of malnutrition. Leaf protein is an example. By processing a ton of wet leaves it is possible to extract up to 39 kg of high-grade protein—enough to provide a 15 g protein supplement to each of 2000 people [37]. Leaf protein concentrate (LPC) is also a rich source of iron, calcium, magnesium, vitamin E, vitamin A, and some of the B vitamins. There are some drawbacks to the production of LPC—the product is often objectionable because of its color and taste. There are also many problems involved in manufacturing the product. One difficulty is the tremendous amounts of energy needed to produce LPC. At present LPC is mainly in the experimental stage.

Another protein source is fish protein concentrate (FPC) made from species of fish usually discarded by commercial fishermen. FPC is relatively inexpensive and its nutritive value is close to that of raw fish. The concentrate can be added to baked products or to food mixtures. Its potential is great, but FPC is not yet used in significant amounts. Part of the difficulty lies in the fact that there is no guarantee that fish supplies will hold out. Marketing of FPC is hard to maintain on a large scale, partly because of antagonistic attitudes toward consumption of unconventional forms of fish [38]. The successful use of such novel protein sources must take local food preferences into account when planning the use of new foods.

Single cell protein (SCP) is a term used to describe proteins obtained from bacteria, yeasts, mold, and algae. SCP can be grown from different organisms using a variety of substrates such as crude petroleum, oil waste, molasses, starch, and sewage. Organisms that produce SCP grow very rapidly—yeast and bacteria, for example, need 0.3 to 2 hours to double their weight; in contrast plants need 1

A CLOSER LOOK

Some food mixes are commercially available—Incaparina, a special high-protein food mix, for example, is widely available in South America. However, many of these commercial foods are very expensive, and may not even reach those who need them most. These foods have been termed "commerciogenic nutritious foods"; critics have charged that in some cases they actually aggravate the problem of malnutrition, not because of the quality of the foods themselves, but because of their expense and the way they are marketed. They can be compared to infant formulas in that they are often too costly for the very poor, but because they are often so aggressively advertised the poor may be persuaded to sacrifice money that could actually be used to purchase less expensive but equally nutritious food [36].

to 2 weeks, chicks need 2 to 4 weeks, and cattle need 2 to 4 months to double their weight [39].

Advantages of SCP include its rapid production, the fact that few skilled laborers are needed, and that only limited resources such as land and water are required. But production costs are high and there are acceptability problems.

The nutritive value of SCP is similar to that of soybeans; the methionine content tends to be low. Kidney and digestive problems are sometimes associated with SCP. Nevertheless, SCP can be used to fortify foods in limited amounts. If the gastrointestinal and kidney problems resulting from its use can be removed, SCP has potential for use in infant foods, in beverages, as an extender for ground meat, and in fabricated foods similar to those currently made from soy fibers [40].

Health and Education Programs   Some of the most successful programs designed to reduce malnutrition are those that combine health, education, and socioeconomic improvements. Sometimes called applied nutrition programs, they are comprehensive health and education measures aimed at improving food production and use. Often these programs are funded by international relief programs or other aid programs [41].

These types of programs involve training local people in agricultural practices, in principles of food and nutrition, health, and sanitation. Resources such as seeds, fertilizers, and gardening equipment as well as films, slides, and audiovisual materials are supplied. Children are given health care, immunizations, and deworming services. The local trained community workers then pass along their newly learned skills to others in the community.

A number of variations of applied nutrition programs can be found in several developing countries. For example, there are Mothercraft Centers in Haiti, Brazil, Colombia, Guatemala, and the Philippines, while Under-Five Clinics are conducted in various African nations.

How are these programs operated? In a typical program, health workers select the most severely malnourished children and treat them for 2 to 3 months, while the mothers receive instruction in rehabilitating their children. Once the children are well enough to go home, the mothers are able to continue treatment there. Mothers learn how to use locally available nutritious foods and often take turns spending time at the clinic and helping to care for the children there. Health workers discuss principles of nutrition, selection and preparation of food, and health and sanitation measures. Thus, the mothers receive a type of on-the-job training. Strengths of the program include the broad focus on health, nutrition, and education; the use of trained local workers who can organize and administer the programs; and the general community acceptance and support of the concept and operation of the program [42].

Foreign Aid   The initiative for solving problems of poverty and malnutrition should rest with the developing countries themselves, but the more affluent developed nations can play a great role in initiating the process of development. Different types of foreign aid can help alleviate malnutrition [43]:

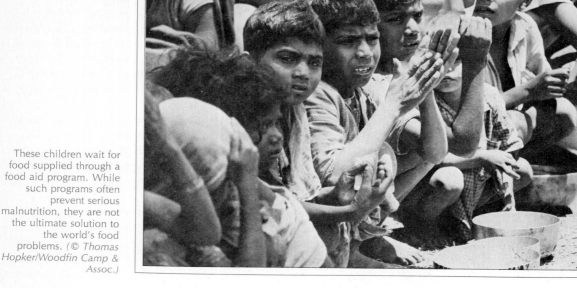

These children wait for food supplied through a food aid program. While such programs often prevent serious malnutrition, they are not the ultimate solution to the world's food problems. (© Thomas Hopker/Woodfin Camp & Assoc.)

1. Grain reserves can protect poor nations during emergencies resulting from unstable climates or poor harvests.
2. Aid in research and training can provide the poor with expertise needed to encourage their growth and development.
3. Financial aid can help poor nations to begin the process of development.

Many people think that the easy solution to world hunger is to take food from the places where there is plenty and transport it to places where there is little. In other words, food aid programs are the solution. However, it isn't that easy. There are many problems with food aid, apart from the fact that it is often used as a political weapon. These problems include [44]:

- Food is heavy and difficult to transport. Many foods also spoil easily and may actually be worthless when they reach the poor for whom they were intended. For example, in Guatemala it has been estimated that costs of transporting, storing, and handling U.S. food aid are almost 90 percent of the value of the food itself. Thus, food is a very inefficient type of aid.
- Distributing food in developing nations is not only costly, it is also difficult in areas with poor communication and transportation problems.
- Food must travel through long lines of intermediate dealers and thus may be appropriated by people for whom it was not intended.
- In supplementary feeding programs it is difficult to incorporate nutrition

education because the foods used may not be familiar to the mothers and cannot be obtained outside the program.

Food aid may also take away the incentive to produce food locally. It may also hold down local food prices.

There are many reasons for food aid other than to help the poor for humanitarian purposes. In some situations, the primary rationale for aid is to further an affluent nation's self-interest to achieve a desired foreign policy, world security, or economic objectives. For example, U.S. food shipments to Europe after World War II had political as well as humanitarian objectives. These political uses of food aid are not necessarily "bad" but they should be recognized as such.

The most effective type of international assistance is an international climate that gives first priority to human aspects of growth, rather than to political advantages and power. Food aid and financial aid should be seen as only interim, not permanent, measures. Food aid is needed in cases of famine and disaster, for example. The long-term goal is that countries should no longer need outside assistance, or at least that they possess the resources to buy the food and supplies they need.

Thus, while food aid is vital, it is only part of a very complex combination of trade policies, investment, and technical assistance aid. Through cooperation and research programs, the developing nations can be helped to increase their food production capacity, make more efficient use of fertilizer, improve pest management activities, improve food distribution systems, and address problems of local poverty.

DEALING WITH WORLD FOOD PROBLEMS: WHOSE RESPONSIBILITY?

Who influences decisions of food production, distribution, and consumption? Who can address these problems of hunger and malnutrition? The tasks to be addressed require the commitment and cooperation of all nations. Many countries are active in providing assistance to individual nations. France, for example, gives aid to some of her former colonies; Canada provides aid to Asian nations. But the United States, because of its great wealth and power, must recognize a particular role—its actions affect the lives and well-being of billions of people throughout the world.

We are becoming increasingly aware of the fact that our American domestic concerns of inflation, unemployment, energy, and immigration are not unrelated to the developing nations of the world. These countries now play very important roles in the global economic system. Many of these countries control large amounts of oil; others provide us with inexpensive goods; they represent markets for our exports; they supply important raw materials to us; and they are becoming more and more involved in the world financial system. Thus, it is not only because of a moral obligation, or because of our desire to safeguard our security interests, but it is also because of these countries' influence on the U.S. economy that the United States must recognize and take steps to eliminate world hunger [45].

The United States currently maintains a variety of efforts aimed at combating hunger and malnutrition. Under the Agricultural Trade Development and Assistance Act of 1954, commonly referred to as Public Law 480, over $1 billion annually is spent in overseas aid. The Agency for International Development (AID) maintains various programs designed to aid developing nations. For example, AID provides policy guidance on such matters as land reform and mobilization of capital; it provides financial assistance to increase food production; it offers education, technical assistance, and training programs. Some AID programs directly or indirectly support land reform which allows the landless poor to receive land to help them feed themselves and their families. In addition to its development projects, AID participates directly with various governments in improving the problems of hunger and poverty [46]. AID also sponsors grant programs to help developing nations monitor the nutritional status of young children and combat problems of iron deficiency, anemia, and vitamin A deficiency.

The United States has usually taken the initiative among nations in directing food aid activities, largely because of great excess U.S. food stocks. In the whole process of aid programs, multilateral relationships evolved and international agencies such as the United Nations have become active participants in decision making.

The concept of multilateral food aid began in 1943 when FAO and the United Nations Relief and Rehabilitation Administration (UNRRA) were established. In 1962 the World Food Program (WFP) began. The United States supplies a large proportion of the aid distributed by this program. Food is distributed to the governments which handle projects such as school feeding and mother-child nutrition programs [47].

PROSPECTS FOR THE FUTURE

In 1980 the first U.S. government effort to study population, resources, and the environment from a long-term global perspective was published. The report, called the *Global 2000 Report*, made the following projections for our entry into the twenty-first century [7].

The world is expected to be very different in many respects. There will be more people, for one thing. For every two people on earth in 1975, there will be three people at the start of the twenty-first century. An increasing number will be poor, and there will be a greater gap between the incomes of the richest and the poorest.

We will have fewer resources to distribute among the increased population. Where there was about two-fifths of a hectare of arable land per person in 1975, there will be only one-fourth hectare per person in 2000. Over the next quarter-century, our available petroleum resources are expected to decline by 50 percent, and the per capita water supplies will decline by 35 percent because of increased population.

The prices of many of our most vital resources will continue to rise. Food production will be more vulnerable to problems of tight energy supplies.

If present population growth continues unchanged, we could reach a world population of 10 billion by 2030, and almost 30 billion by the end of the twenty-first century. A population of 10 billion has been estimated to be the maximum that a very well managed world could sustain with any comfort.

As the Report concluded, we are running out of time to prevent sure disaster. Individuals as well as nations must take creative and decisive action to improve social and economic conditions, to reduce the population growth rate, to better manage resources, and to protect the environment, or we can "expect a troubled entry into the twenty-first century."

SUMMARY

1   Malnutrition may take many forms. In addition to protein and kilocalorie malnutrition, numerous vitamin and mineral deficiencies are serious health problems.

2   Malnutrition is found among populations in the industrialized as well as underdeveloped nations, but is of greater magnitude in underdeveloped countries.

3   Food production and food distribution are key factors determining what food is available to people. Factors influencing food production include: land availability, water, energy, fertilizer, climate, and technology. Wise use of resources as well as recognition of the importance of aiding people to produce their own food are important for the enhancement of food production.

4   In many areas of the world burgeoning populations means insufficient food supplies. Family planning programs are important in curbing population growth.

5   Cultural factors may restrict equitable distribution of available food supplies, and may also restrict diets of all members of a specific culture. Most frequent victims are pregnant and lactating women, infants, and young children.

6   Elimination of global hunger requires programs that will enhance food production, improve food distribution, and improve the health and nutritional status of groups who are especially vulnerable to malnutrition.

7   Various nutrition intervention measures can reduce malnutrition on a short-term basis. These include supplementary feeding programs, food fortification, use of food mixtures, and novel food sources.

8   Some of the most successful programs designed to reduce malnutrition are those that combine health, education, and socioeconomic improvement. These programs aim to promote self-help among local populations.

FOR DISCUSSION AND APPLICATION

1   Both Chapters 1 and 18 make the point that large amounts of energy are required to produce the American food supply. To increase your awareness of energy costs of food production, divide foods into the following categories: beverages, meats, vegetables, fruits, grains and cereals, milk and milk products, snack foods, and condiments. For each category list types of products that require greater vs. lesser amounts of energy in their production. Consider type of packaging, extent of processing, energy costs of storage, distance covered to transport food to your local markets, etc. Visit supermarkets, small food cooperatives, and farmer's markets when compiling your list. Compare your lists in class and discuss them.

2   At times when gasoline prices fall, should we relax and assume that energy availability is not a problem in this country, and that we need not be concerned about energy required to produce food? Why or why not?

3   Think over the suggestions made in this chapter for preventing or alleviating food problems in underdeveloped or developing countries. Which of these may come into conflict with value systems in some countries? How might local governments handle some of these problems? Should the United States offer assistance only to those countries that control their population growth? What are the issues involved in this question?

4   What are the responsibilities of developed countries, such as the United States, to help relieve food problems in underdeveloped countries?

SUGGESTED READINGS

Hensley, Elizabeth S., *Basic Concepts of World Nutrition*, Springfield, Ill.: Charles C Thomas, 1981. A multidisciplinary approach to world nutrition. This book approaches international nutrition from social, anthropological, geographical, psychological, and economic frameworks.

Food Monitor. This is a bimonthly publication devoted to increasing people's awareness of hunger problems in an effort to stimulate change. It may be ordered from Food Monitor, P.O. Box 1975, Garden City, N.Y., 11530.

Agenda. This is published 10 times a year by The Agency for International Development. It is free on request to the U.S. public. It covers various aspects of international development, including health and nutrition. Publications Division, Office of Public Affairs, Agency for International Development, Washington, D.C. 20523.

Gussow, J. D., *The Feeding Web: Issues in Nutritional Ecology*, Palo Alto, Calif.: Bull Publishing Co., 1978. This is a compilation of readings and interpretations of these readings. It examines biological, technical, social, scientific, and commercial influences on food production and consumption.

Nicholson, H. J., and R. L. Nicholson, *Distant Hunger: Agriculture, Food, and Human Values,* West Lafayette, Ind.: Purdue Research Foundation, 1979. A paperback book emphasizing that human values are critical in determining the extent of the world food problem and in deciding what we will do about it.

BIBLIOGRAPHY

INTRODUCTION

1 Maloney, L., and J. Thornton: "America's Great New Food Craze." *U.S. News and World Report,* December 7, 1981, pp. 60–63.
2 Belloc, N. B.: "Relationship of Health Practices and Mortality." *Preventive Medicine,* 2:67, 1973.
3 Breslow, L.: "A Positive Strategy for the Nation's Health." *Journal of the American Medical Association,* 242:2093, 1979.
4 Belloc, N. B., and L. Breslow: "Relationship of Physical Health Status and Health Practices." *Preventive Medicine,* 1:409, 1972.

CHAPTER 1

1 Loomis, R. S.: "Agricultural Systems." *Scientific American,* 235(3):99, 1976.
2 Thompson, L. M.: "Weather Variability, Climatic Change and Grain Production." *Science* 188:535, 1975.
3 Dando, W. A.: *The Geography of Famine.* New York: John Wiley & Sons, 1980.
4 Heady, E. O.: "The Agriculture of the U.S." *Scientific American,* 235(3):107, 1976.
5 Walsh, J.: "U.S. Agribusiness and Agricultural Trends." *Science,* 188:531, 1975.

6 Pimentel, D., and J. Hawthorn: "Energy Costs of Food and Nutrition Systems." *Progress in Clinical and Biological Research,* 77:1005, 1981.
7 1980 Handbook of Agricultural Charts. Agriculture Handbook No. 574, USDA. Washington, D.C., 1980.
8 Gallo, A. E., and J. M. Connor: "Packaging in Food Marketing." *National Food Review,* Economics and Statistics Service, USDA, spring 1981, p. 10.
9 Steinhart, J. S., and C. E. Steinhart: "Energy Use in the U.S. Food System." *Science,* 184:307, 1974.
10 Pimentel, D., L. E. Hurd, A. C. Belloti, M. J. Forster, I. N. Oka, O. D. Sholes, and R. J. Whitman: "Food Production and the Energy Crisis." *Science,* 182:443, 1973.
11 Brown, L. R.: "Human Food Production as a Process in the Biosphere." In: *Food,* Readings from Scientific American, San Francisco: W. H. Freeman and Co., 1973, p. 205.
12 Carter, L. J.: "Soil Erosion: The Problem Persists Despite the Billions Spent on It." *Science,* 196:409, 1977.
13 McDonald, T., and G. Coffman: *Fewer, Larger U.S. Farms by Year*

2000—and Some Consequences. National Economics Division, Economics and Statistics Service, USDA, Agriculture Information Bulletin No. 439, Washington, D.C., 1980.
14 *A Time to Choose.* Summary Report on the Structure of Agriculture. Washington, D.C.: USDA, 1981.
15 Connor, J. M.: *The U.S. Food and Tobacco Manufacturing Industries: Market Structure, Structural Change, and Economic Performance.* Agricultural Economic Report No. 451. Washington, D.C.: USDA, 1980.
16 Wonnacott, P. and R. Wonnacott: *Economics.* New York: McGraw-Hill Book Co., 1979, p. 480.
17 SNE Communicator. *Newsletter of the Society for Nutrition Education,* 12(4):4, 1981.
18 USDA Study Team on Organic Farming. Report and Recommendations on Organic Farming. Washington, D.C.: USDA, 1980.
19 "Position Paper on Food and Nutrition Misinformation on Selected Topics." *Journal of the American Dietetic Association,* 66:277, 1975.
20 *Webster's Third International Dictionary.* Springfield, Mass.: G & C Merriam Co., 1976, p. 1590.
21 Herman, L., R. Carlson, T. Gold-

farb, and B. Commoner: The New York Metropolitan Area Product Market: A New Opportunity to Preserve Long Island Farmland. Center for the Biology of Natural Systems, Queens College, CUNY, Flushing, N.Y., July 1982.

22 Gallo, A. E.: "Food Advertising." *National Food Review,* Economics and Statistics Service, USDA, Washington, D.C., winter 1981, p. 7.

23 Gallo, A. E., J. M. Connor, and W. T. Boehm: "Mass Media Food Advertising." *National Food Review,* Economics and Statistics Service, USDA, Washington, D.C., winter 1980, pp. 10–13.

24 Gallo, A. E.: "Food Spending and Income." *National Food Review,* Economics and Statistics Service, USDA, Washington, D.C., winter 1982, p. 25.

25 Popkin, B. M., and P. S. Haines: "Factors Affecting Food Selection: The Role of Economics." *Journal of the American Dietetic Association,* 79:419, 1981.

26 Skelly, G. U.: "Where Do Food Stamp Recipients Shop for Food?" *National Food Review,* Economics, Statistics and Cooperatives Services, USDA, spring 1980, p. 16.

27 Foster, G. M.: *Traditional Cultures: The Impact of Technological Change.* New York: Harper & Row, 1962.

28 Mead, M.: "Food and the Family." In: *Food and People.* New York: UNESCO, United Nations, 1953, p. 7.

29 Mead, M.: "Dietary Patterns and Food Habits." *Journal of the American Dietetic Association,* 19:1, 1943.

30 Jelliffe, D. B.: *The Assessment of the Nutritional Status of the Community.* WHO Monograph Series No. 53, Geneva, World Health Organization, 1966.

31 Desor, J. A., O. Maller, and L. S. Greene: "Preference for Sweet in Humans: Infants, Children and Adults." In: Weiffenbach, J. M. (ed.), *Taste and Development, The Genesis of Sweet Preference.* Fogarty International Center Proceedings No. 32, Bethesda, Md, National Institutes of Health, 1977, p. 161.

32 Laird, D. A., and W. J. Breen: "Sex and Age Alterations in Taste Preferences." *Journal of the American Dietetic Association,* 15:549, 1939.

33 Uchendu, V. C.: "Cultural and Economic Factors Influencing Food Habit Patterns in Sub-Saharan Africa." *Proceedings of the Third International Congress of Food Science and Technology,* Washington, D.C., 1970.

34 Packard, V.: *The Status Seekers.* New York: David McKay Company, Inc., 1959, p. 146.

35 Ritchie, J.: *Learning Better Nutrition.* FAO Nutritional Studies, 20. Rome: FAO, 1967.

36 Ogbeide, O.: "Nutritional Hazards of Food Taboos and Preferences in Mid-West Nigeria." *American Journal of Clinical Nutrition,* 27:213, 1974.

37 Herbert, V., and S. Barrett: *Vitamins and "Health" Foods: The Great American Hustle.* New York: G. F. Stickley, 1981.

38 Erhard, D.: "The New Vegetarians. Part Two. The Zen Macrobiotic Movement and Other Cults Based on Vegetarianism." *Nutrition Today,* January/February 1974.

39 Wolff, R. J.: "Who Eats for Health?" *American Journal of Clinical Nutrition,* 26:438, 1973.

CHAPTER 2

1 U.S. Senate, Select Committee on Nutrition and Human Needs, *Dietary Goals for the United States,* Washington, D.C.: U.S. Government Printing Office, February 1977.

2 U.S. Senate, Select Committee on Nutrition and Human Needs, *Dietary Goals for the United States,* 2d ed., Washington, D.C.: U.S. Government Printing Office, December 1977.

3 Harper, A. E.: "Dietary Goals—a Skeptical View." *American Journal of Clinical Nutrition,* 31:310, 1978.

4 Olson, R. E.: "Are Professionals Jumping the Gun with the 'Goals'?" *Journal of the American Dietetic Association,* 74:543, 1979.

5 Turner, R. W. D.: "Perspectives on Coronary Prevention." *Postgraduate Medical Journal,* 54:141, 1978.

6 U.S. Department of Health Education and Welfare, *Healthy People.* The Surgeon General's Report on Health Promotion and Disease Prevention. DHEW (PHS) Publ. No. 79–55071, Washington, D.C.: U.S. Government Printing Office, July 1979.

7 U.S. Department of Agriculture and U.S. Department of Health, Education and Welfare, *Nutrition and Your Health, Dietary Guidelines for Americans.* Washington, D.C.: U.S. Government Printing Office, February 1980.

8 Food and Nutrition Board, *Toward Healthful Diets.* National Research Council, National Academy of Science, Washington, D.C., 1980.

9 McGinnis, J. M., Deputy Assistant Secretary for Health, Department of Health and Human Services. Testimony before the Committee on Appropriations, Subcommittee on Agriculture and Related Agencies, U.S. Senate, July 16, 1980.

10 Hegsted, D. M.: "Dietary Goals—a Progressive View." *American Journal of Clinical Nutrition,* 31:1504, 1978.

11 Johnson, G. T.: 1980 Chicago Tribune. N.Y. News Syndicate, Inc.

12 Committee on Diet, Nutrition and Cancer, Assembly of Life Sciences, National Research Council, National Academy of Sciences. *Diet, Nutrition and Cancer,* Washington, D.C.: National Academy Press, 1982.

13 King, J. C., S. H. Cohenour, C. G. Corruccini, and P. Schneeman: "Evaluation and Modification of

the Basic Four Food Guide." *Journal of Nutrition Education,* 10:27, 1978.

14 U.S. Department of Agriculture: *Food.* Home and Garden Bulletin No. 228, U.S. Government Printing Office, 1979.

15 Supplement to Exchange Lists for Meal Planning. Vegetarian Cookery, American Diabetes Association, Washington, D.C. Area Affiliate, Food and Nutrition Comm., 1978.

16 So, Betty, D. Chew, and E. Bright-See: "Dietetic Counselling of Chinese Diabetic Patients." *Canadian Dietetic Association Journal,* 39:46, 1978.

CHAPTER 3

1 Paul, P. C., and H. H. Palmer: *Food Theory and Applications.* New York: John Wiley & Sons, Inc., 1972.

2 Crapo, P. A., and J. M. Olefsky: "Fructose—Its Characteristics, Physiology, and Metabolism." *Nutrition Today,* 15(4):10, 1980.

3 Vuilleumier, S.: "Corn Sweetener Outlook." Agricultural Outlook Conference, USDA, Washington, D.C., Nov. 17–20, 1980, session no. 13.

4 Cummings, J. H.: What Is Fiber?" In: Spiller, G. A., and R. J. Amen (eds.): *Fiber In Human Nutrition.* New York: Plenum Press, 1976.

5 West, K. M.: "Diabetes Mellitus." In: Schneider, H. A., C. E. Anderson, and D. B. Coursin (eds.), *Nutritional Support of Medical Practice.* New York: Harper & Row, 1977.

6 Expert Panel on Food Safety and Nutrition, Institute of Food Technologists: "Sugars and Nutritive Sweeteners in Processed Foods." *Food Technology,* 33:101, 1979.

7 Van Soest, P.: "The Secret My Friends is the Fiber." *Cornell*

Human Ecology Forum, 6(4):1–4, 1976.

8 Page, L., and B. Friend: "Level of Use of Sugars in the United States." In: Sipple, H. L., and K. W. McNutt, *Sugars in Nutrition.* New York: Academic Press, 1974.

9 Spiro, H. M.: *Clinical Gastroenterology,* 2d ed. New York: Macmillan Co., 1977.

10 Oser, B. L. (ed.): *Hawk's Physiological Chemistry,* 14th ed. New York: McGraw-Hill Book Co., 1965.

11 Ingelfinger, F. J.: "Gastrointestinal Absorption." *Nutrition Today,* 2(1):2, 1967.

12 Gray, G. M.: "Absorption and Malabsorption of Dietary Carbohydrate." In: Winick, M. (ed.), *Nutrition and Gastroenterology.* New York: John Wiley & Sons, 1980.

13 Turner, S. J., T. Daly, J. A. Hourigan, A. G. Rand, and W. R. Thayer, Jr.: "Utilization of Low-Lactose Milk." *American Journal of Clinical Nutrition,* 29:739, 1976.

14 American Academy of Pediatrics, Committee on Nutrition: "The Practical Significance of Lactose Intolerance in Children." *Pediatrics,* 62:240, 1978.

15 Levine, R.: "Carbohydrates." In: Goodhart, R. S., and M. E. Shils (eds.), *Modern Nutrition in Health and Disease,* 5th ed. Philadelphia: Lea & Febiger, 1973.

16 Vitousek, S. H.: "Is More Better?" *Nutrition Today,* 14:10, 1979.

17 American Dietetic Association: "Nutrition and Physical Fitness." *Journal of the American Dietetic Association,* 76:437, 1980.

18 Forgac, M. T.: "Carbohydrate Loading. A Review." *Journal of the American Dietetic Association,* 75:42, 1979.

19 Food and Nutrition Board: *Recommended Dietary Allowances,* 9th ed. National Research Council, National Academy of Sciences, Washington, D.C., 1980.

20 Kraft, D. P.: "College Students and Alcohol: The 50 + 12 Project." *Alcohol Health and Research World,* DHEW Publication No.

(ADM) 76–157, Washington, D.C., 1976.

21 Roe, D. A.: "Nutritional Concerns in the Alcoholic." *Journal of the American Dietetic Association,* 78:17, 1981.

22 Roe, D. A.: *Alcohol and the Diet.* Westport, Conn.: Avi Publishing Co., Inc., 1979.

23 Lieber, C. S.: "The Metabolism of Alcohol." *Scientific American,* 234(3):25, 1976.

CHAPTER 4

1 Davenport, H. W.: *Physiology of the Digestive Tract.* Chicago, Ill.: Year Book Medical Publishers, 1961.

2 Roels, O. A., M. Trout, and R. Dujacquier: "Carotene Balances on Boys in Ruanda where Vitamin A Deficiency is Prevalent." *Journal of Nutrition,* 65:115, 1958.

3 Holman, R. T., S. B. Johnson, and T. F. Hatch: "A Case of Human Linolenic Acid Deficiency Involving Neurological Abnormalities." *American Journal of Clinical Nutrition,* 35:617, 1982.

4 Kannel, W. B.: "Status of Coronary Heart Disease Risk Factors." *Journal of Nutrition Education,* 10:10, 1978.

5 Thomas, L. H., P. R. Jones, J. A. Winter, and H. Smith: "Hydrogenated Oils and Fats: The Presence of Chemically-Modified Fatty Acids in Human Adipose Tissue." *American Journal of Clinical Nutrition,* 34:877, 1981.

6 Paul, P. C., and H. H. Palmer: *Food Theory and Applications.* New York: John Wiley & Sons, Inc., 1972.

7 Alfin-Slater, R. B., and L. Aftergood: "Lipids." In: Goodhart, R. S., and M. E. Shils (eds.), *Modern Nutrition in Health and Disease,* 6th ed. Philadelphia: Lea & Febiger, 1980, p. 113.

8 Makhlouf, G. M.: "Function of the Gallbladder." *Nutrition Today,* 17(1):10, 1982.

9 Dayton, S., S. Hashimoto, W. Dixon, and M. L. Pearce: "Composition of Lipids in Human Serum

and Adipose Tissue during Prolonged Feeding of a Diet High in Unsaturated Fat." *Journal of Lipid Research,* 7:103, 1966.

10 Gordon, T., W. P. Castelli, M. C. Hjortland, W. B. Kannel, and T. R. Dawber: "Predicting Coronary Heart Disease in Middle-aged and Older Persons." *Journal of the American Medical Association,* 238:497, 1977.

11 Gotto, Jr., A. M., J. Shepherd, L. W. Scott, and E. Manis: "Primary Hyperlipidemia and Dietary Management. In: Levy, R. I., B. M. Rifkind, B. H. Dennis, and N. Ernst (eds.), *Nutrition, Lipids and Coronary Heart Disease.* New York: Raven Press, 1979, p. 247.

12 Welsh, S. O., and R. Marston: "Review of Trends in Food Use in the United States, 1909 to 1980." *Journal of the American Dietetic Association,* 81:120, 1982.

13 U.S. Senate, Select Committee on Nutrition and Human Needs, *Dietary Goals for the United States,* 2d ed., Washington, D.C.: U.S. Government Printing Office, December 1977.

14 Committee on Diet, Nutrition and Cancer, Assembly of Life Sciences, National Research Council, National Academy of Sciences. *Diet, Nutrition and Cancer.* Washington, D.C.: National Academy Press, 1982.

CHAPTER 5

1 Levy, R. I., and J. Moskowitz: "Cardiovascular Research: Decades of Progress, a Decade of Promise." *Science,* 217:121, 1982.

2 Levy, R. I.: "Declining Mortality in Coronary Heart Disease." *Atherosclerosis,* 1:312, 1981.

3 Kannel, W. B.: "The Disease of Living." *Nutrition Today,* 6(3):2, 1971.

4 Krehl, W. A.: "The Nutritional Epidemiology of Cardiovascular Disease." *Annals of the New York Academy of Sciences,* 300:335, 1977.

5 Kannel, W. B.: "Status of Coronary Heart Disease Risk Factors." *Journal of Nutrition Education,* 10:10, 1978.

6 Glueck, C. J.: "Dietary Fat and Atherosclerosis." *American Journal of Clinical Nutrition,* 32:2703, 1979.

7 McGill, Jr., H. C.: "The Relationship of Dietary Cholesterol to Serum Cholesterol Concentration and to Atherosclerosis in Man." *American Journal of Clinical Nutrition,* 32:2664, 1979.

8 Stamler, J.: "Population Studies." In: Levy, R. I., B. M. Rifkind, B. H. Dennis, and N. Ernst, *Nutrition, Lipids, and Coronary Heart Disease.* New York: Raven Press, 1979.

9 Roberts, S. L., M. P. McMurry, and W. E. Connor: "Does Egg Feeding (i.e., Dietary Cholesterol) Affect Plasma Cholesterol Levels in Humans? The Results of a Double-Blind Study." *American Journal of Clinical Nutrition,* 34:2092, 1981.

10 Keys, A., J. T. Anderson, and F. Grande: "Prediction of Serum Cholesterol Responses of Man to Change of Fat in the Diet." *Lancet,* 2:959, 1957.

11 Hegsted, D. M., R. B. McGandy, M. L. Myers, and F. J. Stare: "Quantitative Effects of Dietary Fat on Serum Cholesterol in Man." *American Journal of Clinical Nutrition,* 17:281, 1965.

12 McGandy, R. B., and D. M. Hegsted: "Quantitative Effects of Dietary Fat and Cholesterol in Man." In: Vergroesen, A. J. (ed.), *The Role of Fat in Human Nutrition.* New York: Academic Press, 1975.

13 Flynn, M. A., G. B. Nolph, T. C. Flynn, R. Kahrs, and G. Krause: "Effect of Dietary Egg on Human Serum Cholesterol and Triglycerides." *American Journal of Clinical Nutrition,* 32:1051, 1979.

14 Porter, M. W., W. Yamanaka, S. Carlson, and M. Flynn: "Effect of Dietary Egg on Serum Cholesterol and Triglycerides of Human Males." *American Journal of Clinical Nutrition,* 30:490, 1977.

15 Connor, W. E., R. E. Hodges, and R. E. Bleiler: "The Serum Lipids in Men Receiving High Cholesterol and Cholesterol-free Diets." *Journal of Clinical Investigation,* 40:894, 1961.

16 Glueck, C. J., and W. E. Connor: "Diet–Coronary Heart Disease Relationships Reconnoitered." *American Journal of Clinical Nutrition,* 31:727, 1978.

17 Hjermann, I., K. Velve Byre, I. Holme, and P. Leren: "Effect of Diet and Smoking Intervention on the Incidence of Coronary Heart Disease." *Lancet,* 2:1303, 1981.

18 Multiple Risk Factor Intervention Trial Research Group. Multiple Risk Factor Intervention Trial. "Risk Factor Changes and Mortality Results." *Journal of the American Medical Association,* 248:1465, 1982.

19 Carroll, K. K.: "Soya Protein and Atherosclerosis." *Journal of the American Oil Chemists' Society,* 58:416, 1981.

20 Little, J. A., V. McGuire, and A. Derksen: "Available Carbohydrates." In: Levy, R. I., B. M. Rifkind, B. H. Dennis, and N. Ernst: *Nutrition, Lipids and Coronary Heart Disease.* New York: Raven Press, 1979.

21 Seelig, M. S., and H. A. Heggtveit: "Magnesium Interrelationships in Ischemic Heart Disease: A Review." *American Journal of Clinical Nutrition,* 27:59, 1974.

22 Klevay, L. M.: "Coronary Heart Disease. The Zinc/Copper Hypothesis." *American Journal of Clinical Nutrition,* 28:764, 1975.

23 Bierenbaum, M. L., A. I. Fleischman, and R. I. Raichelson: "Long-Term Human Studies of the Lipid Effects of Oral Calcium." *Lipids,* 7:202, 1972.

24 Kramsch, D. M., A. J. Aspen, and L. L. Rozler: "Atherosclerosis: Prevention by Agents not Affecting Ab-

normal Levels of Blood Lipids." *Science,* 213:1511, 1981.

25 Schroeder, H. A., A. P. Nason, and I. H. Tipton: "Chromium Deficiency as a Factor in Atherosclerosis." *Journal of Chronic Diseases,* 23:123, 1970.

26 Luoma, H., S. K. J. Helminen, H. Runta, I. Rytoma, and J. H. Meurman: "Relationship Between the Fluoride and Magnesium Concentrations in Drinking Water and Some Components in Serum Related to Cardiovascular Disease in Men from Four Rural Districts in Finland." *Scandinavian Journal of Clinical and Laboratory Investigation,* 32:217, 1973.

27 Senate Select Committee on Nutrition and Human Needs: *Dietary Goals for the United States,* 2d ed. U.S. Government Printing Office, Washington, D.C., December 1977.

28 *Nutrition and Health. Dietary Guidelines for Americans.* USDA, DHEW, Washington, D.C., February 1980.

29 Harper, A. E.: "Dietary Goals—A Skeptical View." *American Journal of Clinical Nutrition,* 31:310, 1978.

30 Hegsted, D. M.: "Dietary Goals—a Progressive View." *American Journal of Clinical Nutrition,* 31:1504, 1978.

31 Grundy, S. M.: "Saturated Fats and Coronary Heart Disease." In: Winick, M. (ed.), *Nutrition and the Killer Diseases.* New York: John Wiley & Sons, 1981.

32 Hegsted, D. M.: "Rationale for Change in the American Diet." *Food Technology,* 32(9):44, 1978.

33 Reiser, R.: "Oversimplification of Diet: Coronary Heart Disease Relationships and Exaggerated Diet Recommendations." *American Journal of Clinical Nutrition,* 31:865, 1978.

34 Pearce, M. L., and S. Dayton: "Incidence of Cancer in Men on a Diet High in Polyunsaturated Fat." *Lancet,* 1:464, 1971.

35 Sturdevant, R. A. L., M. L. Pearce, and S. Dayton: "Increased Prevalence of Cholelithiasia in Men Ingesting a Serum-Cholesterol-Lowering Diet." *New England Journal of Medicine,* 288:24, 1973.

36 Ederer, F., P. Leren, O. Turpeinen, and I. D. Frantz: "Cancer Among Men on Cholesterol-Lowering Diets: Experience From Five Clinical Trials." *Lancet,* 2:203, 1971.

37 *Health United States.* USDHHS, PHS, Hyattsville, Md., December 1980.

38 Hentges, D. J.: "Does Diet Influence Human Fecal Microflora Composition?" *Nutrition Reviews,* 38:329, 1980.

39 Wynder, E. L.: "Dietary Habits and Cancer Epidemiology." *Cancer,* 43(suppl):1955, 1979.

40 Lilienfeld, A. M.: "The Humean Fog: Cancer and Cholesterol." *American Journal of Epidemiology,* 114:1, 1981.

41 "Cholesterol and Noncardiovascular Mortality." From the NIH. *Journal of the American Medical Association,* 246:731, 1981.

42 Committee on Diet, Nutrition and Cancer, Assembly of Life Sciences, National Research Council, National Academy of Sciences. *Diet, Nutrition and Cancer.* Washington, D.C.: National Academy Press, 1982.

43 National Caries Program: DHEW: Status Report. NIH Publication No. 73–394, Washington, D.C., 1972.

44 Alfano, M. C.: "Dental Caries: The Nature of the Problem." *Cereal Foods World* 26:5, 1981.

45 Sweeney, E. A.: *The Food that Stays: An Update on Nutrition, Diet, Sugar and Caries.* New York: Medcom, Inc., 1977.

46 DePaola, D. P., and M. C. Alfano: "Diet and Oral Health." *Nutrition Today,* 12:6, 1977.

47 Russell, A. L.: "World Epidemiology and Oral Health." In: *Environmental Variables in Oral Disease.* Publication No. 81:21–39. Washington, D.C.: American Association for the Advancement of Science, 1966.

48 Sanders, H. J.: "Tooth Decay." *Chemical Engineering News,* 58(8):30, 1980.

49 Holloway, P. J., et al.: "Dental Disease in Tristan da Cunha." *British Dental Journal,* 115:19, 1963.

50 Taylor, A. G.: "Dental Conditions Among the Inhabitants of Easter Island." *Journal Canadian Dental Association,* 32:286, 1966.

51 Gustafson, B. E., et al.: "The Vipeholm Dental Caries Study. The Effect of Different Levels of Carbohydrate Intake on Dental Caries in 436 Individuals Observed for Five Years." *Acta Odontologica Scandinavica,* 11:232, 1954.

52 Newbrun, E.: "Sugar and Dental Caries: A Review of Human Studies." *Science,* 217:418, 1982.

53 Campbell, G. D.: "Diabetes in Asians and Africans in and around Durban." *South African Medical Journal,* 37:1195, 1963.

54 Reiser, S., and J. Hallfrisch: "Insulin Sensitivity and Adipose Tissue Weight of Rats Fed Starch or Sucrose Diets Ad Libitum or in Meals." *Journal of Nutrition,* 107:147, 1977.

55 Cohen, A. M., A. Teitelbaum, S. Briller, L. Yanko, E. Rosenmann, and E. Schafria: "Experimental Models of Diabetes." In: Sipple, H. L., and K. W. McNutt (eds.), *Sugars in Nutrition.* New York: Academic Press, 1974.

56 West, K. M.: "Prevention and Therapy of Diabetes Mellitus." *Nutrition Reviews,* 33:193, 1975.

57 Yudkin, J.: "Diet and Coronary Thrombosis." *Lancet,* 2:155, 1957.

58 Grande, F.: "Sugar and Cardiovascular Disease." *World Review of Nutrition and Dietetics,* 22:248, 1975.

59 Bierman, E. L.: "Carbohydrate and Sucrose Intake in the Causation of Atherosclerotic Heart Disease, Diabetes Mellitus, and Dental Caries." *American Journal of Clinical Nutrition,* 32:2644, 1979.

60 Reiser, S., J. G. Hallfrisch, O. E. Michaelis IV, F. L. Lazan, R. E.

Martin, and E. S. Prather: "Isocaloric Exchange of Dietary Starch and Sucrose in Humans. I. Effects on Levels of Fasting Blood Lipids." *American Journal of Clinical Nutrition,* 32:1659, 1979.

61 Gotto, Jr., A. M., J. Shepherd, L. W. Scott, and E. Manis: "Primary Hyperlipidemia and Dietary Management." In: Levy, R. I., B. M. Rifkind, B. H. Dennis, and N. D. Ernst (eds.), *Nutrition, Lipids, and Coronary Heart Disease.* New York: Raven Press, 1979, p. 247.

62 Burkitt, D. P., and H. C. Trowell (eds.): *Refined Carbohydrates and Disease.* New York: Academic Press, 1975.

63 Gear, J. S. S., A. Ware, P. Fursdon, et al.: "Symptomless Diverticular Disease and Intake of Dietary Fiber." *Lancet,* 1:511, 1979.

64 Brodribb, A. J. M.: "Dietary Fiber in Diverticular Disease of the Colon." In: Spiller, G. A., and R. M. Kay (eds.), *Medical Aspects of Dietary Fiber.* New York: Plenum Medical Book Co., 1980.

65 Kelsay, J. L.: "A Review of Research on Effects of Fiber Intake on Man." *American Journal of Clinical Nutrition,* 31:142, 1978.

66 Spiller, G. A., and H. J. Freeman: "Recent Advances in Dietary Fiber and Colorectal Diseases." *American Journal of Clinical Nutrition,* 34:1145, 1981.

67 Jenkins, D. J. A., A. R. Leeds, C. Newton, and J. H. Cummings: "Effect of Pectin, Guar Gum and Wheat Fiber on Serum Cholesterol." *Lancet,* 1:1116, 1975.

68 Kirby, R. W., J. W. Anderson, B. Sieling, E. D. Rees, W. J. L. Chen, R. E. Miller, and R. M. Kay: "Oat–Bran Intake Selectively Lowers Serum Low-Density Lipoprotein Cholesterol Concentrations of

Hypercholesterolemic Men." *American Journal of Clinical Nutrition,* 34:824, 1981.

69 Chen, W. J. L., and J. W. Anderson: "Soluble and Insoluble Plant Fiber in Selected Cereals and Vegetables." *American Journal of Clinical Nutrition,* 34:1077, 1981.

70 Van Itallie, T. B.: "Dietary Fiber and Obesity." *American Journal of Clinical Nutrition,* 31(suppl):43, 1978.

71 Anderson, J. W., and W. J. L. Chen: "Plant Fiber, Carbohydrate and Lipid Metabolism." *American Journal of Clinical Nutrition,* 32:346, 1979.

72 Jenkins, D. J. A., T. M. S. Wolever, S. Bacon, R. Nineham, R. Lees, R. Rowden, M. Love, and T. D. R. Hockaday: "Diabetic Diets: High Carbohydrate Combined with High Fiber." *American Journal of Clinical Nutrition,* 33:1729, 1980.

73 Anderson, J. W., and K. Ward: "High-Carbohydrate, High Fiber Diets for Insulin-Treated Men with Diabetes Mellitus." *American Journal of Clinical Nutrition,* 32:2312, 1979.

74 Jenkins, D. J. A., D. Reynolds, A. R. Leeds, A. L. Waller, and J. H. Cummings: "Hypocholesterolemic Action of Dietary Fiber Unrelated to Fecal Bulking Effect." *American Journal of Clinical Nutrition,* 32:2430, 1979.

75 Cummings, J. H.: "Nutritional Implications of Dietary Fiber." *American Journal of Clinical Nutrition,* 31(suppl):21, 1978.

CHAPTER 6

1 Hegsted, D. M.: "Protein Needs and Possible Modifications of the American Diet." *Journal of the American Dietetic Association,* 68:317, 1976.

2 Welsh, S. O., and R. M. Marston: "Review of Trends in Food Use in the United States, 1909 to 1980." *Journal of the American Dietetic Association,* 81:120, 1982.

3 Mayer, L. H.: *Food Chemistry.* New York: Reinhold Publ. Corp., 1960.

4 Albanese, A. A., and L. A. Orto: "The Proteins and Amino Acids." In: Goodhart, R. S., and M. E. Shils (eds.). *Modern Nutrition in Health and Disease,* 5th ed. Philadelphia: Lea & Febiger, 1973.

5 Crim, M. C., and H. N. Munro: "Protein." In: *Present Knowledge in Nutrition.* The Nutrition Foundation, 1976.

6 Committee on Dietary Allowances, Food and Nutrition Board. *Recommended Dietary Allowances,* 9th ed. National Research Council, National Academy of Sciences, 1980.

7 Bentivegna, A., E. J. Kelley, and A. Kalanek: "Diet, Fitness and Athletic Performance." *The Physician and Sportsmedicine,* 7(10):99, 1979.

8 Von Liebig, J.: *Letters on Chemistry.* London: 1851, p. 361.

9 Durnin, J.: "Protein Requirements and Physical Activity." In: Parizkova, J., and V. A. Rogozkin (eds.), *Nutrition, Physical Fitness and Health,* Baltimore, Md.: University Park Press, 1978.

10 Vitousek, S. H.: "Is More Better?" *Nutrition Today,* 14(6):10, 1979.

11 Edington, D. W., and V. R. Edgerton: *The Biology of Physical Fitness.* Boston: Houghton-Mifflin, 1976.

12 Consolazio, C. F., H. L. Johnson, R. A. Nelson, J. G. Dramie, and J. H. Skala: "Protein Metabolism During Intensive Physical Training in the Young Adult." *American Journal of Clinical Nutrition,* 28:29, 1975.

13 Rasch, P. J., J. W. Hamby, and H. J. Burns, Jr.: "Protein Dietary Supplementation and Physical Performance." *Medicine & Science in Sports,* 1:195, 1969.

14 Hegsted, D. M., A. G. Tsongas, D. B. Abbott, and F. J. Stare: "Protein Requirements of Adults." *Journal of Laboratory & Clinical Medicine,* 31:261, 1946.

15 Hardinge, M. G., H. Crooks, and F. J. Stare: "Nutritional Studies of Vegetarians. IV. Dietary Fatty Acids and Serum Cholesterol Levels."

American Journal of Clinical Nutrition, 10:516, 1962.

16 Kirkeby, K.: "Blood Lipids, Lipoproteins and Proteins in Vegetarians." *Acta Medica Scandinavica,* 179:(suppl)443:7, 1966.

17 Leverton, R. M., and M. R. Gram: "Nitrogen Excretion of Women Related to the Distribution of Animal Protein in Daily Meals." *Journal of Nutrition,* 39:57, 1949.

18 Robertson, L., C. Flinders, and B. Godfrey: *Laurel's Kitchen.* Petaluma; Calif.: Nilgiri Press, 1976.

19 A.D.A. Reports: "Position Paper on the Vegetarian Approach to Eating." *Journal of the American Dietetic Association,* 77:61, 1980.

20 Ohlson, M. A., W. D. Brewer, L. Jackson, P. P. Swanson, P. H. Roberts, M. Mangel, R. M. Leverton, M. Chaloupka, M. R. Gram, M. S. Reynolds, and R. Lutz: "Intakes and Retentions of Nitrogen, Calcium and Phosphorus by 136 Women Between 30 and 85 Years of Age." *Federation Proceedings,* 11:775, 1952.

21 Mayer, J.: "The Dimensions of Human Hunger." *Scientific American,* 235:40, 1976.

22 Viteri, F. E., and B. Torun: "Protein-Calorie Malnutrition." In: Goodhart, R. S., and M. E. Shils (eds.), *Modern Nutrition in Health and Disease,* 6th ed., Philadelphia: Lea & Febiger, 1980.

23 Gopalan, C.: "Protein Versus Calories in the Treatment of Protein-Calorie Malnutrition: Metabolic and Population Studies in India." In: R. E. Olson (ed.), *Protein-Calorie Malnutrition.* New York: Academic Press, 1975.

24 Latham, M. C.: "Diet and Infection in Relation to Malnutrition in the United States." *New York State Journal of Medicine,* 70:558, 1970.

25 Bengoa, J. M.: "Prevention of Protein-Calorie Malnutrition." In: R. E. Olson (ed.), *Protein-Calorie Malnutrition.* New York: Academic Press, 1975.

CHAPTER 7

1 Grande, F., and A. Keys: "Body Weight, Body Composition and Calorie Status." In: Goodhart, R. S., and M. E. Shils (eds.), *Modern Nutrition in Health and Disease,* 6th ed., Philadelphia: Lea & Febiger, 1980.

2 Cunningham, J. J.: "A Reanalysis of the Factors Influencing Basal Metabolic Rate in Normal Adults." *American Journal of Clinical Nutrition,* 33:2372, 1980.

3 Cunningham, J. J.: "Body Composition and Resting Metabolic Rate: The Myth of Feminine Metabolism." *American Journal of Clinical Nutrition,* 36:721, 1982.

4 Watkin, D. M.: "The Physiology of Aging." *American Journal of Clinical Nutrition,* 36(suppl):750, 1982.

5 Keys, A., J. Brozek, A. Hanschel, O. Michelson, and H. L. Taylor: *The Biology of Human Starvation.* Minneapolis, Minn.: University of Minnesota Press, 1950.

6 Benedict, F. G., W. R. Miles, P. Roth, and M. Smith: *Human Vitality and Efficiency Under Prolonged Restricted Diet.* Carnegie Institution of Washington, Publication 280, 1919.

7 DuBois, E. F.: *Fever and the Regulation of Body Temperature.* Springfield, Ill.: Charles C Thomas Co., 1948.

8 Consolazio, C. F., J. E. Shapiro, J. E. Masterson, and P. S. L. McKinzie: "Energy Requirements of Men in Extreme Heat." *Journal of Nutrition,* 73:126, 1961.

9 Food and Nutrition Board: *Recommended Dietary Allowances.* National Research Council, National Academy of Sciences, Washington, D.C., 1980.

10 Katch, F. I., and W. D. McArdle: *Nutrition, Weight Control, and Exercise.* Boston: Houghton Mifflin Co., 1977.

11 DuBois, E. F.: *Basal Metabolism in Health and Disease,* 3d ed. Philadelphia: Lea Publishers, 1936.

12 Garrow, J. S.: *Energy Balance and Obesity in Man.* New York: American Elsevier Publ. Co., Inc., 1974.

13 Kleiber, M.: *The Fire of Life.* Huntington, N.Y.: Robert E. Kreiger Publ. Co., 1975.

14 Durnin, J. V. G. A., and R. Passmore: *Energy, Work and Leisure.* London: Heinemann, 1967.

15 Swift, R. W. : "Food Energy." In: *The Yearbook of Agriculture.* U.S. Dept. of Agriculture, Washington, D.C., 1959.

16 Taylor, C. M., and O. F. Pye: *Foundations of Nutrition,* 6th ed. New York: The Macmillan Co., 1966.

17 Vitousek, S. H.: "Is More Better?" *Nutrition Today,* 14(6):10, 1979.

CHAPTER 8

1 Hannon, B., and T. Lohman: "The Energy Cost of Overweight in the United States." *American Journal of Public Health,* 68:765, 1978.

2 Eckholm, E., and F. Record: *The Two Faces of Malnutrition.* Worldwatch Paper 9, Worldwatch Institute, Washington, D.C., December 1976.

3 United States Public Health Service, Division of Chronic Diseases: *Obesity and Health.* Public Health Service Publication 1485, U.S. Government Printing Office, Washington, D.C., 1966.

4 Abraham, S., and C. L. Johnson: "Prevalence of Severe Obesity in Adults in the United States." *American Journal of Clinical Nutrition,* 33(suppl):364, 1980.

5 Bray, G. A., M. B. Davidson, and E. J. Drenick: "Obesity: A Serious Symptom." *Annals of Internal Medicine,* 77:979, 1972.

6 Beller, A. S.: *Fat and Thin, A Natural History of Obesity.* New York: Farrar, Straus and Giroux, 1977, p. 261.

7 Van Itallie, T. B.: "Obesity: Adverse Effects on Health and Longevity." *American Journal of Clinical Nutrition,* 32:2723, 1979.

8 Keys, A.: "Overweight, Obesity,

Coronary Heart Disease and Mortality." *Nutrition Reviews,* 38:297, 1980.

9 Check, W., and J. Elliott: "Medical News. Obesity May Reduce Survival, Increase Risk, in Breast Cancer." *Journal of the American Medical Association,* 244:419, 1980.

10 Fomon, S. J.: *Nutritional Disorders of Children. Prevention, Screening, and Followup.* Rockville, Md.: DHEW Publication No. (HSA) 77–5104, 1977.

11 Mayer, J.: "Obesity." In: R. S. Goodhart, and M. S. Shils (eds.), *Nutrition in Health and Disease,* 6th ed. Philadelphia: Lea & Febiger, 1980.

12 Van Itallie, T. B.: "Obesity: The American Disease." *Food Technology,* 33(12):43, 1979.

13 United States Department of Health, Education and Welfare: *Ten State Nutrition Survey.* DHEW Publication No. (HSM) 73–7804. Washington, D.C., 1972.

14 Ginsberg-Fellner, F., L. A. Jagendorf, H. Carmel, and T. Harris: "Overweight and Obesity in Preschool Children in New York City." *American Journal of Clinical Nutrition,* 34:2236, 1981.

15 Abraham, S., C. Collins, and M. Nordsieck: "Relationship of Childhood Weight Status to Morbidity in Adults." *Public Health Reports,* 86:273, 1971.

16 Johnson, F. E., and R. W. Mack: "Obesity in Urban Black Adolescents of High and Low Relative Weight at One Year of Age." *American Journal of Diseases of Children,* 132:862, 1978.

17 Poskitt, E.: "Overfeeding and Overweight in Infancy and Their Relation to Body Size in Early Childhood." *Nutrition and Metabolism,* 21:54, 1977.

18 Garrow, J. S.: "Infant Feeding and Obesity of Adults." *Bibliotheca Nutritio et Dieta,* 26:29, 1978.

19 Stunkard, A. J.: *The Pain of Obesity.* Palo Alto, Calif.: Bull Publishing Co., 1976.

20 Bruch, H.: *Eating Disorders.* New York: Basic Books, Inc., 1973.

21 Mayer, J.: "Obesity During Childhood." In: M. Winick (ed.), *Childhood Obesity.* New York: John Wiley & Sons, 1975.

22 Lebow, M.: "Can Lighter Become Thinner?" *Addictive Behaviors,* 2:87, 1977.

23 Hirsch, J.: "Cell Number and Size as a Determinant of Subsequent Obesity." In: M. Winick (ed.), *Childhood Obesity.* New York: John Wiley & Sons, 1975.

24 Winick, M.: *Childhood Obesity.* New York: John Wiley & Sons, 1975.

25 Ashwell, M. A., P. Priest, and M. Bondoux: "Adipose Tissue Cellularity in Obese Women. I. Relation to Age and Onset of Obesity. II. Relation to the Behaviour of the Fat Site on Weight Gain and Loss." In: Howard, A. M. (ed.), *Recent Advances in Obesity Research,* vol. I. Westport, Conn.: Technomic, 1975.

26 Hirsch, J., and B. Batchelor: "Adipose Tissue Cellularity in Human Obesity." *Clinics in Endocrinology and Metabolism,* 5:299, 1976.

27 Chumlea, W. C., A. F. Roche, R. M. Siervogel, J. L. Knittle, and P. Webb: "Adipocytes and Adiposity in Adults." *Americal Journal of Clinical Nutrition,* 34:1798, 1981.

28 Roche, A. F.: "The Adipocyte-Number Hypothesis." *Child Development,* 52:31, 1981.

29 Kirtland, J., and M. I. Gurr: "Adipose Tissue Cellularity: A Review. 2. The Relationship Between Cellularity and Obesity." *International Journal of Obesity,* 3:15, 1979.

30 Roncari, D. A. K., and R. L. R. Van: "Adipose Tissue Cellularity and Obesity: New Perspectives." *Clinical and Investigative Medicine,* 1:71, 1978.

31 Mayer, J.: "Physiology of Hunger and Appetite." In: R. S. Goodhart and M. S. Shils (eds.), *Modern Nutrition in Health and Disease,* 6th ed. Philadelphia: Lea & Febiger, 1980.

32 Thompson, C. I.: *Controls of Eating.* New York: S. P. Medical & Scientific Books, 1980.

33 Hamilton, C. L.: "Physiologic Control of Food Intake." *Journal of the American Dietetic Association,* 62:35, 1973.

34 Heaton, J. M.: "The Distribution of Brown Adipose Tissue in the Human." *Journal of Anatomy,* 112:35, 1972.

35 Elliott, J.: "Medical News. Blame It All on Brown Fat Now." *Journal of the American Medical Association,* 243:1983, 1980.

36 Hegsted, D. M.: "Energy Needs and Energy Utilization." *Nutrition Reviews,* 32:33, 1974.

37 DeLuise, M., G. L. Blackburn, and J. S. Flier: "Reduced Activity of the Red-Cell Sodium-Pump in Human Obesity." *New England Journal of Medicine,* 303:1017, 1980.

38 Norgan, N. G., and J. V. G. A. Durnin: "The Effect of 6 Weeks of Overfeeding on the Body Weight, Body Composition, and Energy Metabolism of Young Men." *American Journal of Clinical Nutrition,* 33:978, 1980.

39 Van Itallie, T. B., Interviewed by W. Stockton: "Conspiracy against Fatness." *Psychology Today,* October 1978, pp. 97–106.

40 Coates, T. J., and C. E. Thoresen: "Treating Obesity in Children and Adolescents: A Review." *American Journal of Public Health,* 68:143, 1978.

41 Bray, G. A.: *The Obese Patient.* Philadelphia: W. B. Saunders Co., 1976.

42 United States Department of Health, Education and Welfare, FDA: *FDA Consumer Memo.* HEW Publication No. (FDA) 77–3035, 1977.

43 Food and Drug Administration: "Liquid Protein and Sudden Cardiac Deaths—An Update." *FDA Drug Bulletin,* May–June 1978.

44 Pennington, A. W.: "Treatment of Obesity with Calorically Unrestric-

ted Diets." *American Journal of Clinical Nutrition,* 1:343, 1953.

45 Taller, H.: *Calories Don't Count.* New York: Simon & Schuster, Inc., 1961.

46 Jameson, G., and E. Williams: *The Drinking Man's Diet.* San Francisco: Cameron and Co., 1964.

47 Stillman, I. M., and S. S. Baker: *The Doctor's Quick Weight Loss Diet.* Englewood Cliffs, N.J.: Prentice-Hall, Inc., 1967.

48 Atkins, R. C.: *Dr. Atkin's Diet Revolution: The High Calorie Way to Stay Thin Forever.* New York: David McKay, Inc., 1972.

49 Tarnower, H., and S. S. Baker: *The Complete Scarsdale Medical Diet.* New York: Bantam Books, 1979.

50 American Medical Association, Council on Foods and Nutrition: "A Critique of Low-Carbohydrate Ketogenic Weight Reduction Regimens." *Journal of the American Medical Association,* 224(10):1415, 1973.

51 Yang, M. U., and T. B. Van Itallie: "Composition of Weight Loss during Short-Term Weight Reduction: Metabolic Responses of Obese Subjects to Starvation and Low-Calorie Ketogenic and Nonketogenic Diets." *Journal of Clinical Investigation,* 58:722, 1976.

52 Van Itallie, T. B.: "Dietary Fiber and Obesity." *American Journal of Clinical Nutrition,* 31(suppl):S-43, 1978.

53 Brownell, K. D.: "The psychological and medical sequelae of nonprescription weight reduction programs." Paper presented at annual meeting of the American Psychological Association, Toronto, August 1978.

54 Katch, F. I., and W. D. McArdle: *Nutrition, Weight Control, and Exercise.* Boston: Houghton Mifflin Co., 1977.

55 Gwinup, G.: "Effect of Exercise Alone on the Weight of Obese Women." *Archives of Internal Medicine,* 135:676, 1975.

56 Sidney, K. H., R. J. Shephard, and J. E. Harrison: "Endurance Training and Body Composition of the Elderly." *American Journal of Clinical Nutrition,* 30:326, 1977.

57 Gwinup, G., R. Chelvam, and T. Steinberg: "Thickness of Subcutaneous Fat and Activity of Underlying Muscles." *Annals of Internal Medicine,* 74:408, 1971.

58 Franklin, B. A., and M. Rubenfire: "Losing Weight through Exercise." *Journal of the American Medical Association,* 244:377, 1980.

59 Konishi, F.: "Food and Energy Equivalents of Various Activities." *Journal of the American Dietetic Association,* 46:187, 1965.

60 Mahan, L. K.: "Obesity: New Knowledge and Current Treatment." In: *Contemporary Developments in Nutrition.* B. Worthington-Roberts, St. Louis: C. V. Mosby Co., 1981.

61 Leon, G. R.: (Letter) "Is It Bad Not To Be Thin?" *American Journal of Clinical Nutrition,* 33:174, 1980.

62 Katz, J. L., et al.: "Toward an Elucidation of the Psycho-endocrinology of Anorexia Nervosa." In: Sacher, E. J. (ed.), *Hormones, Behavior and Psychopathology.* New York: Raven Press, 1976.

63 Bruch, H.: "Anorexia Nervosa." *Nutrition Today,* 13:14, 1978.

64 Krause, M. V., and L. K. Mahan: *Food, Nutrition and Diet Therapy.* Philadelphia: W. B. Saunders Co., 1979.

65 Pyle, R., J. Mitchell, and E. Eckert: "Bulimia: A Report of 34 Cases." *Journal of Clinical Psychiatry,* 42:60, 1981.

66 Lucas, A.: "Bulimia and Vomiting Syndrome." *Contemporary Nutrition,* 6(4), April 1981.

CHAPTER 9

1 Pauling, L.: *Vitamin C and the Common Cold.* San Francisco: W. H. Freeman & Co., 1970.

2 Herbert, V.: "Laetrile: The Cult of Cyanide. Promoting Poison for Profit." *American Journal of Clinical Nutrition,* 32:1121, 1979.

3 Moertel, C. G., T. R. Fleming, J. Rubin, L. K. Kvols, G. Sarna, R. Koch, V. E. Currie, C. W. Young, S. E. Jones, and J. P. Davignon: "A Clinical Trial of Amygdalin (Laetrile) in the Treatment of Human Cancer." *The New England Journal of Medicine,* 306:201, 1982.

4 Herbert, V.: "Pangamic Acid (Vitamin B_{15})." *American Journal of Clinical Nutrition,* 32:1534, 1979.

5 Herbert, V., A. Gardner, and N. Colman: "Mutagenicity of Dichloroacetate, an Ingredient of Some Formulations of Pangamic Acid (Trade-Named Vitamin B_{15})." *American Journal of Clinical Nutrition,* 33:1179, 1980.

6 Weininger, J., and G. M. Briggs: "Bioflavonoids." In: Goodhart, R. S., and M. E. Shils (eds.), *Modern Nutrition in Health and Disease,* 6th ed. Philadelphia: Lea & Febiger, 1980.

7 Hodges, R. E.: "Ascorbic Acid." In: *Modern Nutrition in Health and Disease.* Goodhart, R. S., and M. E. Shils (eds.), 6th ed. Philadelphia: Lea & Febiger, 1980.

8 Lind, J.: *A Treatise on Scurvy.* London: A. Millar, 1753. Republished by Stewart, C. P., and D. Guthrie (eds.), *Lind's Treatise on Scurvy.* Edinburgh: University Press, 1953.

9 Editorial. "Captain James Cook (1728–1779)." *Journal of the American Medical Association,* 209:1217, 1969.

10 Priestley, R.: "Inexpressible Island." *Nutrition Today,* 4:18, 1969.

11 Funk, C.: "The Etiology of Deficiency Diseases." *The Journal of State Medicine,* 20:341, 1912. Reprinted in Goldblith, S. A., and M. A. Joslyn, *Milestones in Nutrition.* Westport, Conn.: The AVI Publishing Co., Inc., 1964, p. 145.

12 Szent-Györgyi, A., and W. N. Haworth: (Letter). "Hexuronic Acid (Ascorbic Acid) as the Antiscorbutic Factor." *Nature,* 131:24, 1933.

13 Waugh, W. A., and C. G. King: "Isolation and Identification of Vi-

tamin C." *The Journal of Biological Chemistry,* 97:325, 1932.

14 "The Role of Ascorbic Acid in the Hydroxylation of Peptide-bound Proline." *Nutrition Reviews,* 37:26, 1979.

15 Barnes, M. J.: "Function of Ascorbic Acid in Collagen Metabolism." *Annals of the New York Academy of Sciences,* 258:264, 1975.

16 Ryer III, R., M. I. Grossman, T. E. Friedemann, W. R. Best, F. Consolazio, W. J. Kuhl, W. Insull, Jr., and F. T. Hatch: "The Effect of Vitamin Supplementation on Soldiers Residing in a Cold Environment. Part I. Physical Performance and Response to Cold Exposure." *Journal of Clinical Nutrition,* 2:97, 1954.

17 Ryer III, R., M. I. Grossman, T. E. Friedemann, W. R. Best, F. Consolazio, W. J. Kuhl, W. Insull, Jr., and F. T. Hatch: "The Effect of Vitamin Supplementation on Soldiers Residing in a Cold Environment. Part II. Psychological, Biochemical and Other Measurements." *Journal of Clinical Nutrition,* 2:179, 1954.

18 Robinson, C. H., and M. R. Lawler: *Normal and Therapeutic Nutrition,* 16th ed. New York: MacMillan Publishing Co., Inc., 1982, p. 594.

19 Conrad, M. E., and S. G. Schade: "Ascorbic Acid Chelates in Iron Absorption: A Role for Hydrochloric Acid and Bile." *Gastroenterology,* 55:35, 1968.

20 Lynch, S. R., and J. D. Cook: "Interactions of Vitamin C and Iron." *Annals of the New York Academy of Sciences,* 355:32, 1980.

21 Hornig, D.: "Distribution of Ascorbic acid, Metabolites and Analogues in Man and Animals." *Annals of the New York Academy of Sciences,* 258:103, 1975.

22 Hodges, R. E., J. Hood, J. E. Canham, H. E. Sauberlich, and E. M. Baker: "Clinical Manifestations of Ascorbic Acid Deficiency in Man." *American Journal of Clinical Nutrition,* 24:432, 1971.

23 Food and Nutrition Board: *Recommended Dietary Allowances,* 9th ed. National Academy of Sciences, Washington, D.C., 1980.

24 Hodges, R. E.: "Vitamin C." In: *Nutrition and the Adult. Micronutrients,* R. B. Alfin-Slater and D. Kritchevsky (eds.) New York: Plenum Press, 1980.

25 Kallner, A. B., D. Hartmann, and D. H. Hornig: "On the Requirements of Ascorbic Acid in Man: Steady-State Turnover and Body Pool in Smokers." *American Journal of Clinical Nutrition,* 34:1347, 1981.

26 Thorp, V. J.: "Effect of Oral Contraceptive Agents on Vitamin and Mineral Requirements." *Journal of the American Dietetic Association,* 76:581, 1980.

27 Wilson, C. W. M.: "Clinical Pharmacological Aspects of Ascorbic Acid." *Annals of the New York Academy of Sciences,* 258:355, 1975.

28 Visagie, M. E., J. P. DuPlessis, and N. F. Laubscher: "Effect of Vitamin C Supplementation on Black Mineworkers." *South African Medical Journal,* 49:889, 1975.

29 Anderson, T. W.: "New Horizons for Vitamin C." *Nutrition Today,* 12(1):6, 1977.

30 Anderson, T. W., A. Szent-Györgyi, R. Passmore, L. C. Pauling, C. F. Enloe, Jr., and H. L. Hartley: "To Dose or Megadose: A Debate about Vitamin C." *Nutrition Today,* 13:6, 1978.

31 Kykes, M. H. M., and P. Meier: "Ascorbic Acid and the Common Cold. Evaluation of its Efficacy and Toxicity." *Journal of the American Medical Association,* 231:1073, 1975.

32 Anderson, T. W., G. Suranyi, and G. H. Beaton: "The Effect on Winter Illness of Large Doses of Vitamin C." *Canadian Medical Association Journal,* 111:31, 1974.

33 Cameron, E., and L. Pauling: "Supplemental Ascorbate in the Supportive Treatment of Cancer: Prolongation of Survival Times in Terminal Human Cancer." *Proceedings of the National Academy of Sciences,* 73:3685, 1976.

34 Creagan, E. T., C. G. Moertel, J. R. O'Fallon, A. J. Schutt, M. J. O'Connell, J. Rubin, and S. Frytak: "Failure of High-Dose Vitamin C (Ascorbic Acid) Therapy to Benefit Patients with Advanced Cancer." *The New England Journal of Medicine,* 301:687, 1979.

35 Mirvish, S. S., L. Wallcave, M. Eagen, and P. Shubik: "Ascorbate-Nitrite Reaction: Possible Means of Blocking the Formation of Carcinogenic N-Nitroso Compounds." *Science,* 177:65, 1972.

36 Passmore, R.: "How Vitamin C Deficiency Injures the Body." *Nutrition Today,* 12:6, 1977.

37 Briggs, M.: (Letter) "Vitamin-C Induced Hyperoxaluria." *Lancet,* 1:154, 1976.

38 Barness, L. A.: "Safety Considerations with High Ascorbic Acid Dosage." *Annals of the New York Academy of Sciences,* 258:523, 1975.

39 Marcus, M., M. Prabhudesai, and S. Wassef: "Stability of Vitamin B_{12} in the Presence of Ascorbic Acid in Food and Serum: Restoration by Cyanide of Apparent Loss." *American Journal of Clinical Nutrition,* 33:137, 1980.

CHAPTER 10

1 Kamil, A.: "How Natural are Those (Natural) Vitamins?" *Journal of Nutrition Education,* 4:92, 1972.

2 Goldsmith, G. A.: "The B Vitamins: Thiamine, Riboflavin, Niacin." In: Beaton, G. H., and E. W. McHenry (eds.), *Nutrition, A Comprehensive Treatise,* vol. II. New York: Academic Press, 1964.

3 Katsura, E., and T. Oiso: "Beriberi." In: Beaton, G. H., and J. M. Bengoa (eds.), *Nutrition in Preventive Medicine.* Geneva, Switzerland: World Health Organization, 1976.

4 Vimokesant, S. L., D. M. Hilker, S. Nakornchai, K. Rungruangsak, and S. Dhanamitta: "Effects of Betel Nut and Fermented Fish on the Thiamin Status of Northeastern Thais." *American Journal of Clinical Nutrition,* 28:1458, 1975.

5 Tomasulo, P. A., R. M. Kater, and F. L. Iber: "Impairment of Thiamine Absorption in Alcoholism." *American Journal of Clinical Nutrition,* 21:1340, 1968.

6 Leevy, C. M., and H. M. Baker: "Vitamins and Alcoholism." *American Journal of Clinical Nutrition,* 21:1325, 1968.

7 Food and Nutrition Board: *Recommended Dietary Allowances,* 9th ed. National Research Council, National Academy of Sciences, Washington, D.C., 1980.

8 Sebrell, Jr., W. H., and R. E. Butler: "Riboflavin Deficiency in Man. A Preliminary Note." *Public Health Reports,* 53:2282, 1938.

9 Horwitt, M. K., C. C. Harvey, O. W. Hills, and E. Liebert: "Correlation of Urinary Excretion of Riboflavin with Dietary Intake and Symptoms of Ariboflavinosis." *Journal of Nutrition,* 41:247, 1950.

10 Horwitt, M. K.: "Riboflavin. Deficiency Effects in Man." In: Sebrell, W. H., Jr., and R. S. Harris (eds.), *The Vitamins,* 2d ed., vol. V. New York: Academic Press, 1972.

11 Darby, W. J., K. W. McNutt, and E. N. Todhunter: "Niacin." *Nutrition Reviews,* 33:289, 1975.

12 Elvehjem, C. A., R. J. Madden, S. M. Strong, and D. W. Wooley: "Relation of Nicotinic acid and Nicotinic Acid Amide to Canine Black Tongue." Communication to the editor. *Journal of the American Chemical Society,* 59:1767, 1937.

13 Elvehjem, C. A., R. J. Madden, S. M. Strong, and D. W. Wooley: "Isolation and Identification of Anti-Black Tongue Factor." *Journal of Biological Chemistry,* 123:137, 1938.

14 Coronary Drug Project Research Group: "Clofibrate and Niacin in Coronary Heart Disease." *Journal of the American Medical Association,* 231:360, 1975.

15 Ban, T. A., and H. E. Lehmann: "Nicotinic Acid in the Treatment of Schizophrenia." Canadian Mental Health Association Collaborative Study: Progress Report II. *Canadian Psychiatric Association Journal,* 20:103, 1975.

16 Coursin, D. B.: "Convulsive Seizures in Infants with Pyridoxine-Deficient Diet." *Journal of the American Medical Association,* 154:406, 1954.

17 Sauberlich, H. E., and J. E. Canham: "Vitamin B_6." In: Goodhart, R. S., and M. E. Shils (eds.), *Modern Nutrition in Health and Disease,* 6th ed. Philadelphia: Lea & Febiger, 1980.

18 Robson, L. C., M. R. Schwarz, and W. D. Perkins: "Vitamin B_6 and Immunity." In: National Research Council, *Human Vitamin B_6 Requirements.* Washington, D.C.: National Academy of Sciences, 1978, p. 162.

19 Rose, D. P.: "Oral Contraceptives and Vitamin B_6." In: National Research Council, *Human Vitamin B_6 Requirements.* Washington, D.C.: National Academy of Sciences, 1978, p. 193.

20 Li, Ting-Kai: "Factors Influencing Vitamin B_6 Requirement in Alcoholism." In: National Research Council, *Human Vitamin B_6 Requirements.* Washington, D.C.: National Academy of Sciences, 1978, p. 210.

21 Bauernfeind, J. C., and O. N. Miller: "Vitamin B_6: Nutritional and Pharmaceutical Usage, Stability, Bioavailability, Antagonists, and Safety." In: *Human Vitamin B_6 Requirements.* Washington, D.C.: National Academy of Sciences, 1978, p. 104.

22 Williams, R. J., C. M. Lyman, G. H. Goodyear, J. H. Truesdail, and D. Holaday: "Pantothenic Acid, a Growth Determinant of Universal Biological Occurrence." *Journal of the American Chemical Society,* 55:2912, 1933.

23 Hodges, R. E., W. B. Bean, M. A. Ohlson, and B. Bleiler: "Human Pantothenic Acid Deficiency Produced by Omega-Methyl Pantothenic Acid." *Journal of Clinical Investigation;* 38:1421, 1959.

24 Fry, P. C., H. M. Fox, and H. G. Tao: "Metabolic Response to a Pantothenic Acid Deficient Diet in Humans." *Journal of Nutritional Science and Vitaminology,* 22:339, 1976.

25 Johnson, N. E., and S. Nitzke: "Nutritional Adequacy of Diets of a Selected Group of Low-Income Women: Identification of Some Related Factors." *Home Economics Research Journal,* 3:241, 1975.

26 Cohenour, S. H., and D. H. Calloway: "Blood, Urine and Dietary Pantothenic Acid Levels of Pregnant Teenagers." *American Journal of Clinical Nutrition,* 25:512, 1972.

27 Harris, R. S., and S. Lepkovsky: "Pantothenic Acid." In: Sebrell, W. H., Jr., and R. S. Harris (eds.), *The Vitamins,* vol. 2, New York: Academic Press, 1954.

28 Wills, L., P. W. Clutterbuck, and B. D. F. Evans: "A New Factor in the Production and Cure of Macrocytic Anemias and its Relation to Other Haemopoietic Principles Curative in Pernicious Anemia." *Biochemical Journal,* 31:2136, 1937.

29 Herbert, V., N. Colman, and E. Jacob: "Folic Acid and Vitamin B_{12}." In: Goodhart, R. S., and M. E. Shils (eds.), *Modern Nutrition in Health and Disease,* 6th ed. Philadelphia: Lea & Febiger, 1980.

30 Editorial. "Folate Deficiency and the Nervous System." *British Medical Journal,* 2(6027):71, July 10, 1976.

31 Goldsmith, G. A.: "Curative Nutrition: Vitamins." In: Schneider, H. A., C. E. Anderson, and D. B. Coursin (eds.), *Nutritional Support*

in Medical Practice. New York: Harper & Row, 1977.

32 Rodriquez, M. S.: "A Conspectus of Research on Folacin Requirements of Man." *Journal of Nutrition,* 108:1983, 1978.

33 Theuer, R. C., and J. J. Vitale: "Drug and Nutrient Interactions." In: Schneider, H. A., C. E. Anderson, and D. B. Coursin (eds.), *Nutritional Support in Medical Practice.* New York: Harper & Row, 1977.

34 Check, W. A.: "Medical News. Folate for Oral Contraceptive Users May Reduce Cervical Cancer Risk." *Journal of the American Medical Association,* 244:633, 1980.

35 Ek, J., and E. Magnus: "Plasma and Red Cell Folacin in Cow's Milk-fed Infants and Children during the First Two Years of Life: The Significance of Boiling Pasteurized Cow's Milk." *American Journal of Clinical Nutrition,* 33:1220, 1980.

36 Addison, T.: *On the Constitutional and Local Effects of Disease of the Suprarenal Capsules.* London: S. Highley, 1855.

37 Minot, G. R., and W. P. Murphy: "Treatment of Pernicious Anemia by a Special Diet." *Journal of the American Medical Association,* 87:470, 1926.

38 Castle, W. B., W. C. Townsend, C. W. Heath, and M. B. Strauss: "Observations on the Etiologic Relationship of Achylia Gastrica to Pernicious Anemia." *Journal of the American Medical Association,* 178:748 and 764, 1929; 180:305, 1930; 182:741, 1931.

39 Albert, M. J., V. I. Mathan, and S. J. Baker: "Vitamin B_{12} Synthesis by Human Small Intestinal Bacteria." *Nature,* 283:781, 1980.

40 Ericson, L. E., and Z. G. Banhidi: "Bacterial Growth Factors Related to Vitamin B_{12} and Folinic Acid in Some Brown and Red Seaweed." *Acta Chemica Scandinavica,* 7:167, 1953.

41 Harris, R. S., and E. Karmas: *Nutritional Evaluation of Food Processing,* 2d ed. Westport, Conn.: The Avi Publishing Co., 1975.

42 Sydenstricker, V. P., S. A. Singel, A. P. Briggs, N. M. DeVaughn, and H. Isbell: "Observations of the 'Egg White Injury' in Man and Its Cure with a Biotin Concentrate." *Journal of the American Medical Association,* 118:1199, 1942.

43 Sauberlich, H. E.: "Interactions of Thiamin, Riboflavin and other B-Vitamins." *Annals of the New York Academy of Sciences,* 355:80, 1980.

44 Appel, J. A., and G. M. Briggs: "Choline." In: Goodhart, R. S., and M. E. Shils (eds.), *Modern Nutrition in Health and Disease,* 6th ed. Philadelphia: Lea & Febiger, 1980.

CHAPTER 11

1 McCollum, E. V., and M. Davis: "The Nature of the Dietary Deficiencies of Rice." *Journal of Biological Chemistry,* 23:181, 1915.

2 Drummond, J. C.: "The Nomenclature of the So-called Accessory Food Factors (Vitamins)." *Biochemical Journal,* 14:660, 1920.

3 McCollum, E. V.: *History of Nutrition.* Boston: Houghton Mifflin Co., 1957.

4 Bernard, R. A., and B. P. Halpern: "Taste Changes in Vitamin A Deficiency." *Journal of General Physiology,* 52:444, 1968.

5 Lui, Nan Sen Tseng, and O. A. Roels: "Vitamin A and Carotene." In: Goodhart, R. S., and M. E. Shils (eds.), *Modern Nutrition in Health and Disease,* 6th ed. Philadelphia, Lea & Febiger, 1980.

6 Smith, F. R., R. Suskind, O. Thanangkul, C. Leitzmann, D. S. Goodman, and R. E. Olson: "Plasma Vitamin A, Retinol-binding Protein and Prealbumin Concentrations in Protein-Calorie Malnutri-

tion. III. Response to Varying Dietary Treatments." *American Journal of Clinical Nutrition,* 28:732, 1975.

7 Tarwotjo, I., A. Sommer, T. Soegiharto, D. Susanto, and Muhilal: "Dietary Practices and Xerophthalmia among Indonesian Children." *American Journal of Clinical Nutrition,* 35:574, 1982.

8 Sweeney, J. P., and A. C. Marsh: "Effect of Processing on Provitamin A in Vegetables." *Journal of the American Dietetic Association,* 59:238, 1971.

9 Yaffe, S. J., and L. J. Filer, Jr.: "The Use and Abuse of Vitamin A." *Nutrition Reviews,* 32(suppl 1):41, 1974.

10 Quan, M. A., W. M. Rodney, and R. A. Strick: "Treatment of Acne Vulgaris." *Journal of Family Practice,* 11:1041, 1980.

11 Kligman, A. M., O. H. Mills, Jr., J. J. Leyden, P. R. Gross, H. B. Allen, and R. I. Rudolph: "Oral Vitamin A in Acne Vulgaris." *International Journal of Dermatology,* 20:278, 1981.

12 Peck, G. L., T. G. Olson, F. W. Yoder, J. S. Strauss, D. T. Downing, M. Pandya, D. Butkus, and J. Arnaud-Battandier: "Prolonged Remissions of Cystic and Conglobate Acne with 13-*Cis*-Retinoic Acid." *New England Journal of Medicine,* 300:329, 1979.

13 Jones, H., D. Blanc, and W. J. Cunliffe: "13-Cis-Retinoic Acid and Acne." *Lancet,* 2(8203):1048, 1980.

14 Christiansen, J. V., E. Gadborg, K. Ludivigsen, C. H. Meier, A. Norholm, P. E. Osmundsen, D. Pederson, K. A. Rasmussen, H. Reiter, F. Reymann, N. Rosman, B. Sylvest, P. Unna, R. Wehnert, B. Aastrup, B. Andersen, and P. Holm: "Topical Vitamin A Acid and Systemic Oxytetracycline in the Treatment of Acne Vulgaris." *Dermatologica,* 149:121, 1974.

15 Kligman, A. M., O. H. Mills, K. J. McGinley, and J. J. Leyden: "Acne Therapy with Tretinoin in Combination with Antibiotics."

Acta Dermato-Venereologica, suppl 74:111, 1975.

16 Michaelsson, G., A. Vahlquist, and L. Juklin: "Serum Zinc and Retinol-binding Protein in Acne." *British Journal of Dermatology,* 96:283, 1977.

17 Verma, K. C., A. S. Saini, and S. K. Dhamija: "Oral Zinc Sulphate Therapy in Acne Vulgaris: A Double-Blind Trial." *Acta Dermato-Venereologica,* 60:337, 1980.

18 Food and Nutrition Board: *Recommended Dietary Allowances,* 9th ed. National Academy of Sciences, Washington, D.C., 1980.

19 Wolf, G.: "Vitamin A." In: Alfin-Slater, R. B., and D. Kritchevsky, (eds.), *Human Nutrition. Nutrition and the Adult, Micronutrients,* vol. 3B, New York: Plenum, 1980.

20 Nettsheim, P., and M. L. Williams: "The Influence of Vitamin A on the Susceptibility of the Rat Lung to 3-Methylcholanthreme." *International Journal of Cancer,* 17:351, 1976.

21 Newberne, P. M., and A. E. Rogers: "Rat Colon Carcinomas Associated with Aflatoxin and Marginal Vitamin A." *Journal of the National Cancer Institute,* 50:439, 1973.

22 Bjelke, E.: "Dietary Vitamin A and Human Lung Cancer." *International Journal of Cancer,* 15:561, 1975.

23 Basu, T. K., D. Donaldson, M. Jenner, D. C. Williams, and A. Sakula: "Plasma Vitamin A in Patients with Bronchial Carcinoma." *British Journal of Cancer,* 33:119, 1976.

24 DeLuca, H. F.: "Vitamin D." In: Alfin-Slater, R. B., and D. Kritchevsky (eds.), *Human Nutrition,* vol. 3B, *Nutrition and the Adult, Micronutrients.* New York: Plenum, 1980.

25 Sandstead, H. H.: "Clinical Manifestations of Certain Classical Deficiency Diseases." In: Goodhart, R. S., and M. E. Shils (eds.), *Modern Nutrition in Health and Disease,* 6th ed. Philadelphia: Lea & Febiger, 1980.

26 "Vitamin D Deficient Rickets, Revisited." *Nutrition Reviews,* 38:116, 1980.

27 American Academy of Pediatrics, Committee on Nutrition, "The Prophylactic Requirement and the Toxicity of Vitamin D." *Pediatrics,* 31:512, 1963.

28 American Academy of Pediatrics, Committee on Nutrition, "The Relationship between Infantile Hypercalcemia and Vitamin D—Public Health Implications in North America." *Pediatrics,* 40:1050, 1967.

29 Machlin, L. J., and M. Brin: "Vitamin E." In: Alfin-Slater, R. B., and D. Kritchevsky (eds.), *Human Nutrition,* vol. 3B, *Nutrition and the Adult, Micronutrients.* New York: Plenum, 1980.

30 Horwitt, M. K.: "Vitamin E." In: Goodhart, R. S., and M. E. Shils (eds.), *Modern Nutrition in Health and Disease,* 6th ed. Philadelphia: Lea & Febiger, 1980.

31 Horwitt, M. K.: "Therapeutic Uses of Vitamin E in Medicine." *Nutrition Reviews,* 38:105, 1980.

32 Koehler, H. H., H. C. Lee, and M. Jacobson: "Tocopherols in Canned Entrees and Vended Sandwiches." *Journal of the American Dietetic Association,* 70:616, 1977.

33 Bauernfeind, J. C.: "Food Sources of the Tocopherols." In: Machlin, L. J. (ed.), *Vitamin E,* New York: Marcel Dekker, 1980.

34 Williams, H. T. G., D. Fenna, and R. A. Macbeth: "Alpha-Tocopherol in the Treatment of Intermittent Claudication." *Surgery, Gynecology and Obstetrics,* 132:662, 1971.

35 Haeger, K.: "Long-Time Treatment of Intermittent Claudication with Vitamin E." *American Journal of Clinical Nutrition,* 27:1179, 1974.

36 Johnson, L., D. Schaffer, and T. R. Boggs, Jr.: "The Premature Infant, Vitamin E Deficiency and Retrolental Fibroplasia." *American Journal of Clinical Nutrition,* 27:1158, 1974.

37 Weiter, J. J.: Editorial. "Retrolental Fibroplasia. An Unsolved Problem." *New England Journal of Medicine,* 305:1404, 1981.

38 Ehrenkranz, R. A., B. W. Bonta, R. C. Ablow, and J. B. Warshaw: "Amelioration of Bronchopulmonary Dysplasia after Vitamin E Administration." *New England Journal of Medicine,* 299:564, 1978.

39 Ehrenkranz, R. A., R. C. Ablow, and J. B. Warshaw: "Prevention of Bronchopulmonary Dysplasia with Vitamin E Administration during the Acute Stages of Respiratory Distress Syndrome." *Journal of Pediatrics,* 95:873, 1979.

40 Anderson, T. W., and D. B. W. Reid: "A Double-Blind Trial of Vitamin E in Angina Pectoris." *American Journal of Clinical Nutrition,* 27:1174, 1974.

41 Tappel, A. L.: "Vitamin E." *Nutrition Today,* 8(4):4, 1973.

42 Draper, H. H., J. G. Bergan, M. Chiri, A. S. Csallany, and A. V. Boaro: "A Further Study of the Specificity of the Vitamin E Requirement for Reproduction." *Journal of Nutrition,* 84:395, 1964.

43 Fletcher, B. L., and A. L. Tappel: "Protective Effects of Dietary α-Tocopherol in Rats Exposed to Toxic Levels of Ozone and Nitrogen Dioxide." *Environmental Research,* 6:165, 1973.

44 Tappel, A., B. Fletcher, and D. Deamer: "Effects of Antioxidants and Nutrients on Lipid Peroxidation Fluorescent Products and Aging." *Journal of Gerontology,* 28:415, 1973.

45 Olson, R. E.: "Vitamin K." In: Goodhart, R. S., and M. E. Shils (eds.), *Modern Nutrition in Health and Disease,* 6th ed. Philadelphia: Lea & Febiger, 1980.

CHAPTER 12

1 Grande, F., and A. Keys: "Body Weight, Body Composition, and

Calorie Status." In: Goodhart, R. S., and M. E. Shils (eds.), *Modern Nutrition in Health and Disease,* 6th ed. Philadelphia: Lea & Febiger, 1980.

2 Randall, H. T.: "Water, Electrolytes and Acid-Base Balance." In: Goodhart, R. S., and M. E. Shils (ed.), *Modern Nutrition in Health and Disease,* 6th ed. Philadelphia: Lea & Febiger, 1980.

3 Smith, N. J.: *Food For Sport.* Palo Alto, Calif.: Bull Publishing Co., 1976.

4 Food and Nutrition Board: *Recommended Dietary Allowances,* 9th ed. National Academy of Sciences, Washington, D.C., 1980.

5 Food and Nutrition Board: *Toward Healthful Diets.* National Academy of Sciences, Washington, D.C., 1980.

6 Tobian, L.: "The Relationship of Salt to Hypertension." *American Journal of Clinical Nutrition,* 32:2739, 1979.

7 Fisher, K. D.: In: *Evaluation of the Health Aspects of Sodium Chloride and Potassium Chloride as Food Ingredients.* SCOGS–102, Federation of American Societies for Experimental Medicine, Bethesda, Md., 1979.

8 Altschul, A. M., and J. K. Grommet: "Sodium Intake and Sodium Sensitivity." *Nutrition Reviews,* 38:393, 1980.

9 Kolata, G.: "Should Hypertensives Take Potassium?" *Science,* 218:361, 1982.

10 Yap, V., A. Patel, and J. Thomsen: "Hyperkalemia with Cardiac Arrhythmia: Introduction by Salt Substitutes, Spironolactone, and Azotemia." *Journal of the American Medical Association,* 236:2775, 1976.

11 Kolata, G.: "Value of Low-Sodium Diets Questioned." *Science,* 216:38, 1982.

12 Meneely, G. R., and H. D. Battarbee: "Sodium and Potassium." *Nutrition Reviews,* 34:225, 1976.

13 Kesteloot, H., B. C. Park, C. S. Lee, E. Brems-Heyns, and J. V. Joossens: In: Kesteloot, H., and J. V. Joossens (eds.), *Epidemiology of Arterial Blood Pressure.* The Hague: Martinus Nijhoff, 1980.

14 Grim, C. E., F. C. Luft, J. Z. Miller, G. R. Meneely, H. D. Battarbee, C. G. Hames, and L. K. Dahl: "Racial Differences in Blood Pressure in Evans County, Georgia: Relationship to Sodium and Potassium Intake and Plasma Renin Activity." *Journal of Chronic Disease,* 33:87, 1980.

15 Luft, G. C., C. E. Grim, N. S. Fineberg, and W. H. Weinberger: "Effects of Volume Expansion and Contraction in Normotensive Whites, Blacks and Subjects of Different Ages." *Circulation,* 59:643, 1979.

16 Bulpitt, C. J.: "Is There a New Member in the High Blood Pressure Mafia?" *Nutrition Today,* 17(2):6, 1982.

17 Kark, R. M., and J. H. Oyama: "Nutrition, Hypertension and Kidney Disease." In: Goodhart, R. S., and M. E. Shils (eds.), *Modern Nutrition in Health and Disease,* 6th ed. Philadelphia: Lea & Febiger, 1980.

18 Committee on Nutrition, American Academy of Pediatrics: "Salt Intake and Eating Patterns of Infants and Children in Relation to Blood Pressure." *Pediatrics,* 53:115, 1974.

19 Roy, S., III, and B. S. Arant, Jr.: (Letter). "Alkalosis from Chloride-deficient Neo-Mull-Soy." *New England Journal of Medicine,* 301:615, 1979.

20 Simopoulos, A. P., and F. C. Bartter: "The Metabolic Consequences of Chloride Deficiency." *Nutrition Reviews,* 38:201, 1980.

21 "Study of Infants Fed Chloride-deficient Formulas." *FDA Drug Bulletin,* 11:8, 1981.

22 DeLuca, H. F.: "Vitamin D." In: Goodhart, R. S., and M. E. Shils (eds.), *Modern Nutrition in Health*

and Disease, 6th ed. Philadelphia: Lea & Febiger, 1980.

23 Avioli, L. V.: "Major Minerals: Calcium and Phosphorus." In: Goodhart, R. S., and M. E. Shils (eds.), *Modern Nutrition in Health and Disease,* 6th ed. Philadelphia: Lea & Febiger, 1980.

24 Wilkinson, R.: "Absorption of Calcium, Phosphorus and Magnesium." In: Nordin, B. E. C. (ed.), *Calcium, Phosphate and Magnesium Metabolism.* New York: Churchill Livingstone, 1976.

25 Allen, L. H., E. A. Oddoye, and S. Margen: "Protein-induced Hypercalciuria: A Longer-Term Study." *American Journal of Clinical Nutrition,* 32:741, 1979.

26 FAO Nutrition Meetings Report. *Calcium Requirements.* Series no. 30, Rome, 1962.

27 Page, L., and B. Friend: "The Changing United States Diet." *Bio Science,* 28:192, 1978.

28 LSRO (Life Sciences Research Office): "Evaluation of the Health Aspects of Phosphates as Food Ingredients." SCOGS 32. Federation of American Societies for Experimental Biology, Bethesda, Md., 1975.

29 Shils, M. E.: "Magnesium." In: Goodhart, R. S., and M. E. Shils (eds.), *Modern Nutrition in Health and Disease,* 6th ed. Philadelphia: Lea & Febiger, 1980.

30 Roberts, H. J.: (Letter) "Dolomite as a Source of Toxic Metals." *New England Journal of Medicine,* 304:423, 1981.

CHAPTER 13

1 Cotzias, G. C.: In: Proceedings of the First Annual Conference on Trace Substances and Environmental Health, Columbia, Missouri, 1965, p. 5.

2 White, H. S.: "Iron-Hemoglobin." In: Alfin-Slater, R. B., and D. Kritchevsky (eds.), *Human Nutrition: A Comprehensive Treatise,* vol. 3B. New York: Plenum Press, 1980.

3 Monsen, E. R., L. Hallberg, M. Layrisse, D. M. Hegsted, J. D. Cook, W. Mertz, and C. A. Finch: "Estimation of Available Dietary

Iron." *American Journal of Clinical Nutrition*, 31:134, 1978.

4 Monsen, E. R., and J. D. Cook: "Food Iron Absorption in Human Subjects. IV. The Effects of Calcium and Phosphate Salts on the Absorption of Nonheme Iron." *American Journal of Clinical Nutrition*, 29:1142, 1976.

5 Beutler, E.: "Iron." In: Goodhart, R. S., and M. E. Shils (eds.), *Modern Nutrition in Health and Disease*, 6th ed. Philadelphia: Lea & Febiger, 1980.

6 Joint FAO/WHO Expert Group: "Requirements of Ascorbic Acid, Vitamin D, Vitamin B$_{12}$, Folate and Iron." WHO Technical Report Series, No. 452, 1970.

7 Monsen, E. R., and J. L. Balintfy: "Calculating Dietary Iron Bioavailability. Refinement and Computerization." *Journal of the American Dietetic Association*, 80:307, 1982.

8 Hallberg, L., L. Rossander, H. Persson, and E. Svahn: "Deleterious Effects of Prolonged Warming of Meals on Ascorbic Acid Content and Iron Absorption." *American Journal of Clinical Nutrition*, 36:846, 1982.

9 Crosby, W. H.: "Prescribing Iron? Think Safety." *Archives of Internal Medicine*, 128:766, 1978.

10 Solomons, N. W.: "Factors Affecting the Bioavailability of Zinc." *Journal of the American Dietetic Association*, 80:115, 1982.

11 Prasad, A. S., A. Miale, Jr., Z. Farid, H. H. Sandstead, and A. R. Schulert: "Zinc Metabolism in Patients with the Syndrome of Iron Deficiency Anemia, Hepatosplenomegaly, Dwarfism, and Hypogonadism." *Journal of Laboratory and Clinical Medicine*, 61:537, 1963.

12 Hambidge, K. M., C. Hambidge, M. Jacobs, and J. D. Baum: "Low Levels of Zinc in Hair, Anorexia, Poor Growth, and Hypogeusia in Children." *Pediatric Research*, 6:868, 1972.

13 Hambidge, K. M., P. A. Walravens, R. M. Brown, J. Webster, S. White, M. Autbouy, and M. L. Roth: "Zinc Nutrition of Preschool Children in the Denver Head Start Program." *American Journal of Clinical Nutrition*, 29:734, 1976.

14 Hambidge, K. M.: "Trace Elements in Pediatric Nutrition." *Advances in Pediatrics*, 24:191, 1977.

15 "Infections and Undernutrition." *Nutrition Reviews*, 40:119, 1982.

16 Walravens, P. A., and K. M. Hambidge: "Growth of Infants Fed a Zinc Supplemented Formula." *American Journal of Clinical Nutrition*, 29:1114, 1976.

17 King, J. C., T. Stein, and M. Doyle: "Effect of Vegetarianism on the Zinc Status of Pregnant Women." *American Journal of Clinical Nutrition*, 34:1049, 1981.

18 Anderson, B. M., R. S. Gibson, and J. H. Sabry: "The Iron and Zinc Status of Long-Term Vegetarian Women." *American Journal of Clinical Nutrition*, 34:1042, 1981.

19 Food and Nutrition Board: *Recommended Dietary Allowances*, 9th ed. National Research Council, National Academy of Sciences, Washington, D.C., 1980.

20 Hooper, P. L., L. Visconti, P. J. Garry, and G. E. Johnson: "Zinc Lowers High-Density Lipoprotein-Cholesterol Levels." *Journal of the American Medical Association*, 244:1960, 1980.

21 Klevay, L. M.: "The Ratio of Zinc to Copper of Diets in the United States." *Nutrition Reports International*, 11:237, 1975.

22 Kimball, O. P., and D. Marine: "The Prevention of Simple Goiter in Man." *Archives of Internal Medicine*, 22:41, 1918.

23 Cavalieri, R. R.: "Trace Elements." In: Goodhart, R. S., and M. E. Shils (eds.), *Modern Nutrition in Health and Disease*, 6th ed. Philadelphia: Lea & Febiger, 1980.

24 Taylor, F.: "Iodine." *FDA Consumer*, April 1981.

25 Nagataki, S.: "Effect of Excess Quantities of Iodine." In: *Handbook of Physiology. III. Endocrinology*. American Physiological Society, Bethesda, Md.

26 LSRO (Life Sciences Research Office): "Iodine in Foods: Chemical Methodology and Sources of Iodine in the Human Diet." Federation of American Societies for Experimental Biology, Bethesda, Md.

27 Mertz, W.: "Effects and Metabolism of Glucose Tolerance Factor." *Nutrition Reviews*, 33:129, 1975.

28 Anderson, R. A., M. M. Polansky, N. A. Bryden, E. E. Roginski, K. Y. Patterson, C. Veillon, and W. Glinsmann: "Urinary Chromium Excretion of Human Subjects: Effects of Chromium Supplementation and Glucose Loading." *American Journal of Clinical Nutrition*, 36:1184, 1982.

29 Gurson, C. T., and G. Saner: "Effect of Chromium on Glucose Utilization in Marasmic Protein-Calorie Malnutrition." *American Journal of Clinical Nutrition*, 24:1313, 1971.

30 Doisy, R. J., D. H. Streeten, J. M. Freiberg, and A. J. Schneider: "Chromium Metabolism in Man and Biochemical Effects." In: Prasad, A. S., and D. Oberleas (eds.), *Trace Elements in Human Health and Disease*, II. New York: Academic Press, 1976.

31 Tipton, I. H., H. A. Schroeder, H. M. Perry, and M. J. Cook: "Trace Elements in Human Tissue. III. Subjects from Africa, the Near and Far East and Europe." *Health Physics*, 11:403, 1965.

32 Schroeder, H. A.: "The Role of Chromium in Mammalian Nutrition." *American Journal of Clinical Nutrition*, 21:230, 1968.

33 Toepfer, E. W., W. Mertz, E. E. Roginski, and M. M. Polansky: "Chromium in Foods in Relation to Biological Activity." *Journal of Agricultural and Food Chemistry*, 21:69, 1973.

34 Walsh, D. C.: "Fluoridation: Slow Diffusion of a Proved Preventive Measure." *New England Journal of Medicine*, 296:1118, 1977.

35 Shaw, J. H., and E. A. Sweeney: "Nutrition in Relation to Dental

Medicine." In: Goodhart, R. S., and M. E. Shils (eds.), *Modern Nutrition in Health and Disease*, 6th ed. Philadelphia: Lea & Febiger, 1980.

36 Bernstein, D. S., N. Sadowsky, D. M. Hegsted, C. D. Guri, and F. J. Stare: "Prevalence of Osteoporosis in High- and Low-Fluoride Areas in North Dakota." *Journal of the American Medical Association*, 198:499, 1966.

37 Center for Disease Control: "How Does Your State Stand on Fluoridation?" *Morbidity and Mortality Weekly Report*, 26(27):1, 1977.

38 Leverett, D. H.: "Fluorides and the Changing Prevalence of Dental Caries." *Science*, 217:26, 1982.

39 Committee on Biologic Effects of Atmospheric Pollutants, National Research Council: *Fluorides*. National Academy of Sciences, Washington, D.C., 1971.

40 Singer, L., R. H. Ophaug, and B. F. Harland: "Fluoride Intake of Young Male Adults in the United States." *American Journal of Clinical Nutrition*, 33:328, 1980.

41 Watkin, D. M.: "Nutrition for the Aging and the Aged." In: Goodhart, R. S., and M. E. Shils (eds.), *Modern Nutrition in Health and Disease*, 6th ed. Philadelphia: Lea & Febiger, 1980.

42 Cook-Mozaffari, P., and R. Doll: "Fluoridation of Water Supplies and Cancer Mortality. II. Mortality Trends after Fluoridation." *Journal of Epidemiology and Community Health*, 35:233, 1981.

43 Mason, K. E.: A Conspectus of Research on Copper Metabolism and Requirements of Man." *Journal of Nutrition*, 109:1979, 1979.

44 Prasad, A. S.: *Trace Elements and Iron in Human Metabolism*. New York: Plenum Medical Book Co., 1978.

45 Al-Rashid, R. A., and J. Spangler: "Neonatal Copper Deficiency." *New England Journal of Medicine*, 285:841, 1971.

46 Cordano, A., J. M. Baertl, and G. G. Graham: "Copper Deficiency in Infancy." *Pediatrics*, 34:324, 1964.

47 Klevay, L. M., S. J. Reck, R. A. Jacob, G. M. Logan, Jr., J. M. Munoz, and H. H. Sandstead: "The Human Requirement for Copper. I. Healthy Men Fed Conventional, American Diets." *American Journal of Clinical Nutrition*, 33:45, 1980.

48 Hurt, H. D., E. E. Cary, and W. J. Visek: "Growth, Reproduction, and Tissue Concentration of Selenium in the Selenium-Depleted Rat." *Journal of Nutrition*, 101:761, 1971.

49 Frost, D. V., and P. M. Lish: "Selenium in Biology." *Annual Review of Pharmacology and Toxicology*, 15:259, 1975.

50 Gunby, P.: "Medical News. Selenium May Act as Cancer Inhibitor." *Journal of the American Medical Association*, 246:1510, 1981.

51 Burk, R. F., Jr., W. N. Pearson, R. P. Wood II, and F. Viteri: "Blood-Selenium Levels in Vitro Red Blood Cell Uptake of ^{75}Se in Kwashiorkor." *American Journal of Clinical Nutrition*, 20:723, 1967.

52 Thomson, C. D., and M. F. Robinson: "Selenium in Human Health and Disease with Emphasis on Those Aspects Peculiar to New Zealand." *American Journal of Clinical Nutrition*, 33:303, 1980.

53 Commentary. "Are selenium supplements needed (by the general public)?" *Journal of the American Dietetic Association*, 70:249, 1977.

54 Hambidge, K. M.: "Hair Analyses: Worthless for Vitamins, Limited for Minerals." *American Journal of Clinical Nutrition*, 36:943, 1982.

55 Roe, D. A.: *Alcohol and the Diet*. Westport, Conn.: Avi Publishing Co., 1979.

56 Shaw, S., and C. S. Lieber: "Nutrition and Alcoholism." In: Goodhart, R. S., and M. E. Shils (eds.),

Modern Nutrition in Health and Disease, 6th ed. Philadelphia: Lea & Febiger, 1980.

57 Roe, D. A.: "Nutritional Concerns in the Alcoholic." *Journal of the American Dietetic Association*, 78:17, 1981.

CHAPTER 14

1 Pitkin, R. M.: "Assessment of Nutritional Status of Mother, Fetus and Newborn." *American Journal of Clinical Nutrition*, 34(suppl):658, 1981.

2 Food and Nutrition Board: *Recommended Dietary Allowances*. National Academy of Sciences, Washington, D.C., 1980.

3 Lind, T.: "Nutrient Requirements during Pregnancy." *American Journal of Clinical Nutrition*, 34:669, 1981.

4 Achari, K., and U. Rani: "Maternal Anemia and the Fetus." *Journal of Obstetrics and Gynecology, India*, 21:305, 1971.

5 Garn, S. M., M. T. Keating, and F. Falkner: (Letter) "Hematological status and pregnancy outcomes." *American Journal of Clinical Nutrition*, 34:115, 1981.

6 Herbert, V., N. Colman, M. Spivack, E. Ocasio, V. Ghanta, K. Kimonel, L. Brenner, J. Freundlich, and J. Scott: "Folic Acid Deficiency in the United States: Folate Assays in a Prenatal Clinic." *American Journal of Obstetrics and Gynecology*, 123:175, 1975.

7 Page, E. W., and E. P. Page: "Leg Cramps in Pregnancy: Etiology and Treatment." *Obstetrics and Gynecology*, 1:94, 1953.

8 Abrams, J., and G. E. Aponte: "The Leg Cramp Syndrome during Pregnancy. The Relationship to Calcium and Phosphorus Metabolism." *American Journal of Obstetrics and Gynecology*, 76:432, 1957.

9 Holden, J. M., N. R. Wolf, and N. Mertz: "Zinc and Copper in Self-Selected Diets." *Journal of the American Dietetic Association*, 75:23, 1979.

10 Stange, L., K. Carlstrom, and M. Eriksson: "Hypervitaminosis A in

Early Human Pregnancy and Malformations of the Central Nervous System." *Acta Obstetrica Scandinavica,* 57:289, 1978.

11 Cochrane, W. A.: "Overnutrition in Prenatal and Neonatal Life: A Problem?" *Canadian Medical Association Journal,* 93:893, 1965.

12 Hillman, R. W., P. G. Cabaud, D. E. Nilsson, P. D. Arpin, and R. J. Tufano: "Pyridoxine Supplementation during Pregnancy. Clinical and Laboratory Observations." *American Journal of Clinical Nutrition,* 12:427, 1963.

13 Roepke, J. L. B., and A. Kirksey: "Vitamin B_6 Nutrition during Pregnancy and Lactation. II. The Effect of Long-Term Use of Oral Contraceptives." *American Journal of Clinical Nutrition,* 32:2257, 1979.

14 Rosso, P.: "Nutrition and Maternal-Fetal Exchange." *American Journal of Clinical Nutrition,* 34:744, 1981.

15 Robson, E. B.: "The Genetics of Birthweight." In: Falkner, F., and J. M. Tanner (eds.), *Human Growth,* vol. I. New York: Plenum, 1978, p. 285.

16 Johnson, S., R. Knight, D. J. Marmer, and R. W. Steele: "Immune Deficiency in Fetal Alcohol Syndrome." *Pediatric Research,* 15:908, 1981.

17 Hanson, J. N., A. P. Streissgurth, and D. N. Smith: "The Effects of Moderate Alcohol Consumption during Pregnancy on Fetal Growth and Morphogenesis." *Journal of Pediatrics,* 92:457, 1978.

18 Little, R. E., A. P. Streissgurth, H. M. Barr, and C. S. Herman: "Decreased Birth Weight in Infants of Alcoholic Women who Abstained during Pregnancy." *Journal of Pediatrics,* 96:974, 1980.

19 Hanson, J. N., K. L. Jones, and D. N. Smith: "Fetal Alcohol Syndrome." *Journal of the American Medical Association,* 235:1458, 1976.

20 Hook, E. B.: "Dietary Cravings and Aversions during Pregnancy." *American Journal of Clinical Nutrition,* 31:1355, 1978.

21 Kitay, D. Z., and R. A. Harbort: "Iron and Folic Acid Deficiency in Pregnancy." *Clinics in Perinatology,* 2:255, 1975.

22 Crosby, W. H.: "Pica." *Journal of the American Medical Association,* 235:2765, 1976.

23 Coltman, C. A.: "Pagophagia and Iron Lack." *Journal of the American Medical Association,* 207:513, 1969.

24 Oldham, H., and B. B. Sheft: "Effect of Caloric Intake on Nitrogen Utilization during Pregnancy." *Journal of the American Dietetic Association,* 27:847, 1951.

25 Choudry, V. P., O. P. Ghai, and A. K. Saraya: "Hemopoietic Nutrients in Anemia of Infancy and Childhood with Suggestive Vitamin B_{12} and Folic Acid Deficiency." *Indian Pediatrics,* 10:435, 1973.

26 Stone, S. C., and R. P. Dickey: "Management of Nursing and Non-Nursing Mothers." *Clinical Obstetrics and Gynecology,* 18:139, 1975.

27 Lawrence, R. A.: *Breast-Feeding: A Guide for the Medical Profession.* St. Louis: C. V. Mosby Co., 1980.

28 Yoshida, H.: "Electrophoresis of Sera of Breast-fed Infants and its Relation to Nutritional Dystrophy of Their Mothers." *Tohuku Journal of Experimental Medicine,* 63:69, 1955.

CHAPTER 15

1 Beal, V.: *Nutrition in the Life Span.* New York: John Wiley & Sons, 1980.

2 Winick, M.: *Year One: Nutrition, Growth, Health.* New York: Medcom for Ross Laboratories, Columbus, Ohio, 1975.

3 Food and Nutrition Board: *Recommended Dietary Allowances.* Washington, D.C.: National Academy of Sciences, 1980.

4 Committee on Nutrition, AAP, American Academy of Pediatrics: "Vitamin and Mineral Supplement Needs in Normal Children in the United States." *Pediatrics,* 66:1015, 1980.

5 Fineberg, L.: Editorial. "Human Milk Feeding and Vitamin D Supplementation—1981." *Journal of Pediatrics,* 99:228, 1981.

6 Greer, F. R., M. Ho, D. Dodson, and R. C. Taang: "Lack of 25-Hydroxyvitamin D and 1,25-Dihydroxyvitamin D in Human Milk." *Journal of Pediatrics,* 99:233, 1981.

7 Hollis, B. W., B. A. Roos, H. H. Draper, and P. W. Lambert: "Occurrence of Vitamin D Sulfate in Human Milk Whey." *Journal of Nutrition,* 111:384, 1981.

8 Leerbeck, E., and H. Sondergaard: "The Total Content of Vitamin D in Human Milk and Cow's Milk." *British Journal of Nutrition,* 44:7, 1980.

9 Myres, A. W.: "Breast-feeding—A Rational Priority for Infant Health." *Journal of the Canadian Dietetic Association,* 42:130, 1981.

10 American Academy of Pediatrics: "The Promotion of Breast Feeding." *Pediatrics,* 69:654, 1982.

11 Fallot, M. E., J. L. Boyd III, and F. A. Oski: "Breast-feeding Reduces Incidence of Hospital Admissions for Infection in Infants." *Pediatrics,* 65:1121, 1980.

12 Fomon, S. J., and S. J. Filer: "Milk and Formula." In: S. J. Fomon, *Infant Nutrition,* 2d ed. Philadelphia: W. B. Saunders Co., 1974.

13 Sackett, W. W., Jr.: *Bringing Up Babies.* New York: Harper & Row, Publishers, 1962.

14 Committee on Nutrition, American Academy of Pediatrics: *Pediatric Nutrition Handbook,* P.O. Box 1034, Evanston, IL 60204, 1979.

15 Grunwaldt, E., T. Bates, and D. Guthrie, Jr.: "The Onset of Sleeping Through the Night in Infancy." *Pediatrics,* 26:667, 1960.

16 Anderson, T. A.: "Commercial Infant Foods: Content and Composi-

tion." *Pediatric Clinics of North America,* 24:37, 1977.

17 Food and Nutrition Board, Food Protection Committee: *Safety and Suitability of Salt for Use in Baby Foods.* Washington, D.C.: National Academy of Sciences, 1970.

18 Papalia, D., and S. Olds: *A Child's World. Infancy through Adolescence.* New York: McGraw-Hill Book Company, 1982.

19 Davis, C. M.: "Self-Selection of Diets. An Experiment with Infants." *The Trained Nurse and Hospital Rev.,* vol. 86, May 1931.

20 Beyer, N. R., and P. Morris: "Food Attitudes and Snacking Patterns of Young Children." *Journal of Nutrition Education,* 6:131, 1974.

21 Feingold, B. F.: *Why Your Child is Hyperactive.* New York: Random House, 1975.

22 Marino, D., and J. King: "Nutritional Concerns during Adolescence." *Pediatric Clinics of North America,* 27(1):125, 1980.

23 Irwin, M. I., and E. W. Kienholz: "A Conspectus of Research on Calcium Requirements of Man." *Journal of Nutrition,* 103:1019, 1973.

24 Dwyer, J.: "Nutritional Requirements of Adolescence." *Nutrition Reviews* 39(2):56, 1981.

25 Forbes, G. B. "Biological Implications of the Adolescent Growth Process: Body Composition." In: McKigney, J. I., and H. N. Munro (eds), *Nutrient Requirements in Adolescence.* Cambridge, Mass.: MIT Press, 1976, p. 57.

26 USDHEW: *Ten State Nutrition Survey,* 1968–1970. DHEW Publication No. (HSM) 72–8134 CDC HSMHA, Atlanta, Ga., 1972.

27 National Center for Health Statistics: *Preliminary Findings, First Health and Nutrition Examination Survey.* United States. 1971–1972. Dietary Intake and Biochemical Findings, DHEW Publication No. (HRA) 74–1219-1. HRA, PHS, USDHEW. Rockville, Md., 1974.

28 Jakobovits, C., P. Halstead, L. Kelley, D. Roe, and C. Young: "Eating Habits and Nutrient Intakes of College Women over a Thirty-Year Period." *Journal of the American Dietetic Association,* 71:405–411, 1977.

29 Truswell, A. S., and I. Darnton-Hill: "Food Habits of Adolescents." *Nutrition Reviews,* 39(2):73, 1981.

30 Greger, J. L., L. Divibliss, and S. K. Aschenbeck: "Dietary Habits of Adolescent Females." *Ecology of Food and Nutrition,* 7:213, 1979.

31 Brown, P. T., J. G. Bergan, and C. G. Murgo: "Current Trends in Food Habits and Dietary Intakes of Home Economics Students in Three Junior High Schools in Rhode Island." *Home Economics Research Journal,* 7:324, 1979.

32 Reinhold, R.: "Leveling Off of Drug Use Found Among Students." *The New York Times,* February 19, 1981, p. A1.

33 Rachel, J. V., L. L. Guess, R. L. Hubbard, S. A. Maisto, E. R. Cavanaugh, R. Waddell, and C. H. Benrud: *Adolescent Drinking Behavior,* vol. 1. *The Extent and Nature of Adolescent Alcohol and Drug Use.* Research Triangle Park, N.C.: Research Triangle Institute, 1980.

34 Michaelsson, G.: "Diet and Acne." *Nutrition Reviews,* 39(2):104, 1981.

CHAPTER 16

1 Carlson, A. D.: *In the Fullness of Time.* Chicago, Ill.: Contemporary Books, Inc., 1977, p. 108.

2 The Top 25 Americans over 50." *50 Plus.* December 1981, pp. 18–23.

3 Kuhn, M.: In: Dychtwald, K. (ed.), "Liberating Aging." *New Spirit,* 1(3):17, April 1979.

4 U.S. Bureau of the Census, Statistical Abstract of the United States: 1980, 101st ed. Washington, D.C., 1980.

5 Mayer, J.: "Aging and Nutrition." *Geriatrics,* 29:57, 1974.

6 Pekkanen, J.: "Secrets of Eternal Youth." *The Washingtonian,* May 1980.

7 Krehl, W. A.: "The Influence of Nutritional Environment on Aging." *Geriatrics,* 29:65, 1974.

8 Weg, R. B.: *Nutrition and the Later Years.* Los Angeles: University of Southern California Press, 1978.

9 McCay, C. M., M. F. Crowell, and L. A. Maynard: "The Effect of Retarded Growth upon the Length of Lifespan and upon the Ultimate Body Size." *Journal of Nutrition,* 10:63, 1935.

10 Ross, M. H., and G. Bras: "Dietary Preference and Diseases of Age." *Nature,* 250:834, 1974.

11 Leaf, A.: "Observations of a Peripatetic Gerontologist." *Nutrition Today,* 8(5):4, 1973.

12 Staff Report: "Paradise Lost." *Nutrition Today,* 13(3):6, 1978.

13 Food and Nutrition Board: *Recommended Dietary Allowances,* 9th ed. Washington, D.C.: National Research Council, National Academy of Sciences, 1980.

14 Sidney, K. H., R. J. Shephard, and J. E. Harrison: "Endurance Training and Body Composition of the Elderly." *American Journal of Clinical Nutrition,* 30:326, 1977.

15 Jowsey, J.: "Prevention and Treatment of Osteoporosis." In: M. Winick (ed.), *Nutrition and Aging.* New York: John Wiley & Sons, 1976.

16 Ahrens, E. H., Jr.: "The Use of Liquid Formula Diets in Metabolic Studies: 15 Years' Experience." In: R. Levine, and R. Luft (eds.) *Advances in Metabolic Disorders,* vol. 4. New York: Academic Press, 1970, p. 297.

17 U.S. Department of Health, Education and Welfare: Ten State Nutrition Survey, 1968-70. Vol. 1-5. DHEW Publication No. (HSM) 72–8130-8133.

18 Uanz, R., N. S. Scrimshaw, and V. R. Young: "Human Protein Requirements: Nitrogen Balance Response to Graded Levels of Egg

Protein in Elderly Men and Women." *American Journal of Clinical Nutrition*, 31:779, 1978.

19 Zanni, E., O. H. Callaway, and A. Zezulka: "Protein Requirements of Elderly Men." *Journal of Nutrition*, 109:513, 1979.

20 Roe, D. A.: *Drug-Induced Nutritional Deficiencies*, Westport, Conn.: The Avi Publishing Co., Inc., 1976.

21 Lutwak, L.: "Continuing Need for Dietary Calcium Throughout Life." *Geriatrics*, 29:171, 1974.

22 Garn, S. N., C. G. Rothmann, and B. Wagner: "Bone Loss as a General Phenomenon in Man." *Federation Proceedings*, 26:1729, 1967.

23 Lutwak, L.: "Periodontal Disease." In: M. Winick (ed.), *Nutrition and Aging*. New York: John Wiley & Sons, 1976. p. 145.

24 Winick, M.: "Nutrition and Aging." *Contemporary Nutrition*, 2(6). June 1977.

25 Whedon, G. D.: Editorial. "Osteoporosis." *New England Journal of Medicine*, 305:397, 1981.

26 Korcok, M.: "Medical News. Add Exercise to Calcium in Osteoporosis Prevention." *Journal of the American Medical Association*, 247:1106, 1982.

27 Allen, L. H., E. A. Oddoye, and S. Margen: "Protein-induced Hypercalciuria: A Longer Term Study." *American Journal of Clinical Nutrition*, 32:741, 1979.

28 Hegsted, M., S. A. Schuette, M. B. Zemel, and H. M. Linkswiler: "Urinary Calcium and Calcium Balance in Young Men as Affected by Level of Protein and Phosphorus Intake." *Journal of Nutrition*, 111:553, 1981.

29 Fletcher, A. J.: "A Multi-Centre Study of Potassium Deficiency in the Elderly." *Scottish Medical Journal*, 19(3):142, 1974.

30 Schroeder, H. A.: "Nutrition." In: E. V. Dowdry, F. U. Steinberg (eds.), *The Care of the Geriatric Patient*. St. Louis: C. V. Mosby, 1971.

31 Kart, C. S., E. S. Metress, and J. F. Metress: *Aging and Health: Biologic and Social Perspectives*. Menlo Park, California: Addison-Wesley Publications Company, 1978.

32 Schiffman, S.: "Changes in Taste and Smell in Old Persons." *Advances in Research*, vol. 2. Fall 1978, pp. 1–6. Duke University Center for the Study of Aging and Human Development.

33 Dell, R. A. (ed.): "Drug-Food Interaction." *Nutrition in Disease*. Columbus, Ohio: Ross Laboratories, May 1977.

34 Lambert, M. L.: "Drug and Diet Interactions." *American Journal of Nursing*, 75(3):402, 1975.

35 Lehmann, P.: "Food and Drug Interactions." *FDA Consumer*. HEW Publication No. (FDA) 78–3070, March 1978.

36 Roe, D.: "Drugs, Diet and Nutrition." *Contemporary Nutrition*, 3(6), June 1978.

37 *Physicians' Desk Reference*. Oradell, New Jersey: Medical Economics, 1982.

38 Johnson, G. S.: Food intake patterns and the relative positions of factors affecting ingestion of nutrients of selected elderly adults in Akron, Ohio area. Master's thesis. Kent State University, Kent, Ohio, 1971.

39 Derby, G., R. Bleyer, and J. M. Martin: "Nutrition of the Elderly." *Journal of Human Nutrition*, 31:195, 1977.

40 U.S. Department of Health, Education and Welfare: Preliminary Findings of the First Health and Nutrition Examination Survey (HANES). U.S. 1971–72. Dietary Intakes and Biochemical Findings. DHEW Publication No. (HRA) 74–1219-1.

41 Rowe, D.: "Aging—A Jewel in the Mosaic of Life." *Journal of the American Dietetic Association*, 72:478, 1978.

CHAPTER 17

1 Forbes, A. L.: "Nutrition Labeling from the Government Point of View." *Food Technology*, 32:37, 1978.

2 Larsen, L.: Personal Communication. Division of Nutrition, Bureau of Foods, Food and Drug Administration, Department of Health and Human Services, 1982.

3 Schrayer, D. U.: "Consumer Response to Nutrition Labeling." *Food Technology*, 32:42, 1978.

4 Vratanina, D. L.: "Labeling: Understanding the Issues." *School Food Service Journal*, 35:27, 1981.

5 FDA Consumer Memo. Some questions and answers about food additives. DHEW Publication No. (FDA) 74–2056. May 1974.

6 Mayer, J.: "Experts are Divided about Food Additives." *Family Health/Today's Health*, July 1976. pp. 36–38.

7 Lehmann, T.: "More Than You Ever Thought You Would Know about Food Additives." *FDA Consumer*, April 1979, pp. 10–16.

8 Middlekauff, R. D.: "Concerning Food Additives." *Food Technology*, 28:42, 1974.

9 Wodicka, V.: "FDA's Objectives in Food Today, 27 CCH." *Drug Cosmetic Law Journal*, 59, 1972.

10 Strong, F. M.: "Toxicants Occurring Naturally in Foods." In: *Present Knowledge in Nutrition*, 4th ed. Washington, D.C.: Nutrition Foundation, 1976.

11 Federal Food, Drug and Cosmetic Act, as amended October, 1976. Sec.409(C)(3)(A).Washington,D.C.: U.S. Government Printing Office.

12 Food Protection Committee: *The Use of Chemicals in Food Production, Processing, Storage and Distribution*. Washington, D.C.: National Academy of Sciences, 1973.

13 Food Additives Amendment of 1958: An Act to Protect the Public Health by Amending the Federal Food, Drug and Cosmetic Act to Prohibit the Use in Food of Additives Which Have Not Been Tested to Establish Their Safety. 72 Stat. 1784.

14 Seligsohn, N.: "Is GRAS Safe?" *Food Engineering,* 52:20, 1980.

15 FASEB: Federation of American Societies for Experimental Biology. Evaluation of GRAS Monographs (Scientific Literature Review). No. PB80203789. Springfield, Va.: National Technical Information Service, 1981.

16 Crocco, S. C.: "Nitrosamines in Beer. Questions and Answers." *Journal of the American Medical Association,* 245:968, 1981.

17 Committee on Diet, Nutrition and Cancer, National Academy of Sciences: *Diet, Nutrition and Cancer.* Washington, D.C.: National Academy Press, 1982.

18 Gray, J. L., and C. J. Randall: "The Nitrite/n-Nitrosamine Problem in Meats: An Update." *Journal of Food Protection,* 42(2):168, 1979.

19 National Academy of Sciences: *The Health Effects of Nitrate, Nitrite and N-Nitroso Compounds.* Part 1 of a two-part study by the Committee on Nitrite and Alternative Curing Agents in Food. Washington, D.C.: National Academy Press, 1981.

20 Tannenbaum, S. R.: "Ins and Outs of Nitrites." *The Sciences,* p. 7, January 1980.

21 *Nitrite.* Nitrite Safety Council, October 1978.

22 Williams, D. L. H.: "Comparison of the Efficiencies of Ascorbic Acid and Sulphamic Acid as Nitrite Traps." *Cosmetic Toxicology,* 16:365, 1978.

23 Lecos, C.: "The Sweet and Sour History of Saccharin, Cyclamate, Aspartame." *FDA Consumer* 15(7):8–11, September 1981.

24 Whitehorn, W. V.: Chronology of Significant Events Relating to Saccharin (Attachment to Consumer Letter). April 8, 1972. Washington, D.C. FDA 1977.

25 Howe, G. R., J. O. Burch, and A. B. Miller: "Artificial Sweeteners and Human Bladder Cancer." *Lancet,* 2:578, 1977.

26 Federal Register 19996. April 15, 1977.

27 Committee for the Study of Saccharin and Food Safety Policy. Saccharin: Technical Assessment of Risks and Benefits. Washington, D.C.: National Academy of Sciences, 1978.

28 Morrison, A. B.: "How Sweet It Is." *Journal of the Canadian Dietetic Association,* 38:282, 1978.

29 Kletz, T. A.: "The Risk Questions: What Risks Should We Run?" *New Scientist,* 74:320, 1977.

30 Miller, S. A.: "Risk/Benefit, No-Effect Levels, and Delaney: Is the Message Getting Through? *Food Technology,* 32:93, 1978.

31 Marshall, E.: "Health Committee Investigates Farm Drugs." *Science,* 209:481, 1980.

32 Novick, R. P.: "Antibiotics: Wonder Drugs or Chicken Feed." *The Sciences,* pp.14–17, July/August 1979.

CHAPTER 18

1 Hopcraft, A.: *Born to Hunger.* London: Pan Books Ltd., 1968, pp. 94–95.

2 Abelson, P. H.: Editorial. "Malnutrition, learning and behavior." *Science,* 164:17, 1969.

3 Lien, N. M., K. K. Meyer, and M. Winick: "Early Malnutrition and 'Adoption': A Study of Their Effects on the Development of Korean Orphans Adopted into American Families." *American Journal of Clinical Nutrition,* 30:1734, 1977.

4 Levitsky, D. A.: "Malnutrition and the Undernourished Curiosity." *Human Ecology Forum,* 6:12, 1974.

5 Poleman, T. T.: "Quantifying the Nutrition Situation in Developing Countries." *Food Research Institute Studies,* 18(1):1, 1981.

6 Poleman, T. T.: "A Reappraisal of the Extent of World Hunger." *Food Policy,* 6(4):236, 1981.

7 Global 2000 Report to the President. President's Council on Environmental Quality. Washington, D.C., 1980 (July).

8 Scrimshaw, N., and L. Taylor: "Food." *Scientific American,* 243:78, 1980.

9 Bradley, C. C.: "Human Water Needs and Water Use in America." *Science,* 138:489, 1962.

10 Goodman, R.: "Managing the Demand for Energy in the Developing World." *Finance and Development,* 17(4):9, 1980.

11 Wade, N.: "Green Revolution: A Just Technology, Often Unjust in Use." *Science,* 186:1983, 1974.

12 Wharton, C.: "The Green Revolution: Cornucopia or Pandora's Box?" *Foreign Affairs,* 47:464, 1969.

13 United Nations University. World Hunger Programme. Tokyo, Japan, 1976.

14 Scott, D.: "Hunger in the Eighties." *Ceres,* 14(3): 17, 1981.

15 Schatan, J.: "Food Marketing: An Introduction." *PAG Bulletin,* V(4):1, 1975.

16 Harrison, P.: "The Inequalities That Curb Potential." *Ceres,* 14(3):22, 1981.

17 Johnston, B. V.: "Alternate Foods —A Hope in the Coming Crisis." *Agenda,* 2(3):8, 1979.

18 Ehrlich, P.: *The Population Bomb.* New York: Ballantine Books, 1970, p. 17.

19 Brown, L.: "Population and Affluence: Growing Pressure on World Food Resources." In: *How Many People, A Symposium.* The Foreign Policy Association, No. 218. New York City, December 1973, p. 32.

20 Mauldin, W. P.: "Family Planning Programs and Fertility Declines in Developing Countries." *Family Planning Perspective,* 7(1):32, 1975.

21 Ritchie, J.: "Learning Better Nutrition." *FAO Nutritional Studies,* 20. Rome: FAO, 1967.

22 Fonaroff, A.: "Undernutrition." *Journal of the American Medical Association,* 237:1825, 1977.

23 Garson, B.: "The Bottle Baby Scandal." In: Gussow, J. D. (ed.), *The*

Feeding Web. Palo Alto: Bull Publishing Co., 1978, p. 238.

24 Jelliffe, E. F. P.: "The Impact of the Food Industry on the Nutritional Status of Infants and Preschool Children in Developing Countries." In: J. Mayer (ed.), *Priorities in Child Nutrition in the Developing Countries.* U.N. Economic and Social Council. E/ICEF/L. 1328, vol. 2, 1975, p. 253.

25 Latham, M. C.: "Introduction." In: T. Greiner (ed.), *Regulation and Education: Strategies for Solving the Bottle Feeding Problem.* Cornell International Nutrition Monograph Ser. 4. Ithaca, New York: Cornell University, 1977, pp. i–xiv.

26 Jelliffe, D. B., and E. F. P. Jelliffe: "Human Milk, Nutrition and the Resource Crisis." *Science,* 188:557, 1975.

27 Berg, A.: *The Nutrition Factor.* Washington, D.C.: Brookings Institution, 1973.

28 Astrachan, A.: "Milking the Third World." *The Progressive,* July 1976, pp. 34–37.

29 Monckeberg, F.: "Factors Conditioning Malnutrition in Latin America with Special Reference to Chile: Advice for Volunteer Action." In: P. Gyorgy, and O. L. Kline (eds.), *Malnutrition is a Problem of Ecology.* New York: S. Karger, 1979, p. 30.

30 Puffer, R. R., and C. V. Serrano: *Patterns of Mortality in Childhood.* Pan American Health Organization Scientific Publication 262, 1973.

31 Brown, R. E.: "Breast-Feeding in Modern Times." *American Journal of Clinical Nutrition,* 26:556, 1973.

32 United Nations World Health Organization: *WHO Code of Marketing Breastmilk Substitutes.* Geneva, World Health Organization, 1981.

33 Hinds, M.: "Nestle's New Formula Policy." *The New York Times,* March 17, 1982.

34 Food and Agriculture Organization: "Food and Nutrition Strategies in National Development." Ninth Report of the Joint FAO/WHO Expert Committee on Nutrition, *Technical Report Series,* 584. Geneva: World Health Organization, 1976.

35 Allan, D. A.: "Focus on Food Mixtures." *UNICEF News,* 71:23, March 1972.

36 Popkin, B. M., and M. C. Latham: "The Limitations and Dangers of Commerciogenic Nutritious Foods." *American Journal of Clinical Nutrition,* 26:1015, 1973.

37 Martin, C.: "Leaf Protein Child Feeding Trial." *League for International Food Education Newsletter,* March 1975.

38 Rawitscher, M., and J. Mayer: "Nutritional Outputs and Energy Inputs in Seafoods." *Science,* 198:261, 1977.

39 Watson, J.: "New Protein Food." *Nutrition,* 28:249, 1974.

40 Food and Agriculture Organization: "PAG Ad Hoc Working Group Meeting on Single Cell Protein." *PAG Bulletin,* VI(2):1–5, 1976.

41 McNaughton, J.: "Applied Nutrition Programmes." *Food and Nutrition,* 1(3):17, 1975.

42 Childers, E.: "Some Notes on Planning Communications Support for an Applied Nutrition Program." *PAG Bulletin,* VI(1):14, 1976.

43 Mellor, J. W.: "The Agriculture of India." *Scientific American,* 235(3):154, 1976.

44 Fryer, J.: "Food for Thought—The Use and Abuse of Food Aid." *Development Forum,* October 1981, p. 15.

45 Sewell, J. A.: "Which Costs More: Aid Or No Aid?" *Agenda,* 4(2):19, 1981.

46 Sommer, J. G.: "Does Foreign Aid Really Help the Poor?" *Agenda,* 4(3):28, 1981.

47 Wallerstein, M. B.: *Food for War—Food for Peace: United States Aid in a Global Content.* Cambridge, Mass., and London: MIT Press, 1980.

GLOSSARY

Absorption that process by which products of digestion cross intestinal mucosal cells and enter the blood circulation.

Acetylcholine a neurotransmitter in the brain.

Acid-base balance maintenance of pH of the blood at a slightly alkaline pH between 7.35 and 7.45.

Acid chyme the fluid leaving the stomach after a meal. It is acid by virtue of having mixed with the digestive juices of the stomach.

Actin a structural protein of muscles.

Active transport the process by which nutrients cross the membrane of the intestinal mucosal cell when the concentration of nutrient is greater within than outside the cell. The process requires special protein carriers and energy.

Acyl carrier protein a coenzyme form of pantothenic acid.

Addisonian pernicious anemia disease resulting from a genetic defect that prevents secretion of intrinsic factor (IF) by the stomach, resulting in inability to absorb vitamin B_{12}.

Adenosine triphosphate (ATP) adenosine triphosphate is a compound having high-energy bonds, and is the useful form of energy in the body. When energy is needed, en-

zymes can break the high-energy bonds, releasing the energy for use in driving chemical reactions.

Albumin blood protein synthesized by the liver. It aids in maintaining the normal distribution of fluid within and outside body cells.

Aldosterone hormone secreted by the adrenal glands when a critical amount of water is lost from the blood. It causes the kidneys to reabsorb sodium, which is accompanied by water.

Alkalosis a condition in which the blood becomes more alkaline than is normal.

Alpha-tocopherol equivalents (in mg) unit for expressing the RDA for vitamin E.

Amino acid pattern amounts of amino acids present in a protein relative to one another.

Amniotic fluid fluid held within a sac in which the developing fetus floats. Amniotic fluid protects the fetus from injury and helps to maintain an even temperature.

Amylopectin a form of starch in which glucose molecules form a straight chain linked at carbons 1 and 4, with branches occurring along the chain in which glucose units are linked at carbons 1 and 6 by alpha bonds.

Amylose a form of starch in which glucose molecules are linked so as to form a straight chain with glucose units linked at carbons 1 and 4 by alpha bonds.

Anabolism the building up or synthesis of compounds or structures.

Aneurysm ballooning out of an artery resulting from weakness in artery wall.

Angina pectoris chest pain, especially upon exertion, resulting from partial blockage of an artery supplying blood to the heart muscle.

Anions ions having negative charges.

a disorder seen particularly among adolescent girls in affluent countries and characterized by refusal to eat until serious underweight results.

Antibiotic a chemical compound which acts as an antagonist to specific forms of life, usually a disease-producing substance.

Antibodies proteins synthesized in the body that protect against bacteria, viruses, and other hazards.

Antidiuretic hormone (ADH) hormone secreted by the brain when a critical amount of water is lost from the blood. It causes the kidneys to reabsorb rather than excrete water.

Antioxidant a substance that protects

another from oxidative destruction by itself becoming oxidized.

Aorta large artery coming from the left ventricle of the heart and passing downward through the center of the trunk.

Appetite a desire for food not necessarily accompanied by hunger, or physiological need for food. Appetite can be triggered by sight, smell, or taste of food, or by reading about or thinking about food.

Arachidonic acid a polyunsaturated fatty acid having 20 carbons and 4 double bonds which the body synthesizes from linoleic acid.

Arteriosclerosis disorder in which arteries thicken and become inelastic.

Atherosclerosis specific type of hardening of the arteries characterized by plaque buildup in artery walls. The plaques contain cholesterol, triglycerides, phospholipids, fibrin, connective tissue, and large numbers of smooth muscle cells.

Avidin a protein in raw egg white that combines with biotin and prevents its absorption.

Basal conditions the status of lying down, awake but completely relaxed mentally, emotionally, and physically in a room of comfortable temperature 12 to 18 hours after eating.

Basal metabolism (*or basal metabolic rate, BMR*) the energy required to support the vital functions of the body while at physical, mental, and emotional rest in a room of comfortable temperature, 12 to 18 hours after eating.

Behavior modification a technique used to teach people to analyze external cues or environmental factors that influence their eating behavior or physical activity.

Beriberi disease resulting from lack of thiamine.

Beta-carotene the carotenoid convert-ed most efficiently to vitamin A by body tissues.

Bile secretion of the liver that is stored in the gallbladder and is required for fat digestion.

Bioflavonoids ("vitamin P") substances isolated from plants having some antioxidant effects but which are not vitamins because the body synthesizes needed amounts.

Black tongue disease in dogs due to a niacin deficiency.

Bran the outer layer of whole grains that includes dietary fiber and several vitamins and minerals. The bran is removed when white flour is obtained from whole wheat.

Brown fat a special kind of fat that produces large amounts of heat.

Body mass index Weight/height^2.

Body pool the total amount of a nutrient held by all the body tissues.

Buffer a solution of substances which prevents a change in pH by either removing hydrogen ions or releasing them as needed to prevent a pH change.

Bulimia insatiable craving for food, followed by binge eating in which huge quantities of food are consumed, often at one sitting.

Calcitonin a hormone released by the thyroid gland when blood calcium begins to rise too high. It stops the action of PTH (*see* parathyroid hormone).

Cancer an abnormal overgrowth of cells which crowds out and destroys healthy tissue.

Carbohydrate loading a procedure by which more than the normal amount of glycogen is stored in muscles in an attempt to prolong the endurance of athletes.

Carcinogen a substance that causes cancer.

Carcinogenic cancer causing.

Cardiac output amount of blood pumped by the heart per minute.

Cardiovascular disease (CVD) disease of the heart and blood vessels.

Cariogenic causes tooth decay.

Carotenoids substances in plants, some of which the body cells convert to vitamin A.

Catabolism the breakdown of com-pounds or structures into simpler substances.

Cations ions having positive charges.

Cellulose a component of dietary fiber.

Cementum place of attachment for ligaments and fibers that fasten the tooth to the jaw tissues.

Ceroid pigments (lipofuscin) fluorescent pigments thought to be end products of damaged cell membranes that accumulate in tissues of vitamin E-deficient animals.

Ceruloplasmin the protein in the blood that transports copper and also performs certain enzymatic functions.

Cheilosis a condition in which the lips become inflamed, and cracks or fissures occur at the corners of the mouth. Occurs in riboflavin deficiency.

Chelating agent substance that bonds chemically with a metal ion in such manner that the ion appears to be held by a claw.

Chlorophyll the pigment in green plants, essential in the process of photosynthesis.

Cholecalciferol vitamin D$_3$, synthesized in animals when 7-dehydrocholesterol in the skin is exposed to ultraviolet light.

Cholecystokinin-pancreozymin (CCK-PZ) a hormone secreted in the small intestines when acid chyme containing fat or protein reaches the intestines; it slows stomach motility, causes release of bile from the gallbladder, and stimulates secretion of pancreatic enzymes.

Cholesterol a lipid used by the liver to form bile salts, which are necessary for fat digestion. Cholesterol is also required in the structure of cellular membranes and nervous tissue, is used to form the precursor to vitamin D in the body and to form certain hormones.

Cholesterol esterase a pancreatic enzyme that attacks cholesterol esters, breaking the bond between cholesterol and the fatty acid. This frees cholesterol for absorption.

Choline part of the structure of lecithin and of acetylcholine. Whether or not choline is a dietary essential is unknown.

Chylomicrons the lipoproteins synthesized by intestinal mucosal cells that transport triglycerides and cholesterol from the intestinal mucosal cells to the blood via the lymphatic route.

Cobalamin vitamin B_{12}.

Cobamides the coenzyme forms of vitamin B_{12}.

Coenzyme A coenzyme containing pantothenic acid as part of its structure.

Coenzymes small organic molecules (usually containing one of the B vitamins) required by specific enzymes for activity.

Cofactor an activator of enzymes (often containing a mineral).

Collagen a protein found in connective tissue in skin, bones, ligaments, and cartilage.

Colostrum first milk secreted by the mother either before or after the birth of a baby.

Complementary proteins proteins that, when combined, supply all the essential amino acids. Amino acids that are low in one protein are supplied by the other.

Condensation formation of a larger molecule from two smaller ones during which process water is eliminated.

Conjunctiva membrane lining the eyelids and covering the white portion of the eye.

Cornea colored portion of the eye.

Coronary arteries arteries that nourish the heart muscle.

Coronary heart disease disease in which the arteries that nourish the heart muscle become clogged due to atherosclerosis. Complete blockage of the blood flow in one of these arteries causes a heart attack.

Covalent bonds bonds between two atoms in which electrons are shared.

Cretinism a disorder in which the individual has little or no functioning thyroid tissue, resulting in stunted growth and mental retardation.

Critical growth period a time during growth when a given event will have its greatest impact.

Crude fiber the fraction remaining after plant foods are treated with fat solvents, acid, and alkali. The process destroys a large portion of dietary fiber; hence crude fiber is a poor estimate of dietary fiber.

Culture a learned way of living shared by a group of people which encompasses their attitudes, beliefs, social institutions, motivations, and tools and techniques used to provide their needs and wants.

Daily food guide a guide developed by the U.S. Department of Agriculture which advocates daily consumption of specified numbers of servings from four groups of foods: (1) Vegetables and Fruits, (2) Bread and Cereals, (3) Meats, Poultry, Fish, and Beans, and (4) Milk and Cheese.

Deamination removal of the amino group ($-NH_2$) from an amino acid.

                       one of the active forms of vitamin C.

Delaney Amendment legislation that forbids any additive to be used that is found to cause cancer in animals or in human beings.

Denaturation the uncoiling of a protein molecule, changing its shape or spatial configuration without breaking peptide bonds.

Dental caries tooth decay.

Dental plaque a sticky material produced by oral bacteria that adheres to teeth, allowing the bacteria to multiply rapidly, and producing acid which etches the tooth enamel.

Dentin principal component of the inner tooth core.

Deoxyribonucleic Acid (DNA) molecule synthesized in the cell nucleus containing genetic information that directs synthesis of the cell's proteins.

Dermatitis inflammation of the skin.

Dextrins breakdown products of starch consisting of glucose molecules linked together to form a molecule only about one-fifth the size of the starch molecule from which it came.

Diabetes mellitus a metabolic disorder characterized by an inadequate production of insulin or an inability to use insulin properly.

Dietary fiber components of the plant cell wall and other plant polysaccharides that resist digestion in the upper intestinal tract.

Dietary Goals for the United States goals set by the Senate Select Committee on Nutrition and Human Needs in 1977.

Dietary Guidelines for Americans guidelines set by the U.S. Department of Agriculture and the U.S. Department of Health, Education and Welfare, 1980.

Dietary thermogenesis production of body heat resulting from food consumption. This term is used to mean the Specific Dynamic Action of food (SDA) as well as to designate the postulate that some thin people may lose more body heat after consuming a specified amount of food than some fat people, who may be more efficient in converting food to fat.

Differentiated products similar products that retain some distinctive differences.

Differentiation the process of cell and tissue specialization during development of the embryo.

Diglyceride a compound in which two fatty acid molecules are attached to one glycerol molecule.

Dipeptide a compound made up of two amino acids joined by one peptide bond.

Direct calorimetry method of determining energy expenditure by measuring heat given off.

Disaccharide a sugar whose molecule is made up of two monosaccharide molecules linked together chemically after removal of a water molecule.

Diuretics drugs used to induce urinary excretion of sodium and water. They also result in excretion of potassium and magnesium.

Edema abnormal accumulation of fluid between body cells, which may or may not result in puffiness of the skin.

Elastin the fibrous protein in elastic structures of the body, such as the large blood vessels.

Electrolytes those substances that separate into ions when placed in water.

Embryo term used for the baby-to-be from conception to the end of the first 8 weeks of pregnancy.

Emulsifier (*or* **emulsifying agent**) a molecule capable of holding two nonmixing liquids together by virtue of having one end of its molecule soluble in lipid and the other end soluble in water.

Enamel outermost part of the tooth.

Endogenous produced within the body proper (not in the gastrointestinal tract).

Endoplasmic reticulum (ER) a system of membranes forming small channels in cells through which nutrients and other substances are transported. The ER is divided into rough and smooth portions. The rough ER is dotted with ribosomes which are centers of protein synthesis.

Endosperm the inner part of grains, consisting chiefly of starch and a lesser amount of protein.

Energy the ability to do work.

Energy balance the relationship of energy consumed to that used up or stored by the body. An individual is in a state of energy balance or equilibrium when the kilocalorie intake equals the expenditure.

Enriched flour white flour to which is added three vitamins, thiamine, riboflavin, and niacin, and one mineral, iron, at levels approximating those in whole wheat. Other nutrients removed in milling are not added back.

Enrichment addition of specific nutrients to foods to replace some of the nutrients lost in processing.

Enterogastrone hormone secreted by the duodenum as food enters the duodenum, which diminishes the movements of the stomach.

Enterohepatic circulation route by which a substance passes from the liver via the bile to the duodenum down to the ileum and is returned to the liver via the portal vein. Bile salts are circulated in this fashion.

Epidemiological studies research in which specified characteristics of large groups of people are studied in relationship to the development of disease.

Epithelial tissues those forming the surface of the skin and the surface layer of mucous membranes of the digestive, respiratory, and genitourinary tracts and of the eyes and glands.

Ergocalciferol vitamin D_2, which is synthesized commercially by exposing its precursor, ergosterol, found in certain strains of yeasts and molds, to ultraviolet light.

Essential amino acids those required in the diet because the body is unable to synthesize sufficient amounts to meet its needs.

Essential fatty acid the fatty acid required for body functions that must be supplied in food because the body cannot synthesize it. Linoleic acid is this fatty acid.

Exchange system a system developed by the American Dietetic Association in which foods are arranged into six groups in such a way that one food may be exchanged for another within a group. A plan can be drawn up calling for a specific number of exchanges from each group, simplifying dietary planning.

Extracellular fluid (ECF) fluid outside the body cells, including that in the blood and between the cells.

Extrinsic factor vitamin B_{12}.

Facilitated diffusion the process not requiring energy by which certain nutrients cross the membrane of the intestinal mucosal cell, using a special protein carrier.

Fallopian tubes tubes leading from the area of the ovaries to the uterus.

Fatty acid one of the basic molecules making up triglycerides. Fatty acids consist of carbon atoms joined together to form chains of varying lengths. All fatty acids have one acid group (—COOH) at one end of their molecule, but vary in the amount of hydrogen (—H) held by each carbon.

Feeding center that part of the hypothalamus (in the brain) situated on either side of the central portion which appears to trigger eating when the proper signals are received.

Ferric ion ionic form of iron carrying three positive charges (Fe^{3+}).

Ferritin a storage form of iron found in the liver, spleen, and bone marrow. Normally, small amounts also circulate in the blood.

Ferrous ion ionic form of iron carrying two positive charges (Fe^{2+}).

Fetal alcohol syndrome (FAS) a disorder in infants whose mothers were chronic severe alcoholics during pregnancy. An infant with full-blown FAS has specific facial aberrations, small head size, and is retarded both physically and mentally.

Fetus term applied to the baby-to-be from the beginning of the ninth week of pregnancy until birth.

Fibrin clotting substance of blood.

Fibrinogen a plasma protein synthesized by the liver that, when acted upon by thrombin, produces fibrin which is required for blood clotting.

Flavin adenine dinucleotide (FAD) one of the coenzyme (active) forms of riboflavin.

Flavin mononucleotide (FMN) one of the coenzyme (active) forms of riboflavin.

Flavoproteins enzymes requiring either FAD or FMN, the coenzyme forms of riboflavin.

Food additives substances directly added to food (intentional additives), or substances which may become part of food because of contact through equipment or packaging (unintentional additives), or substances used in food processing that affect food without actually becoming part of it.

Fortification addition of specific nutrients to foods in amounts greater than those naturally present in the food.

Free radicals atoms or molecules having one or more unpaired electrons. They are highly reactive and can seriously damage cells.

Gastric inhibitory peptide (GIP) a hormone secreted by the mucosa of the duodenum and jejunum when fat or carbohydrates reach the intestines.

It inhibits gastric motility and stimulates insulin release by the pancreas.

Germ (of grains) that part of a whole grain that is responsible for the germination or reproduction of the seed. The germ contains fatty acids, and many vitamins and minerals.

Gerontology the study of aging.

Gestation period of pregnancy.

Gestational diabetes diabetes that develops during pregnancy.

Glucagon a hormone secreted by the pancreas which raises the blood glucose level as it begins to reach a low level.

Gluconeogenesis the process by which the liver forms glucose from non-carbohydrate sources (certain amino acids, glycerol from fat catabolism, and lactic acid from muscle exercise).

Glucose tolerance factor (GTF) the organic form of chromium thought to be the physiologically active form.

Glucostatic hypothesis suggests that hunger results when the rate of utilization of glucose in the feeding center of the hypothalamus falls below a certain level. Satiety, according to this hypothesis, results when the rate of utilization of glucose reaches a certain high level, causing the satiety center to shut off the feeding center.

Glycerol a 3-carbon compound required for the synthesis of triglycerides and phospholipids. The body synthesizes glycerol from glucose.

Glycogen the storage form of carbohydrate in the animal body. Glycogen is a large, highly branched molecule consisting only of glucose molecules that is synthesized by both liver and muscles.

Gram-calorie the amount of heat required to raise the temperature of 1 g of water 1°C. This is the unit of energy used in physics and chemistry.

GRAS additives that are "generally recognized as safe." Such substances are currently being reviewed for safety.

Gums One of the classes of components making up dietary fiber.

Heat of combustion heat given off when a food is burned completely in a bomb calorimeter. This provides the kilocalorie value of the food before it is consumed.

Heme iron that form of iron found in meat, poultry, and fish. Heme is a portion of the hemoglobin molecule.

Hemicellulose a component of dietary fiber.

Hemochromatosis a genetic disorder in which intestinal mucosal cells are unable to block the absorption of unneeded iron into the body. The liver, pancreas, and heart eventually become damaged by toxic levels of iron.

Hemoglobin a compound containing iron which is synthesized in the bone marrow and put into red blood cells. It carries oxygen from the lungs to the tissues, and carbon dioxide from the tissues to the lungs.

Hemorrhagic disease of the newborn a bleeding disorder that may develop in newborn infants due to vitamin K deficiency.

Hemosiderin a storage form of iron found in the liver, spleen, and bone marrow.

Hexoses sugars having 6 carbon atoms.

High-density lipoproteins (HDL) lipoproteins thought to carry cholesterol from body cells to the liver for catabolism and excretion as bile salts.

High-quality protein protein having an amino acid pattern similar to that of the body.

Holoenzyme the active enzyme, formed when its required coenzyme combines with the apoenzyme (inactive form of the enzyme).

Homeostasis maintenance of relative constancy of the body's internal environment.

Hunger painful sensation or state indicating a physiological need for food. Symptoms may include stomach "pangs," irritability, light-headedness, and weakness.

Hydrochloric acid acid secreted by stomach cells during digestion.

Hydrogenation the process by which hydrogen is added to fats having some double bonds. The process converts the double to single bonds and increases the degree of saturation of the fat.

Hydrolysis a chemical process by which a compound is broken down with the addition of water in the process.

Hydroxyapatite the crystalline structure of bones, containing chiefly calcium and phosphate ions.

Hydroxylation addition of an —OH group (hydroxyl group) to a compound.

Hyperactivity (*also called* hyperkinesis) a behavior pattern characterized by a short attention span, excessive purposeless activity, hostility, difficulty in relating to others, and difficulty in sleeping.

Hyperglycemia a disorder in which the blood glucose level is higher than normal, resulting in dehydration of (removal of water from) cells. Hyperglycemia is one sign of diabetes.

Hyperplasia growth occurring by means of increase in number of cells.

Hypertension high blood pressure.

Hyperthyroidism a condition in which secretion of thyroxine and triiodothyronine are high, resulting in a high basal metabolic rate.

Hypertrophy growth occurring by enlargement of existing cells.

Hypervitaminosis A toxicity due to excess of vitamin A.

Hypochromic red blood cells those that are unusually pale in color due to low amounts of hemoglobin, as in iron-deficiency anemia.

Hypoglycemia a disorder in which the blood glucose level falls below normal levels, resulting in symptoms of dizziness, nervousness, and fainting.

Hypothyroidism a condition in which secretion of thyroxine and triiodothyronine are low, resulting in a low basal metabolic rate, and sluggish mental and physical activity.

Implantation deposition of the fertilized egg or ovum in the lining of the uterus.

Indirect calorimetry method of determining energy expenditure in which either oxygen consumption or carbon dioxide production or both are measured.

Infancy the period from birth to 1 year of age.

Insulin the hormone secreted by the pancreas whenever blood glucose levels rise above normal; it acts to lower blood glucose levels.

Intestinal lipase an enzyme situated within intestinal mucosal cells which, during absorption, hydrolyzes monoglycerides to glycerol and fatty acids.

Intracellular fluid (ICF) fluid held within body cells.

Intrinsic factor substance secreted by the normal stomach, required for absorption of vitamin B_{12}.

Ion an atom or group of atoms carrying an electrical charge.

Isoniazid a drug used to treat tuberculosis which binds and inactivates vitamin B_6, increasing the dietary need for this vitamin.

Keratin the fibrous, hard protein of hair and nails.

Ketones products of incomplete oxidation of fats in the liver, resulting when insufficient carbohydrates are present in the liver.

Kilocalorie (kcal) the amount of heat required to raise the temperature of 1 kg of water 1°C.

Kinetic (or active) energy that involved in performing work of internal processes, or of the muscles in performing various activities.

Lactase enzyme secreted by the intestinal mucosa that converts lactose to glucose and galactose.

Lacteals small lymph vessels that drain intestinal mucosal cells.

Lactose a disaccharide made up of one molecule of glucose and one of galactose.

Lactose intolerance a disorder involving inadequate secretion of lactase, resulting in inability to digest lactose, characterized by symptoms of bloating, intestinal gas, abdominal pain, and diarrhea.

Laetrile ("vitamin B_{17}") a chemical substance (amygdalin) containing cyanide and viewed by the medical profession as a "fake cancer cure." It is not a vitamin, contrary to claims made for it.

Law of conservation of energy, or first law of thermodynamics the observation that energy cannot ordinarily be created or destroyed, but can only be converted from one form to another.

Lean body mass that portion of the body that is free of fat.

Lecithin a phospholipid containing choline which is used by the body to form the structure of cellular membranes, nervous tissue, and lipoproteins.

Lignin a component of dietary fiber.

Limiting amino acid that amino acid present in a protein or a diet in the least amount relative to the body's need for it.

Linoleic acid a polyunsaturated fatty acid, having 18 carbons and two double bonds, and which is essential in the diet.

Linolenic acid a polyunsaturated fatty acid, having 18 carbons and three double bonds, thought at one time to be essential in the diet, but now assumed not to be.

Lipids substances that do not dissolve in water, but dissolve in ether, chloroform, or other similar solvents.

Lipoprotein lipase an enzyme produced by the lining of blood vessels which catalyzes the release of triglycerides from chylomicrons and very low density lipoproteins (VLDL), and their catabolism to fatty acids and glycerol.

Lipoproteins substances with protein on their exterior which are used by the body to transport triglyceride and cholesterol in the blood.

Lipostatic hypothesis suggestion that some kind of signal (perhaps free fatty acids or prostaglandins) reaches the brain, causing an animal or person to consume enough food to maintain their present level of body fatness. For many people, this is a level of excess body fatness.

Low-density lipoproteins (LDL) lipoproteins that carry chiefly cholesterol to the body cells.

Lumen opening running through the middle of an artery or the gastrointestinal tract or other tube-like structure.

Lysolecithin the compound resulting after one fatty acid has been removed from lecithin.

Lysosomes bags of digestive enzymes in cells that normally destroy dead cells or wornout parts of cells.

Macrocytic anemia anemia in which the blood cells are unusually large and immature. This anemia occurs in either folacin or vitamin B_{12} deficiency.

Major minerals or macronutrient elements those required in the diet in amounts greater than 100 mg per day.

Maltase enzyme secreted by the intestinal mucosa that converts maltose to glucose.

Maltose a disaccharide composed of two molecules of glucose.

Mannitol a sugar alcohol used as a sweetener in some dietetic foods.

Massive or morbid obesity a state of weighing more than 100 percent of desirable weight for height and sex.

Meals on wheels program run by local volunteers in a community who deliver hot meals to homebound elderly, infirm, or handicapped individuals.

Medical model a model in which it is necessary first to find people who have symptoms or are at high risk for developing a disease, then either directing them to obtain medical attention aimed at reducing the risk or treating the disorder.

Megadoses unusually large doses of a nutrient, usually a vitamin, administered in pill or capsule form.

Megaloblasts large, immature red blood cells that occur in the blood in either folacin or vitamin B_{12} deficiency.

Metabolic pool of amino acids those amino acids circulating in the blood and lymph and held as free amino acids in the organs.

Metabolism all those processes in the body by which nutrients become a part of body tissues, are used for energy, or otherwise perform their functions. Additionally, this term encompasses those processes by which body compounds or structures are broken down and their products excreted.

Metabolites compounds resulting from chemical changes of a substance during metabolism.

Microcytic red blood cells those that are abnormally small in size, as in iron-deficiency anemia.

Microflora bacteria that exist in the colon.

Microvilli microscopic projections on the mucosal side of each intestinal cell; also called the brush border.

Mild or moderate obesity a state of weighing 10 to 30 percent above desirable weight.

Mineralization the process by which calcium and phosphorus crystals are embedded in the collagen matrix of bones, hardening them.

Mitochondria (*singular,* mitochondrion) the centers of most of the energy production in the cells.

Monoglyceride a compound in which one fatty acid molecule is attached to one of the carbons of glycerol.

Monosaccharide the basic carbohydrate unit consisting of a single sugar molecule, sometimes called a simple sugar. The most important monosaccharides are glucose, fructose, and galactose.

Mucus a slippery secretion produced by mucous membranes and glands.

Myocardial infarction heart attack; blockage of an artery that supplies blood to the heart.

Myoglobin a compound in muscles that is similar to hemoglobin. It stores oxygen in muscles until needed for energy metabolism.

Myosin a structural protein of muscles.

Negative nitrogen balance the condition in which there is a net loss of body nitrogen, resulting in greater excretion than is taken into the body.

Neurotransmitters the chemical substances in nervous tissue required for sending messages along the nerves and in the brain.

Niacin equivalent (NE), (in mg) term used to express the RDA for niacin. One NE equals either 1 mg of niacin or 60 mg of tryptophan.

Niacytin the bound form of niacin occurring in untreated corn.

Nicotinamide (niacinamide) and nicotinic acid forms of niacin.

Nicotinamide adenine dinucleotide (NAD) a coenzyme (active) form of niacin.

Nicotinamide adenine dinucleotide phosphate (NADP) a coenzyme form of niacin.

Night blindness inability to see in dim light.

Nitrogen equilibrium the condition in which the intake and excretion of nitrogen is equal.

Nitrosamines substances known to produce cancer in animals, which are formed from the reaction of nitrites with certain amines.

Nonessential amino acids those the body can synthesize.

Nonheme iron inorganic forms of iron found in plants.

Nutrient density the extent to which a food provides nutrients relative to the kilocalories it furnishes. A food of *low nutrient density* contains few nutrients relative to the kilocalories it contains, while a food of *high nutrient density* is rich in nutrients relative to its kilocalorie contribution.

Obesity a state of having excessive body fat.

Oligopoly a market in which a small number of companies predominate.

Oral contraceptive agents (OCA) pills consisting of chemicals which are similar to the natural hormones, estrogen or progesterone. They act by preventing ovulation (release of an ovum or egg).

Organically grown foods foods produced by methods using as little fertilizer and pesticides from fossil fuels as possible. Organic farmers use crop rotations, animal manures, mechanical cultivation, and biological pest control methods to help maintain soil productivity.

Osmosis the process of net movement of water across a membrane due to differences in concentration of solute (dissolved substances) on the two sides of the membrane.

Osteomalacia disease in adults due to vitamin D deficiency, resulting in softening and deformity of bones.

Osteoporosis a disease seen usually in later life in which there is excessive loss of bone mass.

Overweight a state of weighing between 10 percent and 20 percent above desirable weight for height.

Oxalate a substance formed in the body from the catabolism of vitamin C. High urinary excretion of oxalate causes kidney stones in susceptible people.

Oxidation the general process by which carbohydrates, proteins, and fats are catabolized for energy in the body. More specifically, oxidation refers to the loss by an atom or molecule of one or more hydrogens or electrons.

Palatability the quality of a diet that makes it agreeable to the sense of taste.

Pancreatic amylase enzyme secreted by the pancreas that converts starch and dextrins to maltose.

Pancreatic lipase an enzyme secreted by the pancreas which catalyzes the breakdown of triglycerides to monoglycerides, fatty acids, and glycerol.

Pancreatic phospholipase an enzyme secreted by the pancreas that breaks a fatty acid off of lecithin, producing lysolecithin.

Pangamic acid ("vitamin B_{15}") a group of substances promoted by some as a cure for many diseases. It is not a vitamin, has never been proved effective in treating any disease, and cannot be sold legally as a dietary supplement or as a drug.

Para-aminobenzoic acid a substance that is not itself a vitamin, but is a constituent of the vitamin folacin.

Parathyroid hormone (PTH) a hormone secreted by the parathyroid glands that raises the concentration of blood calcium when levels fall below a critical concentration.

Pectin a component of dietary fiber.

Pellagra disease resulting from niacin deficiency.

Penicillamine a drug used to treat

rheumatoid arthritis and other diseases which binds and inactivates vitamin B_6, increasing the dietary need for this vitamin.

Peptide bond bond formed between the carboxyl group (—COOH) on one amino acid and the amino group (—NH₂) of another, accompanied by removal of a water molecule. The peptide bond links one amino acid to another in dipeptides, polypeptides, and proteins.

Pernicious anemia anemia due to inability to secrete intrinsic factor, resulting in vitamin B_{12} deficiency.

Pesticides substances including herbicides, rodenticides, fungicides, insecticides, and plant growth regulators that may be used in food production

pH a system of designating degree of acidity or alkalinity in which values below 7.0 indicate acidity, 7.0 indicates neutrality, and values above 7.0 indicate alkalinity.

Phospholipase an enzyme secreted by the pancreas which is able to break off one fatty acid from lecithin, a phospholipid.

Phospholipids lipids containing glycerol, fatty acids, and phosphoric acid. Lecithin is one of the phospholipids.

Photophobia abnormal sensitivity of the eyes to light.

Photosynthesis the process by which chlorophyll in green plants uses light energy from the sun together with carbon dioxide from the air and water from air and soil to synthesize carbohydrates.

Physiological anemia of pregnancy normal decrease in concentration of hemoglobin and hematocrit that occurs in weeks 24 to 32 of pregnancy, due to relatively greater expansion of blood plasma volume than of red cell mass.

Physiological fuel value that portion of the energy present per gram of carbohydrate, fat, protein, or alcohol that is available for use in the body. The general figures for the mixture of foods making up the usual American diet are 4, 9, 4, and 7 kcal/g for carbohydrates, fats, protein, and alcohol, respectively.

Phytates organic forms of phosphates found in whole grains. (Organic compounds are simply those containing carbon.)

Point of unsaturation the position in a carbon chain at which a double bond occurs. The carbons sharing a double bond will be attached to fewer hydrogens (—H) than those sharing single bonds.

Polypeptide a chain of amino acids joined by peptide bonds, containing 10 or more amino acid units.

Polysaccharide a carbohydrate made up of a great many sugar units linked together. The chief polysaccharides are starches, glycogen, and most components of dietary fiber (see *Dietary fiber*).

Polyunsaturated fatty acids those fatty acids having two or more double bonds in their molecules.

Portal vein blood vessel carrying water-soluble nutrients from the intestinal tract to the liver.

Positive energy balance the state of consuming more kilocalories than one expends, leading to obesity.

Positive nitrogen balance the condition in which there is a net gain of nitrogen in the body, with less being excreted than is consumed.

Potential energy energy stored in glycogen, body fat, or in ATP or other high-energy compounds.

Placenta organ attached on one side to the wall of the uterus, and on the other to the fetus via the umbilical cord. Oxygen and nutrients cross from maternal to fetal blood in the placenta, while carbon dioxide and other waste pass from fetal to maternal blood.

Plaque fatty deposits which build up in the artery walls. Plaques contain cholesterol, triglycerides, phospholipids, fibrin, connective tissue, and smooth muscle cells.

Prealbumin a protein synthesized in the liver, required for transport of vitamin A in the blood.

Precursor a substance which is itself nonfunctional as a nutrient but which body tissues convert to a nutrient. Beta-carotene, for example, is a precursor to vitamin A.

Premature infant an infant born before the 37th week of gestation.

Protein-calorie malnutrition a disease common in many less-developed countries among infants and small children. It is due to inadequate intakes of kilocalories and protein, complicated by repeated infections.

Prostaglandins the hormone-like substances synthesized by the body from arachidonic acid.

Prothrombin a plasma protein synthesized by the liver that, in concert with fibrinogen, is necessary for blood clotting.

P/S ratio a ratio in which grams of polyunsaturated fat in a food or a diet are divided by grams of saturated fat in the same food or diet. An optimal ratio is thought to be 1, while a lower ratio indicates a relative excess of saturated fat.

Pteroylglutamic acid (PGA) folic acid, the parent compound from which coenzyme forms of folacin are synthesized.

Public health model a model in which a group of experts, after evaluating all the current evidence concerning a disease, decides upon recommendations believed to benefit the population as a whole, without causing harm.

Pulp soft interior portion of tooth containing blood vessels, lymph, and nerves.

Pyridoxine, pyridoxal, and pyridoxamine the three forms of vitamin B_6.

Recommended Dietary Allowances amounts of calories, proteins, vitamins, and minerals judged by the Food and Nutrition Board, of the National Academy of Sciences, to meet the needs of nearly all healthy people in the U.S. population.

Reduction gain by an atom or molecule of one or more hydrogens or electrons.

Requirement (or minimal requirement) minimal amount of a nutrient needed by the body below which normal tissue functions cannot be maintained, resulting eventually in a deficiency state.

Resting metabolic rate (RMR) the average minimal metabolism for the night and periods of the day when there is no exposure to cold and no physical exercise. The RMR includes the specific dynamic action (SDA) of food.

Retinoids synthetic derivatives of vitamin A being studied experimentally for cancer prevention.

Retinol vitamin A alcohol, the form of vitamin A found in animal foods.

Retinol binding protein (RBP) a protein synthesized by the liver required to transport vitamin A from its liver storage site into the blood.

Retinol equivalent (RE) means of expressing the vitamin A value of foods. One retinol equivalent is equal to 1 μg of retinol or 6 μg of beta-carotene.

Rhodopsin (visual purple) a pigment in cells of the retina of the eye containing vitamin A which permits vision in dim light.

Ribonucleic acid (RNA) molecule that functions with DNA in protein synthesis in cells.

Ribosomes particles in cells associated with the rough endoplasmic reticulum that are the centers of protein synthesis.

Rickets disease in children due to vitamin D deficiency, resulting in failure of bone mineralization.

Risk factor a factor that increases one's chances, statistically, of developing a disease.

Salivary amylase enzyme secreted by the salivary glands that converts starch to dextrins and maltose.

Satiety the state of feeling that one's desire for food has been satisfied.

Satiety value the ability of a food or a mixture of foods to cause one to feel satisfied that enough has been consumed.

Saturated fatty acid a fatty acid having only single covalent bonds between the carbon atoms. Each carbon atom holds all the hydrogen of which it is capable.

Saturation state in which body tissues hold all they can of a water-soluble vitamin; amounts beyond this "ceiling" are excreted in the urine.

Scurvy the disease due to a deficiency of vitamin C.

Serotonin a neurotransmitter in the brain.

Serum iron that form of iron in the blood that is being transported from one part of the body to another. It travels in the blood attached to transferrin, a protein.

Severe obesity a state of weighing 30 to 100 percent more than desirable weight for height and sex.

Skinfold thickness measurements of the width of a double layer of skin and subcutaneous fat made with standard calipers.

Small-for-date (or small-for-gestational-age) infant an infant whose body weight is inappropriately low for his or her gestational age. For full-term infants (birth at 40 weeks or later), inappropriate weight is less than 2500 g (5 ½ lb).

Smoke point the temperature at which a fat decomposes chemically, giving off visible fumes (or smoke).

Sorbitol a sugar alcohol derived from sucrose used as a sweetener in some dietetic foods and gum.

Specific dynamic action (SDA) of foods the extra heat given off when an individual under basal conditions consumes some food. Also called the calorigenic effect of food or dietary thermogenesis.

Starch a large molecule (a polysaccharide) composed only of glucose molecules.

Sucrase enzyme secreted by the intestinal mucosa that catalyzes the conversion of sucrose to glucose and fructose.

Sucrose a disaccharide made up of one molecule of glucose and one of fructose. Sucrose is common table sugar.

Synergist a substance that works along with or boosts the action of another.

Tetany a muscle disorder characterized by twitching, cramps, and convulsions.

Thermostatic hypothesis suggestion that people eat to produce heat to maintain the body temperature. This hypothesis is known not to be the only mechanism controlling hunger and satiety, but is thought to play a role in the normal control of food intake.

Thiaminase an enzyme present in raw fish which destroys thiamine.

Thiamine pyrophosphate (TPP) the coenzyme (active) form of thiamine.

Thoracic duct large lymph vessel into which fat-soluble nutrients flow during absorption from the intestines. These nutrients are carried via this duct to the subclavian vein in the neck region, and there enter the circulation.

Thyroxine (T_4) and triiodothyronine (T_3) hormones containing iodine, which are secreted by the thyroid gland and used to regulate the rate of energy metabolism.

Total vegetarians those who consume no foods of animal origin (also called *strict* or *pure* vegetarians).

Trabeculae storage sites for calcium located on the inner surfaces at the ends of the long bones.

Trace minerals or micronutrient elements those required in the diet in amounts smaller than 100 mg per day.

Transaminases enzymes requiring vitamin B_6 coenzymes that catalyze reactions in which some nonessential amino acids are produced.

Trans fatty acids fatty acids having one or more double bonds, but having a different physical shape than those occurring naturally in the body.

Transferrin a protein synthesized in the liver which is used to transport serum iron.

Triglycerides molecules made of three fatty acids and one glycerol molecule.

Trimester a 3-month period. The 9

months of pregnancy are divided into three trimesters.

Tripeptide a compound made up of three amino acids joined by two peptide bonds.

Turnover rate time required for the cycle of synthesis and breakdown of a compound to occur.

Underweight the state of weighing 15 to 20 percent below desirable weight for height and sex.

United States Recommended Daily Allowances (U.S. RDA) standards, based on the 1968 RDAs, developed by the Food and Drug Administration for labeling foods according to their nutritive contents.

Universal Product Code a series of lines and numbers on label products which allow a computer to identify the product and price at supermarket checkout counters.

Unsaturated fatty acid a fatty acid having one or more double covalent bonds between its carbons.

Urea the chief nitrogen-containing end product of protein catabolism in the body.

U.S. food system the system furnishing Americans with their food supply.

Utilization (of a nutrient) usage of a nutrient in the body's metabolism.

Valence electrons the outermost electrons circling around the nucleus of each atom. These electrons determine how the atom will combine with others in chemical reactions.

Variables factors that can change or vary—that is, either increase or decrease.

Very low density lipoprotein (VLDL) lipoproteins that carry chiefly triglyceride from the liver and intestines to body tissues.

Villi small projections of the intestinal lining (mucosa) that effectively increase the surface area of the mucosa. Each villus is covered on the mucosal side with cells into which the products of digestion must pass as absorption occurs.

Vitamin A activity (or vitamin A value) the combined contributions to the diet of vitamin A and carotenoids.

Vitamins organic compounds (other than amino acids, fatty acids or carbohydrates) required in the diet in small amounts for normal growth, maintenance and development.

Weaning the transition from breast-feeding or bottle-feeding of a child to other forms of feeding.

Xerophthalmia a serious eye disease caused by vitamin A deficiency in which epithelial tissues in the eye become ulcerated, resulting in loss of the lens, deterioration of the entire eyeball, and consequent blindness.

Xylitol a sugar alcohol used in some "sugarless" gums.

APPENDIXES

APPENDIX

APPENDIX A

RECOMMENDED DIETARY ALLOWANCES (RDAs) FOR THE UNITED STATES

TABLE 1. FOOD AND NUTRITION BOARD, NATIONAL ACADEMY OF SCIENCES–NATIONAL RESEARCH COUNCIL RECOMMENDED DAILY DIETARY ALLOWANCES,[a] Revised 1980

Designed for the maintenance of good nutrition of practically all healthy people in the U.S.A.

	Age (years)	Weight (kg)	Weight (lb)	Height (cm)	Height (in)	Protein (g)	Vitamin A (μg RE)[b]	Vitamin D (μg)[c]	Vitamin E (mg α-TE)[d]	Vitamin C (mg)	Thiamine (mg)	Riboflavin (mg)	Niacin (mg NE)[e]	Vitamin B6 (mg)	Folacin (μg)[f]	Vitamin B12 (μg)	Calcium (mg)	Phosphorus (mg)	Magnesium (mg)	Iron (mg)	Zinc (mg)	Iodine (μg)
Infants	0.0–0.5	6	13	60	24	kg × 2.2	420	10	3	35	0.3	0.4	6	0.3	30	0.5[g]	360	240	50	10	3	40
	0.5–1.0	9	20	71	28	kg × 2.0	400	10	4	35	0.5	0.6	8	0.6	45	1.5	540	360	70	15	5	50
Children	1–3	13	29	90	35	23	400	10	5	45	0.7	0.8	9	0.9	100	2.0	800	800	150	15	10	70
	4–6	20	44	112	44	30	500	10	6	45	0.9	1.0	11	1.3	200	2.5	800	800	200	10	10	90
	7–10	28	62	132	52	34	700	10	7	45	1.2	1.4	16	1.6	300	3.0	800	800	250	10	10	120
Males	11–14	45	99	157	62	45	1000	10	8	50	1.4	1.6	18	1.8	400	3.0	1200	1200	350	18	15	150
	15–18	66	145	176	69	56	1000	10	10	60	1.4	1.7	18	2.0	400	3.0	1200	1200	400	18	15	150
	19–22	70	154	177	70	56	1000	7.5	10	60	1.5	1.7	19	2.2	400	3.0	800	800	350	10	15	150
	23–50	70	154	178	70	56	1000	5	10	60	1.4	1.6	18	2.2	400	3.0	800	800	350	10	15	150
	51+	70	154	178	70	56	1000	5	10	60	1.2	1.4	16	2.2	400	3.0	800	800	350	10	15	150
Females	11–14	46	101	157	62	46	800	10	8	50	1.1	1.3	15	1.8	400	3.0	1200	1200	300	18	15	150
	15–18	55	120	163	64	46	800	10	8	60	1.1	1.3	14	2.0	400	3.0	1200	1200	300	18	15	150
	19–22	55	120	163	64	44	800	7.5	8	60	1.1	1.3	14	2.0	400	3.0	800	800	300	18	15	150
	23–50	55	120	163	64	44	800	5	8	60	1.0	1.2	13	2.0	400	3.0	800	800	300	18	15	150
	51+	55	120	163	64	44	800	5	8	60	1.0	1.2	13	2.0	400	3.0	800	800	300	10	15	150
Pregnant						+30	+200	+5	+2	+20	+0.4	+0.3	+2	+0.6	+400	+1.0	+400	+400	+150	h	+5	+25
Lactating						+20	+400	+5	+3	+40	+0.5	+0.5	+5	+0.5	+100	+1.0	+400	+400	+150	h	+10	+50

[a] The allowances are intended to provide for individual variations among most normal persons as they live in the United States under usual environmental stresses. Diets should be based on a variety of common foods in order to provide other nutrients for which human requirements have been less well defined. See Table 3 for suggested average energy intakes.

[b] Retinol equivalents. 1 retinol equivalent = 1 μg retinol or 6 μg β carotene. See text for calculation of vitamin A activity of diets as retinol equivalents.

[c] As cholecalciferol. 10 μg cholecalciferol = 400 IU of vitamin D.

[d] α-tocopherol equivalents. 1 mg d-α tocopherol = 1 α-TE.

[e] 1 NE (niacin equivalent) is equal to 1 mg of niacin or 60 mg of dietary tryptophan.

[f] The folacin allowances refer to dietary sources as determined by *Lactobacillus casei* assay after treatment with enzymes (conjugases) to make polyglutamyl forms of the vitamin available to the test organism.

[g] The recommended dietary allowance for vitamin B-12 in infants is based on the average concentration of the vitamin in human milk. The allowances after weaning are based on energy intake (as recommended by the American Academy of Pediatrics) and consideration of other factors, such as intestinal absorption; see text.

[h] The increased requirement during pregnancy cannot be met by the iron content of habitual American diets nor by the existing iron stores of many women; therefore the use of 30–60 mg of supplemental iron is recommended. Iron needs during lactation are not substantially different from those of nonpregnant women, but continued supplementation of the mother for 2–3 months after parturition is advisable in order to replenish stores depleted by pregnancy.

SOURCE: *Recommended Dietary Allowances*, 9th edition, Committee on Dietary Allowances, Food and Nutrition Board, National Academy of Sciences, Washington, D.C., 1980.

TABLE 2. ESTIMATED SAFE AND ADEQUATE DAILY DIETARY INTAKES OF SELECTED VITAMINS AND MINERALS[a]

| | Age (years) | VITAMINS | | |
		Vitamin K (µg)	Biotin (µg)	Pantothenic Acid (mg)
Infants	0–0.5	12	35	2
	0.5–1	10–20	50	3
Children	1–3	15–30	65	3
and	4–6	20–40	85	3–4
Adolescents	7–10	30–60	120	4–5
	11+	50–100	100–200	4–7
Adults		70–140	100–200	4–7

| | Age (years) | TRACE ELEMENTS[b] | | | | | |
		Copper (mg)	Manganese (mg)	Fluoride (mg)	Chromium (mg)	Selenium (mg)	Molybdenum (mg)
Infants	0–0.5	0.5–0.7	0.5–0.7	0.1–0.5	0.01–0.04	0.01–0.04	0.03–0.06
	0.5–1	0.7–1.0	0.7–1.0	0.2–1.0	0.02–0.06	0.02–0.06	0.04–0.08
Children	1–3	1.0–1.5	1.0–1.5	0.5–1.5	0.02–0.08	0.02–0.08	0.05–0.1
and	4–6	1.5–2.0	1.5–2.0	1.0–2.5	0.03–0.12	0.03–0.12	0.06–0.15
Adolescents	7–10	2.0–2.5	2.0–3.0	1.5–2.5	0.05–0.2	0.05–0.2	0.10–0.3
	11+	2.0–3.0	2.5–5.0	1.5–2.5	0.05–0.2	0.05–0.2	0.15–0.5
Adults		2.0–3.0	2.5–5.0	1.5–4.0	0.05–0.2	0.05–0.2	0.15–0.5

| | Age (years) | ELECTROLYTES | | |
		Sodium (mg)	Potassium (mg)	Chloride (mg)
Infants	0–0.5	115–350	350–925	275–700
	0.5–1	250–750	425–1275	400–1200
Children	1–3	325–975	550–1650	500–1500
and	4–6	450–1350	775–2325	700–2100
Adolescents	7–10	600–1800	1000–3000	925–2775
	11+	900–2700	1525–4575	1400–4200
Adults		1100–3300	1875–5625	1700–5100

[a] Because there is less information on which to base allowances, these figures are not given in the main table of RDAs and are provided here in the form of ranges of recommended intakes.

[b] Since the toxic levels for many trace elements may be only several times usual intakes, the upper levels for the trace elements given in this table should not be habitually exceeded.

SOURCE: *Recommended Dietary Allowances*, 9th edition, Committee on Dietary Allowances, Food and Nutrition Board, National Academy of Sciences, Washington, D.C., 1980.

TABLE 3. MEAN HEIGHTS AND WEIGHTS AND RECOMMENDED ENERGY INTAKE[a]

CATEGORY	AGE (years)	WEIGHT (kg)	WEIGHT (lb)	HEIGHT (cm)	HEIGHT (in)	ENERGY NEEDS (WITH RANGE) (kcal)		ENERGY NEEDS (WITH RANGE) (MJ)
Infants	0.0–0.5	6	13	60	24	kg x 115	(95–145)	kg x 0.48
	0.5–1.0	9	20	71	28	kg x 105	(80–135)	kg x 0.44
Children	1–3	13	29	90	35	1300	(900–1800)	5.5
	4–6	20	44	112	44	1700	(1300–2300)	7.1
	7–10	28	62	132	52	2400	(1650–3300)	10.1
Males	11–14	45	99	157	62	2700	(2000–3700)	11.3
	15–18	66	145	176	69	2800	(2100–3900)	11.8
	19–22	70	154	177	70	2900	(2500–3300)	12.2
	23–50	70	154	178	70	2700	(2300–3100)	11.3
	51–75	70	154	178	70	2400	(2000–2800)	10.1
	76+	70	154	178	70	2050	(1650–2450)	8.6
Females	11–14	46	101	157	62	2200	(1500–3000)	9.2
	15–18	55	120	163	64	2100	(1200–3000)	8.8
	19–22	55	120	163	64	2100	(1700–2500)	8.8
	23–50	55	120	163	64	2000	(1600–2400)	8.4
	51–75	55	120	163	64	1800	(1400–2200)	7.6
	76+	55	120	163	64	1600	(1200–2000)	6.7
Pregnancy						+300		
Lactation						+500		

[a] The data in this table have been assembled from the observed median heights and weights of children, together with desirable weights for adults and for the mean heights of men (70 in) and women (64 in) between the ages of 18 and 34 years as surveyed in the U.S. population (HEW/NCHS data).

The energy allowances for the young adults are for men and women doing light work. The allowances for the two older age groups represent mean energy needs over these age spans, allowing for a 2-percent decrease in basal (resting) metabolic rate per decade and a reduction in activity of 200 kcal/day for men and women between 51 and 75 years, 500 kcal for men over 75 years, and 400 kcal for women over 75 years. The customary range of daily energy output is shown in parentheses for adults and is based on a variation in energy needs of ±400 kcal at any one age, emphasizing the wide range of energy intakes appropriate for any group of people.

Energy allowances for children through age 18 are based on median energy intakes of children of these ages followed in longitudinal growth studies. The values in parentheses are 10th and 90th percentiles of energy intake, to indicate the range of energy consumption among children of these ages.

SOURCE: *Recommended Dietary Allowances*, 9th edition, Committee on Dietary Allowances, Food and Nutrition Board, National Academy of Sciences, Washington, D.C., 1980.

APPENDIX B

THE EXCHANGE LISTS

The Exchange System divides foods into six major exchange lists. No foods containing added sugar are listed. The number of kilocalories and the number of grams of carbohydrate, protein, and fat are given for one exchange in each list. Within a list, one food may be exchanged for another.

List 1. Milk Exchanges. One exchange of milk contains 12 g of carbohydrate, 8 g of protein, a trace of fat, and 80 kcal. This list shows the kinds and amounts of milk to use for one milk exchange. Those which appear in **bold type** are **non-fat.** Low-fat and whole milk contain saturated fat.

Non-Fat Fortified Milk
  Skim or non-fat milk   1 cup
  Powdered (non-fat dry, before adding liquid) $^1/_3$ cup
  Canned, evaporated—skim milk $^1/_2$ cup
  Buttermilk made from skim milk   1 cup
  Yogurt made from skim milk (plain, unflavored)   1 cup

Low-Fat Fortified Milk
  1% fat fortified milk   1 cup
    (omit $^1/_2$ fat exchange)
  2% fat fortified milk   1 cup
    (omit 1 fat exchange)
  Yogurt made from 2% fortified milk (plain, unflavored)   1 cup
    (omit 1 fat exchange)

Whole Milk (omit 2 fat exchanges)
  Whole milk   1 cup
  Canned, evaporated whole milk $^1/_2$ cup
  Buttermilk made from whole milk   1 cup
  Yogurt made from whole milk (plain, unflavored)   1 cup

List 2. Vegetable Exchanges (nonstarchy vegetables). One exchange of vegetables contains about 5 g of carbohydrate, 2 g of protein, and 25 kcal. This list shows the kinds of **vegetables** to use for one vegetable exchange. One exchange is 1/2 cup.

Asparagus	Greens:
Bean sprouts	Mustard
Beets	Spinach
Broccoli	Turnips
Brussels sprouts	Mushrooms
Cabbage	Okra
Carrots	Onions
Cauliflower	Rhubarb
Celery	Rutabaga
Eggplant	Sauerkraut
Green pepper	String beans, green or yellow
Greens:	Summer squash
Beet	Tomatoes
Chards	Tomato juice
Collards	Turnips
Dandelion	Vegetable juice cocktail
Kale	Zucchini

The following **raw vegetables** may be used as desired:

Chicory	Lettuce
Chinese cabbage	Parsley
Cucumbers	Pickles, dill
Endive	Radishes
Escarole	Watercress

Starchy vegetables are found in the Bread Exchange List.

List 3. Fruit Exchanges. One exchange of fruit contains 10 g of carbohydrate and 40 kcal. This list shows the kinds and amounts of **fruits** to use for one fruit exchange.

Apple	1 small	Mango	1/2 small
Apple juice	1/3 cup	Melon	
Applesauce (unsweetened)	1/2 cup	Cantaloupe	1/4 small
Apricots, fresh	2 medium	Honeydew	1/8 medium
Apricots, dried	4 halves	Watermelon	1 cup
Banana	1/2 small	Nectarine	1 small
Berries		Orange	1 small
Blackberries	1/2 cup	Orange juice	1/2 cup
Blueberries	1/2 cup	Papaya	3/4 cup
Raspberries	1/2 cup	Peach	1 medium
Strawberries	3/4 cup	Pear	1 small
Cherries	10 large	Persimmon, native	1 medium
Cider	1/3 cup	Pineapple	1/2 cup
Dates	2	Pineapple juice	1/3 cup
Figs, fresh	1	Plums	2 medium
Figs, dried	1	Prunes	2 medium
Grapefruit	1/2	Prune juice	1/4 cup
Grapefruit juice	1/2 cup	Raisins	2 tbsp
Grapes	12	Tangerine	1 medium
Grape juice	1/4 cup		

Cranberries may be used as desired if no sugar is added.

List 4. Bread Exchanges (includes bread, cereal, and starchy vegetables). One exchange of bread contains 15 g of carbohydrate, 2 g of protein, and 70 kcal. This list shows the kinds and amounts of **Breads, cereals, starchy vegetables,** and prepared foods to use for one bread exchange. Those which appear in **bold type** are **low-fat.**

Bread

White (including French and Italian)	1 slice
Whole wheat	1 slice
Rye or pumpernickel	1 slice
Raisin	1 slice
Bagel, small	$1/2$
English muffin, small	$1/2$
Plain roll, bread	1
Frankfurter roll	$1/2$
Hamburger bun	$1/2$
Dried bread crumbs	3 tbsp
Tortilla, 6"	1

Cereal

Bran flakes	$1/2$ cup
Other ready-to-eat unsweetened cereal	$3/4$ cup
Puffed cereal (unfrosted)	1 cup
Cereal (cooked)	$1/2$ cup
Grits (cooked)	$1/2$ cup
Rice or barley (cooked)	$1/2$ cup
Pasta (cooked), spaghetti, noodles, macaroni	$1/2$ cup
Popcorn (popped, no fat added, large kernel)	3 cups
Cornmeal (dry)	2 tbsp
Flour	$2^1/2$ tbsp
Wheat germ	$1/4$ cup

Crackers

Arrowroot	3
Graham, $2^1/2"$ sq.	2
Matzoth, 4" x 6"	$1/2$
Oyster	20
Pretzels, $3^1/8"$ long x $1/8"$ dia.	25
Rye wafers, 2" x $3^1/2"$	3
Saltines	6
Soda, $2^1/2"$ sq.	4

Dried Beans, Peas and Lentils

Beans, peas, lentils (dried and cooked)	$1/2$ cup
Baked beans, no pork (canned)	$1/4$ cup

Starchy Vegetables

Corn	$1/3$ cup
Corn on cob	1 small
Lima beans	$1/2$ cup
Parsnips	$2/3$ cup
Peas, green (canned or frozen)	$1/2$ cup
Potato, white	1 small
Potato (mashed)	$1/2$ cup
Pumpkin	$3/4$ cup
Winter squash, acorn or butternut	$1/2$ cup
Yam or sweet potato	$1/4$ cup

Prepared Foods

Biscuit 2" dia. (omit 1 fat exchange)	1
Corn bread, 2" x 2" x 1" (omit 1 fat exchange)	1
Corn muffin, 2" dia. (omit 1 fat exchange)	1
Crackers, round butter-type (omit 1 fat exchange)	5
Muffin, plain small (omit 1 fat exchange)	1
Potatoes, french fried, length 2" to $3^1/2"$ (omit 1 fat exchange)	8
Potato or corn chips (omit 2 fat exchanges)	15
Pancake, 5" x $1/2"$ (omit 1 fat exchange)	1
Waffle, 5" x $1/2"$ (omit 1 fat exchange)	1

List 5. Meat Exchanges. *Lean meat.* One exchange of lean meat (1 oz) contains 7 g of protein, 3 g of fat, and 55 kcal. This list shows the kinds and amounts of **lean meat** and other protein-rich foods to use for one low-fat meat exchange. **Trim off all visible fat.**

Beef:	Baby beef (very lean), chipped beef, chuck, flank steak, tenderloin, plate ribs, plate skirt steak, round (bottom, top), all cuts rump, spare ribs, tripe	1 oz
Lamb:	Leg, rib, sirloin, loin (roast and chops), shank, shoulder	1 oz
Pork:	Leg (whole rump, center shank), ham, smoked (center slices)	1 oz
Veal:	Leg, loin, rib, shank, shoulder, cutlets	1 oz
Poultry:	Meat *without skin* of chicken, turkey, Cornish hen, guinea hen, pheasant	1 oz
Fish:	Any fresh or frozen	1 oz
	Canned salmon, tuna, mackerel, crab and lobster,	1/4 cup
	clams, oysters, scallops, shrimp,	5 or 1 oz
	sardines, drained	3
Cheeses containing less than 5% butterfat		1 oz
Cottage cheese, dry and 2% butterfat		1/4 cup
Dried beans and peas (omit 1 bread exchange)		1/2 cup

Medium-fat meat. One exchange of medium-fat meat (1 oz) contains 7 g of protein, 5 g of fat, and 75 kcal. This list shows the kinds and amounts of medium-fat meat and other protein-rich foods to use for one medium-fat meat exchange. **Trim off all visible fat.**

Beef:	Ground (15% fat), corned beef (canned), rib eye, round (ground commercial)	1 oz
Pork:	Loin (all cuts tenderloin), shoulder arm (picnic), shoulder blade, Boston butt, Canadian bacon, boiled ham	1 oz
Liver, heart, kidney and sweetbreads (these are high in cholesterol)		1 oz
Cottage cheese, creamed		1/4 cup
Cheese:	Mozzarella, ricotta, farmer's cheese, Neufchatel,	1 oz
	parmesan	3 tbsp
Egg (high in cholesterol)		1
Peanut butter (omit 2 additional fat exchanges)		2 tbsp

High-fat meat. One exchange of high-fat meat (1 oz) contains 7 g of protein, 8 g of fat, and 100 kcal. This list shows the kinds and amounts of high-fat meat and other protein-rich foods to use for one high-fat meat exchange. **Trim off all visible fat.**

Beef:	Brisket, corned beef (brisket), ground beef (more than 20% fat), hamburger (commercial), chuck (ground commercial), roasts (rib), steaks (club and rib)	1 oz
Lamb:	Breast	1 oz
Pork:	Spare ribs, loin (back ribs), pork (ground), country style ham, deviled ham	1 oz

Veal:	Breast	1 oz
Poultry:	Capon, duck (domestic), goose	1 oz
Cheese:	Cheddar types	1 oz
Cold cuts		4 1/2" x 1/8" slice
Frankfurter		1 small

List 6. Fat Exchanges. One exchange of fat contains 5 g of fat and 45 kcal. This list shows the kinds and amounts of fat-containing foods to use for one fat exchange. To plan a diet low in saturated fat select only those exchanges which appear in **bold type**. They are **polyunsaturated**.

Margarine, soft, tub or stick*	1 tsp
Avocado (4″ in diameter)†	1/8
Oil, corn, cottonseed, safflower, soy, sunflower	1 tsp
Oil, olive†	1 tsp
Oil, peanut†	1 tsp
Olives†	5 small
Almonds†	10 whole
Pecans†	2 large whole
Peanuts†	
Spanish	20 whole
Virginia	10 whole
Walnuts	6 small
Nuts, other†	6 small
Margarine, regular stick	1 tsp
Butter	1 tsp
Bacon fat	1 tsp
Bacon, crisp	1 strip
Cream, light	2 tbsp
Cream, sour	2 tbsp
Cream, heavy	1 tbsp
Cream cheese	1 tbsp
French dressing‡	1 tbsp
Italian dressing‡	1 tbsp
Lard	1 tsp
Mayonnaise‡	1 tsp
Salad dressing, mayonnaise type‡	2 tsp
Salt pork	3/4 inch cube

*Made with corn, cottonseed, safflower, soy, or sunflower oil only.
†Fat content is primarily monounsaturated.
‡If made with corn, cottonseed, safflower, soy, or sunflower oil can be used on fat-modified diet.

SOURCE: *The American Diabetes Assn/The American Dietetic Assn* by The American Diabetic Assn and The American Dietetic Assn. Copyright 1980. Published by Prentice-Hall, Inc. The Exchange Lists are based on material in the *Exchange Lists for Meal Planning* prepared by Committees of the American Diabetes Associations, Inc. and The American Dietetic Association in cooperation with the National Institute of Arthritis, Metabolism and Digestive Diseases and the National Heart and Lung Institute, National Institutes of Health, Public Health Service, U.S. Department of Health, Education and Welfare.

APPENDIX C

NUTRITIVE VALUE OF FOODS COMMONLY CONSUMED

The following table shows the amounts of the energy nutrients, total saturated fatty acids, two unsaturated fatty acids, four minerals, and five vitamins in 730 foods commonly consumed. Values are for those portions of the food commonly eaten; for example, values for meat are for the flesh without the bone.

Foods listed are grouped under the headings:

Dairy products
Eggs
Fats and oils
Fish, shellfish, meat, and poultry
Fruits and fruit products
Grain products
Legumes (dry), nuts, and seeds
Sugars and sweets
Vegetables and vegetable products
Miscellaneous items

Values for other vitamins and minerals in foods are in Appendix D, while information on sugar and cholesterol content of foods can be found in Appendix E and F, respectively. The nutrient composition of fast foods appears in Appendix G.

DAIRY PRODUCTS (CHEESE, CREAM, IMITATION CREAM, MILK; RELATED PRODUCTS)

Butter. See Fats, oils; related products, items 103–108.

Item No. (A)	Foods, approximate measures, units, and weight (edible part unless footnotes indicate otherwise) (B)	Grams	Water (C) Per cent	Food energy (D) Calories	Protein (E) Grams	Fat (F) Grams	Fatty Acids Saturated (total) (G) Grams	Unsaturated Oleic (H) Grams	Linoleic (I) Grams	Carbohydrate (I) Grams	Calcium (K) Milligrams	Phosphorus (L) Milligrams	Iron (M) Milligrams	Potassium (N) Milligrams	Vitamin A value (O) International units	Thiamine (P) Milligrams	Riboflavin (Q) Milligrams	Niacin (R) Milligrams	Ascorbic acid (S) Milligrams
	Cheese:																		
	Natural:																		
1	Blue, 1 oz	28	42	100	6	8	5.3	1.9	0.2	1	150	110	0.1	73	200	0.01	0.11	0.3	0
2	Camembert (3 wedges per 4-oz container), 1 wedge	38	52	115	8	9	5.8	2.2	.2	Trace	147	132	.1	71	350	.01	.19	.2	0
	Cheddar:																		
3	Cut pieces, 1 oz	28	37	115	7	9	6.1	2.1	.2	Trace	204	145	.2	28	300	.01	.11	Trace	0
4	1 cu in	17.2	37	70	4	6	3.7	1.3	.1	Trace	124	88	.1	17	180	Trace	.06	Trace	0
5	Shredded, 1 cup	113	37	455	28	37	24.2	8.5	.7	1	815	579	.8	111	1,200	.03	.42	.1	0
	Cottage (curd not pressed down):																		
	Creamed (cottage cheese, 4% fat):																		
6	Large curd, 1 cup	225	79	235	28	10	6.4	2.4	.2	6	135	297	.3	190	370	.05	.37	.3	Trace
7	Small curd, 1 cup	210	79	220	26	9	6.0	2.2	.2	6	126	277	.3	177	340	.04	.34	.3	Trace
8	Low fat (2%), 1 cup	226	79	205	31	4	2.8	1.0	.1	8	155	340	.4	217	160	.05	.42	.3	Trace
9	Low fat (1%), 1 cup	226	82	165	28	2	1.5	.5	.1	6	138	302	.3	193	80	.05	.37	.3	Trace
10	Uncreamed (cottage cheese dry curd, less than 1/2% fat):																		
11	Cream, 1 oz	28	54	100	2	10	6.2	2.4	.2	1	23	30	.3	34	400	Trace	.06	Trace	0
	Mozzarella, made with—																		
12	Whole milk, 1 oz	28	48	90	6	7	4.4	1.7	.2	1	163	117	.1	21	260	Trace	.08	Trace	0
13	Part skim milk, 1 oz	28	49	80	8	5	3.1	1.2	.1	1	207	149	.1	27	180	.01	.10	Trace	0
	Parmesan, grated:																		
14	Cup, not pressed down, 1 cup	100	18	455	42	30	19.1	7.7	.3	4	1,376	807	1.0	107	700	.05	.39	.3	0
15	Tablespoon, 1 tbsp	5	18	25	2	2	1.0	.4	Trace	Trace	69	40	Trace	5	40	Trace	.02	Trace	0
16	Ounce, 1 oz	28	18	130	12	9	5.4	2.2	.1	1	390	229	.3	30	200	.01	.11	.1	0
17	Provolone, 1 oz	28	41	100	7	8	4.8	1.7	.1	1	214	141	.1	39	230	.01	.09	Trace	0
	Ricotta, made with—																		
18	Whole milk, 1 cup	246	72	430	28	32	20.4	7.1	.7	7	509	389	.9	257	1,210	.03	.48	.3	0
19	Part skim milk, 1 cup	246	74	340	28	19	12.1	4.7	.5	13	669	449	1.1	308	1,060	.05	.46	.2	0
20	Romano, 1 oz	28	31	110	9	8	—	—	—	1	302	215	—	—	160	—	.11	Trace	0
21	Swiss, 1 oz	28	37	105	8	8	5.0	1.7	.2	1	272	171	Trace	31	240	.01	.10	Trace	0
	Pasteurized process cheese:																		
22	American, 1 oz	28	39	105	6	9	5.6	2.1	.1	Trace	174	211	.1	46	340	.01	.10	Trace	0
23	Swiss, 1 oz	28	42	95	7	7	4.5	1.7	.1	1	219	216	.2	61	230	Trace	.08	Trace	0
24	Pasteurized process cheese food, American, 1 oz	28	43	95	6	7	4.4	1.7	.1	2	163	130	.2	79	260	.01	.13	Trace	0
25	Pasteurized process cheese spread, American, 1 oz	28	48	80	5	6	3.8	1.5	.1	2	159	202	.1	69	220	.01	.12	Trace	0
	Cream, sweet:																		
26	Half-and-half (cream and milk), 1 cup	242	81	315	7	28	17.3	7.0	.6	10	254	230	.2	314	260	.08	.36	.2	2
27	1 tbsp	15	81	20	Trace	2	1.1	.4	Trace	1	16	14	Trace	19	20	.01	.02	Trace	2
28	Light, coffee, or table, 1 cup	240	74	470	6	46	28.8	11.7	1.0	9	231	192	.1	292	1,730	.08	.36	.1	2
29	1 tbsp	15	74	30	Trace	3	1.8	.7	.1	1	14	12	Trace	18	110	Trace	.02	Trace	Trace
	Whipping, unwhipped (volume about double when whipped):																		

NUTRIENTS IN INDICATED QUANTITY

Item No. (A)	Foods, approximate measures, units, and weight (edible part unless footnotes indicate otherwise) (B)	(Grams)	Water (C) Percent	Food energy (D) Calories	Protein (E) Grams	Fat (F) Grams	Fatty Acids Saturated (total) (G) Grams	Unsaturated Oleic (H) Grams	Unsaturated Linoleic (I) Grams	Carbohydrate (I) Grams	Calcium (K) Milligrams	Phosphorus (L) Milligrams	Iron (M) Milligrams	Potassium (N) Milligrams	Vitamin A value (O) International units	Thiamine (P) Milligrams	Riboflavin (Q) Milligrams	Niacin (R) Milligrams	Ascorbic acid (S) Milligrams
	DAIRY PRODUCTS (CHEESE, CREAM, IMITATION CREAM, MILK; RELATED PRODUCTS)—Con.																		
	Cheese—Continued																		
	Natural—Continued																		
30	Light .... 1 cup	239	64	700	5	74	46.2	18.3	1.5	7	166	146	0.1	231	2,690	0.06	0.30	0.1	1
31	1 tbsp	15	64	45	Trace	5	2.9	1.1	.1	Trace	10	9	Trace	15	170	Trace	.02	Trace	Trace
32	Heavy .... 1 cup	238	58	820	5	88	54.8	22.2	2.0	7	154	149	.1	179	3,500	.05	.26	.1	1
33	1 tbsp	15	58	80	Trace	6	3.5	1.4	.1	Trace	10	9	Trace	11	220	Trace	.02	Trace	Trace
34	Whipped topping, (pressurized) ... 1 cup	60	61	155	2	13	8.3	3.4	.3	7	61	54	Trace	88	550	.02	.04	Trace	0
35	1 tbsp	3	61	10	Trace	1	.4	.2	Trace	Trace	3	3	Trace	4	30	Trace	Trace	Trace	0
36	Cream, sour .... 1 cup	230	71	495	7	48	30.0	12.1	1.1	10	268	195	.1	331	1,820	.08	.34	Trace	2
37	1 tbsp	12	71	25	Trace	3	1.6	.6	.1	1	14	10	Trace	17	90	Trace	.02	Trace	Trace
	Cream products, imitation (made with vegetable fat):																		
	Sweet:																		
	Creamers:																		
38	Liquid (frozen) .. 1 cup	245	77	335	2	24	22.8	.3	Trace	28	23	157	.1	467	[1]220	0	0	0	0
39	1 tbsp	15	77	20	Trace	1	1.4	Trace	0	2	1	10	Trace	29	[1]10	0	0	0	0
40	Powdered .... 1 cup	94	2	515	5	33	30.6	.9	Trace	52	21	397	.1	763	[1]190	0	[1].16	0	0
41	1 tsp	2	2	10	Trace	1	.7	Trace	0	1	Trace	8	Trace	16	[1]Trace	0	[1]Trace	0	0
	Whipped topping:																		
42	Frozen .... 1 cup	75	50	240	1	19	16.3	1.0	.2	17	5	6	.1	14	[1]650	0	0	0	0
43	1 tbsp	4	50	15	Trace	1	.9	.1	Trace	1	Trace	Trace	Trace	1	[1]30	0	0	0	0
44	Powdered, made with whole milk 1 cup	80	67	150	3	10	8.5	.6	.1	13	72	69	Trace	121	[1]290	.02	.09	Trace	1
45	1 tbsp	4	67	10	Trace	1	.4	Trace	Trace	1	4	3	Trace	6	[1]10	Trace	Trace	Trace	Trace
46	Pressurized .... 1 cup	70	60	185	1	16	13.2	1.4	.2	11	4	13	Trace	13	[1]330	0	0	0	Trace
47	1 tbsp	4	60	10	Trace	1	.8	.1	Trace	1	Trace	1	Trace	1	[1]20	0	0	0	0
48	Sour dressing (imitation sour cream) made with nonfat dry milk. 1 cup	235	75	415	8	39	31.2	4.4	1.1	11	266	205	.1	380	[1]20	.09	.38	.2	2
49	1 tbsp	12	75	20	Trace	2	1.6	.2	.1	1	14	10	Trace	19	[1]Trace	.01	.02	Trace	Trace
	Ice cream. See Milk desserts, frozen (items 75–80).																		
	Ice milk. See Milk desserts, frozen (items 81–83).																		
	Milk:																		
	Fluid:																		
50	Whole (3.3% fat): 1 cup	244	88	150	8	8	5.1	2.1	.2	11	291	228	.1	370	[2]310	.09	.40	.2	2
	Lowfat (2%):																		
51	No milk solids added: 1 cup	244	89	120	8	5	2.9	1.2	.1	12	297	232	.1	377	500	.10	.40	.2	2
	Milk solids added:																		
52	Label claim less than 10 g of protein per cup. 1 cup	245	89	125	9	5	2.9	1.2	.1	12	313	245	.1	397	500	.10	.42	.2	2
53	Label claim 10 or more grams of protein per cup (protein fortified). 1 cup	246	88	135	10	5	3.0	1.2	.1	14	352	276	.1	447	500	.11	.48	.2	3
	Lowfat (1%):																		
54	No milk solids added: 1 cup	244	90	100	8	3	1.6	.7	.1	12	300	235	.1	381	500	.10	.41	.2	2
	Milk solids added:																		
55	Label claim less than 10 g of protein per cup. 1 cup	245	90	105	9	2	1.5	.6	.1	12	313	245	.1	397	500	.10	.42	.2	2

Item	Food, approximate measure	Measure	Grams	Water (%)	Food energy (cal)	Protein (g)	Fat (g)	Saturated (g)	Oleic (g)	Linoleic (g)	Carbohydrate (g)	Calcium (mg)	Phosphorus (mg)	Iron (mg)	Potassium (mg)	Vitamin A (IU)	Thiamin (mg)	Riboflavin (mg)	Niacin (mg)	Ascorbic acid (mg)
56	Label claim 10 or more grams of protein per cup (protein fortified).	1 cup	246	89	120	10	3	1.8	0.7	0.1	14	349	273	0.1	444	500	0.11	0.47	0.2	3
	Nonfat (skim):																			
57	No milk solids added.	1 cup	245	91	85	8	Trace	.3	.1	Trace	12	302	247	.1	406	500	.09	.34	.2	2
	Milk solids added:																			
58	Label claim less than 10 g of protein per cup.	1 cup	245	90	90	9	1	0.4	0.1	Trace	12	316	255	0.1	418	500	0.10	0.43	0.2	2
59	Label claim 10 or more grams of protein per cup (protein fortified).	1 cup	246	89	100	10	1	.4	.1	Trace	14	352	275	.1	446	500	.11	.48	.2	3
60	Buttermilk	1 cup	245	90	100	8	2	1.3	.5	Trace	12	285	219	.1	371	[3]80	.08	.38	.1	2
	Canned:																			
	Evaporated, unsweetened:																			
61	Whole milk	1 cup	252	74	340	17	19	11.6	5.3	0.4	25	657	510	.5	764	[3]610	.12	.80	.5	5
62	Skim milk	1 cup	255	79	200	19	1	.3	.1	Trace	29	738	497	.7	845	[4]1,000	.11	.79	.4	3
63	Sweetened, condensed	1 cup	306	27	980	24	27	16.8	6.7	.7	166	868	775	.6	1,136	[3]1,000	.28	1.27	.6	8
	Dried:																			
	Buttermilk																			
64	Buttermilk	1 cup	120	3	465	41	7	4.3	1.7	.2	59	1,421	1,119	.4	1,910	[3]260	.47	1.90	1.1	7
	Nonfat instant:																			
65	Envelope, net wt., 3.2 oz[5]	1 envelope	91	4	325	32	1	.4	.1	Trace	47	1,120	896	.3	1,552	[6]2,160	.38	1.59	.8	5
66	Cup[7]	1 cup	68	4	245	24	Trace	.3	.1	Trace	35	837	670	.2	1,160	[6]1,610	.28	1.19	.6	4
	Milk beverages:																			
	Chocolate milk (commercial):																			
67	Regular	1 cup	250	82	210	8	8	5.3	2.2	.2	26	280	251	.6	417	[3]300	.09	.41	.3	2
68	Lowfat (2%)	1 cup	250	84	180	8	5	3.1	1.3	.1	26	284	254	.6	422	500	.10	.42	.3	2
69	Lowfat (1%)	1 cup	250	85	160	8	3	1.5	.7	.1	26	287	257	.6	426	500	.10	.46	.3	2
70	Eggnog (commercial)	1 cup	254	74	340	10	19	11.3	5.0	.6	34	330	278	.5	420	890	.09	.48	.3	4
	Malted milk, home-prepared with 1 cup of whole milk and 2 to 3 heaping tsp of malted milk powder (about 3/4 oz):																			
71	Chocolate	1 cup of milk plus 3/4 oz of powder.	265	81	235	9	9	5.5	—	—	29	304	265	.5	500	330	.14	.43	.7	2
72	Natural	1 cup of milk plus 3/4 oz of powder.	265	81	235	11	10	6.0	—	—	27	347	307	.3	529	380	.20	.54	1.3	2
	Shakes, thick:[8]																			
73	Chocolate, container, net wt., 10.6 oz.	1 container	300	72	355	9	8	5.0	2.0	.2	63	396	378	.9	672	260	.14	.67	.4	0
74	Vanilla, container, net wt., 11 oz.	1 container	313	74	350	12	9	5.9	2.4	.2	56	457	361	.3	572	360	.09	.61	.5	0
	Milk desserts, frozen:																			
	Ice cream:																			
	Regular (about 11% fat):																			
75	Hardened	1/2 gal	1,064	61	2,155	38	115	71.3	28.8	2.6	254	1,406	1,075	1.0	2,052	4,340	.42	2.63	1.1	6
76		1 cup	133	61	270	5	14	8.9	3.6	.3	32	176	134	.1	257	540	.05	.33	.1	1
77		3-fl oz container	50	61	100	2	5	3.4	1.4	.1	12	66	51	Trace	96	200	.02	.12	.1	Trace
78	Soft serve (frozen custard)	1 cup	173	60	375	7	23	13.5	5.9	.6	38	236	199	.4	338	790	.08	.45	.2	1
79	Rich (about 16% fat), hardened.	1/2 gal	1,188	59	2,805	33	190	118.3	47.8	4.3	256	1,213	927	.8	1,771	7,200	.36	2.27	.9	5
80		1 cup	148	59	350	4	24	14.7	6.0	.5	32	151	115	.1	221	900	.04	.28	.1	1
	Ice milk:																			
81	Hardened (about 4.3% fat)	1/2 gal	1,048	69	1,470	41	45	28.1	11.3	1.0	232	1,409	1,035	1.5	2,117	1,710	.61	2.78	.9	6
82		1 cup	131	69	185	5	6	3.5	1.4	.1	29	176	129	.1	265	210	.08	.35	.1	1
83	Soft serve (about 2.6% fat)	1 cup	175	70	225	8	5	2.9	1.2	.1	38	274	202	.3	412	180	.12	.54	.2	1
84	Sherbet (about 2% fat)	1/2 gal	1,542	66	2,160	17	31	19.0	7.7	.7	469	827	594	2.5	1,585	1,480	.26	.71	1.0	31
85		1 cup	193	66	270	4	4	2.4	.8	.1	59	103	74	.3	198	190	.03	.09	.1	4

[1] Vitamin A value is largely from β-carotene used for coloring. Riboflavin value for items 40–41 apply to products with added riboflavin.

[2] Applies to product without added vitamin A. With added vitamin A, value is 500 International Units (I.U.).

[3] Applies to product without added vitamin A.

[4] Applies to product with added vitamin A. Without added vitamin A, value is 20 International Units (I.U.).

[5] Yields 1 qt of fluid milk when reconstituted according to package directions.

[6] Applies to product with added vitamin A.

[7] Weight applies to product with label claim of 1 1/3 cups equal 3.2 oz.

[8] Applies to products made from thick shake mixes and that do not contain added ice cream. Products made from thick shake mixes are higher in fat and usually contain added ice cream.

Item No. (A)	Foods, approximate measures, units, and weight (edible part unless footnotes indicate otherwise) (B)	(grams)	Water (C) Percent	Food energy (D) Calories	Protein (E) Grams	Fat (F) Grams	Fatty Acids Saturated (total) (G) Grams	Unsaturated Oleic (H) Grams	Unsaturated Linoleic (I) Grams	Carbohydrate (J) Grams	Calcium (K) Milligrams	Phosphorus (L) Milligrams	Iron (M) Milligrams	Potassium (N) Milligrams	Vitamin A value (O) International units	Thiamine (P) Milligrams	Riboflavin (Q) Milligrams	Niacin (R) Milligrams	Ascorbic acid (S) Milligrams
	DAIRY PRODUCTS (CHEESE, CREAM, IMITATION CREAM, MILK: RELATED PRODUCTS)—Con.																		
	Milk desserts, other:																		
86	Custard, baked · 1 cup	265	77	305	14	15	6.8	5.4	.7	29	297	310	1.1	387	930	.11	.50	.3	1
	Puddings:																		
	From home recipe:																		
	Starch base:																		
87	Chocolate · 1 cup	260	66	385	8	12	7.6	3.3	.3	67	250	255	1.3	445	390	.05	.36	.3	1
88	Vanilla (blancmange) · 1 cup	255	76	285	9	10	6.2	2.5	.2	41	298	232	Trace	352	410	.08	.41	.3	2
89	Tapioca cream · 1 cup	165	72	220	8	8	4.1	2.5	.5	28	173	180	.7	223	480	.07	.30	.2	2
	From mix (chocolate) and milk:																		
90	Regular (cooked) · 1 cup	260	70	320	9	8	4.3	2.6	.2	59	265	247	.8	354	340	.05	.39	.3	2
91	Instant · 1 cup	260	69	325	8	7	3.6	2.2	0.3	63	374	237	1.3	335	340	.08	.39	0.3	2
	Yogurt:																		
	With added milk solids:																		
	Made with lowfat milk:																		
92	Fruit-flavored[9] · 1 container, net wt., 8 oz	227	75	230	10	3	1.8	.6	.1	42	343	269	.2	439	[10]120	.08	.40	.2	1
93	Plain · 1 container, net wt., 8 oz	227	85	145	12	4	2.3	.8	.1	16	415	326	.2	531	[10]150	.10	.49	.3	2
94	Made with nonfat milk · 1 container, net wt., 8 oz	227	85	125	13	Trace	.3	.1	Trace	17	452	355	.2	579	[10]20	.11	.53	.3	2
	Without added milk solids:																		
95	Made with whole milk · 1 container, net wt., 8 oz	227	88	140	8	7	4.8	1.7	.1	11	274	215	.1	351	280	.07	.32	.2	1
	EGGS																		
	Eggs, large (24 oz per dozen):																		
	Raw:																		
96	Whole, without shell · 1 egg	50	75	80	6	6	1.7	2.0	.6	1	28	90	1.0	65	260	.04	.15	Trace	0
97	White · 1 white	33	88	15	3	Trace	0	0	0	Trace	4	4	Trace	45	0	Trace	.09	Trace	0
98	Yolk · 1 yolk	17	49	65	3	6	1.7	2.1	.6	Trace	26	86	.9	15	310	.04	.07	Trace	0
	Cooked:																		
99	Fried in butter · 1 egg	46	72	85	5	6	2.4	2.2	.6	1	26	80	.9	58	290	.03	.13	Trace	0
100	Hard-cooked, shell removed · 1 egg	50	75	80	6	6	1.7	2.0	.6	1	28	90	1.0	65	260	.04	.14	Trace	0
101	Poached · 1 egg	50	74	80	6	6	1.7	2.0	.6	1	28	90	1.0	65	260	.04	.13	Trace	0

FATS, OILS; RELATED PRODUCTS

No.	Food	Measure																		
102	Scrambled (milk added) in butter. Also omelet.	1 egg	64	76	95	6	7	2.8	2.3	.6	1	47	97	.9	85	310	.04	.16	Trace	0
	Butter:																			
	Regular (1 brick or 4 sticks per lb):																			
103	Stick (1/2 cup)	1 stick	113	16	815	1	92	57.3	23.1	2.1	Trace	27	26	.2	29	3,470[9]	.01	.04	Trace	0
104	Tablespoon (about 1/8 stick)	1 tbsp	14	16	100	Trace	12	7.2	2.9	.3	Trace	3	3	Trace	4	430[10]	Trace	Trace	Trace	0
105	Pat (1 in square, 1/3 in high; 90 per lb)	1 pat	5	16	35	Trace	4	2.5	1.0	.1	Trace	1	1	Trace	1	150[10]	Trace	Trace	Trace	0
	Whipped (6 sticks or two 8-oz containers per lb):																			
106	Stick (1/2 cup)	1 stick	76	16	540	1	61	38.2	15.4	1.4	Trace	18	17	.1	20	2,310[12]	Trace	.03	Trace	0
107	Tablespoon (about 1/8 stick)	1 tbsp	9	16	65	Trace	8	4.7	1.9	.2	Trace	2	2	Trace	2	290[11]	Trace	Trace	Trace	0
108	Pat (1 1/4 in square, 1/3 in high; 120 per lb)	1 pat	4	16	25	Trace	3	1.9	.8	.1	Trace	1	1	Trace	1	120[11]	0	Trace	Trace	0
109	Fats, cooking (vegetable shortenings).	1 cup	200	0	1,770	0	200	48.8	88.2	48.4	0	0	0	0	0	—	0	0	0	0
110		1 tbsp	13	0	110	0	13	3.2	5.7	3.1	0	0	0	0	0	—	0	0	0	0
111	Lard	1 cup	205	0	1,850	0	205	81.0	83.8	20.5	0	0	0	0	0	0	0	0	0	0
112		1 tbsp	13	0	115	0	13	5.1	5.3	1.3	0	0	0	0	0	0	0	0	0	0
	Margarine:																			
	Regular (1 brick or 4 sticks per lb):																			
113	Stick (1/2 cup)	1 stick	113	16	815	1	92	16.7	42.9	24.9	Trace	27	26	.2	29	3,750[13]	.01	.04	Trace	0
114	Tablespoon (about 1/8 stick)	1 tbsp	14	16	100	Trace	12	2.1	5.3	3.1	Trace	3	3	Trace	4	470[12]	Trace	Trace	Trace	0
115	Pat (1 in square, 1/3 in high; 90 per lb)	1 pat	5	16	35	Trace	4	.7	1.9	1.1	Trace	1	1	Trace	1	170[12]	Trace	Trace	.1	0
116	Soft, two 8-oz containers per lb.	1 container	227	16	1,635	1	184	32.5	71.5	65.4	Trace	53	52	.4	59	7,500[12]	.01	.08	.1	0
117		1 tbsp	14	16	100	Trace	12	2.0	4.5	4.1	Trace	3	3	Trace	4	470[12]	Trace	Trace	Trace	0
	Whipped (6 sticks per lb):																			
118	Stick (1/2 cup)	1 stick	76	16	545	Trace	61	11.2	28.7	16.7	Trace	18	17	.1	20	2,500[12]	Trace	.03	Trace	0
119	Tablespoon (about 1/8 stick)	1 tbsp	9	16	70	Trace	8	1.4	3.6	2.1	Trace	2	2	Trace	2	310[12]	Trace	Trace	Trace	0
	Oils, salad or cooking:																			
120	Corn	1 cup	218	0	1,925	0	218	27.7	53.6	125.1	0	0	0	0	0	—	0	0	0	0
121		1 tbsp	14	0	120	0	14	1.7	3.3	7.8	0	0	0	0	0	—	0	0	0	0
122	Olive	1 cup	216	0	1,910	0	216	30.7	154.4	17.7	0	0	0	0	0	—	0	0	0	0
123		1 tbsp	14	0	120	0	14	1.9	9.7	1.1	0	0	0	0	0	—	0	0	0	0
124	Peanut	1 cup	216	0	1,910	0	216	37.4	98.5	67.0	0	0	0	0	0	—	0	0	0	0
125		1 tbsp	14	0	120	0	14	2.3	6.2	4.2	0	0	0	0	0	—	0	0	0	0
126	Safflower	1 cup	218	0	1,925	0	218	20.5	25.9	159.8	0	0	0	0	0	—	0	0	0	0
127		1 tbsp	14	0	120	0	14	1.3	1.6	10.0	0	0	0	0	0	—	0	0	0	0
128	Soybean oil, hydrogenated (partially hardened)	1 cup	218	0	1,925	0	218	31.8	93.1	75.6	0	0	0	0	0	—	0	0	0	0
129	Soybean-cottonseed oil blend, hydrogenated.	1 tbsp	14	0	120	0	14	2.0	5.8	4.7	0	0	0	0	0	—	0	0	0	0
130		1 cup	218	0	1,925	0	218	38.2	63.0	99.6	0	0	0	0	0	—	0	0	0	0
131		1 tbsp	14	0	120	0	14	2.4	3.9	6.2	0	0	0	0	0	—	0	0	0	0
	Salad dressings:																			
	Commercial:																			
	Blue cheese:																			
132	Regular	1 tbsp	15	32	75	1	8	1.6	1.7	3.8	1	12	11	Trace	6	30	Trace	.02	Trace	Trace
133	Low calorie (5 Cal per tsp)	1 tbsp	16	84	10	Trace	1	.5	.3	Trace	1	10	8	Trace	5	30	Trace	.01	Trace	Trace
	French:																			
134	Regular	1 tbsp	16	39	65	Trace	6	1.1	1.3	3.2	3	2	2	.1	13	—	—	—	—	—
135	Low calorie (5 Cal per tsp)	1 tbsp	16	77	15	Trace	1	.1	.1	.4	2	2	2	.1	13	—	—	—	—	—

[9] Content of fat, vitamin A, and carbohydrate varies. Consult the label when precise values are needed for special diets.

[10] Applies to product made with milk containing no added vitamin A.

[11] Based on year-round average.

[12] Based on average vitamin A content of fortified margarine. Federal specifications for fortified margarine require a minimum of 15,000 International Units (I.U.) of vitamin A per pound.

NUTRIENTS IN INDICATED QUANTITY

Item No. (A)	Foods, approximate measures, units, and weight (edible part unless footnotes indicate otherwise) (B)		Grams	Water (C) Per-cent	Food energy (D) Cal-ories	Pro-tein (E) Grams	Fat (F) Grams	Fatty Acids Satu-rated (total) (G) Grams	Unsaturated Oleic (H) Grams	Unsaturated Lino-leic (I) Grams	Car-bohy-drate (J) Grams	Cal-cium (K) Milli-grams	Phos-phorus (L) Milli-grams	Iron (M) Milli-grams	Potas-sium (N) Milli-grams	Vitamin A value (O) Inter-national units	Thia-mine (P) Milli-grams	Ribo-flavin (Q) Milli-grams	Niacin (R) Milli-grams	Ascor-bic acid (S) Milli-grams
	FATS, OILS; RELATED PRODUCTS—Con.																			
	Salad dressings:																			
	Italian:																			
136	Regular	1 tbsp	15	28	85	Trace	9	1.6	1.9	4.7	1	2	1	Trace	2		Trace	Trace	Trace	—
137	Low calorie (2 Cal per tsp)	1 tbsp	15	90	10	Trace	1	.1	.1	.4	Trace	2	1	Trace	2	Trace	Trace	Trace	Trace	—
138	Mayonnaise	1 tbsp	14	15	100	Trace	11	2.0	2.4	5.6	Trace	3	4	.1	5	40	Trace	.01	Trace	—
	Mayonnaise type:																			
139	Regular	1 tbsp	15	41	65	Trace	6	1.1	1.4	3.2	2	2	4	Trace	1	30	Trace	Trace	Trace	—
140	Low calorie (8 Cal per tsp)	1 tbsp	16	81	20	Trace	2	.4	.4	1.1	2	3	4	Trace	1	40	Trace	Trace	Trace	—
141	Tartar sauce, regular	1 tbsp	14	34	75	Trace	8	1.5	1.8	4.1	1	3	4	.1	11	30	Trace	Trace	Trace	Trace
	Thousand Island:																			
142	Regular	1 tbsp	16	32	80	Trace	8	1.4	1.7	4.0	2	2	3	.1	18	50	Trace	Trace	Trace	Trace
143	Low calorie (10 Cal per tsp)	1 tbsp	15	68	25	Trace	2	.4	.4	1.0	2	2	3	.1	17	50	Trace	Trace	Trace	Trace
	From home recipe:																			
144	Cooked type[13]	1 tbsp	16	68	25	1	2	.5	.6	.3	2	14	15	.1	19	80	.01	.03	Trace	Trace
	FISH, SHELLFISH, MEAT, POULTRY; RELATED PRODUCTS																			
	Fish and shellfish:																			
145	Bluefish, baked with butter or margarine.	3 oz	85	68	135	22	4	—	—	—	0	25	244	.6	—	40	.09	.08	1.6	—
	Clams:																			
146	Raw, meat only	3 oz	85	82	65	11	1	—	—	—	2	59	138	5.2	154	90	.08	.15	1.1	8
147	Canned, solids and liquid	3 oz	85	86	45	7	1	—	Trace	Trace	2	47	116	3.5	119	—	.01	.09	.9	—
148	Crabmeat (white or king), canned, not pressed down.	1 cup	135	77	135	24	3	0.2	0.4	0.1	1	61	246	1.1	149	—	.11	.11	2.6	—
149	Fish sticks, breaded, cooked, frozen (stick, 4 by 1 by 1/2 in).	1 fish stick or 1oz	28	66	50	5	3	—	—	—	2	3	47	.1	—	0	.01	.02	.5	—
150	Haddock, breaded, fried[14]	3 oz	85	66	140	17	5	1.4	2.2	1.2	5	34	210	1.0	296	—	.03	.06	2.7	2
151	Ocean perch, breaded, fried[14]	1 fillet	85	59	195	16	11	2.7	4.4	2.3	6	28	192	1.1	242	—	.10	.10	1.6	—
152	Oysters, raw, meat only (13-19 medium Selects).	1 cup	240	85	160	20	4	1.3	.2	.1	8	226	343	13.2	290	740	.34	.43	6.0	—
153	Salmon, pink, canned, solids and liquid.	3 oz	85	71	120	17	5	.9	.8	.1	0	[15]167	243	.7	307	60	.03	.16	6.8	—
154	Sardines, Atlantic, canned in oil, drained solids.	3 oz	85	62	175	20	9	3.0	2.5	.5	0	372	424	2.5	502	190	.02	.17	4.6	—
155	Scallops, frozen, breaded, fried, reheated.	6 scallops	90	60	175	16	8	—	—	—	9	—	—	—	—	—	—	—	—	—
156	Shad, baked with butter or margarine, bacon.	3 oz	85	64	170	20	10	—	—	—	0	20	266	.5	320	30	.11	.22	7.3	—
	Shrimp:																			
157	Canned meat	3 oz	85	70	100	21	1	.1	.1	Trace	1	98	224	2.6	104	50	.01	.03	1.5	—
158	French fried[16]	3 oz	85	57	190	17	9	2.3	3.7	2.0	9	61	162	1.7	195	—	.03	.07	2.3	—
159	Tuna, canned in oil, drained solids.	3 oz	85	61	170	24	7	1.7	1.7	.7	0	7	199	1.6	—	70	.04	.10	10.1	—
160	Tuna salad[17]	1 cup	205	70	350	30	22	4.3	6.3	6.7	7	41	291	2.7	—	590	.08	.23	10.3	2
	Meat and meat products:																			
161	Bacon, (20 slices per lb, raw), broiled or fried, crisp.	2 slices	15	8	85	4	8	2.5	3.7	.7	Trace	2	34	.5	35	0	.08	.05	.8	—

Item	Food	Measure	Grams	Water (%)	Food energy (cal)	Protein (g)	Fat (g)	Saturated (g)	Oleic (g)	Linoleic (g)	Carbohydrate (g)	Calcium (mg)	Phosphorus (mg)	Iron (mg)	Potassium (mg)	Vitamin A (IU)	Thiamin (mg)	Riboflavin (mg)	Niacin (mg)	Ascorbic acid (mg)
	Beef,[18] cooked:																			
	Cuts braised, simmered, or pot roasted:																			
162	Lean and fat (piece, 2 1/2 by 2 1/2 by 3/4 in)	3 oz	85	53	245	23	16	6.8	6.5	.4	0	10	114	2.9	184	30	.04	.18	3.6	—
163	Lean only from item 162	2.5 oz	72	62	140	22	5	2.1	1.8	.2	0	10	108	2.7	176	10	.04	.17	3.3	—
	Ground beef, broiled:																			
164	Lean with 10% fat	3 oz or patty 3 by 5/8 in	85	60	185	23	10	4.0	3.9	.3	0	10	196	3.0	261	20	.08	.20	5.1	—
165	Lean with 21% fat	2.9 oz or patty 3 by 5/8 in	82	54	235	20	17	7.0	6.7	0.4	0	9	159	2.6	221	30	0.07	0.17	4.4	—
	Roast, oven cooked, no liquid added:																			
	Relatively fat, such as rib:																			
166	Lean and fat (2 pieces, 4 1/8 by 2 1/4 by 1/4 in).	3 oz	85	40	375	17	33	14.0	13.6	.8	0	8	158	2.2	189	70	.05	.13	3.1	—
167	Lean only from item 166	1.8 oz	51	57	125	14	7	3.0	2.5	.3	0	6	131	1.8	161	10	.04	.11	2.6	—
	Relatively lean, such as heel of round:																			
168	Lean and fat (2 pieces, 4 1/8 by 2 1/4 by 1/4 in).	3 oz	85	62	165	25	7	2.8	2.7	.2	0	11	208	3.2	279	10	.06	.19	4.5	—
169	Lean only from item 168	2.8 oz	78	65	125	24	3	1.2	1.0	.1	0	10	199	3.0	268	Trace	.06	.18	4.3	—
	Steak:																			
	Relatively fat-sirloin, broiled:																			
170	Lean and fat (piece, 2 1/2 by 2 1/2 by 3/4 in).	3 oz	85	44	330	20	27	11.3	11.1	.6	0	9	162	2.5	220	50	.05	.15	4.0	—
171	Lean only from item 170	2 oz	56	59	115	18	4	1.8	1.6	.2	0	7	146	2.2	202	10	.05	.14	3.6	—
	Relatively lean-round, braised:																			
172	Lean and fat (piece, 4 1/8 by 2 1/4 by 1/2 in).	3 oz	85	55	220	24	13	5.5	5.2	.4	0	10	213	3.0	272	20	.07	.19	4.8	—
173	Lean only from item 172	2.4 oz	68	61	130	21	4	1.7	1.5	.2	0	9	182	2.5	238	10	.05	.16	4.1	—
	Beef, canned:																			
174	Corned beef	3 oz	85	59	185	22	10	4.9	4.5	.2	0	17	90	3.7	—	—	.01	.20	2.9	—
175	Corned beef hash	1 cup	220	67	400	19	25	11.9	10.9	.5	24	29	147	4.4	440	—	.02	.20	4.6	—
176	Beef, dried, chipped	2 1/2-oz jar	71	48	145	24	4	2.1	2.0	.1	0	14	287	3.6	142	—	0.05	0.23	2.7	0
177	Beef and vegetable stew	1 cup	245	82	220	16	11	4.9	4.5	.2	15	29	184	2.9	613	2,400	.15	.17	4.7	17
178	Beef potpie (home recipe), baked[19] (piece, 1/3 of 9-in diam. pie).	1 piece	210	55	515	21	30	7.9	12.8	6.7	39	29	149	3.8	334	1,720	.30	.30	5.5	6
179	Chili con carne with beans, canned.	1 cup	255	72	340	19	16	7.5	6.8	.3	31	82	321	4.3	594	150	.08	.18	3.3	—
180	Chop suey with beef and pork (home recipe).	1 cup	250	75	300	26	17	8.5	6.2	.7	13	60	248	4.8	425	600	.28	.38	5.0	33
181	Heart, beef, lean, braised	3 oz	85	61	160	27	5	1.5	1.1	.6	1	5	154	5.0	197	20	.21	1.04	6.5	1
	Lamb, cooked:																			
	Chop, rib (cut 3 per lb with bone), broiled:																			
182	Lean and fat	3.1 oz	89	43	360	18	32	14.8	12.1	1.2	0	8	139	1.0	200	—	.11	.19	4.1	—
183	Lean only from item 182	2 oz	57	60	120	16	6	2.5	2.1	.2	0	6	121	1.1	174	—	.09	.15	3.4	—
	Leg, roasted:																			
184	Lean and fat (2 pieces, 4 1/8 by 2 1/4 by 1/4 in).	3 oz	85	54	235	22	16	7.3	6.0	.6	0	9	177	1.4	241	—	.13	.23	4.7	—
185	Lean only from item 184	2.5 oz	71	62	130	20	5	2.1	1.8	.2	0	9	169	1.4	227	—	.12	.21	4.4	—
	Shoulder, roasted:																			
186	Lean and fat (3 pieces, 2 1/2 by 2 1/2 by 1/4 in).	3 oz	85	50	285	18	23	10.8	8.8	.9	0	9	146	1.0	206	—	.11	.20	4.0	—

[13] Fatty acid values apply to product made with regular-type margarine.
[14] Dipped in egg, milk or water, and breadcrumbs; fried in vegetable shortening.
[15] If bones are discarded, value for calcium will be greatly reduced.
[16] Dipped in egg, breadcrumbs, and flour or batter.
[17] Prepared with tuna, celery, salad dressing (mayonnaise type), pickle, onion, and egg.
[18] Outer layer of fat on the cut was removed to within approximately 1/2 in. of the lean. Deposits of fat within the cut were not removed.
[19] Crust made with vegetable shortening and enriched flour.

Item No. (A)	Foods, approximate measures, units, and weight (edible part unless footnotes indicate otherwise) (B)	Grams	Water (C) Per cent	Food energy (D) Calories	Protein (E) Grams	Fat (F) Grams	Fatty Acids Saturated (total) (G) Grams	Oleic (H) Grams	Linoleic (I) Grams	Carbohydrate (I) Grams	Calcium (K) Milligrams	Phosphorus (L) Milligrams	Iron (M) Milligrams	Potassium (N) Milligrams	Vitamin A value (O) International units	Thiamine (P) Milligrams	Riboflavin (Q) Milligrams	Niacin (R) Milligrams	Ascorbic acid (S) Milligrams
	FISH, SHELLFISH, MEAT, POULTRY; RELATED PRODUCTS—Con.																		
	Meat and meat products—Continued																		
	Lamb, cooked—Continued																		
	Shoulder, roasted—Continued																		
187	Lean only from item 186. 2.3 oz	64	61	130	17	6	3.6	2.3	.2	0	8	140	1.0	193	—	.10	.18	3.7	—
188	Liver, beef, fried[20] (slice, 6 1/2 by 2 3/8 by 3/8 in). 3 oz	85	56	195	22	9	2.5	3.5	.9	5	9	405	7.5	323	[21]45,390	.22	3.56	14.0	23
	Pork, cured, cooked:																		
189	Ham, light cure, lean and fat, roasted (2 pieces, 4 1/8 by 2 1/4 by 1/4 in).[22] 3 oz	85	54	245	18	19	6.8	7.9	1.7	0	8	146	2.2	199	0	.40	.15	3.1	—
	Luncheon meat:																		
190	Boiled ham, slice (8 per 8-oz pkg.). 1 oz	28	59	65	5	5	1.7	2.0	.4	0	3	47	.8	—	0	.12	.04	.7	—
	Canned, spiced or unspiced:																		
191	Slice, approx. 3 by 2 by 1/2 in. 1 slice	60	55	175	9	15	5.4	6.7	1.0	1	5	65	1.3	133	0	.19	.13	1.8	—
	Pork, fresh,[18] cooked:																		
	Chop, loin (cut 3 per lb with bone), broiled:																		
192	Lean and fat. 2.7 oz	78	42	305	19	25	8.9	10.4	2.2	0	9	209	2.7	216	0	.75	.22	4.5	—
193	Lean only from item 192. 2 oz	56	53	150	17	9	3.1	3.6	.8	0	7	181	2.2	192	0	.63	.18	3.8	—
194	Roast, oven cooked, no liquid added: Lean and fat (piece, 2 1/2 by 2 1/2 by 3/4 in). 3 oz	85	46	310	21	24	8.7	10.2	2.2	0	9	218	2.7	233	0	.78	.22	4.8	—
195	Lean only from item 194. 2.4 oz	68	55	175	20	10	3.5	4.1	.8	0	9	211	2.6	224	0	.73	.21	4.4	—
196	Lean and fat (3 pieces, 2 1/2 by 2 1/2 by 1/4 in). 3 oz	85	46	320	20	26	9.3	10.9	2.3	0	9	118	2.6	158	0	.46	0.21	4.1	—
197	Lean only from item 196. 2.2 oz	63	60	135	18	6	2.2	2.6	.6	0	8	111	2.3	146	0	.42	.19	3.7	—
	Sausages (see also Luncheon meat (items 190–191)):																		
198	Bologna, slice (8 per 8-oz pkg.). 1 slice	28	56	85	3	8	3.0	3.4	.5	Trace	2	36	.5	65	—	.05	.06	.7	—
199	Braunschweiger, slice (6 per 6-oz pkg.). 1 slice	28	53	90	4	8	2.6	3.4	.8	1	3	69	1.7	—	1,850	.05	.41	2.3	—
200	Brown and serve (10–11 per 8-oz pkg.), browned. 1 link	17	40	70	3	6	2.3	2.8	.7	Trace	—	—	—	—	—	—	—	—	—
201	Deviled ham, canned. 1 tbsp	13	51	45	2	4	1.5	1.8	.4	0	1	12	.3	—	0	.02	.01	.2	—
202	Frankfurter (8 per 1-lb pkg.), cooked (reheated). 1 frankfurter	56	57	170	7	15	5.6	6.5	1.2	1	3	57	.8	—	—	.08	.11	1.4	—
203	Meat, potted (beef, chicken, turkey), canned. 1 tbsp	13	61	30	2	2	—	—	—	0	—	—	—	—	—	Trace	.03	.2	—
204	Pork link (16 per 1-lb pkg.), cooked. 1 link	13	35	60	2	6	2.1	2.4	.5	Trace	1	21	.3	35	0	.10	.04	.5	—
	Salami:																		
205	Dry type, slice (12 per 4-oz pkg.). 1 slice	10	30	45	2	4	1.6	1.6	.1	Trace	1	28	.4	—	—	.04	.03	.5	—
206	Cooked type, slice (8 per 8-oz pkg.). 1 slice	28	51	90	5	7	3.1	3.0	.2	Trace	3	57	.7	—	—	.07	.07	1.2	—
207	Vienna sausage (7 per 4-oz can). 1 sausage	16	63	40	2	3	1.2	1.4	.2	Trace	1	24	.3	—	—	.01	.02	.4	—
	Veal, medium fat, cooked, bone removed:																		
208	Cutlet (4 1/8 by 2 1/4 by 1/2 in), braised or broiled. 3 oz	85	60	185	23	9	4.0	3.4	.4	0	9	196	2.7	258	—	.06	.21	4.6	—

No.	Food, approximate measure	Measure	Grams	Water (%)	Food energy (cal)	Protein (g)	Fat (g)	Saturated (total) (g)	Oleic (g)	Linoleic (g)	Carbohydrate (g)	Calcium (mg)	Phosphorus (mg)	Iron (mg)	Potassium (mg)	Vitamin A (IU)	Thiamin (mg)	Riboflavin (mg)	Niacin (mg)	Ascorbic acid (mg)
209	Rib (2 pieces, 4 1/8 by 2 1/4 by 1/4 in), roasted.	3 oz	85	55	230	23	14	6.1	5.1	.6	0	10	211	2.9	259	—	.11	.26	6.6	—
	Poultry and poultry products:																			
	Chicken, cooked:																			
210	Breast, fried,[23] bones removed, 1/2 breast (3.3 oz with bones).	2.8 oz	79	58	160	26	5	1.4	1.8	1.1	1	9	218	1.3	—	70	.04	.17	11.6	—
211	Drumstick, fried,[23] bones removed (2 oz with bones).	1.3 oz	38	55	90	12	4	1.1	1.3	.9	Trace	6	89	.9	—	50	.03	.15	2.7	—
212	Half broiler, broiled, bones removed (10.4 oz with bones).	6.2 oz	176	71	240	42	7	2.2	2.5	1.3	0	16	355	3.0	483	160	.09	.34	15.5	—
213	Chicken, canned, boneless	3 oz	85	65	170	18	10	3.2	3.8	2.0	0	18	210	1.3	117	200	.03	.11	3.7	3
214	Chicken a la king, cooked (home recipe).	1 cup	245	68	470	27	34	2.7	14.3	3.3	12	127	358	2.5	404	1,130	.10	.42	5.4	12
215	Chicken and noodles, cooked (home recipe).	1 cup	240	71	365	22	18	5.9	7.1	3.5	26	26	247	2.2	149	430	.05	.17	4.3	Trace
	Chicken chow mein:																			
216	Canned	1 cup	250	89	95	7	Trace	—	—	—	18	45	85	1.3	418	150	.05	.10	1.0	13
217	From home recipe	1 cup	250	78	255	31	10	2.4	3.4	3.1	10	58	293	2.5	473	280	.08	.23	4.3	10
218	Chicken potpie (home recipe), baked,[19] piece (1/3 or 9-in diam. pie).	1 piece	232	57	545	23	31	11.3	10.9	5.6	42	70	232	3.0	343	3,090	.34	.31	5.5	5
	Turkey, roasted, flesh without skin:																			
219	Dark meat, piece, 2 1/2 by 1 5/8 by 1/4 in.	4 pieces	85	61	175	26	7	2.1	1.5	1.5	0	—	—	2.0	338	—	.03	.20	3.6	—
220	Light meat, piece, 4 by 2 by 1/4 in.	2 pieces	85	62	150	28	3	.9	.6	.7	0	—	—	1.0	349	—	.04	.12	9.4	—
	Light and dark meat:																			
221	Chopped or diced	1 cup	140	61	265	44	9	2.5	1.7	1.8	0	11	351	2.5	514	—	.07	.25	10.8	—
222	Pieces (1 slice white meat, 4 by 2 by 1/4 in with 2 slices dark meat, 2 1/2 by 1 5/8 by 1/4 in).	3 pieces	85	61	160	27	5	1.5	1.0	1.1	0	7	213	1.5	312	—	.04	.15	6.5	—
	FRUITS AND FRUIT PRODUCTS																			
	Apples, raw, unpeeled, without cores:																			
223	2 3/4-in diam. (about 3 per lb with cores).	1 apple	138	84	80	Trace	1	—	—	—	20	10	14	.4	152	120	.04	.03	.1	6
224	3 1/4 in diam. (about 2 per lb with cores).	1 apple	212	84	125	Trace	1	—	—	—	31	15	21	.6	233	190	.06	.04	.2	8
225	Apple juice, bottled or canned[24]	1 cup	248	88	120	Trace	Trace	—	—	—	30	15	22	1.5	250	—	.02	.05	.2	[25]2
	Applesauce, canned:																			
226	Sweetened	1 cup	255	76	230	1	Trace	—	—	—	61	10	13	1.3	166	100	.05	.03	.1	[25]3
227	Unsweetened	1 cup	244	89	100	Trace	Trace	—	—	—	26	10	12	1.2	190	100	.05	.02	.1	[25]2
	Apricots:																			
228	Raw, without pits (about 12 per lb with pits).	3 apricots	107	85	55	1	Trace	—	—	—	14	18	25	0.5	301	2,890	0.03	0.04	0.6	11
229	Canned in heavy sirup (halves and sirup).	1 cup	258	77	220	2	Trace	—	—	—	57	28	39	.8	604	4,490	.05	.05	1.0	10
	Dried:																			
230	Uncooked (28 large or 37 medium halves per cup).	1 cup	130	25	340	7	1	—	—	—	86	87	140	7.2	1,273	14,170	.01	.21	4.3	16
231	Cooked, unsweetened, fruit and liquid.	1 cup	250	76	215	4	1	—	—	—	54	55	88	4.5	795	7,500	.01	.13	2.5	8
232	Apricot nectar, canned	1 cup	251	85	145	1	Trace	—	—	—	37	23	30	.5	379	2,380	.03	.03	.5	[26]36

[18] Outer layer of fat on the cut was removed to within approximately 1/2 in of the lean. Deposits of fat within the cut were not removed.
[19] Crust made with vegetable shortening and enriched flour.
[20] Regular-type margarine used.
[21] Value varies widely.
[22] About one-fourth of the outer layer of fat on the cut was removed. Deposits of fat within the cut were not removed.
[23] Vegetable shortening used.
[24] Also applies to pasteurized apple cider.
[25] Applies to product without added ascorbic acid. For value of product with added ascorbic acid, refer to label.

Item No. (A)	Foods, approximate measures, units, and weight (edible part unless footnotes indicate otherwise) (B)	Grams	Water (C) Per-cent	Food energy (D) Cal-ories	Pro-tein (E) Grams	Fat (F) Grams	Fatty Acids Satu-rated (total) (G) Grams	Unsaturated Oleic (H) Grams	Lino-leic (I) Grams	Car-bohy-drate (I) Grams	Cal-cium (K) Milli-grams	Phos-phorus (L) Milli-grams	Iron (M) Milli-grams	Potas-sium (N) Milli-grams	Vitamin A value (O) Inter-national units	Thia-mine (P) Milli-grams	Ribo-flavin (Q) Milli-grams	Niacin (R) Milli-grams	Ascor-bic acid (S) Milli-grams
	FRUITS AND FRUIT PRODUCTS—Con.																		
	Avocados, raw, whole, without skins and seeds:																		
233	California, mid- and late-winter (with skin and seed, 3 1/8-in diam.; wt., 10 oz). 1 avocado	216	74	370	5	37	5.5	22.0	3.7	13	22	91	1.3	1,303	630	.24	.43	3.5	30
234	Florida, late summer and fall (with skin and seed, 3 5/8-in diam.; wt., 1 lb). 1 avocado	304	78	390	4	33	6.7	15.7	5.3	27	30	128	1.8	1,836	880	.33	.61	4.9	43
235	Banana without peel (about 2.6 per lb with peel). 1 banana	119	76	100	1	Trace	—	—	—	26	10	31	.8	440	230	.06	.07	.8	12
236	Banana flakes 1 tbsp	6	3	20	Trace	Trace	—	—	—	5	2	6	.2	92	50	.01	.01	.2	Trace
237	Blackberries, raw 1 cup	144	85	85	2	1	—	—	—	19	46	27	1.3	245	290	.04	.06	.6	30
238	Blueberries, raw 1 cup	145	83	90	1	1	—	—	—	22	22	19	1.5	117	150	.04	.09	.7	20
	Cantaloup. See Muskmelons (item 271).																		
	Cherries:																		
239	Sour (tart), red, pitted, canned, water pack. 1 cup	244	88	105	2	Trace	—	—	—	26	37	32	.7	317	1,660	.07	.05	.5	12
240	Sweet, raw, without pits and stems. 10 cherries	68	80	45	1	Trace	—	—	—	12	15	13	.3	129	70	.03	.04	.3	7
241	Cranberry juice cocktail, bottled, sweetened. 1 cup	253	83	165	Trace	Trace	—	—	—	42	13	8	.8	25	Trace	.03	.03	.1	[27]81
242	Cranberry sauce, sweetened, canned, strained. 1 cup	277	62	405	Trace	1	—	—	—	104	17	11	.6	83	60	.03	.03	.1	6
	Dates:																		
243	Whole, without pits 10 dates	80	23	220	2	Trace	—	—	—	58	47	50	2.4	518	40	.07	.08	1.8	0
244	Chopped 1 cup	178	23	490	4	1	—	—	—	130	105	112	5.3	1,153	90	.16	.18	3.9	0
245	Fruit cocktail, canned, in heavy sirup. 1 cup	255	80	195	1	Trace	—	—	—	50	23	31	1.0	411	360	.05	.03	1.0	5
	Grapefruit:																		
	Raw, medium, 3 3/4-in diam. (about 1 lb 1 oz):																		
246	Pink or red 1/2 grapefruit with peel[28]	241	89	50	1	Trace	—	—	—	13	20	20	.5	166	540	.05	.02	.2	44
247	White 1/2 grapefruit with peel[28]	241	89	45	1	Trace	—	—	—	12	19	19	.5	159	10	.05	.02	.2	44
248	Canned, sections with sirup 1 cup	254	81	180	2	Trace	—	—	—	45	33	36	.8	343	30	.08	.05	.5	76
	Grapefruit juice:																		
249	Raw, pink, red, or white 1 cup	246	90	95	1	Trace	—	—	—	23	22	37	.5	399	(29)	.10	.05	.5	93
	Canned, white:																		
250	Unsweetened 1 cup	247	89	100	1	Trace	—	—	—	24	20	35	1.0	400	20	.07	.05	.5	84
251	Sweetened 1 cup	250	86	135	1	Trace	—	—	—	32	20	35	1.0	405	30	.08	.05	.5	78
	Frozen, concentrate, unsweetened:																		
252	Undiluted, 6-fl oz can 1 can	207	62	300	4	1	—	—	—	72	70	124	.8	1,250	60	.29	.12	1.4	286
253	Diluted with 3 parts water by volume. 1 cup	247	89	100	1	Trace	—	—	—	24	25	42	.2	420	20	.10	.04	.5	96
254	Dehydrated crystals, prepared with water (1 lb yields about 1 gal). 1 cup	247	90	100	1	Trace	—	—	—	24	22	40	.2	412	20	.10	.05	.5	91
	Grapes, European type (adherent skin), raw:																		
255	Thompson Seedless 10 grapes	50	81	35	Trace	Trace	—	—	—	9	6	10	.2	87	50	.03	.02	.2	2
256	Tokay and Emperor, seeded types 10 grapes[30]	60	81	40	Trace	Trace	—	—	—	10	7	11	.2	99	60	.03	.02	.2	2

Item No.	Food, approximate measure	Weight (g)	Water (%)	Food energy (Cal)	Protein (g)	Fat (g)	Saturated	Oleic	Linoleic	Carbohydrate (g)	Calcium (mg)	Phosphorus (mg)	Iron (mg)	Potassium (mg)	Vitamin A (IU)	Thiamin (mg)	Riboflavin (mg)	Niacin (mg)	Ascorbic acid (mg)
	Grapejuice:																		
257	Canned or bottled — 1 cup	253	83	165	1	Trace	—	—	—	42	28	30	.8	293	—	.10	.05	.5	Trace[26]
	Frozen concentrate, sweetened:																		
258	Undiluted, 6-fl oz can — 1 can	216	53	395	1	Trace	—	—	—	100	22	32	.9	255	40	.13	.22	1.5	32[31]
259	Diluted with 3 parts water by volume — 1 cup	250	86	135	1	Trace	—	—	—	33	8	10	.3	85	10	.05	.08	.5	10[31]
260	Grape drink, canned — 1 cup	250	86	135	Trace	Trace	—	—	—	35	8	10	.3	88	—	.03[32]	.03[32]	.3	(32)
261	Lemon, raw, size 165, without peel and seeds (about 4 per lb with peels and seeds) — 1 lemon	74	90	20	1	Trace	—	—	—	6	19	12	.4	102	10	.03	.01	.1	39
	Lemon juice:																		
262	Raw — 1 cup	244	91	60	1	Trace	—	—	—	20	17	24	.5	344	50	.07	.02	.2	112
263	Canned, or bottled, unsweetened — 1 cup	244	92	55	1	Trace	—	—	—	19	17	24	.5	344	50	.07	.02	.2	102
264	Frozen, single strength, unsweetened, 6-fl oz can — 1 can	183	92	40	1	Trace	—	—	—	13	13	16	.5	258	40	.05	.02	.2	81
	Lemonade concentrate, frozen:																		
265	Undiluted, 6-fl oz can — 1 can	219	49	425	Trace	Trace	—	—	—	112	9	13	.4	153	40	.05	.06	.7	66
266	Diluted with 4 1/3 parts water by volume — 1 cup	248	89	105	Trace	Trace	—	—	—	28	2	3	.1	40	10	.01	.02	.2	17
	Limeade concentrate, frozen:																		
267	Undiluted, 6-fl oz can — 1 can	218	50	410	Trace	Trace	—	—	—	108	11	13	0.2	129	Trace	.02	.02	.2	26
268	Diluted with 4 1/3 parts water by volume — 1 cup	247	89	100	Trace	Trace	—	—	—	27	3	3	Trace	32	Trace	Trace	Trace	Trace	6
	Lime juice:																		
269	Raw — 1 cup	246	90	65	1	Trace	—	—	—	22	22	27	.5	256	20	.05	.02	.2	79
270	Canned, unsweetened — 1 cup	246	90	65	1	Trace	—	—	—	22	22	27	.5	256	20	.05	.02	.2	52
	Muskmelons, raw, with rind, without seed cavity:																		
271	Cantaloup, orange-fleshed (with rind and seed cavity, 5-in diam., 2 1/3 lb) — 1/2 melon with rind[33]	477	91	80	2	Trace	—	—	—	20	38	44	1.1	682	9,240	.11	.08	1.6	90
272	Honeydew (with rind and seed cavity, 6 1/2-in diam., 5 1/4 lb) — 1/10 melon with rind[33]	226	91	50	1	Trace	—	—	—	11	21	24	.6	374	60	.06	.04	.9	34
	Oranges, all commercial varieties, raw:																		
273	Whole, 2 5/8-in diam., without peel and seeds (about 2 1/2 per lb with peel and seeds) — 1 orange	131	86	65	1	Trace	—	—	—	16	54	26	.5	263	260	.13	.05	.5	66
274	Sections without membranes — 1 cup	180	86	90	2	Trace	—	—	—	22	74	36	.7	360	360	.18	.07	.7	90
	Orange juice:																		
275	Raw, all varieties — 1 cup	248	88	110	2	Trace	—	—	—	26	27	42	.5	496	500	.22	.07	1.0	124
276	Canned, unsweetened — 1 cup	249	87	120	2	Trace	—	—	—	28	25	45	1.0	496	500	.17	.05	.7	100
	Frozen concentrate:																		
277	Undiluted, 6-fl oz can — 1 can	213	55	360	5	Trace	—	—	—	87	75	126	.9	1,500	1,620	.68	.11	2.8	360
278	Diluted with 3 parts water by volume — 1 cup	249	87	120	2	Trace	—	—	—	29	25	42	.2	503	540	.23	.03	.9	120
279	Dehydrated crystals, prepared with water (1 lb yields about 1 gal) — 1 cup	248	88	115	1	Trace	—	—	—	27	25	40	.5	518	500	.20	.07	1.0	109
	Orange and grapefruit juice: Frozen concentrate:																		
280	Undiluted, 6-fl oz can — 1 can	210	59	330	4	1	—	—	—	78	61	99	.8	1,308	800	.48	.06	2.3	302
281	Diluted with 3 parts water by volume — 1 cup	248	88	110	1	Trace	—	—	—	26	20	32	.2	439	270	.15	.02	.7	102
282	Papayas, raw, 1/2-in cubes — 1 cup	140	89	55	1	Trace	—	—	—	14	28	22	.4	328	2,450	.06	.06	.4	78

[26] Based on product with label claim of 45% of U.S. RDA in 6 fl oz.

[27] Based on product with label claim of 100% of U.S. RDA in 6 fl oz.

[28] Weight includes peel and membranes between sections. Without these parts, the weight of the edible portion is 123 g for item 246 and 118 g for item 247.

[29] For white-fleshed varieties, value is about 20 International Units (I.U.) per cup; for red-fleshed varieties, 1,080 I.U.

[30] Weight includes seeds. Without seeds, weight of the edible portion is 57 g.

[31] Applies to product without added ascorbic acid. With added ascorbic acid, based on claim that 6 fl oz of reconstituted juice contain 45% or 50% of the U.S. RDA, value in milligrams is 108 or 120 for a 6-fl oz can (item 258), 36 or 40 for 1 cup of diluted juice (item 259).

[32] For products with added thiamin and riboflavin but without added ascorbic acid, values in milligrams would be 0.60 for thiamin, 0.80 for riboflavin, and trace for ascorbic acid. For products with only ascorbic acid added, value varies with the brand. Consult the label.

[33] Weight includes rind. Without rind, the weight of the edible portion is 272 g for item 271 and 149 g for item 272.

Item No.	Foods, approximate measures, units, and weight (edible part unless footnotes indicate otherwise)	Grams	Water Per-cent	Food energy Cal-ories	Pro-tein Grams	Fat Grams	Fatty Acids Satu-rated (total) Grams	Unsaturated Oleic Grams	Lino-leic Grams	Car-bohy-drate Grams	Cal-cium Milli-grams	Phos-phorus Milli-grams	Iron Milli-grams	Potas-sium Milli-grams	Vitamin A value Inter-national units	Thia-mine Milli-grams	Ribo-flavin Milli-grams	Niacin Milli-grams	Ascor-bic acid Milli-grams
(A)	(B)		(C)	(D)	(E)	(F)	(G)	(H)	(I)	(J)	(K)	(L)	(M)	(N)	(O)	(P)	(Q)	(R)	(S)
	FRUITS AND FRUIT PRODUCTS—Con.																		
	Peaches:																		
	Raw:																		
283	Whole, 2 1/2-in diam., peeled, pitted (about 4 per lb with peels and pits). 1 peach	100	89	40	1	Trace	-	-	-	10	9	19	.5	202	[34]1,330	.02	.05	1.0	7
284	Sliced 1 cup	170	89	65	1	Trace	-	-	-	16	15	32	.9	343	[34]2,26-	.03	.09	1.7	12
	Canned, yellow-fleshed, solids and liquid (halves or slices):																		
285	Sirup pack 1 cup	256	79	200	1	Trace	-	-	-	51	10	31	.8	333	1,100	.03	.05	1.5	8
286	Water pack 1 cup	244	91	75	1	Trace	-	-	-	20	10	32	.7	334	1,100	.02	.07	1.5	7
	Dried:																		
287	Uncooked 1 cup	160	25	420	5	1	-	-	-	109	77	187	9.6	1,520	6,240	.02	.30	8.5	29
288	Cooked, unsweetened, halves and juice. 1 cup	250	77	205	3	1	-	-	-	54	38	93	4.8	743	3,050	.01	.15	3.8	5
	Frozen, sliced, sweetened:																		
289	10-oz container 1 container	284	77	250	1	Trace	-	-	-	64	11	37	1.4	352	1,850	.03	.11	2.0	[35]116
290	Cup 1 cup	250	77	220	1	Trace	-	-	-	57	10	33	1.3	310	1,630	.03	.10	1.8	[35]103
	Pears:																		
	Raw, with skin, cored:																		
291	Bartlett, 2 1/2-in diam. (about 2 1/2 per lb with cores and stems). 1 pear	164	83	100	1	1	-	-	-	25	13	18	.5	213	30	.03	.07	.2	7
292	Bosc, 2 1/2-in diam. (about 3 per lb with cores and stems). 1 pear	141	83	85	1	1	-	-	-	22	11	16	.4	83	30	.03	.06	.1	6
293	D'Anjou, 3-in diam. (about 2 per lb with cores and stems). 1 pear	200	83	120	1	1	-	-	-	31	16	22	.6	260	40	.04	.08	.2	8
294	Canned, solids and liquid, sirup pack, heavy (halves or slices). 1 cup	255	80	195	1	1	-	-	-	50	13	18	.5	214	10	.03	.05	.3	3
	Pineapple:																		
295	Raw, diced 1 cup	155	85	80	1	Trace	-	-	-	21	26	12	.8	226	110	.14	.05	.3	26
	Canned, heavy sirup pack, solids and liquid:																		
296	Crushed, chunks, tidbits 1 cup	255	80	190	1	Trace	-	-	-	49	28	13	.8	245	130	.20	0.05	0.5	18
	Slices and liquid:																		
297	Large 1 slice; 2 1/4 tbsp liquid.	105	80	80	Trace	Trace	-	-	-	20	12	5	.3	101	50	.08	.02	.2	7
298	Medium 1 slice; 1 1/4 tbsp liquid.	58	80	45	Trace	Trace	-	-	-	11	6	3	.2	56	30	.05	.01	.1	4
299	Pineapple juice, unsweetened, canned. 1 cup	250	86	140	1	Trace	-	-	-	34	38	23	.8	373	130	.13	.05	.5	[27]80
	Plums:																		
	Raw, without pits:																		
300	Japanese and hybrid (2 1/8-in diam., about 6 1/2 per lb with pits). 1 plum	66	87	30	Trace	Trace	-	-	-	8	8	12	.3	112	160	.02	.02	.3	4
301	Prune type (1 1/2-in diam., about 15 per lb with pits). 1 plum	28	79	20	Trace	Trace	-	-	-	6	3	5	.1	48	80	.01	.01	.1	1
	Canned, heavy sirup pack (Italian prunes), with pits and liquid:																		
302	Cup 1 cup[36]	272	77	215	1	Trace	-	-	-	56	23	26	2.3	367	3,130	.05	.05	1.0	5
303	Portion 3 plums; 2 3/4 tbsp liquid[36]	140	77	110	1	Trace	-	-	-	29	12	13	1.2	189	1,610	.03	.03	.5	3

No.	Food	Measure	Grams	Water %	Food energy (cal)	Protein (g)	Fat (g)	Saturated	Oleic	Linoleic	Carbohydrate (g)	Calcium (mg)	Phosphorus (mg)	Iron (mg)	Potassium (mg)	Vitamin A (I.U.)	Thiamin (mg)	Riboflavin (mg)	Niacin (mg)	Ascorbic acid (mg)
	Prunes, dried, "softenized," with pits:																			
304	Uncooked	4 extra large or 5 large prunes[36]	49	28	110	Trace	Trace	–	–	–	29	22	34	1.7	298	690	.04	.07	.7	1
305	Cooked, unsweetened, all sizes, and liquid.	1 cup[36]	250	66	255	1	1	–	–	–	67	51	79	3.8	695	1,590	.07	.15	1.5	2
306	Prune juice, canned or bottled	1 cup	256	80	195	1	Trace	–	–	–	49	36	51	1.8	602	–	.03	.03	1.0	5
	Raisins, seedless:																			
307	Cup, not pressed down	1 cup	145	18	420	4	Trace	–	–	–	112	90	146	5.1	1,106	30	.16	.12	.7	1
308	Packet, 1/2 oz (1 1/2 tbsp)	1 packet	14	18	40	Trace	Trace	–	–	–	11	9	14	.5	107	Trace	.02	.01	.1	Trace
	Raspberries, red:																			
309	Raw, capped, whole	1 cup	123	84	70	1	1	–	–	–	17	27	27	1.1	207	160	.04	.11	1.1	31
310	Frozen, sweetened, 10-oz container	1 container	284	74	280	2	1	–	–	–	70	37	48	1.7	284	200	.06	.17	1.7	60
	Rhubarb, cooked, added sugar:																			
311	From raw	1 cup	270	63	380	1	Trace	–	–	–	97	211	41	1.6	548	220	.05	.14	.8	16
312	From frozen, sweetened	1 cup	270	63	385	1	1	–	–	–	98	211	32	1.9	475	190	.05	.11	.5	16
	Strawberries:																			
313	Raw, whole berries, capped	1 cup	149	90	55	1	1	–	–	–	13	31	31	1.5	244	90	.04	.10	.9	88
	Frozen, sweetened:																			
314	Sliced, 10-oz container	1 container	284	71	310	1	1	–	–	–	79	40	48	2.0	318	90	.06	.17	1.4	51
315	Whole, 1-lb container (about 1 3/4 cups).	1 container	454	76	415	2	1	–	–	–	107	59	73	2.7	472	140	.09	.27	2.3	49
316	Tangerine, raw, 2 3/8-in diam., size 176, without peel (about 4 lb with peels and seeds).	1 tangerine	86	87	40	1	Trace	–	–	–	10	34	15	.3	108	360	.05	.02	.1	27
317	Tangerine juice, canned, sweetened.	1 cup	249	87	125	1	Trace	–	–	–	30	44	35	.5	440	1,040	.15	.05	.2	54
318	Watermelon, raw, 4 by 8 in wedge with rind and seeds (1/16 of 32 2/3-lb melon, 10 by 16 in).	1 wedge with rind and seeds[37]	926	93	110	2	1	–	–	–	27	30	43	2.1	426	2,510	.13	.13	.9	30
	GRAIN PRODUCTS																			
	Bagel, 3-in diam.:																			
319	Egg	1 bagel	55	32	165	6	2	0.5	0.9	0.8	28	9	43	1.2	41	30	.14	.10	1.2	0
320	Water	1 bagel	55	29	165	6	1	.2	.4	.6	30	8	41	1.2	42	0	.15	.11	1.4	0
321	Barley, pearled, light, uncooked	1 cup	200	11	700	16	2	.3	.2	.8	158	32	378	4.0	320	0	.24	.10	6.2	0
	Biscuits, baking powder, 2-in diam. (enriched flour, vegetable shortening):																			
322	From home recipe	1 biscuit	28	27	105	2	5	1.2	2.0	1.2	13	34	49	.4	33	Trace	.08	.08	.7	Trace
323	From mix	1 biscuit	28	29	90	2	3	.6	1.1	.7	15	19	65	.6	32	Trace	.09	.08	.8	Trace
324	Breadcrumbs (enriched):[38] Dry, grated	1 cup	100	7	390	13	5	1.0	1.6	1.4	73	122	141	3.6	152	Trace	.35	.35	4.8	Trace
	Breads:																			
325	Boston brown bread, canned, slice, 3 1/4 by 1/2 in.[38]	1 slice	45	45	95	2	1	.1	.2	.2	21	41	72	.9	131	[39]0	.06	.04	.7	0
	Cracked-wheat bread (3/4 enriched wheat flour, 1/4 cracked wheat):[38]																			
326	Loaf, 1 lb	1 loaf	454	35	1,195	39	10	2.2	3.0	3.9	236	399	581	9.5	608	Trace	1.52	1.13	14.4	Trace

Based on product with label claim of 100% of U.S. RDA in 6 fl oz.

Represents yellow-fleshed varieties. For white-fleshed varieties, value is 50 International Units (I.U.) for 1 peach, 90 I.U. for 1 cup of slices.

Value represents products without added ascorbic acid. For products with added ascorbic acid, value in milligrams is 116 for a 10-oz container, 103 for 1 cup.

Weight includes pits. After removal of the pits, the weight of the edible portion is 258 g for item 302, 133 g for item 303, 43 g for item 304, and 213 g for item 305.

Weight includes rind and seeds. Without rind and seeds, weight of the edible portion is 426 g.

[38] Made with vegetable shortening.

Item No. (A)	Foods, approximate measures, units, and weight (edible part unless footnotes indicate otherwise) (B)		Water (C) Per-cent	Food energy (D) Cal-ories	Pro-tein (E) Grams	Fat (F) Grams	Fatty Acids Satu-rated (total) (G) Grams	Unsaturated Oleic (H) Grams	Unsaturated Lino-leic (I) Grams	Car-bohy-drate (J) Grams	Cal-cium (K) Milli-grams	Phos-phorus (L) Milli-grams	Iron (M) Milli-grams	Potas-sium (N) Milli-grams	Vitamin A value (O) Inter-national units	Thia-mine (P) Milli-grams	Ribo-flavin (Q) Milli-grams	Niacin (R) Milli-grams	Ascor-bic acid (S) Milli-grams
		Grams																	
	GRAIN PRODUCTS—Con.																		
	Breads—Continued																		
	Cracked-wheat bread (3/4 enriched wheat flour, 1/4 cracked wheat):[38]—Continued																		
327	Slice (18 per loaf)	1 slice	25	35	65	2	1	0.1	0.2	0.2	13	22	32	0.5	34	Trace	0.08	0.06	0.8	Trace
328	French or vienna bread, enriched:[38] Loaf, 1 lb		454	31	1,315	41	14	3.2	4.7	4.6	251	195	386	10.0	408	Trace	1.80	1.10	15.0	Trace
	Slice:																		
329	French (5 by 2 1/2 by 1 in)	1 slice	35	31	100	3	1	.2	.4	.4	19	15	30	.8	32	Trace	.14	.08	1.2	Trace
330	Vienna (4 3/4 by 4 by 1/2 in)	1 slice	25	31	75	2	1	.2	.3	.3	14	11	21	.6	23	Trace	.10	.06	.8	Trace
	Italian bread, enriched:																		
331	Loaf, 1 lb		454	32	1,250	41	4	.6	.3	1.5	256	77	349	10.0	336	0	1.80	1.10	15.0	0
332	Slice, 4 1/2 by 3 1/4 by 3/4 in.	1 slice	30	32	85	3	Trace	Trace	Trace	.1	17	5	23	.7	22	0	.12	.07	1.0	0
	Raisin bread, enriched:[38]																		
333	Loaf, 1 lb		454	35	1,190	30	13	3.0	4.7	3.9	243	322	395	10.0	1,057	Trace	1.70	1.07	10.7	Trace
334	Slice (18 per loaf)	1 slice	25	35	65	2	1	.2	.3	.2	13	18	22	.6	58	Trace	.09	.06	.6	Trace
	Rye bread:																		
	American, light (2/3 enriched wheat flour, 1/3 rye flour):																		
335	Loaf, 1 lb		454	36	1,100	41	5	.7	.5	2.2	236	340	667	9.1	658	0	1.35	.98	12.9	0
336	Slice (4 3/4 by 3 3/4 by 7/16 in).	1 slice	25	36	60	2	Trace	Trace	Trace	.1	13	19	37	.5	36	0	.07	.05	.7	0
	Pumpernickel (2/3 rye flour, 1/3 enriched wheat flour):																		
337	Loaf, 1 lb		454	34	1,115	41	5	.7	.5	2.4	241	381	1,039	11.8	2,059	0	1.30	.93	8.5	0
338	Slice (5 by 4 by 3/8 in)	1 slice	32	34	80	3	Trace	.1	Trace	.2	17	27	73	.8	145	0	.09	.07	.6	0
	White bread, enriched:[38]																		
	Soft-crumb type:																		
339	Loaf, 1 lb		454	36	1,225	39	15	3.4	5.3	4.6	229	381	440	11.3	476	Trace	1.80	1.10	15.0	Trace
340	Slice (18 per loaf)	1 slice	25	36	70	2	1	.2	.3	.3	13	21	24	.6	26	Trace	.10	.06	.8	Trace
341	Slice, toasted	1 slice	22	25	70	2	1	.2	.3	.3	13	21	24	.6	26	Trace	.08	.06	.8	Trace
342	Slice (22 per loaf)	1 slice	20	36	55	2	1	.2	.2	.2	10	17	19	.5	21	Trace	.08	.05	.7	Trace
343	Slice, toasted	1 slice	17	25	55	2	1	.2	.2	.2	10	17	19	.5	21	Trace	.06	.05	.7	Trace
344	Loaf, 1 1/2 lb		680	36	1,835	59	22	5.2	7.9	6.9	343	571	660	17.0	714	Trace	2.70	1.65	22.5	Trace
345	Slice (24 per loaf)	1 slice	28	36	75	2	1	.2	.3	.3	14	24	27	.7	29	Trace	.11	.07	.9	Trace
346	Slice, toasted	1 slice	24	25	75	2	1	.2	.3	.3	14	24	27	.7	29	Trace	.09	.07	.9	Trace
347	Slice (28 per loaf)	1 slice	24	36	65	2	1	.2	.3	.3	12	20	23	.6	25	Trace	.10	.06	.8	Trace
348	Slice, toasted	1 slice	21	25	65	2	1	.2	.3	.3	12	20	23	.6	25	Trace	.08	.06	.8	Trace
349	Cubes	1 cup	30	36	80	3	1	.2	.3	.3	15	25	29	.8	32	Trace	.12	.07	1.0	Trace
350	Crumbs	1 cup	45	36	120	4	1	.3	.5	.5	23	38	44	1.1	47	Trace	.18	.11	1.5	Trace
	Firm-crumb type:																		
351	Loaf, 1 lb		454	35	1,245	41	17	3.9	5.9	5.2	228	435	463	11.3	549	Trace	1.80	1.10	15.0	Trace
352	Slice (20 per loaf)	1 slice	23	35	65	2	1	.2	.3	.3	12	22	23	.6	28	Trace	.09	.06	.8	Trace
353	Slice, toasted	1 slice	20	24	65	2	1	.2	.3	.3	12	22	23	.6	28	Trace	.07	.06	.8	Trace
354	Loaf, 2 lb		907	35	2,495	82	34	7.7	11.8	10.4	455	871	925	22.7	1,097	Trace	3.60	2.20	30.0	Trace
355	Slice (34 per loaf)	1 slice	27	35	75	2	1	.2	.3	.3	14	26	28	.7	33	Trace	.11	.06	.9	Trace
356	Slice, toasted	1 slice	23	24	75	2	1	.2	.3	.3	14	26	28	.7	33	Trace	.09	.06	.9	Trace
	Whole-wheat bread:																		
	Soft-crumb type:[38]																		
357	Loaf, 1 lb		454	36	1,095	41	12	2.2	2.9	4.2	224	381	1,152	13.6	1,161	Trace	1.37	.45	12.7	Trace
358	Slice (16 per loaf)	1 slice	28	36	65	3	1	.1	.2	.2	14	24	71	.8	72	Trace	.09	.03	.8	Trace

Item No.	Food, approximate measure, and weight	Measure	Weight (g)	Water (%)	Food energy (cal)	Protein (g)	Fat (g)	Fatty acids Saturated (g)	Oleic (g)	Linoleic (g)	Carbohydrate (g)	Calcium (mg)	Phosphorus (mg)	Iron (mg)	Potassium (mg)	Vitamin A (I.U.)	Thiamin (mg)	Riboflavin (mg)	Niacin (mg)	Ascorbic acid (mg)
359	Slice, toasted	1 slice	24	24	65	3	1	.1	.2	.2	14	24	71	.8	72	Trace	.07	.03	.6	Trace
	Firm-crumb type:[38]																			
360	Loaf, 1 lb	1 loaf	454	36	1,100	48	14	2.5	3.3	4.9	216	449	1,034	13.6	1,238	Trace	1.17	.54	12.7	Trace
361	Slice (18 per loaf)	1 slice	25	36	60	3	1	.1	.2	.3	12	25	57	.8	68	Trace	.06	.03	.7	Trace
362	Slice, toasted	1 slice	21	24	60	3	1	.1	.2	.3	12	25	57	.8	68	Trace	.05	.03	.7	Trace
	Breakfast cereals:																			
	Hot type, cooked:																			
	Corn (hominy) grits, degermed:																			
363	Enriched	1 cup	245	87	125	3	Trace	Trace	Trace	.1	27	2	25	.7	27	[40]Trace	.10	.07	1.0	0
364	Unenriched	1 cup	245	87	125	3	Trace	Trace	Trace	.1	27	2	25	.2	27	[40]Trace	.05	.02	.5	0
365	Farina, quick-cooking, enriched.	1 cup	245	89	105	3	Trace	Trace	Trace	.1	22	147	[41]113	[42]	25	0	.12	.07	1.0	0
366	Oatmeal or rolled oats	1 cup	240	87	130	5	2	.4	.8	.9	23	22	137	1.4	146	0	.19	.05	.2	0
367	Wheat, rolled	1 cup	240	80	180	5	1	—	—	—	41	19	182	1.7	202	0	.17	.07	2.2	0
368	Wheat, whole-meal	1 cup	245	88	110	4	1	—	—	—	23	17	127	1.2	118	0	.15	.05	1.5	0
	Ready-to-eat:																			
369	Bran flakes (40% bran), added sugar, salt, iron, vitamins.	1 cup	35	3	105	4	1	—	—	—	28	19	125	5.6	137	1,540	.46	.52	6.2	0
370	Bran flakes with raisins, added sugar, salt, iron, vitamins.	1 cup	50	7	145	4	1	—	—	—	40	28	146	7.9	154	[43]2,200	[44]	[44]	[44]	0
	Corn flakes:																			
371	Plain, added sugar, salt, iron, vitamins.	1 cup	25	4	95	2	Trace	—	—	—	21	[44]	9	[44]	30	[44]	[44]	[44]	[44]	[45]13
372	Sugar-coated, added salt, iron, vitamins.	1 cup	40	2	155	2	Trace	—	—	—	37	1	10	[44]	27	1,760	.53	.60	7.1	[45]21
373	Corn, oat flour, puffed, added sugar, salt, iron, vitamins.	1 cup	20	4	80	2	1	—	—	—	16	4	18	5.7	—	880	.26	.30	3.5	11
374	Corn, shredded, added sugar, salt, iron, thiamin, niacin.	1 cup	25	3	95	2	Trace	—	—	—	22	1	10	.6	—	0	.33	.05	4.4	13
375	Oats, puffed, added sugar, salt, minerals, vitamins.	1 cup	25	3	100	3	1	—	—	—	19	44	102	4.0	—	1,100	.33	.38	4.4	13
	Rice, puffed:																			
376	Plain, added iron, thiamin, niacin.	1 cup	15	4	60	1	Trace	—	—	—	13	3	14	.3	15	0	.07	.01	.7	0
377	Presweetened, added salt, iron, vitamins.	1 cup	28	3	115	1	0	—	—	—	26	3	14	[44]	43	[45]1,240	[44]	[44]	[44]	[45]15
378	Wheat flakes, added sugar, salt, iron, vitamins.	1 cup	30	4	105	3	Trace	—	—	—	24	12	83	4.8	81	1,320	.40	.45	5.3	16
	Wheat, puffed:																			
379	Plain, added iron, thiamin, niacin.	1 cup	15	3	55	2	Trace	—	—	—	12	4	48	.6	51	0	.08	.03	1.2	0
380	Presweetened, added salt, iron, vitamins.	1 cup	38	3	140	3	Trace	—	—	—	33	7	52	[44]	63	1,680	.50	.57	6.7	[45]20
381	Wheat, shredded, plain	1 oblong biscuit or 1/2 cup spoon-size biscuits.	25	7	90	2	1	—	—	—	20	11	97	.9	87	0	.06	.03	1.1	0
382	Wheat germ, without salt and sugar, toasted.	1 tbsp	6	4	25	2	1	—	—	—	3	3	70	.5	57	10	.11	.05	.3	1
383	Buckwheat flour, light, sifted	1 cup	98	12	340	6	1	—	—	—	78	11	86	1.0	314	0	.08	.04	.4	0
384	Bulgur, canned, seasoned	1 cup	135	56	245	8	4	0.2	—	0.4	44	27	263	1.9	151	0	.08	.05	4.1	0
	Cake icings. See Sugars and Sweets (items 532–536).																			
	Cakes made from cake mixes with enriched flour:[46]																			
	Angelfood:																			
385	Whole cake (9 3/4-in diam. tube cake).	1 cake	635	34	1,645	36	1	—	—	—	377	603	756	2.5	381	0	.37	.95	3.6	0

[38] Made with vegetable shortening.
[39] Applies to product made with white cornmeal. With yellow cornmeal, value is 30 International Units (I.U.).
[40] Applies to white varieties. For yellow varieties, value is 150 International Units (I.U.).
[41] Applies to products that do not contain disodium phosphate. If disodium phosphate is an ingredient, value is 162 mg.
[42] Value may range from less than 1 mg to about 8 mg depending on the brand. Consult the label.
[43] Applies to product with added nutrient. Without added nutrient, value is trace.
[44] Value varies with the brand. Consult the label.
[45] Applies to product with added nutrient. Without added nutrient, value is trace.
[46] Excepting angelfood cake, cakes were made from mixes containing vegetable shortening; icings, with butter.

Item No. (A)	Foods, approximate measures, units, and weight (edible part unless footnotes indicate otherwise) (B)	Grams	Water (C) Percent	Food energy (D) Calories	Protein (E) Grams	Fat (F) Grams	Fatty Acids Saturated (total) (G) Grams	Unsaturated Oleic (H) Grams	Unsaturated Linoleic (I) Grams	Carbohydrate (J) Grams	Calcium (K) Milligrams	Phosphorus (L) Milligrams	Iron (M) Milligrams	Potassium (N) Milligrams	Vitamin A value (O) International units	Thiamine (P) Milligrams	Riboflavin (Q) Milligrams	Niacin (R) Milligrams	Ascorbic acid (S) Milligrams
	GRAIN PRODUCTS—Con.																		
	Cakes made from cake mixes with enriched flour[46]—Continued																		
	Coffeecake:																		
386	Piece, 1/12 of cake	53	34	135	3	Trace	–	–	–	32	50	63	.2	32	0	.03	.08	.3	0
387	Whole cake (7 3/4 by 5 5/8 by 1 1/4 in)	430	30	1,385	27	41	11.7	16.3	8.8	225	262	748	6.9	469	690	.82	.91	7.7	1
388	Piece, 1/6 of cake	72	30	230	5	7	2.0	2.7	1.5	38	44	125	1.2	78	120	.14	.15	1.3	Trace
	Cupcakes, made with egg, milk, 2 1/2-in diam.:																		
389	Without icing	25	26	90	1	5	.8	1.2	.7	14	40	59	.3	21	40	.05	.05	.4	Trace
390	With chocolate icing	36	22	130	2	5	2.0	1.6	.6	21	47	71	.4	42	60	.05	.06	.4	Trace
	Devil's food with chocolate icing:																		
391	Whole, 2 layer cake (8- or 9-in diam.)	1,107	24	3,755	49	136	50.0	44.9	17.0	645	653	,162	16.6	1,439	1,660	1.06	1.65	10.1	1
392	Piece, 1/16 of cake	69	24	235	3	8	3.1	2.8	1.1	40	41	72	1.0	90	100	.07	.10	.6	Trace
393	Cupcake, 2 1/2-in diam.	35	24	120	2	4	1.6	1.4	.5	20	21	37	.5	46	50	.03	.05	.3	Trace
	Gingerbread:																		
394	Whole cake (8-in square)	570	37	1,575	18	39	9.7	16.6	10.0	291	513	570	8.6	1,562	Trace	.84	1.00	7.4	Trace
395	Piece, 1/9 of cake	63	37	175	2	4	1.1	1.8	1.1	32	57	63	.9	173	Trace	.09	.11	.8	Trace
	White, 2 layer with chocolate icing:																		
396	Whole cake (8- or 9-in diam.)	1,140	21	4,000	44	122	48.2	46.4	20.0	716	1,129	2,041	11.4	1,322	680	1.50	1.77	12.5	2
397	Piece, 1/16 of cake	71	21	250	3	8	3.0	2.9	1.2	45	70	127	.7	82	40	.09	.11	.8	Trace
	Yellow, 2 layer with chocolate icing:																		
398	Whole cake (8- or 9-in diam.)	1,108	26	3,735	45	125	47.8	47.8	20.3	638	1,008	2,017	12.2	1,208	1,550	1.24	1.67	10.6	2
399	Piece, 1/16 of cake	69	26	235	3	8	3.0	3.0	1.3	40	63	126	.8	75	100	.08	.10	.7	Trace
	Cakes made from home recipes using enriched flour:[47]																		
	Boston cream pie with custard filling:																		
400	Whole cake (8-in diam.)	825	35	,490	41	78	23.0	30.1	15.2	412	553	833	8.2	[8]734	1,730	1.04	1.27	9.6	2
401	Piece, 1/12 of cake	69	35	210	3	6	1.9	2.5	1.3	34	46	70	.7	[48]61	140	.09	.11	.8	Trace
	Fruitcake, dark:																		
402	Loaf, 1-lb (7 1/2 by 2 by 1 1/2 in)	454	18	,720	22	69	14.4	33.5	14.8	271	327	513	11.8	2,250	540	.72	.73	4.9	2
403	Slice, 1/30 of loaf	15	18	55	1	2	.5	1.1	.5	9	11	17	.4	74	20	.02	.02	.2	Trace

No.	Food, approximate measure	Measure	Grams	Water (%)	Cal	Protein	Fat	Sat.	Oleic	Linoleic	Carb.	Ca	P	Fe	K	Vit. A	Thiamin	Riboflavin	Niacin	Ascorbic
	Plain, sheet cake:																			
	Without icing:																			
404	Whole cake (9-in square)	1 cake	777	25	2,830	35	108	29.5	44.4	23.9	434	497	793	8.5	*614	1,320	1.21	1.40	10.2	2
405	Piece, 1/9 of cake	1 piece	86	25	315	4	12	3.3	4.9	2.6	48	55	88	.9	48 68	150	.13	.15	1.1	Trace
	With uncooked white icing:																			
406	Whole cake (9-in square)	1 cake	1,096	21	4,020	37	129	42.2	49.5	24.4	694	548	822	8.2	*669	2,190	1.22	1.47	10.2	2
407	Piece, 1/9 of cake	1 piece	121	21	445	4	14	4.7	5.5	2.7	77	61	91	.8	48 74	240	.14	.16	1.1	Trace
	Pound:[49]																			
408	Loaf, 8 1/2 by 3 1/2 by 3 1/4 in.	1 loaf	565	16	2,725	31	170	42.9	73.1	39.6	273	107	418	7.9	345	1,410	.90	.99	7.3	0
409	Slice, 1/17 of loaf	1 slice	33	16	160	2	10	2.5	4.3	2.3	16	6	24	.5	20	80	.05	.06	.4	0
	Spongecake:																			
410	Whole cake (9 3/4-in diam. tube cake).	1 cake	790	32	2,345	60	45	13	15.8	5.7	427	237	885	13.4	687	3,560	1.10	1.64	7.4	Trace
411	Piece, 1/12 of cake	1 piece	66	32	195	5	4		1.3	.5	36	20	74	1.1	57	300	.09	.14	.6	Trace
	Cookies made with enriched flour:[50][51]																			
	Brownies with nuts:																			
	Home-prepared, 1 3/4 by 1 3/4 by 7/8 in:																			
412	From home recipe	1 brownie	20	10	95	1	6	1.5	3.0	1.2	10	8	30	.4	38	40	.04	.03	.2	Trace
413	From commercial recipe	1 brownie	20	11	85	1	4	.9	1.4	.9	13	9	27	.4	34	20	.03	.02	.2	Trace
414	Frozen, with chocolate icing,[52] 1 1/2 by 1 3/4 by 7/8 in.	1 brownie	25	13	105	1	5	2.0	2.2	.7	15	10	31	.4	44	50	.03	.03	.2	Trace
	Chocolate chip:																			
415	Commercial, 2 1/4-in diam., 3/8 in thick.	4 cookies	42	3	200	2	9	2.8	2.9	2.2	29	16	48	1.0	56	50	.10	.17	.9	Trace
416	From home recipe, 2 1/3-in diam.	4 cookies	40	3	205	2	12	3.5	4.5	2.9	24	14	40	.8	47	40	.06	.06	.5	Trace
417	Fig bars, square (1 5/8 by 1 5/8 by 3/8 in) or rectangular (1 1/2 by 1 3/4 by 1/2 in).	4 cookies	56	14	200	2	3	.8	1.2	.7	42	44	34	1.0	111	60	.04	.14	.9	Trace
418	Gingersnaps, 2-in diam., 1/4 in thick.	4 cookies	28	3	90	2	2	.7	1.0	.6	22	20	13	.7	129	20	.08	.06	.7	0
419	Macaroons, 2 3/4-in diam., 1/4 in thick.	2 cookies	38	4	180	2	9				25	10	32	.3	176	0	.02	.06	.2	0
420	Oatmeal with raisins, 2 5/8-in diam., 1/4 in thick.	4 cookies	52	3	235	3	8	2.0	3.3	2.0	38	11	53	1.4	192	30	.15	.10	1.0	0
421	Plain, prepared from commercial chilled dough, 2 1/2-in diam., 1/4 in thick.	4 cookies	48	5	240	2	12	3.0	5.2	2.9	31	17	35	.6	23	30	.10	.08	.9	0
422	Sandwich type (chocolate or vanilla), 1 3/4-in diam., 3/8 in thick.	4 cookies	40	2	200	2	9	2.2	3.9	2.2	28	10	96	.7	15	0	.06	.10	.7	0
423	Vanilla wafers, 1 3/4-in diam., 1/4 in thick.	10 cookies	40	3	185	2	6				30	16	25	.6	29	50	.10	.09	.8	0
	Cornmeal:																			
424	Whole-ground, unbolted, dry form.	1 cup	122	12	435	11	5	.5	1.0	2.5	90	24	312	2.9	346	53 620	.46	.13	2.4	0
425	Bolted (nearly whole-grain), dry form.	1 cup	122	12	440	11	4	.5	.9	2.1	91	21	272	2.2	303	53 590	.37	.10	2.3	0
	Degermed, enriched:																			
426	Dry form	1 cup	138	12	500	11	2	.2	.4	.9	108	8	137	4.0	166	53 610	.61	.36	4.8	0
427	Cooked	1 cup	240	88	120	3	Trace	Trace	.1	.2	26	2	38	1.0	38	53 140	.14	.10	1.2	0
	Degermed, unenriched:																			
428	Dry form	1 cup	138	12	500	11	2	.2	.4	.9	108	8	137	1.5	166	53 610	.19	.07	1.4	0
429	Cooked	1 cup	240	88	120	3	Trace	Trace	.1	.2	26	2	34	.5	38	53 140	.05	.02	.2	0
	Crackers:[38]																			
430	Graham, plain, 2 1/2-in square	2 crackers	14	6	55	1	1	.3	.5	.3	10	6	21	.5	55	0	.02	.08	.5	0

[38] Made with vegetable shortening.
[46] Excepting angelfood cake, cakes were made from mixes containing vegetable shortening; icings, with butter.
[47] Excepting spongecake, vegetable shortening used for cake portion; butter, for icing. If butter or margarine used for cake portion, vitamin A values would be higher.
[48] Applies to product made with a sodium aluminum-sulfate type baking powder. With a low-sodium type baking powder containing potassium, value would be about twice the amount shown.
[49] Equal weights of flour, sugar, eggs, and vegetable shortening.
[50] Products are commercial unless otherwise specified.
[51] Made with enriched flour and vegetable shortening except for macaroons which do not contain flour or shortening.
[52] Icing made with butter.
[53] Applies to yellow varieties; white varieties contain only a trace.

Item No. (A)	Foods, approximate measures, units, and weight (edible part unless footnotes indicate otherwise) (B)	Grams	Water (C) Per-cent	Food energy (D) Cal-ories	Pro-tein (E) Grams	Fat (F) Grams	Fatty Acids Saturated (total) (G) Grams	Unsaturated Oleic (H) Grams	Unsaturated Linoleic (I) Grams	Car-bohy-drate (I) Grams	Cal-cium (K) Milli-grams	Phos-phorus (L) Milli-grams	Iron (M) Milli-grams	Potas-sium (N) Milli-grams	Vitamin A value (O) Inter-national units	Thia-mine (P) Milli-grams	Ribo-flavin (Q) Milli-grams	Niacin (R) Milli-grams	Ascor-bic acid (S) Milli-grams
	GRAIN PRODUCTS—Con.																		
	Crackers[38]—Continued																		
431	Rye wafers, whole-grain, 1 7/8 by 3 1/2 in. 2 wafers	13	6	45	2	Trace	—	—	—	10	7	50	.5	78	0	.04	.03	.2	0
432	Saltines, made with enriched flour. 4 crackers or 1 packet	11	4	50	1	1	.3	.5	.4	8	2	10	.5	13	0	.05	.05	.4	0
	Danish pastry (enriched flour), plain without fruit or nuts:[54]																		
433	Packaged ring, 12 oz	340	22	1,435	25	80	24.3	31.7	16.5	155	170	371	6.1	381	1,050	.97	1.01	8.6	Trace
434	Round piece, about 4 1/4-in diam. by 1 in. 1 pastry	65	22	275	5	15	4.7	6.1	3.2	30	33	71	1.2	73	200	.18	.19	1.7	Trace
435	Ounce 1 oz	28	22	120	2	7	2.0	2.7	1.4	13	14	31	.5	32	90	.08	.08	.7	Trace
	Doughnuts, made with enriched flour:[38]																		
436	Cake type, plain, 2 1/2-in diam., 1 in high. 1 doughnut	25	24	100	1	5	1.2	2.0	1.1	13	10	48	.4	23	20	.05	.05	.4	Trace
437	Yeast-leavened, glazed, 3 3/4-in diam., 1 1/4 in high. 1 doughnut	50	26	205	3	11	3.3	5.8	3.3	22	16	33	.6	34	25	.10	.10	.8	0
	Macaroni, enriched, cooked (cut lengths, elbows, shells):																		
	Firm stage (hot):																		
438	1 cup	130	64	190	7	1	—	—	—	39	14	85	1.4	103	0	.23	.13	1.8	0
	Tender stage:																		
439	Cold macaroni 1 cup	105	73	115	4	Trace	—	—	—	24	8	53	.9	64	0	.15	.08	1.2	0
440	Hot macaroni 1 cup	140	73	155	5	1	—	—	—	32	11	70	1.3	85	0	.20	.11	1.5	0
	Macaroni (enriched) and cheese:																		
441	Canned[55] 1 cup	240	80	230	9	10	4.2	3.1	1.4	26	199	182	1.0	139	260	.12	.24	1.0	Trace
442	From home recipe (served hot)[56] 1 cup	200	58	430	17	22	8.9	8.8	2.9	40	362	322	1.8	240	860	.20	.40	1.8	Trace
	Muffins made with enriched flour:[38]																		
	From home recipe:																		
443	Blueberry, 2 3/8-in diam., 1 1/2 in high. 1 muffin	40	39	110	3	4	1.1	1.4	.7	17	34	53	.6	46	90	.09	.10	.7	Trace
444	Bran 1 muffin	40	35	105	3	4	1.2	1.4	.8	17	57	162	1.5	172	90	.07	.10	1.7	Trace
445	Corn (enriched degermed cornmeal and flour), 2 3/8-in diam., 1 1/2 in high. 1 muffin	40	33	125	3	4	1.2	1.6	.9	19	42	68	.7	54	[57]120	.10	.10	.7	Trace
446	Plain, 3-in diam., 1 1/2 in high. 1 muffin	40	38	120	3	4	1.0	1.7	1.0	17	42	60	.6	50	40	.09	.12	.9	Trace
	From mix, egg, milk:																		
447	Corn, 2 3/8-in diam., 1 1/2 in high.[58] 1 muffin	40	30	130	3	4	1.2	1.7	.9	20	96	152	.6	44	[57]100	.08	.09	.7	Trace
448	Noodles (egg noodles), enriched, cooked. 1 cup	160	71	200	7	2	—	—	—	37	16	94	1.4	70	110	.22	.13	1.9	0
449	Noodles, chow mein, canned 1 cup	45	1	220	6	11	—	—	—	26	—	—	—	—	—	—	—	—	—
	Pancakes, (4-in diam.)[38]																		
450	Buckwheat, made from mix (with buckwheat and enriched flours), egg and milk added. 1 cake	27	58	55	2	2	.8	.9	.4	6	59	91	.4	66	60	.04	.05	.2	Trace
	Plain:																		
451	Made from home recipe using enriched flour. 1 cake	27	50	60	2	2	.5	.8	.5	9	27	38	.4	33	30	.06	.07	.5	Trace
452	Made from mix with enriched flour, egg and milk added. 1 cake	27	51	60	2	2	.7	.7	.3	9	58	70	.3	42	70	.04	.06	.2	Trace

Pies, piecrust made with enriched flour, vegetable shortening (9-in diam.):

No.	Food	Measure	Grams	Water (%)	Food energy (cal)	Protein (g)	Fat (g)	Saturated (g)	Oleic (g)	Linoleic (g)	Carbohydrate (g)	Calcium (mg)	Phosphorus (mg)	Iron (mg)	Potassium (mg)	Vitamin A (IU)	Thiamin (mg)	Riboflavin (mg)	Niacin (mg)	Ascorbic acid (mg)
	Apple:																			
453	Whole	1 pie	945	48	2,420	21	105	27.0	44.5	25.2	360	76	208	6.6	756	280	1.06	.79	9.3	9
454	Sector, 1/7 of pie	1 sector	135	48	345	3	15	3.9	6.4	3.6	51	11	30	.9	108	40	.15	.11	1.3	2
	Banana cream:																			
455	Whole	1 pie	910	54	2,010	41	85	26.7	33.2	16.2	279	601	746	7.3	1,847	2,280	.77	1.51	7.0	9
456	Sector, 1/7 of pie	1 sector	130	54	285	6	12	3.8	4.7	2.3	40	86	107	1.0	264	330	.11	.22	1.0	1
	Blueberry:																			
457	Whole	1 pie	945	51	2,285	23	102	24.8	43.7	25.1	330	104	217	9.5	614	280	1.03	.80	10.0	28
458	Sector, 1/7 of pie	1 sector	135	51	325	3	15	3.5	6.2	3.6	47	15	31	1.4	88	40	.15	.11	1.4	4
	Cherry:																			
459	Whole	1 pie	945	47	2,465	25	107	28.2	45.0	25.3	363	132	236	6.6	992	4,160	1.09	.84	9.8	Trace
460	Sector, 1/7 of pie	1 sector	135	47	350	4	15	4.0	6.4	3.6	52	19	34	.9	142	590	.16	.12	1.4	Trace
	Custard:																			
461	Whole	1 pie	910	58	1,985	56	101	33.9	38.5	17.5	213	874	1,028	8.2	1,247	2,090	.79	1.92	5.6	0
462	Sector, 1/7 of pie	1 sector	130	58	285	8	14	4.8	5.5	2.5	30	125	147	1.2	178	300	.11	.27	.8	0
	Lemon meringue:																			
463	Whole	1 pie	840	47	2,140	31	86	26.1	33.8	16.4	317	118	412	6.7	420	1,430	.61	.84	5.2	25
464	Sector, 1/7 of pie	1 sector	120	47	305	4	12	3.7	4.8	2.3	45	17	59	1.0	60	200	.09	.12	.7	4
	Mince:																			
465	Whole	1 pie	945	43	2,560	24	109	28.0	45.9	25.2	389	265	359	13.3	1,682	20	.96	.86	9.8	9
466	Sector, 1/7 of pie	1 sector	135	43	365	3	16	4.0	6.6	3.6	56	38	51	1.9	240	Trace	.14	.12	1.4	1
	Peach:																			
467	Whole	1 pie	945	48	2,410	24	101	24.8	43.7	25.1	361	95	274	8.5	1,408	6,900	1.04	.97	14.0	28
468	Sector, 1/7 of pie	1 sector	135	48	345	3	14	3.5	6.2	3.6	52	14	39	1.2	201	990	.15	.14	2.0	4
	Pecan:																			
469	Whole	1 pie	825	20	3,450	42	189	27.8	101.0	44.2	423	388	850	25.6	1,015	1,320	1.80	.95	6.9	Trace
470	Sector, 1/7 of pie	1 sector	118	20	495	6	27	4.0	14.4	6.3	61	55	122	3.7	145	190	.26	.14	1.0	Trace
	Pumpkin:																			
471	Whole	1 pie	910	59	1,920	36	102	37.4	37.5	16.6	223	464	628	7.3	1,456	22,480	.78	1.27	7.0	Trace
472	Sector, 1/7 of pie	1 sector	130	59	275	5	15	5.4	5.4	2.4	32	66	90	1.0	208	3,210	.11	.18	1.0	Trace
473	Piecrust (home recipe) made with enriched flour and vegetable shortening, baked.	1 pie shell, 9-in diam.	180	15	900	11	60	14.8	26.1	14.9	79	25	90	3.1	89	0	.47	.40	5.0	0
474	Piecrust mix with enriched flour and vegetable shortening, 10-oz pkg. prepared and baked.	Piecrust for 2-crust pie, 9-in diam.	320	19	1,485	20	93	22.7	39.7	23.4	141	131	272	6.1	179	0	1.07	.79	9.9	0
475	Pizza (cheese) baked, 4 3/4-in sector; 1/8 of 12-in diam. pie.[19]	1 sector	60	45	145	6	4	1.7	1.5	.6	22	86	89	1.1	67	230	.16	.18	1.6	4
	Popcorn, popped:																			
476	Plain, large kernel	1 cup	6	4	25	1	Trace	Trace	.1	.2	5	1	17	.2	–	–	–	.01	.1	0
477	With oil (coconut) and salt added, large kernel.	1 cup	9	3	40	1	2	1.5	.2	.2	5	1	19	.2	–	–	–	.01	.2	0
478	Sugar coated	1 cup	35	4	135	2	1	.5	.2	.2	30	2	47	.5	–	–	–	.02	.4	0
	Pretzels, made with enriched flour:																			
479	Dutch, twisted, 2 3/4 by 2 5/8 in.	1 pretzel	16	5	60	2	1	–	–	–	12	4	21	.2	21	0	.05	.04	.7	0
480	Thin, twisted, 3 1/4 by 2 1/4 by 1/4 in.	10 pretzels	60	5	235	6	3	–	–	–	46	13	79	.9	78	0	.20	.15	2.5	0
481	Stick, 2 1/4 in long	10 pretzels	3	5	10	Trace	Trace	–	–	–	2	1	4	Trace	4	0	.01	.01	.1	0

Crust made with vegetable shortening and enriched flour.

Made with vegetable shortening.

[54] Contains vegetable shortening and butter.

[55] Made with corn oil.

[56] Made with regular margarine.

[57] Applies to product made with yellow cornmeal.

[58] Made with enriched degermed cornmeal and enriched flour.

Item No. (A)	Foods, approximate measures, units, and weight (edible part unless footnotes indicate otherwise) (B)	Grams	Water (C) Per-cent	Food energy (D) Cal-ories	Pro-tein (E) Grams	Fat (F) Grams	Fatty Acids Satu-rated (total) (G) Grams	Unsaturated Oleic (H) Grams	Unsaturated Lino-leic (I) Grams	Car-bohy-drate (J) Grams	Cal-cium (K) Milli-grams	Phos-phorus (L) Milli-grams	Iron (M) Milli-grams	Potas-sium (N) Milli-grams	Vitamin A value (O) Inter-national units	Thia-mine (P) Milli-grams	Ribo-flavin (Q) Milli-grams	Niacin (R) Milli-grams	Ascor-bic acid (S) Milli-grams
	GRAIN PRODUCTS—Con.																		
	Rice, white, enriched:																		
482	Instant, ready-to-serve, hot 1 cup	165	73	180	4	Trace	Trace	Trace	Trace	40	5	31	1.3	—	0	.21	(59)	1.7	0
	Long grain:																		
483	Raw 1 cup	185	12	670	12	1	.2	.2	.2	149	44	174	5.4	170	0	.81	.06	6.5	0
484	Cooked, served hot 1 cup	205	73	225	4	Trace	.1	.1	.1	50	21	57	1.8	57	0	.23	.02	2.1	0
	Parboiled:																		
485	Raw 1 cup	185	10	685	14	1	.2	.1	.2	150	111	370	5.4	278	0	.81	.07	6.5	0
486	Cooked 1 cup	175	73	185	4	Trace	.1	.1	.1	41	33	100	1.4	75	0	.19	.02	2.1	0
	Rolls, enriched:[38]																		
	Commercial:																		
487	Brown-and-serve (12 per 12-oz pkg.), browned. 1 roll	26	27	85	2	2	.4	.7	.5	14	20	23	.5	25	Trace	.10	.06	.9	Trace
488	Cloverleaf or pan, 2 1/2-in diam., 2 in high. 1 roll	28	31	85	2	2	.4	.6	.4	15	21	24	.5	27	Trace	.11	.07	.9	Trace
489	Frankfurter and hamburger (8 per 11 1/2-oz pkg.). 1 roll	40	31	120	3	2	.5	.8	.6	21	30	34	.8	38	Trace	.16	.10	1.3	Trace
490	Hard, 3 3/4-in diam., 2 in high. 1 roll	50	25	155	5	2	.4	.6	.5	30	24	46	1.2	49	Trace	.20	.12	1.7	Trace
491	Hoagie or submarine, 11 1/2 by 3 by 2 1/2 in. 1 roll	135	31	390	12	4	.9	1.4	1.4	75	58	115	3.0	122	Trace	.54	.32	4.5	Trace
	From home recipe:																		
492	Cloverleaf, 2 1/2-in diam., 2 in high. 1 roll	35	26	120	3	3	.8	1.1	.7	20	16	36	.7	41	30	.12	.12	1.2	Trace
	Spaghetti, enriched, cooked:																		
493	Firm stage, "al dente," served hot 1 cup	130	64	190	7	1	—	—	—	39	14	85	1.4	103	0	.23	.13	1.8	0
494	Tender stage, served hot 1 cup	140	73	155	5	1	—	—	—	32	11	70	1.3	85	0	.20	.11	1.5	0
	Spaghetti (enriched) in tomato sauce with cheese:																		
495	From home recipe 1 cup	250	77	260	9	9	2.0	5.4	.7	37	80	135	2.3	408	1,080	.25	.18	2.3	13
496	Canned 1 cup	250	80	190	6	2	.5	.3	.4	39	40	88	2.8	303	930	.35	.28	4.5	10
	Spaghetti (enriched) with meat balls and tomato sauce:																		
497	From home recipe 1 cup	248	70	330	19	12	3.3	6.3	.9	39	124	236	3.7	665	1,590	.25	.30	4.0	22
498	Canned 1 cup	250	78	260	12	10	2.2	3.3	3.9	29	53	113	3.3	245	1,000	.15	.18	2.3	5
499	Toaster pastries 1 pastry	50	12	200	3	6	—	—	—	36	[60]54	[60]67	1.9	[60]74	500	.16	.17	2.1	(60)
	Waffles, made with enriched flour, 7-in diam.:[38]																		
500	From home recipe 1 waffle	75	41	210	7	7	2.3	2.8	1.4	28	85	130	1.3	109	250	.17	.23	1.4	Trace
501	From mix, egg and milk added 1 waffle	75	42	205	7	8	2.8	2.9	1.2	27	179	257	1.0	146	170	.14	.22	.9	Trace
	Wheat flours:																		
	All-purpose or family flour, enriched:																		
502	Sifted, spooned 1 cup	115	12	420	12	1	.2	.1	.5	88	18	100	3.3	109	0	.74	.46	6.1	0
503	Unsifted, spooned 1 cup	125	12	455	13	1	.2	.1	.5	95	20	109	3.6	119	0	.80	.50	6.6	0
504	Cake or pastry flour, enriched, sifted, spooned. 1 cup	96	12	350	7	1	.1	.1	.3	76	16	70	2.8	91	0	.61	.38	5.1	0
505	Self-rising, enriched, unsifted, spooned. 1 cup	125	12	440	12	1	.2	.1	.5	93	331	583	3.6	—	0	.80	.50	6.6	0
506	Whole-wheat, from hard wheats, stirred. 1 cup	120	12	400	16	2	.4	.2	1.0	85	49	446	4.0	444	0	.66	.14	5.2	0
	LEGUMES (DRY), NUTS, SEEDS; RELATED PRODUCTS																		
	Almonds, shelled:																		
507	Chopped (about 130 almonds) 1 cup	130	5	775	24	70	5.6	47.7	12.8	25	304	655	6.1	1,005	0	.31	1.20	4.6	Trace

No.	Food	Measure	Weight (g)	Water (%)	Food energy (cal)	Protein (g)	Fat (g)	Saturated fat (g)	Oleic (g)	Linoleic (g)	Carbohydrate (g)	Calcium (mg)	Phosphorus (mg)	Iron (mg)	Potassium (mg)	Vitamin A (IU)	Thiamin (mg)	Riboflavin (mg)	Niacin (mg)	Ascorbic acid (mg)
508	Slivered, not pressed down (about 115 almonds).	1 cup	115	5	690	21	62	5.0	42.2	11.3	22	269	580	5.4	889	0	0.28	1.06	4.0	Trace
	Beans, dry:																			
	Common varieties as Great Northern, navy, and others:																			
	Cooked, drained:																			
509	Great Northern	1 cup	180	69	210	14	1	—	—	—	38	90	266	4.9	749	0	.25	.13	1.3	0
510	Pea (navy)	1 cup	190	69	225	15	1	—	—	—	40	95	281	5.1	790	0	.27	.13	1.3	0
	Canned, solids and liquid: White with—																			
511	Frankfurters (sliced)	1 cup	255	71	365	19	18	—	—	—	32	94	303	4.8	668	330	.18	.15	3.3	Trace
512	Pork and tomato sauce	1 cup	255	71	310	16	7	2.4	2.8	.6	48	138	235	4.6	536	330	.20	.08	1.5	5
513	Pork and sweet sauce	1 cup	255	66	385	16	12	4.3	5.0	1.1	54	161	291	5.9	—	—	.15	.10	1.3	—
514	Red kidney	1 cup	255	76	230	15	1	—	—	—	42	74	278	4.6	673	10	.13	.10	1.5	—
515	Lima, cooked, drained	1 cup	190	64	260	16	1	—	—	—	49	55	293	5.9	1,163	—	.25	.11	1.3	—
516	Blackeye peas, dry, cooked (with residual cooking liquid).	1 cup	250	80	190	13	1	—	—	—	35	43	238	3.3	573	30	.40	.10	1.0	—
517	Brazil nuts, shelled (6–8 large kernels).	1 oz	28	5	185	4	19	4.8	6.2	7.1	3	53	196	1.0	203	Trace	.27	.03	.5	—
518	Cashew nuts, roasted in oil	1 cup	140	5	785	24	64	12.9	36.8	10.2	41	53	522	5.3	650	140	.60	.35	2.5	—
	Coconut meat, fresh:																			
519	Piece, about 2 by 2 by 1/2 in	1 piece	45	51	155	2	16	14.0	.9	.3	4	6	43	.8	115	0	.02	.01	.2	1
520	Shredded or grated, not pressed down.	1 cup	80	51	275	3	28	24.8	1.6	.5	8	10	76	1.4	205	0	.04	.02	.4	2
521	Filberts (hazelnuts), chopped (about 60 kernels).	1 cup	115	6	730	14	72	5.1	55.2	7.3	19	240	388	3.9	810	—	.53	—	1.0	Trace
522	Lentils, whole, cooked	1 cup	200	72	210	16	Trace	—	—	—	39	50	238	4.2	498	40	.14	.12	1.2	0
523	Peanuts, roasted in oil, salted (whole, halves, chopped).	1 cup	144	2	840	37	72	13.7	33.0	20.7	27	107	577	3.0	971	—	.46	.19	24.8	0
524	Peanut butter	1 tbsp	16	2	95	4	8	1.5	3.7	2.3	3	9	61	.3	100	80	.02	.02	2.4	0
525	Peas, split, dry, cooked	1 cup	200	70	230	16	1	—	—	—	42	22	178	3.4	592	80	.30	.18	1.8	—
526	Pecans, chopped or pieces (about 120 large halves).	1 cup	118	3	810	11	84	7.2	50.5	20.0	17	86	341	2.8	712	150	1.01	.15	1.1	2
527	Pumpkin and squash kernels, dry, hulled.	1 cup	140	4	775	41	65	11.8	23.5	27.5	21	71	1,602	15.7	1,386	100	.34	.27	3.4	—
528	Sunflower seeds, dry, hulled	1 cup	145	5	810	35	69	8.2	13.7	43.2	29	174	1,214	10.3	1,334	70	2.84	.33	7.8	—
	Walnuts:																			
	Black:																			
529	Chopped or broken kernels	1 cup	125	3	785	26	74	6.3	13.3	45.7	19	Trace	713	7.5	575	380	.28	.14	.9	—
530	Ground (finely)	1 cup	80	3	500	16	47	4.0	8.5	29.2	12	Trace	456	4.8	368	240	.18	.09	.6	—
531	Persian or English, chopped (about 60 halves).	1 cup	120	4	780	18	77	8.4	11.8	42.2	19	119	456	3.7	540	40	.40	.16	1.1	2

SUGARS AND SWEETS

No.	Food	Measure	Weight (g)	Water (%)	Food energy (cal)	Protein (g)	Fat (g)	Saturated fat (g)	Oleic (g)	Linoleic (g)	Carbohydrate (g)	Calcium (mg)	Phosphorus (mg)	Iron (mg)	Potassium (mg)	Vitamin A (IU)	Thiamin (mg)	Riboflavin (mg)	Niacin (mg)	Ascorbic acid (mg)
	Cake icings:																			
	Boiled, white:																			
532	Plain	1 cup	94	18	295	1	0	0	0	0	75	2	2	Trace	17	0	Trace	.03	Trace	0
533	With coconut	1 cup	166	15	605	3	13	11.0	.9	Trace	124	10	50	.8	277	0	.02	.07	.3	0
	Uncooked:																			
534	Chocolate made with milk and butter.	1 cup	275	14	1,035	9	38	23.4	11.7	1.0	185	165	305	3.3	536	580	.06	.28	.6	1
535	Creamy fudge from mix and water.[59]	1 cup	245	15	830	7	16	5.1	6.7	3.1	183	96	218	2.7	238	Trace	.05	.20	.7	Trace
536	White[58]	1 cup	319	11	1,200	2	21	12.7	5.1	.5	260	48	38	Trace	57	860	Trace	.06	Trace	Trace
	Candy:																			
537	Caramels, plain or chocolate	1 oz	28	8	115	1	3	1.6	1.1	.1	22	42	35	.4	54	Trace	.01	.05	.1	Trace
	Chocolate:																			
538	Milk, plain	1 oz	28	1	145	2	9	5.5	3.0	.3	16	65	65	.3	109	80	.02	.10	.1	Trace
539	Semisweet, small pieces (60 per oz).[60]	1 cup or 6-oz pkg	170	1	860	7	61	36.2	19.8	1.7	97	51	255	4.4	553	30	.02	.14	.9	0
540	Chocolate-coated peanuts	1 oz	28	1	160	5	12	4.0	4.7	2.1	11	33	84	.4	143	Trace	.10	.05	2.1	Trace

58 Made with vegetable shortening.
59 Product may or may not be enriched with riboflavin. Consult the label.
60 Value varies with the brand. Consult the label.

SUGARS AND SWEETS—Con.

Item No. (A)	Foods, approximate measures, units, and weight (edible part unless footnotes indicate otherwise) (B)	Grams	Water (C) Per cent	Food energy (D) Calories	Protein (E) Grams	Fat (F) Grams	Fatty Acids Saturated (total) (G) Grams	Unsaturated Oleic (H) Grams	Linoleic (I) Grams	Carbohydrate (J) Grams	Calcium (K) Milligrams	Phosphorus (L) Milligrams	Iron (M) Milligrams	Potassium (N) Milligrams	Vitamin A value (O) International units	Thiamine (P) Milligrams	Riboflavin (Q) Milligrams	Niacin (R) Milligrams	Ascorbic acid (S) Milligrams
	Candy—Continued																		
541	Fondant, uncoated (mints, candy corn, other). 1 oz	28	8	105	Trace	1	.1	.3	.1	25	4	2	.3	1	0	Trace	Trace	Trace	0
542	Fudge, chocolate, plain 1 oz	28	8	115	1	3	1.3	1.4	.6	21	22	24	.3	42	Trace	.01	.03	.1	Trace
543	Gum drops 1 oz	28	12	100	Trace	Trace	—	—	—	25	2	Trace	.1	1	0	0	Trace	Trace	0
544	Hard 1 oz	28	1	110	0	Trace	—	—	—	28	6	2	.5	1	0	0	0	0	0
545	Marshmallows 1 oz	28	17	90	1	Trace	—	—	—	23	5	2	.5	2	0	0	Trace	Trace	0
	Chocolate-flavored beverage powders (about 4 heaping tsp per oz):																		
546	With nonfat dry milk 1 oz	28	2	100	5	1	.5	.3	Trace	20	167	155	.5	227	10	.04	.21	.2	1
547	Without milk 1 oz	28	1	100	1	1	.4	.2	Trace	25	9	48	.6	142	0	.01	.03	.1	0
548	Honey, strained or extracted 1 tbsp	21	17	65	Trace	0	0	0	0	17	1	1	.1	11	0	Trace	.01	.1	Trace
549	Jams and preserves 1 tbsp	20	29	55	Trace	Trace	—	—	—	14	4	2	.2	18	Trace	Trace	.01	Trace	Trace
550	1 packet	14	29	40	Trace	Trace	—	—	—	10	3	1	.1	12	Trace	Trace	.01	Trace	Trace
551	Jellies 1 tbsp	18	29	50	Trace	Trace	—	—	—	13	4	1	.3	14	Trace	Trace	.01	Trace	1
552	1 packet	14	29	40	Trace	Trace	—	—	—	10	3	1	.2	11	Trace	Trace	Trace	Trace	1
	Sirups:																		
	Chocolate-flavored sirup or topping:																		
553	Thin type 1 fl oz or 2 tbsp	38	32	90	1	1	.5	.3	Trace	24	6	35	.6	106	Trace	.01	.03	.2	0
554	Fudge type 1 fl oz or 2 tbsp	38	25	125	2	5	3.1	1.6	.1	20	48	60	.5	107	60	.02	.08	.2	Trace
	Molasses, cane:																		
555	Light (first extraction) 1 tbsp	20	24	50	—	—	—	—	—	13	33	9	.9	183	—	.01	.01	Trace	—
556	Blackstrap (third extraction) 1 tbsp	20	24	45	—	—	—	—	—	11	137	17	3.2	585	—	.02	.04	.4	—
557	Sorghum 1 tbsp	21	23	55	—	—	—	—	—	14	35	5	2.6	—	—	—	.02	Trace	—
558	Table blends, chiefly corn, light and dark. 1 tbsp	21	24	60	0	0	0	0	0	15	9	3	.8	1	0	0	0	0	0
	Sugars:																		
559	Brown, pressed down 1 cup	220	2	820	0	0	0	0	0	212	187	42	7.5	757	0	.02	.07	.4	0
	White:																		
560	Granulated 1 cup	200	1	770	0	0	0	0	0	199	0	0	.2	6	0	0	0	0	0
561	1 tbsp	12	1	45	0	0	0	0	0	12	0	0	Trace	Trace	0	0	0	0	0
562	1 packet	6	1	23	0	0	0	0	0	6	0	0	Trace	Trace	0	0	0	0	0
563	Powdered, sifted, spooned into cup. 1 cup	100	1	385	0	0	0	0	0	100	0	0	.1	3	0	0	0	0	0

VEGETABLE AND VEGETABLE PRODUCTS

Item	Food	Measure	Grams	Water (%)	Food energy	Protein (g)	Fat (g)	Saturated	Oleic	Linoleic	Carbohydrate (g)	Calcium (mg)	Phosphorus (mg)	Iron (mg)	Potassium (mg)	Vitamin A (IU)	Thiamin (mg)	Riboflavin (mg)	Niacin (mg)	Ascorbic acid (mg)
	Asparagus, green:																			
	Cooked, drained:																			
	Cuts and tips, 1 1/2- to 2-in lengths:																			
564	From raw	1 cup	145	94	30	3	Trace	—	—	—	5	30	73	.9	265	1,310	.23	.26	2.0	38
565	From frozen	1 cup	180	93	40	6	Trace	—	—	—	6	40	115	2.2	396	1,530	.25	.23	1.8	41
	Spears, 1/2-in diam. at base:																			
566	From raw	4 spears	60	94	10	1	Trace	—	—	—	2	13	30	.4	110	540	.10	.11	.8	16
567	From frozen	4 spears	60	92	15	2	Trace	—	—	—	2	13	40	.7	143	470	.10	.08	.7	16
568	Canned, spears, 1/2-in diam. at base.	4 spears	80	93	15	2	Trace	—	—	—	3	15	42	1.5	133	640	.05	.08	.6	12
	Beans:																			
	Lima, immature seeds, frozen, cooked, drained:																			
569	Thick-seeded types (Fordhooks)	1 cup	170	74	170	10	Trace	—	—	—	32	34	153	2.9	724	390	.12	.09	1.7	29
570	Thin-seeded types (baby limas)	1 cup	180	69	210	13	Trace	—	—	—	40	63	227	4.7	709	400	.16	.09	2.2	22
	Snap:																			
	Green:																			
	Cooked, drained:																			
571	From raw (cuts and French style).	1 cup	125	92	30	2	Trace	—	—	—	7	63	46	.8	189	680	.09	.11	.6	15
	From frozen:																			
572	Cuts	1 cup	135	92	35	2	Trace	—	—	—	8	54	43	.9	205	780	.09	.12	.5	7
573	French style	1 cup	130	92	35	2	Trace	—	—	—	8	49	39	1.2	177	690	.08	.10	.4	9
574	Canned, drained solids (cuts).	1 cup	135	92	30	2	Trace	—	—	—	7	61	34	2.0	128	630	.04	.07	.4	5
	Yellow or wax:																			
	Cooked, drained:																			
575	From raw (cuts and French style).	1 cup	125	93	30	2	Trace	—	—	—	6	63	46	.8	189	290	.09	.11	.6	16
576	From frozen (cuts)	1 cup	135	92	35	2	Trace	—	—	—	8	47	42	.9	221	140	.09	.11	.5	8
577	Canned, drained solids (cuts).	1 cup	135	92	30	2	Trace	—	—	—	7	61	34	2.0	128	140	.04	.07	.4	7
	Beans, mature. See Beans, dry (items 509–515) and Blackeye peas, dry (item 516).																			
	Bean sprouts (mung):																			
578	Raw	1 cup	105	89	35	4	Trace	—	—	—	7	20	67	1.4	234	20	.14	.14	.8	20
579	Cooked, drained	1 cup	125	91	35	4	Trace	—	—	—	7	21	60	1.1	195	30	.11	.13	.9	8
	Beets:																			
	Cooked, drained, peeled:																			
580	Whole beets, 2-in diam.	2 beets	100	91	30	1	Trace	—	—	—	7	14	23	.5	208	20	.03	.04	.3	6
581	Diced or sliced	1 cup	170	91	55	2	Trace	—	—	—	12	24	39	.9	354	30	.05	.07	.5	10
	Canned, drained solids:																			
582	Whole beets, small	1 cup	160	89	60	2	Trace	—	—	—	14	30	29	1.1	267	30	.02	.05	.2	5
583	Diced or sliced	1 cup	170	89	65	2	Trace	—	—	—	15	32	31	1.2	284	30	.02	.05	.2	5
584	Beet greens, leaves and stems, cooked, drained.	1 cup	145	94	25	2	Trace	—	—	—	5	144	36	2.8	481	7,400	.10	.22	.4	22
	Blackeye peas, immature seeds, cooked and drained:																			
585	From raw	1 cup	165	72	180	13	1	—	—	—	30	40	241	3.5	625	580	.50	.18	2.3	28
586	From frozen	1 cup	170	66	220	15	1	—	—	—	40	43	286	4.8	573	290	.68	.19	2.4	15
	Broccoli, cooked, drained:																			
	From raw:																			
587	Stalk, medium size	1 stalk	180	91	45	6	1	—	—	—	8	158	112	1.4	481	4,500	0.16	0.36	1.4	162
588	Stalks cut into 1/2-in pieces	1 cup	155	91	40	5	Trace	—	—	—	7	136	96	1.2	414	3,880	.14	.31	1.2	140
	From frozen:																			
589	Stalk, 4 1/2 to 5 in long	1 stalk	30	91	10	1	Trace	—	—	—	1	12	17	.2	66	570	.02	.03	.2	22
590	Chopped	1 cup	185	92	50	5	1	—	—	—	9	100	104	1.3	392	4,810	.11	.22	.9	105
	Brussels sprouts, cooked, drained:																			
591	From raw, 7–8 sprouts (1 1/4- to 1 1/2-in diam.).	1 cup	155	88	55	7	1	—	—	—	10	50	112	1.7	423	810	.12	.22	1.2	135
592	From frozen	1 cup	155	89	50	5	Trace	—	—	—	10	33	95	1.2	457	880	.12	.16	.9	126
	Cabbage:																			
	Common varieties:																			
	Raw:																			
593	Coarsely shredded or sliced	1 cup	70	92	15	1	Trace	—	—	—	4	34	20	.3	163	90	.04	.04	.2	33
594	Finely shredded or chopped	1 cup	90	92	20	1	Trace	—	—	—	5	44	26	.4	210	120	.05	.05	.3	42

Item No.	Foods, approximate measures, units, and weight (edible part unless footnotes indicate otherwise)			Water	Food energy	Protein	Fat	Fatty Acids: Saturated (total)	Fatty Acids: Unsaturated: Oleic	Fatty Acids: Unsaturated: Linoleic	Carbohydrate	Calcium	Phosphorus	Iron	Potassium	Vitamin A value	Thiamine	Riboflavin	Niacin	Ascorbic acid
(A)	(B)			(C)	(D)	(E)	(F)	(G)	(H)	(I)	(J)	(K)	(L)	(M)	(N)	(O)	(P)	(Q)	(R)	(S)
			Grams	Percent	Calories	Grams	Grams	Grams	Grams	Grams	Grams	Milligrams	Milligrams	Milligrams	Milligrams	International units	Milligrams	Milligrams	Milligrams	Milligrams
	VEGETABLE AND VEGETABLE PRODUCTS—Con.																			
	Cabbage—Continued																			
595	Cooked, drained	1 cup	145	94	30	2	Trace	—	—	—	6	64	29	.4	236	190	.06	.06	.4	48
596	Red, raw, coarsely shredded or sliced.	1 cup	70	90	20	1	Trace	—	—	—	5	29	25	.6	188	30	.06	.04	.3	43
597	Savoy, raw, coarsely shredded or sliced.	1 cup	70	92	15	2	Trace	—	—	—	3	47	38	.6	188	140	.04	.06	.2	39
598	Cabbage, celery (also called pe-tsai or wongbok), raw, 1-in pieces.	1 cup	75	95	10	1	Trace	—	—	—	2	32	30	.5	190	110	.04	.03	.5	19
599	Cabbage, white mustard (also called bokchoy or pakchoy), cooked, drained.	1 cup	170	95	25	2	Trace	—	—	—	4	252	56	1.0	364	5,270	.07	.14	1.2	26
	Carrots:																			
	Raw, without crowns and tips, scraped:																			
600	Whole, 7 1/2 by 1 1/8 in, or strips, 2 1/2 to 3 in long.	1 carrot or 18 strips	72	88	30	1	Trace	—	—	—	7	27	26	.5	246	7,930	.04	.04	.4	6
601	Grated	1 cup	110	88	45	1	Trace	—	—	—	11	41	40	.8	375	12,100	.07	.06	.7	9
602	Cooked (crosswise cuts), drained	1 cup	155	91	50	1	Trace	—	—	—	11	51	48	.9	344	16,280	.08	.08	.8	9
	Canned:																			
603	Sliced, drained solids	1 cup	155	91	45	1	Trace	—	—	—	10	47	34	1.1	186	23,250	.03	.05	.6	3
604	Strained or junior (baby food)	1 oz (1 3/4 to 2 tbsp)	28	92	10	Trace	Trace	—	—	—	2	7	6	.1	51	3,690	.01	.01	.1	1
	Cauliflower:																			
605	Raw, chopped	1 cup	115	91	31	3	Trace	—	—	—	6	29	64	1.3	339	70	.13	.12	.8	90
	Cooked, drained:																			
606	From raw (flower buds)	1 cup	125	93	30	3	Trace	—	—	—	5	26	53	.9	258	80	.11	.10	.8	69
607	From frozen (flowerets)	1 cup	180	94	30	3	Trace	—	—	—	6	31	68	.9	373	50	.07	.09	.7	74
	Celery, Pascal type, raw:																			
608	Stalk, large outer, 8 by 1 1/2 in, at root end.	1 stalk	40	94	5	Trace	Trace	—	—	—	2	16	11	.1	136	110	.01	.01	.1	4
609	Pieces, diced	1 cup	120	94	20	1	Trace	—	—	—	5	47	34	.4	409	320	.04	.04	.4	11
	Collards, cooked, drained:																			
610	From raw (leaves without stems)	1 cup	190	90	65	7	1	—	—	—	10	357	99	1.5	498	14,820	.21	.38	2.3	144
611	From frozen (chopped)	1 cup	170	90	50	5	1	—	—	—	10	299	87	1.7	401	11,560	.10	.24	1.0	56
	Corn, sweet:																			
	Cooked, drained:																			
612	From raw, ear 5 by 1 3/4 in	1 ear[61]	140	74	70	2	1	—	—	—	16	2	69	.5	151	[62] 310	.09	.08	1.1	7
	From frozen:																			
613	Ear, 5 in long	1 ear[61]	229	73	120	4	1	—	—	—	27	4	121	1.0	291	[62] 440	.18	.10	2.1	9
614	Kernels	1 cup	165	77	130	5	1	—	—	—	31	5	120	1.3	304	[62] 580	.15	.10	2.5	8
	Canned:																			
615	Cream style	1 cup	256	76	210	5	2	—	—	—	51	8	143	1.5	248	[62] 840	.08	.13	2.6	13
	Whole kernel:																			
616	Vacuum pack	1 cup	210	76	175	5	1	—	—	—	43	6	153	1.1	204	[62] 740	.06	.13	2.3	11
617	Wet pack, drained solids	1 cup	165	76	140	4	1	—	—	—	33	8	81	.8	160	[62] 580	.05	.08	1.5	7
	Cowpeas. See Blackeye peas. (items 585–586).																			
	Cucumber slices, 1/8 in thick (large, 2 1/8-in diam.; small, 1 3/4-in diam.):																			

No.	Food, approximate measure	Measure	Grams	Water (%)	Food energy	Protein (g)	Fat (g)	Sat.	Oleic	Linoleic	Carbohydrate (g)	Calcium (mg)	Phosphorus (mg)	Iron (mg)	Potassium (mg)	Vit. A (IU)	Thiamin (mg)	Riboflavin (mg)	Niacin (mg)	Ascorbic acid (mg)
618	With peel	6 large or 8 small slices	28	95	5	Trace	Trace	—	—	—	1	7	8	.3	45	70	.01	.01	.1	3
619	Without peel	6 1/2 large or 9 small pieces.	28	96	5	Trace	Trace	—	—	—	1	5	5	.1	45	Trace	.01	.01	.1	3
620	Dandelion greens, cooked drained	1 cup	105	90	35	2	1	—	—	—	7	147	44	1.9	244	12,290	.14	.17	–	19
621	Endive, curly (including escarole), raw, small pieces.	1 cup	50	93	10	1	Trace	—	—	—	2	41	27	0.9	147	1,650	0.04	0.07	0.3	5
	Kale, cooked, drained:																			
622	From raw (leaves without stems and midribs).	1 cup	110	88	45	5	1	—	—	—	7	206	64	1.8	243	9,130	.11	.20	1.8	102
623	From frozen (leaf style)	1 cup	130	91	40	4	1	—	—	—	7	157	62	1.3	251	10,660	.08	.20	.9	49
	Lettuce, raw:																			
	Butterhead, as Boston types:																			
624	Head, 5-in diam	1 head[63]	220	95	25	2	Trace	—	—	—	4	57	42	3.3	430	1,580	.10	.10	.5	13
625	Leaves	1 outer or 2 inner or 3 heart leaves.	15	95	Trace	Trace	Trace	—	—	—	Trace	5	4	.3	40	150	.01	.01	Trace	1
	Crisphead, as Iceberg:																			
626	Head, 6-in diam	1 head[64]	567	96	70	5	1	—	—	—	16	108	118	2.7	943	1,780	.32	.32	1.6	32
627	Wedge, 1/4 of head	1 wedge	135	96	20	1	Trace	—	—	—	4	27	30	.7	236	450	.08	.08	.4	8
628	Pieces, chopped or shredded	1 cup	55	96	5	Trace	Trace	—	—	—	2	11	12	.3	96	180	.03	.03	.2	3
629	Looseleaf (bunching varieties including romaine or cos), chopped or shredded pieces.	1 cup	55	94	10	1	Trace	—	—	—	2	37	14	.8	145	1,050	.03	.04	.2	10
630	Mushrooms, raw, sliced or chopped	1 cup	70	90	20	2	Trace	—	—	—	3	4	81	.6	290	Trace	.07	.32	2.9	2
631	Mustard greens, without stems and midribs, cooked, drained.	1 cup	140	93	30	3	1	—	—	—	6	193	45	2.5	308	8,120	.11	.20	.8	67
632	Okra pods, 3 by 5/8 in, cooked	10 pods	106	91	30	2	Trace	—	—	—	6	98	43	.5	184	520	.14	.19	1.0	21
	Onions:																			
	Mature:																			
	Raw:																			
633	Chopped	1 cup	170	89	65	3	Trace	—	—	—	15	46	61	.9	267	[65]Trace	.05	.07	.3	17
634	Sliced	1 cup	115	89	45	2	Trace	—	—	—	10	31	41	.6	181	[65]Trace	.03	.05	.5	12
635	Cooked (whole or sliced), drained.	1 cup	210	92	60	3	Trace	—	—	—	14	50	61	.8	231	[65]Trace	.06	.06	.4	15
636	Young green, bulb (3/8 in. diam.) and white portion of top.	6 onions	30	88	15	Trace	Trace	—	—	—	3	12	12	.2	69	Trace	.02	.01	.1	8
637	Parsley, raw, chopped	1 tbsp	4	85	Trace	Trace	Trace	—	—	—	Trace	7	2	.2	25	300	Trace	.01	Trace	6
638	Parsnips, cooked (diced or 2-in lengths).	1 cup	155	82	100	2	1	—	—	—	23	70	96	.9	587	50	.11	.12	.2	16
	Peas, green:																			
	Canned:																			
639	Whole, drained solids	1 cup	170	77	150	8	1	—	—	—	29	44	129	3.2	163	1,170	.15	.10	1.4	14
640	Strained (baby food)	1 oz (1 3/4 to 2 tbsp)	28	86	15	1	Trace	—	—	—	3	3	18	.3	28	140	.02	.03	.3	3
641	Frozen, cooked, drained	1 cup	160	82	110	8	Trace	—	—	—	19	30	138	3.0	216	960	.43	.14	2.7	21
642	Peppers, hot, red, without seeds, dried (ground chili powder, added seasonings).	1 tsp	2	9	5	Trace	Trace	—	—	—	1	5	4	.3	20	1,300	Trace	.02	.2	Trace
	Peppers, sweet (about 5 per lb, whole), stem and seeds removed:																			
643	Raw	1 pod	74	93	15	1	Trace	—	—	—	4	7	16	.5	157	310	.06	.06	.4	94
644	Cooked, boiled, drained	1 pod	73	95	15	1	Trace	—	—	—	3	7	12	.4	109	310	.05	.05	.4	70
	Potatoes, cooked:																			
645	Baked, peeled after baking (about 2 per lb, raw).	1 potato	156	75	145	4	Trace	—	—	—	33	14	101	1.1	782	Trace	.15	.07	2.7	31

[61] Weight includes cob. Without cob, weight is 77 g for item 612, 126 g for item 613.
[62] Based on yellow varieties. For white varieties, value is trace.
[63] Weight includes refuse of outer leaves and core. Without these parts, weight is 163 g.
[64] Weight includes core. Without core, weight is 539 g.
[65] Value based on white-fleshed varieties. For yellow-fleshed varieties, value in International Units (I.U.) is 70 for item 633, 50 for item 634, and 80 for item 635.

VEGETABLE AND VEGETABLE PRODUCTS—Con.

Item No. (A)	Foods, approximate measures, units, and weight (edible part unless footnotes indicate otherwise) (B)		Grams	Water (C) Per-cent	Food energy (D) Cal-ories	Pro-tein (E) Grams	Fat (F) Grams	Fatty Acids Satu-rated (total) (G) Grams	Unsaturated Oleic (H) Grams	Unsaturated Lino-leic (I) Grams	Car-bohy-drate (J) Grams	Cal-cium (K) Milli-grams	Phos-phorus (L) Milli-grams	Iron (M) Milli-grams	Potas-sium (N) Milli-grams	Vitamin A value (O) Inter-national units	Thia-mine (P) Milli-grams	Ribo-flavin (Q) Milli-grams	Niacin (R) Milli-grams	Ascor-bic acid (S) Milli-grams
	Boiled (about 3 per lb, raw):																			
646	Peeled after boiling	1 potato	137	80	105	3	Trace	—	—	—	23	10	72	.8	556	trace	.12	.05	2.0	22
647	Peeled before boiling	1 potato	135	83	90	3	Trace	—	—	—	20	8	57	.7	385	Trace	.12	.05	1.6	22
	French-fried, strip, 2 to 3 1/2 in long:																			
648	Prepared from raw	10 strips	50	45	135	2	7	1.7	1.2	3.3	18	8	56	.7	427	Trace	.07	.04	1.6	11
649	Frozen, oven heated	10 strips	50	53	110	2	4	1.1	.8	2.1	17	5	43	.9	326	Trace	.07	.01	1.3	11
650	Hashed brown, prepared from frozen.	1 cup	155	56	345	3	18	4.6	3.2	9.0	45	28	78	1.9	439	Trace	.11	.03	1.6	12
	Mashed, prepared from—																			
	Raw:																			
651	Milk added	1 cup	210	83	135	4	2	.7	.4	Trace	27	50	103	.8	548	40	.17	.11	2.1	21
652	Milk and butter added	1 cup	210	80	195	4	9	5.6	2.3	.2	26	50	101	.8	525	360	.17	.11	2.1	19
653	Dehydrated flakes (without milk), water, milk, butter, and salt added.	1 cup	210	79	195	4	7	3.6	2.1	.2	30	65	99	.6	601	270	.08	.08	1.9	11
654	Potato chips, 1 3/4 by 2 1/2 in oval cross section.	10 chips	20	2	115	1	8	2.1	1.4	4.0	10	8	28	.4	226	Trace	.04	.01	1.0	3
655	Potato salad, made with cooked salad dressing.	1 cup	250	76	250	7	7	2.0	2.7	1.3	41	80	160	1.5	798	350	.20	.18	2.8	28
656	Pumpkin, canned	1 cup	245	90	80	2	1	—	—	—	19	61	64	1.0	588	15,680	.07	.12	1.5	12
657	Radishes, raw (prepackaged) stem ends, rootlets cut off.	4 radishes	18	95	5	Trace	Trace	—	—	—	1	5	6	.2	58	Trace	.01	.01	.1	5
658	Sauerkraut, canned, solids and liquid.	1 cup	235	93	40	2	Trace	—	—	—	9	85	42	1.2	329	120	.07	.09	.5	33
	Southern peas. See Blackeye peas (items 585–586).																			
	Spinach:																			
659	Raw, chopped	1 cup	55	91	15	2	Trace	—	—	—	2	51	28	1.7	259	4,460	0.06	0.11	0.3	28
	Cooked, drained:																			
660	From raw	1 cup	180	92	40	5	1	—	—	—	6	167	68	4.0	583	14,580	.13	.25	.9	50
	From frozen:																			
661	Chopped	1 cup	205	92	45	6	1	—	—	—	8	232	90	4.3	683	16,200	.14	.31	.8	39
662	Leaf	1 cup	190	92	45	6	1	—	—	—	7	200	84	4.8	688	15,390	.15	.27	1.0	53
663	Canned, drained solids	1 cup	205	91	50	6	1	—	—	—	7	242	53	5.3	513	16,400	.04	.25	.6	29
	Squash, cooked:																			
664	Summer (all varieties), diced, drained.	1 cup	210	96	30	2	Trace	—	—	—	7	53	53	.8	296	820	.11	.17	1.7	21
665	Winter (all varieties), baked, mashed.	1 cup	205	81	130	4	1	—	—	—	32	57	98	1.6	945	8,610	.10	.27	1.4	27
	Sweet potatoes:																			
	Cooked (raw, 5 by 2 in; about 2 1/2 per lb):																			
666	Baked in skin, peeled	1 potato	114	64	160	2	1	—	—	—	37	46	66	1.0	342	9,230	.10	.08	.8	25
667	Boiled in skin, peeled	1 potato	151	71	170	3	1	—	—	—	40	48	71	1.1	367	11,940	.14	.09	.9	26
668	Candied 2 1/2 by 2-in piece	1 piece	105	60	175	1	3	2.0	.8	.1	36	39	45	.9	200	6,620	.06	.04	.4	11
	Canned:																			
669	Solid pack (mashed)	1 cup	255	72	275	5	1	—	—	—	63	64	105	2.0	510	19,890	.13	.10	1.5	36
670	Vacuum pack, piece 2 3/4 by 1 in.	1 piece	40	72	45	1	Trace	—	—	—	10	10	16	.3	80	3,120	.02	.02	.2	6
	Tomatoes:																			
671	Raw, 2 3/5-in diam. (3 per 12 oz pkg.).	1 tomato[66]	135	94	25	1	Trace	—	—	—	6	[65]16	33	.6	300	1,110	.07	.05	.9	[7]28
672	Canned, solids and liquid	1 cup	241	94	50	2	Trace	—	—	—	10	14	46	1.2	523	2,170	.12	.07	1.7	41
673	Tomato catsup	1 cup	273	69	290	5	1	—	—	—	69	60	137	2.2	991	3,820	.25	.19	4.4	41
674		1 tbsp	15	69	15	Trace	Trace	—	—	—	4	3	8	.1	54	210	.01	.01	.2	2
	Tomato juice, canned:																			

No.	Food	Measure	Grams	Water (%)	Food energy (cal)	Protein (g)	Fat (g)	Saturated (g)	Oleic (g)	Linoleic (g)	Carbohydrate (g)	Calcium (mg)	Phosphorus (mg)	Iron (mg)	Potassium (mg)	Vitamin A (IU)	Thiamin (mg)	Riboflavin (mg)	Niacin (mg)	Ascorbic acid (mg)
675	Cup	1 cup	243	94	45	2	Trace	—	—	—	10	17	44	2.2	552	1,940	.12	.07	1.9	39
676	Glass (6 fl oz)	1 glass	182	94	35	2	Trace	—	—	—	8	13	33	1.6	413	1,460	.09	.05	1.5	29
677	Turnips, cooked, diced	1 cup	155	94	35	1	Trace	—	—	—	8	54	37	.6	291	Trace	.06	.08	.5	34
	Turnip greens, cooked, drained:																			
678	From raw (leaves and stems)	1 cup	145	94	30	3	Trace	—	—	—	5	252	49	1.5	—	8,270	.15	.33	.7	68
679	From frozen (chopped)	1 cup	165	93	40	4	Trace	—	—	—	6	195	64	2.6	246	11,390	.08	.15	.7	31
680	Vegetables, mixed, frozen, cooked	1 cup	182	83	115	6	1	—	—	—	24	46	115	2.4	348	9,010	.22	.13	2.0	15
	MISCELLANEOUS ITEMS																			
	Baking powders for home use:																			
	Sodium aluminum sulfate:																			
681	With monocalcium phosphate monohydrate.	1 tsp	3.0	2	5	Trace	0	0	0	0	1	58	87	—	5	0	0	0	0	0
682	With monocalcium phosphate monohydrate, calcium sulfate.	1 tsp	2.9	1	5	Trace	0	0	0	0	1	183	45	—	—	0	0	0	0	0
683	Straight phosphate	1 tsp	3.8	2	5	Trace	0	0	0	0	1	239	—	—	6	0	0	0	0	0
684	Low sodium	1 tsp	4.3	2	5	Trace	0	0	0	0	2	207	314	—	471	0	0	0	0	0
685	Barbecue sauce	1 cup	250	81	230	4	17	2.2	4.3	10.0	20	53	50	2.0	435	900	.03	.03	.8	13
	Beverages, alcoholic:																			
686	Beer	12 fl oz	360	92	150	1	0	0	0	0	14	18	108	Trace	90	—	.01	.11	2.2	—
	Gin, rum, vodka, whisky:																			
687	80-proof	1 1/2-fl oz jigger	42	67	95	—	—	—	—	—	Trace	—	—	—	1	—	—	—	—	—
688	86-proof	1 1/2-fl oz jigger	42	64	105	—	—	—	—	—	Trace	—	—	—	1	—	—	—	—	—
689	90-proof	1 1/2-fl oz jigger	42	62	110	—	—	—	—	—	Trace	—	—	—	1	—	—	—	—	—
	Wines:																			
690	Dessert	3 1/2-fl oz glass	103	77	140	Trace	0	0	0	0	8	8	—	—	77	—	.01	.02	.2	—
691	Table	3 1/2-fl oz glass	102	86	85	Trace	0	0	0	0	4	9	10	.4	94	—	Trace	.01	.1	—
	Beverages, carbonated, sweetened, nonalcoholic:																			
692	Carbonated water	12 fl oz	366	92	115	0	0	0	0	0	29	—	—	—	—	0	0	0	0	0
693	Cola type	12 fl oz	369	90	145	0	0	0	0	0	37	—	—	—	—	0	0	0	0	0
694	Fruit-flavored sodas and Tom Collins mixer.	12 fl oz	372	88	170	0	0	0	0	0	45	—	—	—	—	0	0	0	0	0
695	Ginger ale	12 fl oz	366	92	115	0	0	0	0	0	29	—	—	—	0	0	0	0	0	0
696	Root beer	12 fl oz	370	90	150	0	0	0	0	0	39	—	—	—	0	0	0	0	0	0
	Chili powder. See Peppers, hot, red (item 642).																			
	Chocolate:																			
697	Bitter or baking	1 oz	28	2	145	3	15	8.9	4.9	.4	8	22	109	1.9	235	20	.01	.07	.4	0
	Semisweet, see Candy, chocolate (item 539).																			
698	Gelatin, dry	1, 7-g envelope	7	13	25	6	Trace	0	0	0	0	—	—	—	—	0	0	0	0	—
699	Gelatin dessert prepared with gelatin dessert powder and water.	1 cup	240	84	140	4	0	0	0	0	34	—	—	—	—	0	—	—	—	—
700	Mustard, prepared, yellow	1 tsp or individual serving pouch or cup.	5	80	5	Trace	Trace	—	—	—	Trace	4	4	.1	7	—	—	—	—	—
	Olives, pickled, canned:																			
701	Green	4 medium or 3 extra large or 2 giant[69]	16	78	15	Trace	2	.2	1.2	.1	Trace	8	2	.2	7	40	—	—	—	—
702	Ripe, Mission	3 small or 2 large[69]	10	73	15	Trace	2	.2	1.2	.1	Trace	9	1	.1	2	10	Trace	Trace	—	—
	Pickles, cucumber:																			
703	Dill, medium, whole, 3 3/4 in long, 1 1/4-in diam.	1 pickle	65	93	5	Trace	Trace	—	—	—	1	17	14	.7	130	70	Trace	.01	Trace	4

[66] Weight includes cores and stem ends. Without these parts, weight is 123 g.

[67] Based on year-round average. For tomatoes marketed from November through May, value is about 12 mg; from June through October, 32 mg.

[68] Applies to product without calcium salts added. Value for products with calcium salts added may be as much as 63 mg for whole tomatoes, 241 mg for cut forms.

[69] Weight includes pits. Without pits, weight is 13 g for item 701, 9 g for item 702.

Item No. (A)	Foods, approximate measures, units, and weight (edible part unless footnotes indicate otherwise) (B)	Grams	Water (C) Percent	Food energy (D) Calories	Protein (E) Grams	Fat (F) Grams	Fatty Acids Saturated (total) (G) Grams	Fatty Acids Unsaturated Oleic (H) Grams	Fatty Acids Unsaturated Linoleic (I) Grams	Carbohydrate (J) Grams	Calcium (K) Milligrams	Phosphorus (L) Milligrams	Iron (M) Milligrams	Potassium (N) Milligrams	Vitamin A value (O) International units	Thiamine (P) Milligrams	Riboflavin (Q) Milligrams	Niacin (R) Milligrams	Ascorbic acid (S) Milligrams
	MISCELLANEOUS ITEMS—Con.																		
	Pickles, cucumber—Continued																		
704	Fresh-pack, slices 1 1/2-in diam., 1/4 in thick.	2 slices	79	10	Trace	Trace	—	—	—	3	5	4	.3	—	20	Trace	Trace	Trace	1
705	Sweet, gherkin, small, whole, about 2 1/2 in long, 3/4-in diam.	1 pickle	61	20	Trace	Trace	—	—	—	5	2	2	.2	—	10	Trace	Trace	Trace	1
706	Relish, finely chopped, sweet.	1 tbsp	63	20	Trace	Trace	—	—	—	5	3	2	.1	—	—	—	—	—	—
	Popcorn. See items 475–478.																		
707	Popsicle, 3-fl oz size.	1 popsicle	80	70	0	0	0	0	0	18	0	—	Trace	—	0	0	0	0	0
	Soups:																		
	Canned, condensed:																		
	Prepared with equal volume of milk:																		
708	Cream of chicken	1 cup	85	180	7	10	4.2	3.6	1.3	15	172	152	.5	260	610	.05	.27	.7	2
709	Cream of mushroom	1 cup	83	215	7	14	5.4	2.9	4.6	16	191	169	.5	279	250	.05	.34	.7	1
710	Tomato	1 cup	84	175	7	7	3.4	1.7	1.0	23	168	155	.8	418	1,200	.10	.25	1.3	15
	Prepared with equal volume of water:																		
711	Bean with pork	1 cup	84	170	8	6	1.2	1.8	2.4	22	63	128	2.3	395	650	.13	.08	1.0	3
712	Beef broth, bouillon, consomme.	1 cup	96	30	5	0	0	0	0	3	Trace	31	.5	130	Trace	Trace	.02	1.2	—
713	Beef noodle.	1 cup	93	65	4	3	.6	.7	.8	7	7	48	1.0	77	50	.05	.07	1.0	Trace
714	Clam chowder, Manhattan type (with tomatoes, without milk).	1 cup	92	80	2	3	.5	.4	1.3	12	34	47	1.0	184	880	.02	.02	1.0	—
715	Cream of chicken	1 cup	92	95	3	6	1.6	2.3	1.1	8	24	34	.5	79	410	.02	.05	.5	Trace
716	Cream of mushroom	1 cup	90	135	2	10	2.6	1.7	4.5	10	41	50	.5	98	70	.02	.12	.7	Trace
717	Minestrone	1 cup	90	105	5	3	.7	.9	1.3	14	37	59	1.0	314	2,350	.07	.05	1.0	—
718	Split pea	1 cup	85	145	9	3	1.1	1.2	.4	21	29	149	1.5	270	440	.25	.15	1.5	1
719	Tomato	1 cup	91	90	2	3	.5	.5	1.0	16	15	34	.7	230	1,000	.05	.05	1.2	12
720	Vegetable beef	1 cup	92	80	5	2	—	—	—	10	12	49	.7	162	2,700	.05	.05	1.0	—
721	Vegetarian	1 cup	92	80	2	2	—	—	—	13	20	39	1.0	172	2,940	.05	.05	1.0	—
	Dehydrated:																		
722	Bouillon cube, 1/2 in	1 cube	4	5	1	Trace	—	—	—	Trace	—	—	—	4	—	—	—	—	—
	Mixes:																		
	Unprepared:																		
723	Onion	1 1/2-oz pkg	3	150	6	5	1.1	2.3	1.0	23	42	49	.6	238	30	.05	.03	.3	6
	Prepared with water:																		
724	Chicken noodle	1 cup	95	55	2	1	—	—	—	8	7	19	.2	19	50	.07	.05	.5	Trace
725	Onion	1 cup	96	35	1	1	—	—	—	6	10	12	.2	58	Trace	Trace	Trace	Trace	5
726	Tomato vegetable with noodles.	1 cup	93	65	1	1	—	—	—	12	7	19	.2	29	480	.05	.02	.5	5
727	Vinegar, cider.	1 tbsp	94	Trace	Trace	0	0	0	0	1	1	1	.1	15	—	—	—	—	—
728	White sauce, medium, with enriched flour.	1 cup	73	405	10	31	19.3	7.8	.8	22	288	233	.5	348	1,150	.12	.43	.7	2
	Yeast:																		
729	Baker's, dry, active.	1 pkg	5	20	3	Trace	—	—	—	3	3	90	1.1	140	Trace	.16	.38	2.6	Trace
730	Brewer's, dry.	1 tbsp	5	25	3	Trace	—	—	—	3	[70]17	140	1.4	152	Trace	1.25	.34	3.0	Trace

[70] Value may vary from 6 to 60 mg.

Adams, C. F., and M. Richardson, *Nutritive Values of Food.* Home and Garden Bulletin No. 72, USDA, Washington, D.C., revised April, 1981.

APPENDIX D

SELECTED MINERALS AND VITAMINS IN FOODS

The following table contains values for four minerals (sodium, magnesium, copper, and zinc) and four vitamins (pantothenic acid, vitamin B_6, vitamin B_{12}, and folacin) in 167 foods commonly consumed. Values are for portions of foods commonly eaten and are for household measures. Sources of values are indicated at the end of the table.

SELECTED MINERALS AND VITAMINS IN FOODS

(Values per household measure, edible portion)

ITEM No.	FOOD	SODIUM (mg)	MAGNESIUM (mg)	COPPER (mg)	ZINC (mg)	PANTOTHENIC ACID (mg)	VITAMIN B_6 (mg)	VITAMIN B_{12} (µg)	FOLACIN (µg)
1	Almonds, dried, shelled, 1 cup	6	383	1.2	—	.667	.142	0	136
2	Almonds, salted, 1 cup	311	—	—	—	—	—	—	—
3	Apple, 1–2½ in diameter	1	9	.1	.08	.121	.035	0	9
4	Apple juice, 1 cup	2	10	.49	.27	—	.074	0	—
5	Apricots, raw—3 apricots	1	14	.13	—	.274	.080	0	—
6	Apricots, canned in syrup—1 cup	3	19	.14	—	.253	.149	0	—
7	Asparagus, raw—1 cup	3	27	.15	1.31	.837	.207	0	86
8	Asparagus, canned—1 cup	564	—	.36	—	.472	.133	0	—
9	Avocado, raw—1	9	136	.21	1.30	3.231	1.268	0	—
	BABY FOODS, Items 10-14								
10	Cherry vanilla pudding, junior—1 jar	32	5	—	.066	—	.026	—	.7
11	Chicken with vegetables, junior—1 jar	33	9	—	1.280	.435	.050	.205	1.5
12	Macaroni and cheese dinner, junior—1 jar	163	14	.045	.682	—	.034	.060	3.2
13	Pears, strained—1 jar	3	10	.083	.096	.115	.010	—	4.6
14	Peas, strained—1 jar	5	19	.082	.447	.358	.088	.1	33.2
15	Bacon, raw—2 slices	153	4	.02	.35	.050	.019	0	—
16	Banana, 1 medium	1	58	.30	—	.455	.893	0	49
17	Barley, pearled—1 cup	6	74	1.24	.33	1.006	.448	0	40
18	Barbecue sauce—1 cup	2038	139	—	—	—	.188	0	10
19	Basil—1 tsp	Trace	6	—	0.08	—	—	0	—
	Beans, immature, lima								
20	frozen—1 cup	172	82	—	—	.408	.255	0	53
21	canned—1 cup	401	—	—	—	.221	.153	0	—
	Beans, mature, dry								
22	lima, raw—1 cup	7	324	1.3	5	1.755	1.044	0	203
23	pinto, raw—1 cup	19	—	—	—	1.226	1.010	0	410
24	red, raw—1 cup	19	302	—	—	.925	.816	0	246
25	white, raw—1 cup	34	306	—	—	1.305	1.008	0	232
26	white, canned with tomato sauce, 1 cup	862	—	—	—	.235	—	—	61
	Beans, snap, green								
27	raw—1 cup	8	35	.15	.4	.209	.088	0	48
28	canned—1 cup	319	18	.05	.4	.010	.052	0	—

No.	Food								
29	frozen—1 cup	1	27	—	—	.176	.091	0	43
30	Yellow (wax), raw—1 cup	8	—	—	—	.275	—	0	44
31	canned—1 cup	319	—	—	—	—	.055	0	—
32	frozen—1 cup	1	15	.07	—	.179	.103	0	44
33	Beef, raw—3 oz	55	—	—	3.57	.399	.281	1.2	6
34	corned, canned—3 oz	1105	—	—	1.65	—	—	1.5	—
35	dried, chipped—3 oz	3655	3.2	.233	2.328	—	—	1.5	—
36	Beef gravy, canned—1 cup	117	34	.2	—	.203	.023	.23	126
37	Beets, raw—1 cup	81	26	.24	—	.17	.074	0	—
38	canned—1 cup	401	—	—	—	.17	.085	0	—
	Beverages, alcoholic:								
39	beer—1 cup	17	—	.17	.07	.192	.144	0	—
40	wine—3½ oz	5	—	.11	.10	.031	.041	0	—
41	Biscuit dough, frozen, commercial—1	255	—	—	—	—	—	—	—
42	mix—1 cup	1664	—	—	—	—	—	0	—
43	Blackberries, raw—1 cup	2	43	.23	—	.346	.072	0	—
44	canned, sweetened—1 cup	3	—	—	—	.190	.059	0	9
45	Blueberries, raw—1 cup	1	9	.22	—	.226	.097	0	9
46	canned—1 cup	.6	9	—	—	.156	.090	0	—
47	Bouillon cube—1 cube	960	1.2	.03	—	—	—	0	6
48	Brazil nuts, shelled—1 cup	1	315	2.14	7.1	.323	.238	0	—
	Bread:								
49	cracked wheat—1 slice	132	9	—	—	.152	.023	0	—
50	French—1 slice	203	8	.06	.4	.132	.019	0	—
51	rye, American—1 slice	139	11	.06	.36	.113	.025	0	—
52	pumpernickel—1 slice	182	23	.06	.2	.16	.051	0	—
53	white—1 slice	142	6	.05	.5	.120	.011	Trace	—
54	whole wheat—1 slice	132	19.5	—	.50	.19	.045	0	107
55	Broccoli, raw—1 cup	23	37	.18	.27	1.814	.302	0	—
56	frozen—1 cup	31	39	.08	.59	.833	.278	0	87
57	cooked—1 cup	22	—	—	—	—	—	—	121
58	Brussel sprouts, raw—1 cup	16	45	.12	.56	1.121	.357	0	—
59	frozen—1 cup	25	33	—	.01	.651	.271	0	56
60	cooked—1 cup	16	—	—	—	—	—	—	.42
61	Butter—1 tbsp	140	.3	—	.3	—	0	Trace	59
62	Cabbage, raw—1 cup	18	12	.07	.6	.185	.144	0	26
63	cooked—1 cup	20	9	.13	—	—	—	—	—
64	Carrots, raw—1 cup	52	25	.11	.44	.308	.165	0	35
65	cooked—1 cup	51	—	—	.47	.202	.047	0	—
66	Cashews—1 cup	21	374	—	6.13	1.82 (canned)	(canned)	0	95
67	Cauliflower, raw—1 cup	13	24	.07	.29	1.000	.210	0	—
68	frozen—1 cup	20	23	—	—	.972	.342	0	99

SELECTED MINERALS AND VITAMINS IN FOODS

(Values per household measure, edible portion)

ITEM No.	FOOD	SODIUM (mg)	MAGNESIUM (mg)	COPPER (mg)	ZINC (mg)	PANTOTHENIC ACID (mg)	VITAMIN B6 (mg)	VITAMIN B12 (µg)	FOLACIN (µg)
69	Celery, chopped—1 cup	151	26	.08	.17	.515	.072	0	14
70	Cheese:								
71	natural, blue or bleu—1 oz	396	7	—	.75	.504	.048	.39	10
72	camembert—1 oz	239	6	—	.67	.35	.062	.36	18
73	cheddar—1 oz	196	13	.03	1.12	.14	.022	.28	5
74	cottage—1 cup	423	11	.03	.67	.321	.058	1.46	17
75	mozzarella—1 oz	106	6	—	1.09	.018	.018	.28	2
76	swiss—1 oz	201	10	.03	1.29	.104	.021	.50	2
77	processed American—1 oz	406	6	—	.85	.137	.020	.197	2
78	processed swiss—1 oz	388	8	—	1.02	.073	.012	.34	—
	Cherries, raw, sweet— 10 cherries	2	—	.09	—	—	.024	0	6
79	canned, drained—1 cup	3	24	.16	—	.196	.081	0	—
80	Chickpeas, dry, raw—1 cup	52	—	—	5.4	2.5	1.08	0	398
81	canned, drained—1 cup	—	—	—	1.4	—	—	—	204
82	Chicken gravy, canned—1 cup	1375	—	.238	1.907	—	.024	—	—
83	Chicken, without skin—3 oz	43	19.6	.12	.6	.68	.581	.38	5
84	Cinnamon—1 tsp	1	1	—	.05	—	—	—	—
85	Corn, sweet, canned—1 cup	389	31	—	.8	.363	.33	0	—
86	frozen, kernels off cob—1 cup	2	37	—	—	.726	.363	0	35
87	Cowpeas (black-eyed), dry, raw—1 cup	60	391	1.26	4.9	1.785	.955	0	226
88	canned, drained—1 cup	401	—	—	2.0	.275	.090	0	136
89	Crab, cooked—1 cup	424	39	1.75	4.95	.690	.345	11.5	—
90	Crackers, saltines—4	308	—	—	.06	—	.007	0	—
91	Cranberries—1 cup	2	7.6	.10	—	.208	.033	0	2
92	Dates, chopped—1 cup	2	103	.39	—	1.388	.272	0	37
93	Egg, raw, whole—1 medium	70	5.5	.05	.5	.800	.055	1.0	32
94	Figs, raw—1 medium	1	10	.04	—	.150	.057	0	5
95	Flounder, raw—3 oz	201	25.5	.13	.60	.723	1.445	1.02	—
96	Grapefruit, raw—1/2	1	22	.07	—	.521	.063	0	20
97	juice, canned—1 cup	2	27	.02	.07	.320	.027	0	52
98	Ham, canned—3 oz	1114	—	.03	—	—	.306	—	9
99	Herring, raw—3 oz	63	14	.16	—	.825	.315	8.5	—
100	smoked—3 oz	5296	—	—	—	.791	.272	1.11	—
101	Ice cream, vanilla—1 cup	116	18	—	1.41	.654	.061	.625	3
102	Kale, raw—1 lb	340	168	—	—	4.540	1.362	0	272
103	frozen—1 lb	118	141	—	—	1.707	.840	0	—

104	Lamb, raw—3 oz	64	—	.20	2.6	.468	.234	1.83	36
105	Lentils, dry—1 cup	57	152	—	5.9	2.584	1.14	0	68
106	Lettuce, head—1 cup	7	6	.05	.22	.110	.030	0	20
107	romaine—1 cup	5	—	—	—	—	—	—	98
108	Liver, beef, raw—3 oz	116	11	2.38	3.23	6.545	.714	68	186
109	cooked—3 oz	156	15	—	5.1	—	.638	—	123
110	chicken, raw—3 oz	60	—	.23	2.04	5.100	.638	21	309
111	cooked—3 oz	52	—	—	2.89	—	—	—	204
112	Lobster, raw—3 oz	—	5	—	2.61	2.175	—	.73	—
113	Milk, fresh, whole—1 cup	122	32	.09	.98	.830	.098	.98	12
114	fresh, skim—1 cup	127	34	.05	.98	.903	.102	.98	—
115	nonfat, dry—1 cup	638	149	.50	4.68	3.744	.395	3.33	—
116	Molasses, blackstrap—1 tbsp	19	52	—	—	.070	.040	0	42
117	Oatmeal, dry—1 cup	2	115	.46	2.7	1.200	.112	0	—
118	Olives—4 medium	370	3	.05	.04	.002	—	0	—
119	Orange, raw—1	1	18	.10	.32	.403	.097	0	74
120	juice, frozen, concentrate, diluted—1 cup	2	25	.02	.05	.408	.070	0	137
121	Oysters, raw—1 cup	175	77	41.14	179.28	.600	.120	43.2	—
122	Pancake mix—1 cup	1935	—	—	6.4	—	—	—	—
123	Peanuts, raw, shelled—1 cup	7	297	.89	4.18	4.032	.576	0	153
124	roasted, shelled—1 cup	7	252	—	4.32	3.024	—	0	—
125	roasted, salted—1 cup	602	—	—	—	—	—	—	—
126	Peanut butter—1 tbsp	97	28	.09	.46	—	.053	0	13
127	Peas, immature, seeds, raw 1 cup	3	51	.32	1.3	1.088	.232	0	—
128	frozen—1 cup	187	35	—	1.2	.457	.189	0	77
129	dried, mature seeds—1 cup	70	360	—	6.4	—	—	—	—
130	Pecans, shelled—1 cup	Trace	153	1.23	—	1.845	.120	0	26
131	Pepper, black—1 tsp	1	4	—	.03	—	—	0	—
132	Potatoes, raw 2½ in diameter	3	85	.53	.75	.950	.625	0	48
133	frozen, french fries 10 strips, 4 in	3	25	—	.28	.540	.180	0	—
134	Pretzels, 1 rod—7½ in long	235	3	.02	.15	.076	.003	Trace	—
135	Raisins—1 cup	39	51	.36	.26	.203	.508	0	—
136	Rice, brown—1 cup, raw	17	163	.52	3.33	2.035	1.018	0	30
137	white—1 cup, raw	9	52	.37	2.4	1.018	.315	0	18
138	Salad dressing, Italian—1 tbsp	314	—	.11	.02	—	—	—	—
139	Russian—1 tbsp	130	—	.17	.06	—	—	—	—
140	Salmon, raw—3 oz	—	—	—	—	1.105	.595	3.4	—
141	canned—3 oz	444	25	.06	.77	.425	.255	5.857	17
142	Sausage and lunchmeat bologna, 1 slice	369	2	—	.23	—	.013	—	.65

SELECTED MINERALS AND VITAMINS IN FOODS

(Values per household measure, edible portion)

ITEM No.	FOOD	SODIUM (mg)	MAGNESIUM (mg)	COPPER (mg)	ZINC (mg)	PANTOTHENIC ACID (mg)	VITAMIN B6 (mg)	VITAMIN B12 (µg)	FOLACIN (µg)
143	frankfurter, raw—1 (2 oz)	627	7.5	.05	1.14	.245	.080	.74	2.5
144	Shrimp, canned—3 oz	1955	—	.14	1.8	.179	.051	—	13
145	Soups: commercial, canned, prepared chicken noodle, 1 cup	979	25	.195	.395	—	.125	—	2.2
146	vegetable beef—1 cup, dehydrated	1046	6	.183	1.545	—	.076	—	15
147	beef noodle, prepared—1 cup	420	9	—	.100	—	.035	—	1.6
148	chicken noodle, prepared, 1 cup	578	7	.46	.14	—	.008	—	1.4
149	Soybeans, mature, dry—1 cup	11	557	—	—	3.570	1.701	0	359
150	Spinach, raw—1 cup	39	48	.06	.44	.165	.154	0	106
151	cooked—1 cup	90	—	—	—	—	—	—	164
152	Stuffing mix, cooked—1 cup	1131	—	—	—	—	—	—	—
153	Strawberries—1 cup	1	18	.10	.12	.507	.082	0	24
154	Sunflower seeds, hulled—1 cup	44	55	2.57	—	2.030	1.813	0	—
155	Sweet potato, canned—1 cup	96	—	.12	—	.860	.132	0	100
156	Tomato, ripe, raw—1	3	19	.15	.27	.446	.135	0	53
157	canned—1 cup	313	29	.48	.48	.554	.217	0	—
158	catsup—1 tbsp	158	3	.09	.04	—	.016	0	.75
159	Tuna, canned—3 oz	448	—	.07	.56	.179	.238	1.23	13
160	Turkey, raw—3 oz	37	13	.06	1.26	.481	.247	.226	4.9
161	Wheat flour, whole—1 cup	4	136	.6	2.9	1.32	.408	0	65
162	all purpose—1 cup	3	34	.27	.96	.637	.082	0	29
163	Wheat products, farina, dry—1 cup	4	45	.40	1.0	.927	.121	0	43
164	bran, 100%—1 cup	493	252	.87	5.9	1.740	.492	0	155
165	germ, toasted—1 tbsp	—	20	.14	1.0	.072	.069	0	20
166	Yeast, brewer's—1 tbsp	10	18	—	—	.960	.200	0	313
167	Yogurt—1 cup	125	—	—	1.2	.767	.113	.270	12

SOURCES: Pennington, J. T., and D. H. Calloway, "Copper Content of Foods." *Journal of the American Dietetic Association,* 63:144–149, August 1973. Copyright The American Dietetic Association. Used with permission.

Greger, J. L., S. Marchefka, and A. H. Geissler, "Magnesium Content of Selected Foods." *Journal of Food Science,* 43:1610, 1978. Copyright by Institute of Food Technologists.

Adams, C., *Nutritive Value of American Foods.* Agriculture Handbook No. 456, USDA, Washington, D.C., 1975.

Marsh, A. C., R. N. Klippstein, and S. D. Kaplan, *The Sodium Content of Your Food.* Home and Garden Bulletin No. 233, USDA, Washington, D. C., 1980.

Haeflein, K. A., and A. I. Rasmussen, "Zinc Content of Selected Foods." *Journal of the American Dietetic Association,* 70:612, 1977. Copyright The American Dietetic Association. Used with permission.

Freeland, J. H., and R. J. Cousins, "Zinc Content of Selected Foods." *Journal of the American Dietetic Association,* 68:527, 1976. Copyright The American Dietetic Association. Used with permission.

Murphy, E. W., B. W. Willis, and B. K. Watt, "Provisional Tables on the Zinc Content of Foods." *Journal of the American Dietetic Association,* 66:346, 1975. Copyright The American Dietetic Association. Used with permission.

Watt, B. W., and A. L. Merrill, *Composition of Foods.* Agriculture Handbook No. 8, USDA, 1963.

Orr, M. L., *Pantothenic Acid, Vitamin B_6 and Vitamin B_{12} in Foods.* Home Economics Research Report No. 36, USDA, Washington, D. C., 1969.

Perloff, B. P., and R. R. Butrum, "Folacin in Selected Foods." *Journal of the American Dietetic Association,* 70:161, 1977. Copyright The American Dietetic Association. Used with permission.

APPENDIX E

SUGAR CONTENT OF SELECTED FOODS

The following tables show the percentage of sucrose or total sugars in foods, but in the text we pointed out that the *amount of sugar per serving* is more informative. You can convert percentage sugar to amounts per serving as follows. Look up in Appendix C the food you are interested in—let's say apples. Find the weight in grams of one serving. We find, for example, that a medium apple weighs 138 g. Now look up the percentage of sugars in apples in one of the following tables. You find 3.1 percent sucrose and 11.4 percent total sugars. Multiply 138 g by 0.031 = 4.3 (rounded) g of sucrose; and 138 g multiplied by 0.114 = 15.7 g total sugars. One tsp of sucrose weighs 4 g. Therefore, one medium apple contains the equivalent of about 1 tsp of sucrose, and about 4 tsp of total sugars (assuming their weight is the same as that of sucrose).

When serving sizes are given in ounces (oz), use the relationship of 1 oz = 28 g.

TABLE 1. PERCENTAGE OF SUCROSE AND TOTAL SUGARS IN SOME MINIMALLY PROCESSED AND PROCESSED FOODS

(— indicates lack of data)

	% SUCROSE	% TOTAL SUGARS
FRUITS		
Apple	3.1	11.4
Apple juice	4.2	12.2
Apricots	5.5	7.8
Banana, yellow	8.9	17.3
Cherries	0.1	12.6
Cranberries	0.1	3.5
Grapes, Concord	0.2	9.7
Grapefruit	2.9	6.1
Lemon	0.2	1.5

	% SUCROSE	% TOTAL SUGARS
Melon, cantaloupe	4.4	6.7
Orange	4.6	9.6
Orange juice, frzn., reconst.	3.2	7.8
Peaches	6.6	9.7
Pears, Bartlett	1.5	9.5
Plums, Italian prune	5.4	10.0
Plums, sweet	4.4	11.8
Prunes, unckd.	2.0	49.0
Strawberries	1.4	6.3
Tangerine	9.0	13.8
Tomatoes, seedless, pulp	0.4	6.9
Watermelon	4.0	7.8
VEGETABLES		
Beans, lima	1.4	—
Beans, snap	0.5	2.2
Beets, sugar	12.9	—
Cabbage, raw	0.3	3.7
Carrots	1.7	7.5
Cauliflower	0.3	3.1
Celery	0.3	0.6
Corn	0.3	0.8
Cucumber	0.1	2.6
Eggplant	0.6	2.7
Lettuce	0.2	1.6
Onions	2.9	8.3
Peas, green	5.5	—
White potatoes	0.1	1.1
Pumpkin	0.6	2.8
Radishes	0.3	3.4
Spinach	—	0.2
Squash, butternut	0.4	0.7
Squash, golden crookneck	1.0	3.8
Sweet potato, baked	7.2	21.7
LEGUMES		
Soybeans	7.2	8.8
Garbanzos (chickpeas)	2.4	—
Field pea	6.7	—
Lentils	2.1	—
Soybean flour or meal	6.8	—
MILK PRODUCTS		
Ice cream	16.6	20.2
Sweetened condensed milk	43.5	57.6
NUTS		
Almonds, blanched	2.3	2.5
Chestnuts	3.6	5.8
Macadamia nuts	5.5	5.8
Peanuts	4.5	4.7
Pecans	1.1	—
CEREALS		
Rice, brown	0.8	0.9
Rice, polished	0.4	2.4
Defatted wheat germ	8.3	—
Wheat flour, patent	0.2	2.2

	% SUCROSE	% TOTAL SUGARS
SYRUPS AND OTHER SWEETS		
Chocolate, sweet, dry	56.4	—
Golden syrup	31.0	68.5
Honey	1.9	76.6
Jellies, pectin	52.5	—
Maple syrup	62.9	64.4
Milk chocolate	43.0	51.1
Molasses	53.6	70.4
Blackstrap molasses	36.9	63.8
Carob bean	21.3	32.5

Values from Hardinge, M. G., J. B. Swarner, and H. Crooks, *Carbohydrates in Foods. Journal of the American Dietetics Association*, 46:197, 1965. Copyright The American Dietetic Association. Used with permission.

TABLE 2. PERCENTAGE OF SUCROSE AND TOTAL SUGARS IN READY-TO-EAT BREAKFAST CEREALS

PRODUCT	% SUCROSE	% TOTAL SUGARS
Sugar Smacks	43.0	56.0
Apple Jacks	54.0	54.6
Froot Loops	48.0	48.0
Sugar Corn Pops	39.0	46.0
Super Sugar Crisp	36.0	46.0
Frankenberry	38.0	43.7
Cookie Crisp, Vanilla	43.0	43.5
Cap'n Crunch w/Crunchberries	42.0	43.3
Cocoa Krispies	41.0	43.0
Cocoa Pebbles	42.0	42.6
Fruity Pebbles	42.0	42.5
Lucky Charms	36.0	42.2
Cookie Crisp, Chocolate	40.0	41.0
Sugar Frosted Corn Flakes	39.0	41.0
Quisp	40.0	40.7
Cookie Crisp, Oatmeal	39.0	40.1
Cap'n Crunch	40.0	40.0
Count Chocula	35.0	39.5
Alpha Bits	38.0	38.0
Honey Comb	37.0	37.2
Frosted Rice	35.0	37.0
Trix	33.0	35.9
Cocoa Puffs	32.0	33.3
Cap'n Crunch, Peanut Butter	31.0	32.2
Raisin Bran	15.0	30.4
Golden Grahams	27.0	30.0
Craklin' Bran	27.0	29.0
Kellogg's Raisin Bran	11.0	29.0
Frosted Mini Wheats	26.0	26.0
Life, Cinnamon	21.0	21.0
Nabisco 100% Bran	19.0	21.0
All-Bran	16.0	19.0
Life	16.0	16.0
Team	12.0	14.1

	% SUCROSE	% TOTAL SUGARS
Grape Nuts Flakes	7.0	13.3
40% Bran	10.0	13.0
Buckwheats	10.0	12.2
Product 19	8.1	9.9
Concentrate (Kellogg's)	9.0	9.3
Total	7.0	8.3
Wheaties	7.0	8.2
Rice Krispies	7.0	7.8
Special K	5.0	5.4
Corn Flakes	3.0	5.3
Post Toasties	5.0	3.0
Kix	4.0	4.8
Rice Chex	4.0	4.4
Corn Chex	4.0	4.0
Wheat Chex	2.0	3.5
Cheerios	3.0	3.0
Shredded Wheat	0.6	0.6
Puffed Wheat	0.5	0.5
Puffed Rice	0.1	0.1

SOURCE: *Analysis of Sugar Content of Ready-to-eat Cereals*, Nutrient Composition Laboratory, USDA, 1979.

TABLE 3. PERCENTAGE OF SUCROSE IN SOME BRAND NAME FOODS

	% SUCROSE
BREAKFAST PRODUCTS	
Breakfast bars	26.0 (Average)
Instant Breakfast powders	33.0 (Average)
CANDIES	
French Burnt Peanuts	58.4
Jelly beans	61.3
Peppermints	43.8
Hershey's Milk Chocolate w/Peanuts	52.5
Mr. Goodbar	34.2
M&M's Plain Chocolate Candy	52.2
Snickers	28.0
Almond Joy	20.0
Cracker Jack	14.7
Cadbury Milk Chocolate	32.1
Planter's Peanut Candy Block	21.5
Mints	70.1
Tootsie Roll	21.1
GUM	
Chewing gum	67.0 (Average)
COOKIES	
Chocolate chip cookies	28.6 (Average)
Oatmeal cookies	26.4 (Average)
Macaroons	31.2 (Average)

	% SUCROSE
Fig newtons	23.3
Sugar cookies	27.1 (Average)
Oreo cookies	35.3

COUGH MEDICINES
Cough drops and medicated lozenges	49.3 (Average)
Cough syrup	22.0 (Average)

CRACKERS
Honey Maid Graham Crackers (Nabisco)	16.7
Town House Crackers	6.3
Cheese Nips	2.4
Graham Crackers (Nabisco)	15.8
Ritz Crackers	3.2
Triscuit	0.7
Wheat Thins	4.4

CANNED JUICES
Pineapple juice (Del Monte)	1.4
Apricot nectar (Libby)	6.1
Peach nectar (Libby))	8.1
Pear nectar (Libby)	7.0

ICE CREAM
Chocolate fudge ice cream bar	14.2
Eskimo Pie	20.7
Ice cream sandwich	19.5
Orange sherbet	19.6
Popsicle	11.8
Vanilla ice cream	8.8

SNACK ITEMS
Doritos	1.7
Fritos	0.8
Potato chips	0.9
Apple pie	13.5
Chocolate cupcake, filled	35.5
Frosted Pop-Tarts	19.9
Instant chocolate mix	79.6
Raisins	0.6
Twinkies	32.0
Snack pudding	9.7 (Average)

SOFT DRINKS
Coca Cola	4.2
Dr. Pepper	3.4
Grape Tang	9.8
Hawaiian Punch	6.9
Kool-Aid punch	8.0
Nestea instant tea	2.0
Pepsi-Cola	2.5
7-Up	4.1
Sprite	8.7

SOURCE: Shannon, I. L., *Brand Name Guide to Sugar,* Chicago: Nelson-Hall, 1977.

APPENDIX F

CHOLESTEROL IN FOODS

Cholesterol occurs only in foods of animal origin. Values are given in this table for common serving sizes of foods grouped under headings.

CHOLESTEROL IN FOODS

ITEM	PORTION SIZE	mg CHOLESTEROL
MEATS		
Beef, lean, trimmed of fat, ckd.	3 oz	77
Lamb, lean, trimmed of fat, ckd.	3 oz	85
Pork, lean, trimmed of fat, ckd.	3 oz	75
Veal, lean, trimmed of fat, ckd.	3 oz	84
Liver, beef, ckd.	3 oz	372
FISH AND SHELLFISH		
Crab, meat only, ckd.	3 oz	85
Flounder, flesh only	3 oz	42
Oysters, raw	3 oz	42
Shrimp	3 oz	128
Tuna, canned in oil, drained	3 oz	55
CHICKEN		
Light meat, w/skin, roasted	3 oz	71
Dark meat, w/skin, roasted	3 oz	77
Light meat, no skin, roasted	3 oz	72
Dark meat, no skin, roasted	3 oz	79
Breast, w/skin, roasted	1/2 breast (98 g)	83
Breast, meat only, roasted	1/2 breast (86 g)	73
Drumstick, w/skin, roasted	1 drumstick (52 g)	48
Drumstick, meat only, roasted	1 drumstick (44 g)	41
Liver, raw	1 liver	140

ITEM	PORTION SIZE	mg CHOLESTEROL
TURKEY		
Light meat, w/skin, roasted	3 oz	64
Dark meat, w/skin, roasted	3 oz	76
Light meat, no skin, roasted	3 oz	59
Dark meat, no skin, roasted	3 oz	72
LUNCHMEATS		
Chicken frankfurter	1 frank	45
Turkey frankfurter	1 frank	48
Beef and pork frankfurter	1 frank	22
Bologna, beef and pork	1 oz	16
Sliced ham, 11% fat	1 oz	16
Lunchmeat, beef	1 oz	12
DAIRY PRODUCTS		
Butter, regular	1 tsp	11
Cheddar cheese	1 oz	30
Creamed cottage cheese	1/4 cup	8
Cream cheese	1 tbsp	17
Mozzarella, part skim	1 oz	16
Parmesan, hard	1 oz	19
Ricotta, part skim	1 oz	9
Swiss cheese	1 oz	26
American, pasteurized process	1 oz	18
Coffee, cream, light	1 tbsp	10
Whipping cream, light	1 tbsp	17
Whipping cream, heavy	1 tbsp	21
Sour cream	1 tbsp	5
Ice cream, vanilla, 10% fat	1 cup	59
Ice milk, vanilla	1 cup	18
Whole milk, 3.3% fat	1 cup	33
Skim milk	1 cup	4
Yogurt, plain, whole milk	1 cup	30
Yogurt, plain, skim milk	1 cup	4
Egg, whole	1 egg	274

Values obtained or calculated from:

Feeley, R. M., P. E Criner, and B. K. Watt, "Cholesterol Content of Foods." *Journal of the American Dietetic Association*, 61:134, 1972.

Posati, L. P., *Composition of Foods. Poultry Products.* Agriculture Handbook No. 8-5, USDA, Washington, D.C., 1979.

Richardson, M., L. P. Posati, and B. A. Anderson, *Composition of Foods. Sausages and Luncheon Meats.* Agriculture Handbook No. 8-7, USDA, Washington, D.C., 1980.

Posati, L. P., and M. L. Orr, *Composition of Foods. Dairy and Egg Products.* Agriculture Handbook No. 8-1. USDA, Washington, D.C., 1976.

APPENDIX G

NUTRITIONAL ANALYSES OF FAST FOODS

	WT (g)	ENERGY (kcal)	PRO (g)	CHO (g)	FAT (g)	CHOL (mg)	A (IU)	B₁ (mg)	B₂ (mg)	Nia (mg)	B₆ (mg)	B₁₂ (µg)	C (mg)	D (IU)	Ca (mg)	Cu (mg)	Fe (mg)	K (mg)	Mg (mg)	P (mg)	Na (mg)	Zn (mg)	MOIS-TURE (g)	CRUDE FIBER (g)
ARBY'S®																								
Roast Beef	140	350	22	32	15	45	X	0.30	0.34	5	—	—	X	—	80	—	3.6	—	—	—	880	—	—	—
Beef and Cheese	168	450	27	36	22	55	X	0.38	0.43	6	—	—	X	—	200	—	4.5	—	—	—	1220	—	—	—
Super Roast Beef	263	620	30	61	28	85	X	0.53	0.43	7	—	—	X	—	100	—	5.4	—	—	—	1420	—	—	—
Junior Roast Beef	74	220	12	21	12	35	X	0.15	0.17	3	—	—	X	—	40	—	1.8	—	—	—	530	—	—	—
Ham & Cheese	154	380	23	33	17	60	X	0.75	0.34	5	—	—	X	—	200	—	2.7	—	—	—	1350	—	—	—
Turkey Deluxe	236	510	28	46	24	70	X	0.45	0.34	8	—	—	X	—	80	—	2.7	—	—	—	1220	—	—	—
Club Sandwich	252	560	30	43	30	100	X	0.68	0.43	7	—	—	X	—	200	—	3.6	—	—	—	1610	—	—	—

SOURCE: Consumer Affairs, Arby's, Inc., Atlanta, Georgia. Nutritional analysis by Technological Resources, Camden, New Jersey.

	WT (g)	ENERGY (kcal)	PRO (g)	CHO (g)	FAT (g)	CHOL (mg)	A (IU)	B₁ (mg)	B₂ (mg)	Nia (mg)	B₆ (mg)	B₁₂ (µg)	C (mg)	D (IU)	Ca (mg)	Cu (mg)	Fe (mg)	K (mg)	Mg (mg)	P (mg)	Na (mg)	Zn (mg)	MOIS-TURE (g)	CRUDE FIBER (g)
BURGER CHEF®																								
Hamburger	91	244	11	29	9	27	114	0.17	0.16	2.7	0.16	0.26	1.2	—	45	0.08	2.0	208	9	106	—	1.6	41	0.2
Cheeseburger	104	290	14	29	13	39	267	0.18	0.21	2.8	0.17	0.36	1.2	—	132	0.08	2.2	218	9	202	—	1.9	46	0.2
Double Cheeseburger	145	420	24	30	22	77	431	0.20	0.32	4.4	0.31	0.73	1.2	—	223	0.10	3.2	360	15	355	—	3.6	67	0.2
Fish Filet	179	547	21	46	31	43	400	0.23	0.22	2.7	0.04	0.10	1.0	—	145	0.04	2.2	271	19	302	—	1.2	72	0.4
Super Shef® Sandwich	252	563	29	44	30	105	754	0.31	0.40	6.0	0.45	0.87	9.3	—	205	0.21	4.5	578	25	377	—	4.5	143	0.5
Big Shef® Sandwich	186	569	23	38	36	81	279	0.26	0.31	4.7	0.31	0.63	1.0	—	152	0.05	3.6	382	14	280	—	3.4	80	0.3
TOP Shef® Sandwich	138	661	41	36	38	134	273	0.35	0.47	8.1	0.56	1.16	1.0	—	194	0.13	5.4	612	26	445	—	5.9	91	0.1
Funmeal® Feast	—	545	15	55	30	27	123	0.25	0.21	4.6	0.16	0.26	12.8	—	61	0.24	2.8	688	26	183	—	1.6	70	0.8
Rancher® Platter*	316	640	32	33	42	106	1750*	0.29	0.38	8.6	0.61	1.01	23.5	—	66	0.38	5.3	1237	53	326	—	5.6	209	1.3
Mariner® Platter*	373	734	29	78	34	35	2069*	0.34	0.23	5.2	0.09	0.56	23.5	—	63	0.32	3.3	996	49	397	—	1.2	195	1.8
French Fries, small	68	250	2	20	19	0	0	0.07	0.04	1.7	—	—	11.5	—	9	0.16	0.7	473	16	62	—	<0.1	29	0.6
French Fries, large	85	351	3	28	26	0	0	0.10	0.06	2.4	—	—	16.2	—	13	0.23	0.9	661	22	86	—	<0.1	40	0.9
Vanilla Shake (12 oz)	336	380	13	60	10	40	387	0.10	0.66	0.5	0.1	1.77	0	—	497	—	0.3	622	40	392	—	1.3	—	—
Chocolate Shake (12 oz)	336	403	10	72	9	36	292	0.16	0.76	0.4	0.1	1.07	0	—	449	—	1.1	762	54	429	—	1.6	—	—
Hot Chocolate	—	198	8	23	8	30	288	0.93	0.39	0.3	0.1	0.79	2.1	—	271	0.09	0.7	436	50	245	—	1.1	—	—

*Includes salad.
SOURCE: Burger Chef Systems, Inc., Indianapolis, Indiana. Nutritional analysis from *Handbook No. 8.* Washington: US Dept. of Agriculture.

	WT (g)	ENERGY (kcal)	PRO (g)	CHO (g)	FAT (g)	CHOL (mg)	A (IU)	B₁ (mg)	B₂ (mg)	Nia (mg)	B₆ (mg)	B₁₂ (µg)	C (mg)	D (IU)	Ca (mg)	Cu (mg)	Fe (mg)	K (mg)	Mg (mg)	P (mg)	Na (mg)	Zn (mg)	MOIS-TURE (g)	CRUDE FIBER (g)
CHURCH'S FRIED CHICKEN®																								
White Chicken Portion	100	327	21	10	23	—	160	0.10	0.18	7.2	—	—	0.7	—	94	—	1.00	186	—	—	498	—	45	0.10
Dark Chicken Portion	100	305	22	7	21	—	140	0.10	0.27	5.3	—	—	1.0	—	15	—	1.3	206	—	—	475	—	48	0.20

SOURCE: Church's Fried Chicken, San Antonio, Texas. Nutritional analysis by Medallion Laboratories, Minneapolis, Minnesota.

	WT (g)	ENERGY (kcal)	PRO (g)	CHO (g)	FAT (g)	CHOL (mg)	A (IU)	B₁ (mg)	B₂ (mg)	Nia (mg)	B₆ (mg)	B₁₂ (µg)	C (mg)	D (IU)	Ca (mg)	Cu (mg)	Fe (mg)	K (mg)	Mg (mg)	P (mg)	Na (mg)	Zn (mg)	MOIS-TURE (g)	CRUDE FIBER (g)
DAIRY QUEEN®																								
Frozen Dessert	113	180	5	27	6	20	100	0.09	0.17	X	—	0.6	X	X	150	—	X	—	—	100	—	—	—	—
DQ Cone, small	71	110	3	18	3	10	100	0.03	0.14	X	—	0.4	X	X	100	—	X	—	—	60	—	—	—	—
DQ Cone, regular	142	230	6	35	7	20	300	0.09	0.26	X	—	0.6	X	X	200	—	X	—	—	150	—	—	—	—
DQ Cone, large	213	340	10	52	10	30	400	0.15	0.43	X	—	1.2	X	8	300	—	X	—	—	200	—	—	—	—
DQ Dip Cone, small	78	150	3	20	7	10	100	0.03	0.17	X	—	0.4	X	X	100	—	0.4	—	—	80	—	—	—	—
DQ Dip Cone, regular	156	300	7	40	13	20	300	0.09	0.34	X	—	0.6	X	X	200	—	0.4	—	—	150	—	—	—	—
DQ Sundae, small	106	170	4	30	4	15	100	0.03	0.17	X	—	0.5	X	X	100	—	0.7	—	—	100	—	—	—	—
DQ Sundae, regular	177	290	6	51	7	20	300	0.06	0.26	X	—	0.6	X	X	200	—	1.1	—	—	150	—	—	—	—
DQ Sundae, large	248	400	9	71	9	30	400	0.09	0.43	0.4	—	1.2	X	8	300	—	1.8	—	—	250	—	—	—	—
DQ Malt, small	241	340	10	51	11	30	400	0.06	0.34	0.4	—	1.2	2.4	60	300	—	1.8	—	—	200	—	—	—	—
DQ Malt, regular	418	600	15	89	20	50	750	0.12	0.60	0.8	—	1.8	3.6	100	500	—	3.6	—	—	400	—	—	—	—

DQ Malt, large	588	840	22	125	28	70	750	0.15	0.85	1.2	—	2.4	6	140	600	—	5.4	—	600	—	—
DQ Float	397	330	6	59	8	20	100	0.12	0.17	X	—	0.6	X	X	200	—	X	—	200	—	—
DQ Banana Split	383	540	10	91	15	30	750	0.60	0.60	0.8	—	0.9	18	8	350	—	1.8	—	250	—	—
DQ Parfait	284	460	10	81	11	30	400	0.12	0.43	0.4	—	1.2	X	X	300	—	1.8	—	250	—	—
DQ Freeze	397	520	11	89	13	35	200	0.15	0.34	X	—	1.2	X	X	300	—	X	—	250	—	—
Mr. Misty® Freeze	411	500	10	87	12	35	200	0.15	0.34	X	—	0.12	X	X	300	—	X	—	200	—	—
Mr. Misty® Float	404	440	6	85	8	20	100	0.12	0.17	X	—	0.6	X	X	200	—	X	—	200	—	—
"Dilly"® Bar	85	240	4	22	15	10	100	0.06	0.17	0.4	—	0.5	X	X	100	—	0.4	—	100	—	—
DQ Sandwich	60	140	3	24	4	10	100	0.03	0.14	X	—	0.2	X	X	60	—	0.4	—	60	—	—
Mr. Misty® Kiss	89	70	0	17	0	0	X	X	X	X	X	X	X	X	X	X	X	X	X	—	—
Brazier® Cheese Dog	113	330	15	24	19	—	—	—	0.18	3.3	0.07	1.22	11.0	23	168	0.08	1.6	23	182	939	1.9
Brazier® Chili Dog	128	330	13	25	20	—	—	0.15	0.23	3.9	0.17	1.29	11.0	20	86	0.13	2.0	38	139	868	1.8
Brazier® Dog	99	273	11	23	15	—	—	0.12	0.15	2.6	0.08	1.05	11.0	23	75	0.79	1.5	21	104	868	1.4
Fish Sandwich	170	400	20	41	17	—	tr	0.15	0.26	3.0	0.16	1.20	tr	40	60	0.08	1.1	24	200	—	0.3
Fish Sandwich w/Cheese	177	440	24	39	21	—	100	0.15	0.26	3.0	0.16	1.50	40	44	150	0.08	0.4	24	250	—	0.3
Super Brazier® Dog	182	518	20	41	30	—	tr	0.42	0.44	7.0	0.17	2.09	14.0	44	158	0.18	4.3	37	195	1552	2.8
Super Brazier® Dog w/Cheese	203	593	26	43	36	—	tr	0.43	0.48	8.1	0.18	2.34	14.0	44	297	0.18	4.4	42	312	1986	3.5
Super Brazier® Chili Dog	210	555	23	42	33	—	—	0.42	0.48	8.8	0.27	2.67	18.0	32	158	0.21	4.0	48	231	1640	2.8
Brazier® Fries, small	71	200	2	25	10	—	tr	0.06	tr	0.8	0.16	—	—	16	tr	0.04	0.4	16	100	—	tr
Brazier® Fries, large	113	320	3	40	16	—	tr	0.09	0.03	1.2	0.30	—	4.8	24	tr	0.08	0.4	24	150	—	0.3
Brazier® Onion Rings	85	300	6	33	17	—	tr	0.09	tr	0.4	0.08	—	2.4	8	20	0.08	0.4	16	60	—	0.3

SOURCE: International Dairy Queen, Inc., Minneapolis, Minnesota. Nutritional analysis by Raltech Scientific Services, Inc. (formerly WARF), Madison, Wisconsin. (Nutritional analysis not applicable in the state of Texas.)

JACK IN THE BOX®

Hamburger	97	263	13	29	11	26	49	0.27	0.18	5.6	0.11	0.73	1.1	20	82	0.10	2.3	165	115	566	1.8	43	0.2
Cheeseburger	109	310	16	28	15	32	338	0.27	0.21	5.4	0.12	0.87	<1.1	20	172	0.10	2.6	177	194	877	2.3	47	0.2
Jumbo Jack® Hamburger	246	551	28	45	29	80	246	0.47	0.34	11.6	0.30	2.68	3.7	42	134	0.22	4.5	492	261	1134	4.2	139	0.7
Jumbo Jack® Hamburger w/Ch	272	628	32	45	35	110	734	0.52	0.38	11.3	0.31	3.05	4.9	41	273	0.24	4.6	499	411	1666	4.8	153	0.8
Regular Taco	83	189	8	15	11	22	356	0.07	0.07	1.8	0.14	0.5	<0.9	6	116	0.11	1.2	264	150	460	1.3	47	0.6
Super Taco	146	285	12	20	17	37	599	0.10	0.12	2.8	0.22	0.77	1.6	9	196	0.18	1.9	415	235	968	2.1	92	1.0
Moby Jack® Sandwich	141	455	17	38	26	56	240	0.30	0.21	4.5	0.12	1.1	1.4	24	167	0.08	1.7	246	263	837	1.1	57	0.1
Breakfast Jack® Sandwich	121	301	18	28	13	182	442	0.41	0.47	5.1	0.14	1.1	3.4	51	177	0.11	2.5	190	310	1037	1.8	59	0.1
French Fries	80	270	3	31	15	13	—	0.12	0.02	1.9	0.22	0.17	3.7	<1	19	0.10	0.7	423	88	128	0.3	29	0.6
Onion Rings	85	351	5	32	23	24	—	0.24	0.12	3.1	0.07	0.26	<1.2	<1	26	0.07	1.4	109	69	318	0.4	24	0.3
Apple Turnover	119	411	4	45	24	17	—	0.23	0.12	2.5	0.03	0.17	<1.2	1	11	0.06	1.4	69	33	352	0.2	45	0.2
Vanilla Shake*	317	317	10	57	6	26	11	0.16	0.38	0.5	0.20	1.36	<3.2	41	349	0.06	0.2	599	312	229	1.0	243	0.3
Strawberry Shake*	328	323	11	55	7	26	—	0.16	0.46	0.6	0.15	1.25	<3.3	43	371	0.10	0.6	613	328	241	1.1	253	0.3
Chocolate Shake*	322	325	11	55	7	26	440	0.16	0.64	0.6	0.19	1.55	<3.2	45	348	0.13	0.7	676	328	270	1.1	247	0.3
Vanilla Shake	314	342	10	54	9	36	426	0.16	0.47	0.5	0.18	0.92	3.5	44	349	0.06	0.4	536	318	263	1.0	238	0.3
Strawberry Shake	328	380	11	63	10	33	380	0.16	0.62	0.5	0.18	0.98	<3.2	30	351	0.07	0.3	556	316	268	1.0	242	0.3
Chocolate Shake	317	365	11	59	10	35	—	0.16	0.60	0.6	0.18	0.98	<3.2	38	350	0.16	1.2	633	332	294	1.2	235	0.3
Ham & Cheese Omelette	174	425	21	32	23	355	766	0.45	0.70	3.0	0.18	1.44	<1.7	64	260	0.14	4.0	237	397	975	2.3	94	0.2
Double Cheese Omelette	166	423	19	30	25	370	797	0.33	0.68	2.5	0.14	1.33	1.7	61	276	0.13	3.6	208	370	899	2.1	88	0.2
Ranchero Style Omelette	196	414	20	33	23	343	853	0.33	0.74	2.6	0.18	1.51	<2.0	78	278	0.14	3.8	260	372	1098	2.0	117	0.4
French Toast	180	537	15	54	29	115	522	0.56	0.30	4.4	0.47	1.62	9.2	22	119	0.11	3.0	194	256	1130	1.8	78	0.9
Pancakes	232	626	16	79	27	87	488	0.63	0.44	4.6	0.19	0.56	<26.2	23	105	0.12	2.8	237	633	1670	1.9	104	0.7
Scrambled Eggs	267	719	26	55	44	259	694	0.69	0.56	5.2	0.34	1.31	<12.8	80	257	0.24	5.0	635	483	1110	3.0	137	1.3

*Special formula for shakes sold in California, Arizona, Texas, and Washington.

SOURCE: Jack-in-the-Box, Foodmaker, Inc., San Diego, California. Nutritional analysis by Raltech Scientific Services, Inc. (formerly WARF), Madison, Wisconsin.

	WT (g)	ENERGY (kcal)	PRO (g)	CHO (g)	FAT (g)	CHOL (mg)	A (IU)	B₁ (mg)	B₂ (mg)	Nia. (mg)	B₆ (mg)	B₁₂ (µg)	C (mg)	D (IU)	Ca (mg)	Cu (mg)	Fe (mg)	K (mg)	Mg (mg)	P (mg)	Na (mg)	Zn (mg)	MOIS-TURE (g)	CRUDE FIBER (g)
KENTUCKY FRIED CHICKEN®																								
Original Recipe® Diner*																								
Wing & Rib	322	603	30	48	32	133	25.5	0.22	0.19	10.0	–	–	36.6	–	–	–	–	–	–	–	–	–	–	–
Wing & Thigh	341	661	33	48	38	172	25.5	0.24	0.27	8.4	–	–	36.6	–	–	–	–	–	–	–	–	–	–	–
Drum & Thigh	346	643	35	46	35	180	25.5	0.25	0.32	8.5	–	–	36.6	–	–	–	–	–	–	–	–	–	–	–
Extra Cripsy Dinner*																								
Wing & Rib	349	755	33	60	43	132	25.5	0.31	0.29	10.4	–	–	36.6	–	–	–	–	–	–	–	–	–	–	–
Wing & Thigh	371	812	36	58	48	176	25.5	0.31	0.35	10.3	–	–	36.6	–	–	–	–	–	–	–	–	–	–	–
Drum & Thigh	376	765	38	55	44	183	25.5	0.32	0.38	10.4	–	–	36.6	–	–	–	–	–	–	–	–	–	–	–
Mashed Potatoes	85	64	2	12	1	0	<18	<0.01	0.02	0.8	–	–	4.9	–	–	–	–	–	–	–	–	–	–	–
Gravy	14	23	0	1	2	0	<3	0.00	0.01	0.1	–	–	<0.2	–	–	–	–	–	–	–	–	–	–	–
Cole Slaw	91	122	1	13	8	7	–	–	–	–	–	–	–	–	–	–	–	–	–	–	–	–	–	–
Rolls	21	61	2	11	1	1	<5	0.10	0.04	1.0	–	–	0.3	–	–	–	–	–	–	–	–	–	–	–
Corn (5.5-inch ear)	135	169	5	31	3	X	162	0.12	0.07	1.2	–	–	2.6	–	–	–	–	–	–	–	–	–	–	–

*Includes two pieces of chicken, mashed potato and gravy, cole slaw, and roll.

SOURCE: Kentucky Fried Chicken, Inc., Louisville, Kentucky. Nutritional analysis by Raltech Scientific Services, Inc. (formerly WARF), Madison, Wisconsin.

	WT (g)	ENERGY (kcal)	PRO (g)	CHO (g)	FAT (g)	CHOL (mg)	A (IU)	B₁	B₂	Nia.	B₆	B₁₂	C	D	Ca	Cu	Fe	K	Mg	P	Na	Zn	MOIS-TURE	CRUDE FIBER
LONG JOHN SILVER'S®																								
Fish w/Batter (2 pc)	136	366	22	21	22	229	–	–	–	–	–	–	–	–	–	–	–	–	–	–	–	–	–	–
Fish w/Batter (3 pc)	207	549	32	32	32	13	–	–	–	–	–	–	–	–	–	–	–	–	–	–	–	–	–	–
Treasure Chest®	143	506	30	32	33	47	–	–	–	–	–	–	–	–	–	–	–	–	–	–	–	–	–	–
Chicken Planks® (4 pc)	166	457	27	35	23	43	–	–	–	–	–	–	–	–	–	–	–	–	–	–	–	–	–	–
Peg Legs® w/Batter (5 pc)	125	350	22	26	28	349	–	–	–	–	–	–	–	–	–	–	–	–	–	–	–	–	–	–
Ocean Scallops (6 pc)	120	283	11	30	13	7	–	–	–	–	–	–	–	–	–	–	–	–	–	–	–	–	–	–
Shrimp w/Batter (6 pc)	88	268	8	30	13	7	–	–	–	–	–	–	–	–	–	–	–	–	–	–	–	–	–	–
Breaded Oysters (6 pc)	156	441	13	53	19	86	–	–	–	–	–	–	–	–	–	–	–	–	–	–	–	–	–	–
Breaded Clams	142	617	18	61	34	37	–	–	–	–	–	–	–	–	–	–	–	–	–	–	–	–	–	–
Fish Sandwich	193	337	22	49	31	10	–	–	–	–	–	–	–	–	–	–	–	–	–	–	–	–	–	–
French Fryes	85	288	4	33	16	25	–	–	–	–	–	–	–	–	–	–	–	–	–	–	–	–	–	–
Cole Slaw	113	138	1	16	8	67	–	–	–	–	–	–	–	–	–	–	–	–	–	–	–	–	–	–
Corn on the Cob (1 ear)	150	176	5	29	4	96	–	–	–	–	–	–	–	–	–	–	–	–	–	–	–	–	–	–
Hushpuppies (3)	45	153	3	20	7	47	–	–	–	–	–	–	–	–	–	–	–	–	–	–	–	–	–	–
Clam Chowder (8 oz)	170	107	5	15	3	–	–	–	–	–	–	–	–	–	–	–	–	–	–	–	–	–	–	–

SOURCE: Long John Silver's Food Shoppes, Lexington, Kentucky. Nutritional analysis by L. V. Packett, PhD, The Department of Nutrition and Food Science, University of Kentucky.

	WT (g)	ENERGY (kcal)	PRO (g)	CHO (g)	FAT (g)	CHOL (mg)	A (IU)	B₁ (mg)	B₂ (mg)	Nia. (mg)	B₆ (mg)	B₁₂ (µg)	C (mg)	D (IU)	Ca (mg)	Cu (mg)	Fe (mg)	K (mg)	Mg (mg)	P (mg)	Na (mg)	Zn (mg)	MOIS-TURE (g)	CRUDE FIBER (g)
McDONALD'S®																								
Egg McMuffin®	138	327	19	31	15	229	97	0.47	0.44	3.8	0.21	0.75	<1.4	46	226	0.12	2.9	168	26	322	885	1.9	70.7	0.1
English Muffin, Buttered	63	186	5	30	5	13	164	0.28	0.49	2.6	0.04	0.02	0.8	14	117	0.69	1.5	71	13	74	318	0.5	21.7	0.1
Hotcakes w/Butter & Syrup	214	500	8	94	10	47	257	0.26	0.36	2.3	0.12	0.19	4.7	28	103	0.11	2.2	187	28	501	1070	0.7	97.8	0.2
Sausage (Pork)	53	206	9	tr	19	43	<32	0.27	0.11	2.1	0.18	0.53	0.5	31	16	0.05	0.8	127	9	95	615	1.5	22.9	0.1
Scrambled Eggs	98	180	13	3	13	349	652	0.08	0.47	0.1	0.19	0.93	1.2	65	61	0.06	2.5	135	13	264	205	1.7	68.1	<0.1
Hashbrown Potatoes	55	125	2	14	7	7	<14	0.06	<0.01	0.8	0.13	0.01	4.1	<1	5	0.04	0.4	247	13	67	325	0.2	30.9	0.3
Big Mac®	204	563	26	41	33	86	530	0.39	0.37	6.5	0.27	1.8	2.2	33	157	0.18	4.0	237	38	314	1010	4.7	100.4	0.6
Cheeseburger	115	307	15	30	14	37	345	0.25	0.23	3.8	0.12	0.91	1.6	13	132	0.11	2.4	156	23	205	767	2.6	108.4	0.2
Hamburger	102	255	12	30	10	25	82	0.25	0.18	4.0	0.12	0.81	1.7	12	51	0.10	2.3	142	19	126	520	2.1	48.0	0.3
Quarter Pounder®	166	424	24	33	22	67	133	0.32	0.28	6.5	0.27	1.88	1.7	23	63	0.17	4.1	322	37	249	735	5.1	83.7	0.7
Quarter Pounder® w/Ch	194	524	30	32	31	96	660	0.31	0.37	7.4	0.23	2.15	2.7	25	219	0.18	4.3	341	41	382	1236	5.7	96.0	0.8
Filet-O-Fish®	139	432	14	37	25	47	42	0.26	0.20	2.6	0.10	0.82	<1.4	25	93	0.10	1.7	150	27	229	781	0.9	59.5	0.1

McDonald's Corporation (continued)

Regular Fries	68	220	3	9	26	12	<17	0.12	0.02	2.3	0.22	<0.03	12.5	<1	9	0.03	0.6	564	27	101	109	0.3	25.4	0.5
Apple Pie	85	253	2	12	29	14	<34	0.02	0.02	0.2	0.02	<0.04	<0.8	2	14	0.05	0.6	39	6	27	398	0.2	38.3	0.3
Cherry Pie	88	260	2	13	32	14	114	0.03	0.02	0.4	0.02	<0.02	<0.8	<2	12	0.06	0.6	35	7	27	427	0.2	38.9	0.1
McDonaldland® Cookies	67	308	4	10	49	11	<27	0.23	0.23	2.9	0.03	0.03	0.9	10	12	0.07	1.5	52	11	74	358	0.3	2.2	0.1
Chocolate Shake	291	383	10	30	66	9	349	0.12	0.44	0.5	0.13	1.16	<2.9	44	320	0.19	0.8	580	49	335	300	1.4	203.0	0.3
Strawberry Shake	290	362	9	32	62	9	377	0.12	0.44	0.4	0.14	1.16	4.1	32	322	0.07	0.2	423	31	313	201	1.2	207.9	<0.3
Vanilla Shake	291	352	9	31	60	8	349	0.12	0.70	0.3	0.12	1.19	3.2	26	329	0.09	0.2	422	31	314	201	1.2	211.3	<0.3
Hot Fudge Sundae	164	310		18	46	11	230	0.07	0.31	1.1	0.13	0.7	2.5	16	215	0.13	0.6	410	35	236	175	1.0	97.9	0.2
Caramel Sundae	165	328	7	26	53	10	279	0.07	0.31	1.0	0.05	0.6	3.6	14	200	0.09	0.2	338	30	230	195	0.9	93.2	<0.2
Strawberry Sundae	164	289	7	20	46	9	230	0.07	0.30	1.0	0.05	0.6	2.8	16	174	0.11	0.4	290	28	80	96	0.8	101.0	0.2

SOURCE: McDonald's Corporation, Oak Brook, Illinois. Nutritional analysis by Raltech Scientific Services, Inc. (formerly WARF), Madison, Wisconsin.

TACO BELL®

Bean Burrito	166	343	11	11	48	12	—	1657	0.37	0.22	2.2	—	—	15.2	—	98	—	2.8	235	—	173	272	—	—
Beef Burrito	184	466	30	21	37	21	—	1675	0.30	0.39	7.0	—	—	15.2	—	83	—	4.6	320	—	288	327	—	—
Beefy Tostada	184	291	19	15	21	15	—	3450	0.16	0.27	3.3	—	—	12.7	—	208	—	3.4	277	—	265	138	—	—
Bellbeefer®	123	221	15	7	23	7	—	2961	0.15	0.20	3.7	—	—	10.0	—	40	—	2.6	183	—	140	231	—	—
Bellbeefer® w/Cheese	137	278	19	12	23	12	—	3146	0.16	0.27	3.7	—	—	10.0	—	147	—	2.7	195	—	208	330	—	—
Burrito Supreme®	225	457	21	22	43	22	—	3462	0.33	0.35	4.7	—	—	16.0	—	121	—	3.8	350	—	245	367	—	—
Combination Burrito	175	404	21	16	43	16	—	1666	0.34	0.31	4.6	—	—	15.2	—	91	—	3.7	278	—	230	300	—	—
Enchirito®	207	454	25	21	42	21	—	1178	0.31	0.37	4.7	—	—	9.5	—	259	—	3.8	491	—	338	1175	—	—
Pintos 'N Cheese	158	168	11	5	21	5	—	3123	0.26	0.16	0.9	—	—	9.3	—	150	—	2.3	307	—	210	102	—	—
Taco	83	186	15	8	14	8	—	120	0.09	0.16	2.9	—	—	0.2	—	120	—	2.5	143	—	175	79	—	—
Tostada	138	179	9	6	25	6	—	3152	0.18	0.15	0.8	—	—	9.7	—	191	—	2.3	172	—	186	101	—	—

SOURCES: (1) Menu Item Portions. San Antonio, Texas: Taco Bell Co., July 1976. (2) Adams, C. F.: "Nutritive value of American foods in common units." In Handbook No. 456. Washington: USDA Agricultural Research Service. November 1975. (3) Church E. F., and H. N. Church (eds): Food Values of Portions Commonly Used, 12th ed. Philadelphia: J. B. Lippincott Co. 1975. (4) Valley Baptist Medical Center, Food Service Department: Descriptions of Mexican-American Foods. Fort Atkinson, Wisconsin: NASCO.

WENDY'S®

Single Hamburger	200	470	26	34	26	70	94	0.24	0.36	5.8	—	—	0.6	—	84	—	5.3	239	—	774	—	4.8	110.6	0.8
Double Hamburger	285	670	44	34	40	125	128	0.43	0.54	10.6	—	—	1.5	—	138	—	8.2	364	—	980	—	8.4	162.1	1.1
Triple Hamburger	360	850	65	33	51	205	220	0.47	0.68	14.7	—	—	2.0	—	104	—	10.7	525	—	1217	—	13.5	204.6	1.4
Single w/Cheese	240	580	33	34	34	90	221	0.38	0.43	6.3	—	—	0.7	—	228	—	5.4	315	—	1085	—	5.5	133.4	1.0
Double w/Cheese	325	800	50	41	48	155	439	0.49	0.75	11.4	—	—	2.3	—	177	—	10.2	489	—	1414	—	10.1	179.2	1.3
Triple w/Cheese	400	1040	72	35	68	225	472	0.80	0.84	15.1	—	—	3.4	—	371	—	10.9	712	—	1848	—	14.3	216.4	1.6
Chili	250	230	19	21	8	25	1188	0.22	0.25	3.4	—	—	2.9	—	83	—	4.4	168	—	1065	—	3.7	195.9	2.3
French Fries	120	330	5	41	16	5	40	0.14	0.07	3.0	—	—	6.4	—	16	—	1.2	196	—	112	—	0.5	54.9	1.2
Frosty	250	390	9	54	16	45	355	0.20	0.60	X	X	—	0.7	—	270	—	0.9	278	—	247	—	1.0	169.8	0.0

SOURCE: Wendy's International, Inc., Dublin, Ohio. Nutritional analysis by Medallion Laboratories, Minneapolis, Minnesota.

NUTRITIONAL ANALYSES OF FAST FOODS (Dashes indicate no data available. X = Less than 2% US RDA; tr = trace.)

	WT (g)	ENERGY (kcal)	PRO (g)	CHO (g)	FAT (g)	CHOL (mg)	VITAMINS								MINERALS								CAFFEINE (mg)	SACCHAR. (mg)
							A (IU)	B_1 (mg)	B_2 (mg)	Nia. (mg)	B_6 (mg)	B_{12} (µg)	C (mg)	D (IU)	Ca (mg)	Cu (mg)	Fe (mg)	K (mg)	Mg (mg)	P (mg)	Na (mg)	Zn (mg)		
BEVERAGES																								
Coffee*	180	2	tr	tr	tr	–	0	0	tr	0.5	–	–	0	–	4	–	0.2	65	–	7	2	–	100†	0
Tea*	180	2	tr	–	tr	–	0	0	0.04	0.1	–	–	1	–	5	–	0.2	–	–	4	–	–	40†	0
Orange Juice	183	82	1	20	tr	–	366	0.17	0.02	0.6	–	–	82.4	–	17	–	0.2	340	18	29	2	–	0	0
Chocolate Milk	250	213	9	28	9	9	330	0.08	0.40	0.3	–	–	3.0	–	278	–	0.5	365	–	235	118	–	–	0
Skim Milk	245	88	9	13	tr	tr	10	0.09	0.44	0.2	–	–	2.0	–	296	–	0.1	355	–	233	127	–	–	0
Whole Milk	244	159	9	12	9	27	342	0.07	0.41	0.2	–	–	2.4	100	188	–	tr	351	32	227	122	–	–	0
Coca-Cola®	246	96	0	24	0	0	–	–	–	–	–	–	–	–	–	–	–	–	–	40	20‡	–	28	0
Fanta® Ginger Ale	244	84	0	21	0	0	–	–	–	–	–	–	–	–	–	–	–	–	–	0	30‡	–	0	0
Fanta® Grape	247	114	0	29	0	0	–	–	–	–	–	–	–	–	–	–	–	–	–	0	21‡	–	0	0
Fanta® Orange	248	117	0	30	0	0	–	–	–	–	–	–	–	–	–	–	–	–	–	0	21‡	–	0	0
Fanta® Root Beer	246	103	0	27	0	0	–	–	–	–	–	–	–	–	–	–	–	–	–	0	23‡	–	0	0
Mr. Pibb®	245	95	0	25	0	0	–	–	–	–	–	–	–	–	–	–	–	–	–	29	23‡	–	27	0
Mr. Pibb® w/o Sugar	236	1	0	tr	0	0	–	–	–	–	–	–	–	–	–	–	–	–	–	28	37‡	–	38	76
Sprite®	245	95	0	24	0	0	–	–	–	–	–	–	–	–	–	–	–	–	–	0	42‡	–	0	0
Sprite® w/o Sugar	236	3	0	0	0	0	–	–	–	–	–	–	–	–	–	–	–	–	–	0	42‡	–	0	57
Tab®	236	tr	0	tr	0	0	–	–	–	–	–	–	–	–	–	–	–	–	–	30	30‡	–	30	74
Fresca®	236	2	0	0	0	0	–	–	–	–	–	–	–	–	–	–	–	–	–	0	38	–	0	54

*6-oz serving; all other data are for 8-oz serving. †Caffeine content depends on strength of beverage. ‡Value when bottling water with average sodium content (12 mg/8 oz) is used.

SOURCES: (1) Adams, C. F.: "Nutritive value of American foods in common units." in *Handbook No. 456.* Washington: USDA Agricultural Research Service, November 1975; (2) The Coca-Cola Company, Atlanta, Georgia, January 1977; (3) *American Hospital Formulary Service.* Washington, American Society of Hospital Pharmacists, Section 28:20, March 1978.

SOURCE: Young, E. A., E. H. Brennan, and G. L. Irving, "Update: Nutritional Analysis of Fast Foods." *Dietetic Currents,* 8(2), March–April, 1981. (Ross Laboratories, Columbus, Ohio, 43216.)

APPENDIX H

ENERGY EXPENDITURE FOR PHYSICAL ACTIVITY

The uses and limitations of this table are discussed in Chapter 7.

ENERGY EXPENDITURE FOR PHYSICAL ACTIVITY

ACTIVITY	kcal/min/kg		
Archery	0.065	Cycling	
Badminton	0.097	Leisure, 5.5 mph	0.064
Baking, general (F)	0.035	Leisure, 9.4 mph	0.100
Basketball	0.138	Racing	0.169
Billiards	0.042	Dancing	
Boxing		Ballroom	0.051
In ring	0.222	"Twist," "wiggle"	0.168
Sparring	0.138	Digging trenches	0.145
Canoeing		Dishwashing	0.045
Leisure	0.044	Drawing (standing)	0.036
Racing	0.103	Dressing	0.035
Card playing	0.025	Driving car	0.022
Carpentry, general	0.052	Eating (sitting)	0.023
Carpet sweeping (F)	0.045	Electrical work	0.058
Carpet sweeping (M)	0.048	Farming	
Cleaning (F)	0.062	Barn cleaning	0.135
Cleaning (M)	0.058	Driving tractor	0.037
Climbing hills		Feeding cattle	0.085
With no load	0.121	Feeding animals	0.065
With 5-kg load	0.129	Forking straw bales	0.138
With 10-kg load	0.140	Milking by hand	0.054
With 20-kg load	0.147	Milking by machine	0.023
Cooking	0.045	Shoveling grain	0.085
Croquet	0.059	Field hockey	0.134

ACTIVITY	kcal/min/kg	ACTIVITY	kcal/min/kg
Fishing	0.062	5½ min per mile	0.289
Food shopping (F)	0.062	Scraping paint	0.063
Food shopping (M)	0.058	Scrubbing floors (F)	0.109
Football	0.132	Scrubbing floors (M)	0.108
Gardening		Shoe repair, general	0.045
Digging	0.126	Sitting quietly	0.021
Hedging	0.077	Skiing, hard snow	
Mowing	0.112	Level, moderate speed	0.119
Raking	0.054	Level, walking	0.143
Golf	0.085	Uphill, maximum speed	0.274
Gymnastics	0.066	Skiing, soft snow	
Housework, light	0.045	Leisure (F)	0.111
Horse-grooming	0.128	Leisure (M)	0.098
Horse-racing		Skindiving, with scuba gear	
Galloping	0.137	Considerable motion	0.276
Trotting	0.110	Moderate motion	0.206
Walking	0.041	Snowshoeing, soft snow	0.166
Ironing (F)	0.033	Squash	0.212
Ironing (M)	0.064	Standing quietly (F)	0.025
Judo	0.195	Standing quietly (M)	0.027
Knitting, sewing		Stock clerking	0.054
Locksmithing	0.057	Swimming	
Lying at ease	0.022	Backstroke	0.169
Marching, rapid	0.142	Breast stroke	0.162
Mopping floor (F)	0.062	Crawl, fast	0.156
Mopping floor (M)	0.058	Crawl, slow	0.128
Music playing		Side stroke	0.122
Accordion (sitting)	0.032	Treading, fast	0.170
Cello (sitting)	0.041	Treading, normal	0.062
Conducting	0.039	Table tennis	0.068
Drums (sitting)	0.066	Tailoring	
Flute (sitting)	0.035	Cutting	0.041
Horn (sitting)	0.029	Hand-sewing	0.032
Organ (sitting)	0.053	Machine-sewing	0.045
Piano (sitting)	0.040	Pressing	0.062
Trumpet (standing)	0.031	Talking (sitting)	0.029
Violin (sitting)	0.045	Tennis	0.109
Woodwind (sitting)	0.032	Typing	
Painting, inside	0.034	Electric	0.027
Painting, outside	0.077	Manual	0.031
Planting seedlings	0.070	Volleyball	0.050
Plastering	0.078	Walking	
Printing	0.035	2 mph	0.047
Running, cross-country	0.163	3 mph	0.066
Running, horizontal		4 mph	0.086
11½ min per mile	0.135	Plowed field	0.077
9 min per mile	0.193	Wallpapering	0.048
8 min per mile	0.208	Watch repairing	0.025
7 min per mile	0.228	Window cleaning	0.059
6 min per mile	0.252	Writing (sitting)	0.029

Excerpted from: (1) Katch, F. I., and W. D. McArdle, *Nutrition, Weight Control and Exercise*, 2d ed., Philadelphia: Lea and Febiger, 1983. (2) Durnin, J. V. G. A., and R. Passmore, *Energy, Work and Leisure*, London: Heinemann Educational Books, Ltd., 1967.

APPENDIX I

HEIGHT–WEIGHT TABLES

Two height-weight tables are shown here. Table 1, the Metropolitan Life Insurance Company table published in 1983, is based on statistical studies of correlations between body weight and longevity in over 4 million insured Americans over a 20-year period. The weights for heights in this table are heavier than those in the previous revision of this table, but are still below *average* weights for height and sex.

Although frame size is known to be an important factor in determining body weight, no actual measurements of frame size were taken in gathering data for the table.

TABLE 1. HEIGHT AND WEIGHT TABLES (1983, Metropolitan Life Insurance Company)

| | MEN | | | | WOMEN | | |
HEIGHT	SMALL FRAME	MEDIUM FRAME	LARGE FRAME	HEIGHT	SMALL FRAME	MEDIUM FRAME	LARGE FRAME
5'2"	128–134	131–141	138–150	4'10"	102–111	109–121	118–131
5'3"	130–136	133–143	140–153	4'11"	103–113	111–123	120–134
5'4"	132–138	135–145	142–156	5'0"	104–115	113–126	122–137
5'5"	134–140	137–148	144–160	5'1"	106–118	115–129	125–140
5'6"	136–142	139–151	146–164	5'2"	108–121	118–132	128–143
5'7"	138–145	142–154	149–168	5'3"	111–124	121–135	131–147
5'8"	140–148	145–157	152–172	5'4"	114–127	124–138	134–151
5'9"	142–151	148–160	155–176	5'5"	117–130	127–141	137–155
5'10"	144–154	151–163	158–180	5'6"	120–133	130–144	140–159
5'11"	146–157	154–166	161–184	5'7"	123–136	133–147	143–163
6'0"	149–160	157–170	164–188	5'8"	126–139	136–150	146–167
6'1"	152–164	160–174	168–192	5'9"	129–142	139–153	149–170
6'2"	155–168	164–178	172–197	5'10"	132–145	142–156	152–173
6'3"	158–172	167–182	176–202	5'11"	135–148	145–159	155–176
6'4"	162–176	171–187	181–207	6'0"	138–151	148–162	158–179

Weight at ages 25–59 in shoes (1-in heels) and 5 pounds of indoor clothing.

Weight at ages 29–59 in shoes (1-in heels) and 3 pounds of indoor clothing.

SOURCE: *1979 Build Study,* Society of Actuaries and Association of Life Insurance Medical Directors of America, 1980.

A serious problem with the Metropolitan table is that these weights are not representative of the American population since individuals studied were chiefly middle-class whites. Only about one-third were women.

For those who prefer to use a table showing height without shoes and weight without clothing, refer to Table 3. This table was adapted from the old Metropolitan table, based upon the Build and Blood Pressure Study of 1959, and makes no assumptions about frame size. Weights for height and sex are lower in this table than in the new Metropolitan table.

TABLE 2. RECOMMENDED WEIGHT IN RELATION TO HEIGHT*

HEIGHT		MEN		WOMEN	
FEET	INCHES	AVERAGE	RANGE	AVERAGE	RANGE
4	10	. . . .		102	92–119
4	11	. . . .		104	94–122
5	0	. . . .		107	96–125
5	1	. . . .		110	99–128
5	2	123	112–141	113	102–131
5	3	127	115–144	116	105–134
5	4	130	118–148	120	108–138
5	5	133	121–152	123	111–142
5	6	136	124–156	128	114–146
5	7	140	128–161	132	118–150
5	8	145	132–166	136	122–154
5	9	149	136–170	140	126–158
5	10	153	140–174	144	130–163
5	11	158	144–179	148	134–168
6	0	162	148–184	152	138–173
6	1	166	152–189	. . . .	
6	2	171	156–194	. . . .	
6	3	176	160–199	. . . .	
6	4	181	164–204	. . . .	

*Height without shoes, weight without clothes.

SOURCE: Bray, G. A. (ed.), *Obesity in Perspective.* Fogarty International Center Series on Preventive Medicine, volume 2, Part 1, DHEW Publication No. (NIH) 75–708, 1974, p. 7.

APPENDIX J

LABORATORY TESTS IN NUTRITIONAL ASSESSMENT

TABLE OF CURRENT GUIDELINES FOR CRITERIA OF NUTRITIONAL STATUS FOR LABORATORY EVALUATION

NUTRIENT AND UNITS	AGE OF SUBJECT (years)	CRITERIA OF STATUS		
		DEFICIENT	MARGINAL	ACCEPTABLE
*Hemoglobin	6–23 months	Up to 9.0	9.0– 9.9	10.0+
(gm/100ml)	2–5	Up to 10.0	10.0–10.9	11.0+
	6–12	Up to 10.0	10.0–11.4	11.5+
	13–16M	Up to 12.0	12.0–12.9	13.0+
	13–16F	Up to 10.0	10.0–11.4	11.5+
	16+M	Up to 12.0	12.0–13.9	14.0+
	16+F	Up to 10.0	10.0–11.9	12.0+
	Pregnant (after 6+ months)	Up to 9.5	9.5–10.9	11.0+
*Hematocrit	Up to 2	Up to 28	28–30	31+
(Packed cell volume in percent)	2–5	Up to 30	30–33	34+
	6–12	Up to 30	30–35	36+
	13–16M	Up to 37	37–39	40+
	13–16F	Up to 31	31–35	36+
	16+M	Up to 37	37–43	44+
	16+F	Up to 31	31–37	38+
	Pregnant	Up to 30	30–32	33+

*Adapted from the Ten-State Nutrition Survey.

NUTRIENT AND UNITS	AGE OF SUBJECT (years)	CRITERIA OF STATUS		
		DEFICIENT	MARGINAL	ACCEPTABLE
*Serum Albumin (gm/100mL)	Up to 1	—	Up to 2.5	2.5+
	1–5	—	Up to 3.0	3.0+
	6–16	—	Up to 3.5	3.5+
	16+	Up to 2.8	2.8–3.4	3.5+
	Pregnant	Up to 3.0	3.0–3.4	3.5+
*Serum Protein (gm/100mL)	Up to 1	—	Up to 5.0	5.0+
	1–5	—	Up to 5.5	5.5+
	6–16	—	Up to 6.0	6.0+
	16+	Up to 6.0	6.0–6.4	6.5+
	Pregnant	Up to 6.5	5.5–5.9	6.0+
*Serum Ascorbic Acid (mg/100mL)	All ages	Up to 0.1	0.1–0.19	0.2+
*Plasma vitamin A (mcg/100mL)	All ages	Up to 10	10–19	20+
*Plasma Carotene (mcg/100mL)	All ages	Up to 20	20–39	40+
	Pregnant	—	40–79	80+
*Serum Iron (mcg/100mL)	Up to 2	Up to 30	—	30+
	2–5	Up to 40	—	40+
	6–12	Up to 50	—	50+
	12+M	Up to 60	—	60+
	12+F	Up to 40	—	40+
*Transferrin Saturation (percent)	Up to 2	Up to 15.0	—	15.0+
	2–12	Up to 20.0	—	20.0+
	12+M	Up to 20.0	—	20.0+
	12+F	Up to 15.0	—	15.0+
†Serum Folacin (ng/mL)	All ages	Up to 2.0	2.1–5.9	6.0+
†Serum vitamin B_{12} (pg/mL)	All ages	Up to 100	—	100+

*Adapted from the Ten-State Nutrition Survey.
†Criteria may vary with different methodology.

NUTRIENT AND UNITS	AGE OF SUBJECT (years)	CRITERIA OF STATUS		
		DEFICIENT	MARGINAL	ACCEPTABLE
*Thiamine in Urine (mcg/g creatinine)	1–3	Up to 120	120–175	175+
	4–5	Up to 85	85–120	120+
	6–9	Up to 70	70–180	180+
	10–15	Up to 55	55–150	150+
	16+	Up to 27	27– 65	65+
	Pregnant	Up to 21	21– 49	50+
*Riboflavin in Urine (mcg/g creatinine)	1–3	Up to 150	150–499	500+
	4–5	Up to 100	100–299	300+
	6–9	Up to 85	85–269	270+
	10–16	Up to 70	70–199	200+
	16+	Up to 27	27– 79	80+
	Pregnant	Up to 30	30– 89	90+
**RBC Transketolase-TPP-effect (ratio)	All ages	25+	15– 25	Up to 15
**RBC Glutathione Reductase-FAD-effect (ratio)	All ages	1.2+	—	Up to 1.2
**Tryptophan Load (mg Xanthurenic acid excreted)	Adults (Dose: 100mg/kg body weight)	25+(6 hr) 75+(24 hr)	— —	Up to 25 Up to 75
**Urinary Pyridoxine (mcg/g creatinine)	1–3	Up to 90	—	90+
	4–6	Up to 80	—	80+
	7–9	Up to 60	—	60+
	10–12	Up to 40	—	40+
	13–15	Up to 30	—	30+
	16+	Up to 20	—	20+
*Urinary N'methyl nicotinamide (mg/g creatinine)	All ages	Up to 0.2	0.2–5.59	0.6+
	Pregnant	Up to 0.8	0.8–2.49	2.5+
**Urinary Pantothenic Acid (mcg)	All ages	Up to 200	—	200+
**Plasma vitamin E (mg/100mL)	All ages	Up to 0.2	0.2–0.6	0.6+
**Transaminase Index (ratio)				
†EGOT	Adult	2.0+	—	Up to 2.0
‡EGPT	Adult	1.25+	—	Up to 1.25

*Adapted from the Ten-State Nutrition Survey.
**Criteria may vary with different methodology.
†Erythrocyte Glutamic Oxalacetic Transaminase.
‡Erythrocyte Glutamic Pyruvic Transaminase.

SOURCE: Christakis, G. (ed.), "Nutritional Assessment in Health Programs." *American Journal of Public Health*, 63(suppl):34–35, 1973.

APPENDIX K
CHEMICAL STRUCTURES

In Chapter 3, Figure 3-18, we discussed the Krebs cycle, using numbers to indicate its carbohydrate intermediates. Here we show the chemical structures of those intermediates, numbering them as was done in Figure 3-18.

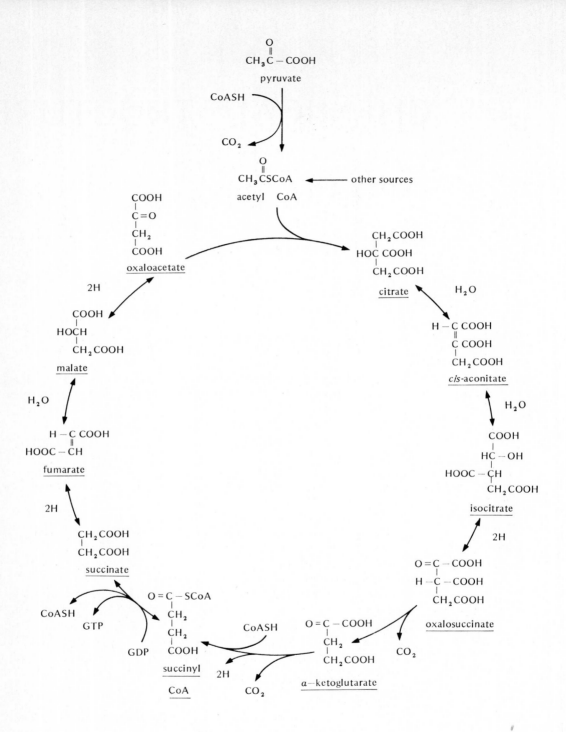

The Krebs, or Tricarboxylic Acid (TCA), Cycle

APPENDIX L

RECORDING AND CALCULATING DIETARY INTAKE

RECORDING AND CALCULATING DIETARY INTAKE

DIRECTIONS FOR RECORDING FOOD INTAKE

1. Choose 3 days during which you anticipate your food intake will be typical. (Don't record a day when you are "dieting.")
2. Record your intake of food and drink (except water) throughout entire period of study.
3. Record foods eaten while eating or as soon afterwards as possible.
4. Do not forget to record sugar, butter, jelly, and dressings added to food.
5. Remember to record all foods or drink consumed between meals.
6. Estimate amounts of foods as follows: (For meals eaten at home, you may want to actually weigh or measure food before eating it.)
   a. Cooked vegetables and fruits, cereals, salad greens, pasta, rice and other grains, and mixed dishes such as casseroles should be estimated in standard measuring cups.
   b. Estimate meats in inches. Note length and width as well as thickness. Meats may be recorded in ounces if you know the weight.
   c. Record beverages in cups or ounces (1 cup = 8 oz).
   d. List sugar, butter, coffee creamer, jelly, honey, syrups in standard teaspoons or tablespoons (3 tsp = 1 tbsp; 16 tbsp = 1 c).
   e. Estimate size of pieces of cake in inches (height, length, width). (Sometimes you can estimate a cake slice, for example, as $1/12$ of a 9-in cake.) Estimate size of pieces of pie as the fraction of the size of pie (giving the diameter).

f. For mixtures of foods such as casseroles, soups, and stews, estimate and record the amounts of different ingredients present.

g. For food prepared at home, indicate whether food was prepared "from scratch," from packaged mix, was canned, frozen, dried, etc. (give brands).

7. To estimate sodium intake: If you do your own cooking or eat at home, use an individual salt shaker for these 3 days. Record the weight of the filled salt shaker at the outset, then salt food during cooking and/or at table from that shaker only. At the end of the 3 days, again record weight of the shaker. Values for the sodium already in foods can be obtained from tables.

8. If you consumed a vitamin or mineral preparation, record the brand name and the nutrients per tablet, and number of tablets consumed.

DIRECTIONS FOR CALCULATING NUTRIENT INTAKE

1. You will need: (a) your 3-day food intake record, (b) a form similar to one shown here (Form A), (c) your text, (d) pencils, (e) ruler, (f) red pencil, and (g) pocket calculator. Use the food composition tables in both Appendix C and other tables if other nutrients are to be calculated.

2. Group foods according to the categories shown in Appendix C. From your 3-day dietary record, total the amount of a given food consumed during the 3-day period. For example, if you consumed 1 c of whole milk on Day 1 and 2 c on Day 2 and 1 c on Day 3, write in "whole milk, 4 c." Then enter 4 times the amount of nutrients listed for whole milk. If you also had skim milk, enter that as a separate item. *Use a ruler in reading the tables to avoid errors. Use a pencil, so you can correct errors.*

3. Check to be sure you calculated *all the foods* on your food intake record.

4. After you have completed recording the nutrients for the foods consumed in a given group, total the nutrients for that group and divide by 3 to obtain the average. Record both the total and the average, *but record the average in red. When recording totals, round figures as follows:*
   a. For energy, round to the nearest kilocalorie.
   b. For protein, fat, and carbohydrates, round to the nearest g.
   c. For fatty acids, round to the nearest 0.1 g.
   d. For calcium and vitamin C, round to the nearest mg.
   e. For vitamin A, round to the nearest IU.
   f. For iron and niacin, round to the nearest 0.1 mg.
   g. For thiamine and riboflavin, round to the nearest 0.01 mg.

5. If you consumed any vitamin or mineral preparations, record the average 3-day intake in the space provided (under "Grand Total").

6. Add the *average* figures from each group (the red figures) to obtain the Grand Total. If you consumed vitamin or mineral pills, record a Grand Total with and without the pills.

7. Record your RDA as follows:
   a. For kilocalories, use the kilocalorie need you calculated for yourself in Chapter 7.
   b. For protein, calculate 0.8 g times your weight in kg.
   c. For vitamins and minerals, use the amount given in the RDA table, Appendix A, for your age and sex.

FORM A

FATTY ACIDS

FOOD	AMOUNT	FOOD ENERGY (kcal)	PRO- TEIN (g)	FAT (g)	SATU- RATED (g)	UNSATURATED		CAR- BOHY- DRATE (g)	CAL- CIUM (mg)	IRON (mg)	VITA- MIN A (IU)	THIA- MINE (mg)	RIBO- FLAVIN (mg)	NIA- CIN (mg)	ASCOR- BIC ACID (mg)	CHO- LES- TEROL (mg)
						OLEIC (g)	LIN- OLEIC (g)									
Dairy products and eggs																
Total																
Average																
Fats and oils																
Total																
Average																
Fish and meats																
Total																
Average																

(additional forms continued in this manner)

APPENDIX M

MEASURING PROTEIN QUALITY

MEASURING PROTEIN QUALITY

In Chapter 6 we noted that the quality of protein in a diet depends upon the amount and pattern of amino acids present relative to the body's need for them. Scientists have long been interested in how to determine dietary protein quality. We briefly consider here the chief methods used, their advantages and limitations.

CHEMICAL OR AMINO ACID SCORE

The concept of chemical or amino acid score arose as scientists realized that for protein synthesis to occur, all the needed amino acids had to be present simultaneously within the cells, and that low amounts of one essential amino acid would limit protein synthesis. They reasoned that if they determined the amino acid composition of protein X, for example, they could ascertain its limiting amino acid (that one present in the least amount relative to the need for it) by comparing its composition with that of a known high-quality protein or of an "ideal pattern." From the most limiting amino acid they could then derive a "chemical" or "amino acid score."

From the analysis of the amino acid composition of the protein, one first expresses the amount of each essential amino acid in terms of its percentage of the total amino acid content. The resulting pattern is then compared with that of an "ideal pattern." In 1973 an expert committee of the WHO/FAO set an ideal pattern based upon the essential amino acid needs of the preschool child [1].

Table 1 shows how chemical score is calculated from the limiting amino acid in a protein. This table shows only those amino acids (lysine, the sulfur amino acids, threonine, and tryptophan) most likely to be limiting; the values are given in terms of their

TABLE 1. CHEMICAL OR AMINO ACID SCORE OF SEVERAL PROTEIN SOURCES

AMINO ACID CONTENT OF PROTEIN

PROTEIN SOURCE	LYSINE	SULFUR AMINO ACIDS	THRE-ONINE	TRYPTO-PHAN	CHEMICAL SCORE	LIMITING AMINO ACIDS
	%	%	%	%		
Ideal pattern	5.5	3.5	4.0	1.0	100	
Cereal	2.4	3.8	3.0	1.1	44	Lysine
Legume	7.2	2.4	4.2	1.4	68	Sulfur amino acids
Milk powder	8.0	2.9	3.7	1.3	83	Sulfur amino acids
Mixture: cereal–legume–milk (65:22:11)	5.1	3.2	3.5	1.2	88	Threonine

SOURCE: Adapted from Munro, H. N., and M. C. Crim, "The Proteins and Amino Acids." In: Goodhart, R. S., and M. E. Shils (eds.), *Modern Nutrition in Health and Diseases*, 6th ed., Philadelphia: Lea & Febiger, 1980, p. 89.

percentage of the total amino acids in each protein. The ideal pattern shown is that of the WHO/FAO set in 1973 [1]. Comparing the percentage of each amino acid in cereal, for example, with the ideal pattern, we see that lysine is the limiting amino acid: $2.4 \div 5.5 \times 100 = 44\%$. Its chemical score is therefore 44, and is low compared with that of milk or legume protein, but a mixture of cereal, legume, and milk protein has a relatively high score (Table 1).

Chemical scoring is an inexpensive method of judging protein quality and allows one to readily perceive how to complement one protein with another. A major disadvantage is that this method tells you nothing about how well the body can digest or utilize the protein, nor the extent to which amino acids are destroyed during the analysis of amino acid composition. These disadvantages prompted investigators to study biological methods of evaluating protein quality.

PROTEIN EFFICIENCY RATIO (PER)

PER has been widely used because it is a relatively simple test to perform. The investigator feeds 10 weanling rats the test protein at 9 percent by weight of their diet for 4 weeks. During this time, their weight gain and food intake are routinely measured. The PER is calculated as:

$$\frac{\text{average total weight gain (g)}}{\text{average amount of protein consumed (g)}}$$

A high-quality protein produces greater weight gain per gram of protein consumed than a poorer quality protein.

Unfortunately, while PER can be used to decide whether or not one protein is better in quality than another, it is incorrect to assume that it is superior by a stated percentage [2]. For example, one cannot say that a protein having a PER of 1.0 has only 33 percent the value of a protein with a PER of 3.0. This is because PER is influenced by factors *other* than the protein quality, such as the amount of food the animal consumes, the amount of protein in the diet, and the composition of the weight gain. Weight gain may be due to fat accumulation rather than to the laying down of new protein tissue, for example. Another problem is that PER fails to take into account that protein being used to meet the maintenance requirement of the animals. Furthermore, different laboratories obtain different PER values of the same protein [2]. Finally, the extent to which PER indicates the quality of protein for human use is uncertain since the amino acid needs of growing rats differ from that of growing or adult humans.

BIOLOGICAL VALUE (BV)

Biological value is defined as the percentage of *absorbed* nitrogen *retained* by body tissues for protein synthesis. A high percentage of the amino acids in a high-quality protein remains within the body cells to participate in protein synthesis because the amino acid pattern is similar to that of body proteins. The amino acids in a poor-quality protein will be retained less well because protein synthesis will be limited by the fact that this protein furnishes inadequate amounts of the limiting amino acid. The remaining amino acids will therefore be catabolized and wasted.

Biological value may be measured in animals or in human subjects using nitrogen balance. For human subjects the procedure is fairly arduous because the contribution to total fecal and urinary nitrogen of endogenous nitrogen must be determined. To accomplish this, subjects must consume a nitrogen-free (protein-free) diet while their nitrogen balance is determined. They are then changed to a diet containing the test protein as data continue to be collected to determine nitrogen balance. The intake of kilocalories, vitamins, and minerals must be kept constant during both the protein-free and the test periods. During the test period the nitrogen intake must be just adequate to maintain nitrogen equilibrium in adults or to permit growth if growing animals are used.

BV is calculated using the following formula [2]:

$$BV = \frac{N_i - (F - F_0) - (U - U_0)}{N_i - (F - F_0)}$$

where: N_i = nitrogen intake of test protein
F = fecal nitrogen when test protein fed
F_0 = fecal nitrogen when protein-free diet fed
U = urinary nitrogen when test protein fed
U_0 = urinary nitrogen when protein-free diet fed

The numerator represents nitrogen kept within the body (retained) for protein synthesis, while the denominator represents nitrogen absorbed; therefore,

$$BV = \frac{\text{retained nitrogen}}{\text{absorbed nitrogen}}$$

This method is expensive to perform when human subjects are used. BV ignores the digestibility of the test protein, although this can be calculated as follows [2]:

$$\text{Percent digestibility} = \frac{N_i - (F - F_0)}{N_i} \times 100$$

One can then calculate the overall nutritive value of the test protein by multiplying its BV by its digestibility. One then obtains a score that should be identical with NPU, discussed next.

NET PROTEIN UTILIZATION (NPU)

NPU can be obtained using the nitrogen balance technique when either animal or human subjects are used. Another technique used with animals involves analyzing the body nitrogen content of animals fed a nitrogen-free diet compared with those fed the test protein.

When the balance technique is used, NPU is calculated as follows [2]:

$$NPU = \frac{N_i - (F - F_0) - (U - U_0)}{N_i}$$

The numerator is the same as for BV, but the denominator is the nitrogen intake rather than absorbed nitrogen. NPU therefore *includes* protein digestibility. It should now be apparent that BV $\times$ digestibility = NPU, and that BV is apt to be higher for a protein than its NPU.

One problem with NPU is that it will be unclear whether a low NPU value is due to poor digestibility of the protein or to a poor amino acid pattern. Other procedures for determining protein quality are currently under investigation. Values obtained for different proteins using the four measures of protein quality discussed are in Table 2.

TABLE 2. PROTEIN QUALITY DETERMINED BY FOUR METHODS

PROTEIN SOURCE	BV[a]	NPU[a]	PER[a]	CHEMICAL SCORE	
				1970[a]	1973[b]
Corn (maize)	59	51	1.12	41	49
Oats	65	66	2.19	57	68
Rice, white	64	57	2.18	56	67
Wheat, whole	65	40	1.53	43	53
Beans (various)	58	40	1.48	34	54
Soybeans	73	61	2.32	47	—
Beef	74	67	2.30	69	100
Egg	94	94	3.92	100	100
Cow's milk	85	82	3.09	60	95

[a] Data obtained from: FAO: "Amino-Acid Content of Foods and Biological Data on Proteins." *FAO Nutrition Studies No. 24*, FAO, Rome, 1970.
[b] Data on chemical score for 1973 from WHO/FAO Report, "Energy and Protein Requirements." *WHO Technical Report Series No. 522*, WHO, Geneva, 1973. (The ideal pattern was changed so that both beef and egg rank 100.)

References:

1. WHO/FAO Report, *Energy and Protein Requirements*. WHO Technical Report Series No. 522. WHO, Geneva, 1973.
2. Hegsted, D. M., "Assessment of Protein Quality." In: *Improvement of Protein Nutriture*. Food and Nutrition Board, National Academy of Sciences, Washington, D.C., 1974.

APPENDIX N

U.S. RDAs

UNITED STATES RECOMMENDED DAILY
ALLOWANCES (U.S. RDAs) For Labeling Purposes
Recommendations for Adults and Children Over 4 Years

MANDATORY NUTRIENTS

Protein		
Quality equal to or greater than casein	45	g
Quality less than casein	65	g
Vitamin A	5,000	IU
Vitamin C	60	mg
Thiamine	1.5	mg
Riboflavin	1.7	mg
Niacin	20	mg
Calcium	1.0	g
Iron	18	mg

OPTIONAL NUTRIENTS

Vitamin D	400	IU
Vitamin E	30	IU
Vitamin B_6	2.0	mg
Folacin (folic acid)	0.4	mg
Vitamin B_{12}	6	μg
Phosphorus	1.0	g
Iodine	150	μg
Magnesium	400	mg
Zinc	15	mg
Copper	2	mg
Biotin	0.3	mg
Pantothenic acid	10	mg

INDEX

Boldfaced page numbers indicate illustrations, diagrams, or tables.